The Natural Pharmacy

Skye Lininger, D.C., Editor-in-Chief
Jonathan Wright, M.D.
Steve Austin, N.D.
Donald Brown, N.D.
Alan Gaby, M.D.

PRIMA HEALTH

A Division of Prima Publishing

Library of Congress Cataloging-in-Publication Data

Lininger, Jr., Schuyler W.
    The natural pharmacy / by Schuyler W. Lininger, Jr.
        p.   cm.
    Includes bibliographic references and index.
    ISBN 0-7615-1227-6
    1. Naturopathy. 2. Homeopathy. 3. Herbs—Therapeutic use. 4. Vitamins—Therapeutic use.
5. Minerals—Therapeutic use. I. Title.
RZ440.L58   1998
615.5—dc21   97-43106
                                                                        CIP

98 99 00 01 02 DD 10 9 8 7 6 5 4 3 2
Printed in the United States of America

How to Order
Single copies may be ordered from Prima Publishing, P.O. Box 1260BK, Rocklin, CA 95677; telephone (916) 632-4400. Quantity discounts are also available. On your letterhead, include information concerning the intended use of the books and the number of books you wish to purchase.

Visit us online at www.primapublishing.com

CONTENTS

PART ONE
Conditions

PART TWO
Nutritional Supplements

PART THREE

Herbs

PART FOUR

Homeopathic Remedies

FOREWORD

I first met and really enjoyed the company of Dr. Skye Lininger on a trip to Costa Rica sponsored by the American Botanical Council. As we rode buses through the mountains, Skye ran a red pencil across the printouts for what would later become the *HealthNotes Online* computer program—and now the book you are holding in your hands. We enjoyed stimulating and animated conversations from the hot coasts of Tortugeuro on the Atlantic to the cloud forests of Monte Verde.

At that time I had the pleasure of reading over some of the pages in the herbal section that had been mostly written by Dr. Don Brown, a noted naturopath and teacher, whom I also respect. I was impressed with how easy the information was to access.

Most of the important information about the herb's use and elusive dosage data, cross-referenced to the condition, including potential side effects and interactions, all make this book especially useful. I'm even more impressed with the information about ninety of the most important herbs, complete with backup citations from the scientific literature (including many articles from German journals).

The fact that Dr. Lininger used some of the foremost experts on herbs, homeopathy, and nutrition makes this reference an excellent source book for help with more than seventy common health conditions. I think you'll find yourself turning to this book often!

Enjoy it in good health. Think green, the green of natural medicines, with which you co-evolved.

Dr. Jim Duke
Economic Botanist, USDA (Retired)

ACKNOWLEDGMENTS

No book of this size and scope comes into existence without the inspiration and help of many people—some of whom labor behind the scenes.

Gratitude for a job well done to all the contributors to this book—especially Drs. Steve Austin and Don Brown, who bore the brunt of the workload and whose integrity has ensured this book will set a new standard for excellence, and to Drs. Jonathan Wright and Alan Gaby, who have served as mentors to us all and whose attention to detail and creative innovation served to midwife this book.

Special thanks to Victoria Dolby for her brilliant job in keeping us all on track as managing editor of the *HealthNotes Online* software and book projects.

Thanks to my wife Jane and daughters Cory and Ciel for their love and putting up with long hours and a travel schedule from beyond endurance; to my staff, Norma Hunt, Cindy Hambly, and Tony Patricelli; to my technical advisor Rick Wilkes (and his team) and the person who brought us together, Thom Hartmann (an expert author of books on ADD and someone who also belongs in the mentor category); to those talented people who helped make the *HealthNotes Online* software a beautiful reality, Marcia Berentine, Loren Jenkins, and Steven Foster; to those who were there at the beginning (and helped inspire, motivate, and create), Michael Peet and his sister Margaret, Cheryl Bottger, and Eileen Brady.

To those at Prima who instantly captured our vision, but especially Ben Dominitz, Jamie Miller, Karen Cook, our editor Debra Venzke, and our copy editor-without-peer Kathy Hashimoto; to Dr. Joe Pizzorno, who surely will one day be recognized as one of the fathers of modern naturopathy; to all the health and natural food stores and departments who offer high-quality supplements; to those pioneers and innovators in natural medicine; and finally, to those brave souls of integrity, unfortunately too numerous to mention, who went to jail or lost their licenses for doing nothing more than trying to care for their patients . . . naturally.

INTRODUCTION

In 1975, when I first became interested in "alternative" medicine, it was hard to sort out the fact from the folklore. While millions of people took supplements to either protect their health or help with a problem their doctors were unable to cure, most were relying on anecdotes and hearsay.

Two decades ago, there were many scientific articles that had been written about most of the vitamins and a few of the herbs, but getting hold of that information was difficult. Most medical doctors were either ignorant about or hostile toward nutritional supplements, and the subject wasn't taught in school. So it was largely left to the health food stores and a few courageous physicians to tend the flame.

In the 1970s, books about supplements were a mixed bag. Despite being poorly referenced and filled with errors, the books provided enough information (which later proved true) to help millions of people with their health problems.

In the early 1980s, a steady stream of articles about antioxidants and other dietary supplements began appearing in the medical literature. By the late 1980s, the stream had become a flood and some 15,000 articles began forming a solid foundation for nutritional therapies. Books appearing in those years began to take advantage of the scientific underpinnings and gradually became more reliable and useful. However, they were still aimed squarely at those who accepted the premise that only natural was good.

By the time we began working on this book, the number of useful scientific articles on the role of vitamins and herbs in human health exceeded 25,000. Our team of researchers combed the libraries of medical schools on a weekly basis to keep up-to-date on breaking research. I can say without reservation that those who contributed to this book are among the most knowledgeable physicians in the world on the subject of natural medicine.

Our team consists of a chiropractor (me), several medical doctors (Wright and Gaby), and a group of naturopaths (Austin, Brown, Yarnell, Reichert, and Hudson). Our goal was to create a book

that stressed an integrated approach to self-care, to create a tool that would let readers assess the pluses and minuses of the use of vitamins, minerals, herbs, homeopathic remedies, and other nutrients for the most common and troublesome health conditions.

This book has other unique characteristics.

- All statements that might be controversial have been documented with a reference from the scientific literature. Thousands of citations are included so the serious reader can retrieve the article and review the material we relied on. In addition, we have used primarily human studies; very little of our information depended on either animal or test tube trials.

- Contraindications, side effects, and possible drug–nutrient interactions are noted. Millions of people who are not "hard-core" health-food-store people are now taking supplements. This mainstream consumer is legitimately concerned about the safety (and efficacy) of these products. The information we provide gives you a way to make sensible choices for yourself and your family.

- All of our key contributors have actually been in practice with real patients. They are not writing theoretically or from an ivory tower— but from real-life experience in their clinics.

In short, we think we have created the most useful, comprehensive, and balanced book that has ever been made available on this topic and that it will be the first place many people will turn for information about complementary or alternative medicine. We have also created a special CD-ROM version of this book. Please look on page 450 for information about how you can obtain a copy.

All the authors join me in wishing you good health.

Dr. Skye Lininger
Portland, Oregon

HOW TO USE THIS BOOK

The Natural Pharmacy is divided into four parts. Each part is easily found by looking for the tabs on the side of the book. Once found, you can flip through the pages to find the specific topic you are looking for, alphabetized within each section. You can also use the table of contents or the index to locate topics. The tables found at the beginning of each part can help you locate an entry by main topic, synonym, or closely related term.

Once you have located the information you want in one of the four parts, you can easily navigate throughout the rest of the book with our unique cross-referencing approach. Next to key words (such as Vitamin C or High Cholesterol) are page number links that direct you to more detailed information. By flipping back and forth in the book using the page number links, you can mimic the ease of use you'd find in a computer hypertext document. We think this feature makes *The Natural Pharmacy* the easiest-to-use reference book we've ever seen.

It is very important to realize this book is provided for information or educational purposes only and should only be used in consultation with a nutritionally oriented physician.

Following is a list of the four sections of the book and information about what you'll find in each one.

Conditions

Look here for information about specific health conditions ranging from acne to yellow nail syndrome. Each entry includes a section that describes the condition, makes dietary recommendations when appropriate, and suggests which nutrients and herbs might be of help. Also included is information about possible side effects or interactions.

At the end of each condition is a summary checklist of the nutritional supplements, herbs, and homeopathic remedies discussed in the text. These items are listed in the order of importance. If you can try only a few nutrients or herbs, try the ones that are listed at the beginning of the list.

Nutritional Supplements

Look here for information about specific vitamins, minerals, amino acids, and other nutrients such as coQ10. Each nutrient entry includes information about where it is found, conditions in which the nutrient might be supportive, suggested dosage ranges, and possible side effects or interactions.

Herbs

Look here for information about some ninety specific herbs. Each herb includes information about where it is found, what part is used, in which conditions the herb might be supportive, information about historical and traditional use, data on the active compounds (if known), suggested dosage ranges, and possible side effects or interactions.

Homeopathic Remedies

Look here if you are interested in homeopathy. Information in this section is found by looking up a specific health condition and then matching symptoms to find the specific homeopathic remedy.

Important Features

This book has many unique features that help make it useful. Take a moment to read over this list to learn how to get the most out of *The Natural Pharmacy*.

- In the Conditions section, supportive nutrients and herbs are listed in the order of importance. The first ones mentioned usually have the most scientific evidence and work the best. In our practices, they are the ones we'd usually have patients use initially.

- In the Conditions section, the most critical potential side effects or interactions for nutrients and herbs are described. However, more complete information about side effects or interactions is described under each specific nutritional supplement or herb. You should carefully read the relevant safety information in all sections of the book.

- In the Conditions section, there is a useful checklist at the end of each condition. This checklist is a very useful reminder of what nutrients, herbs, and homeopathic remedies might be supportive.

- In the Nutritional Supplements and Herbs sections, general information is given. To find out how a particular compound is used for a specific condition, refer to the Condition section that is cross-referenced.

- In the Herbs section, the active ingredient(s) of an herb is described if it is known. Many herbs are available in multiple forms: dried (usually in capsules, tablets, poultice, or tea), liquid (as tinctures or extracts), or standardized (where a particular compound is measured and quantified). We have tried to give you dosages for all the various forms when that information was available.

- In all the sections (except Homeopathic Remedies), we have tried not to make any statements without providing scientific documentation in the form of a footnote. If you or your doctor need to find out more on a particular subject, we hope we have made it easier for you by providing a full citation from the scientific literature. We have used, almost exclusively, human studies from the major medical and scientific journals. We have rarely fallen back on a book or a secondary source.

- In all the sections we have tried to be balanced in our approach to giving you the information. We have tried to avoid overstating the case and have attempted to present information about any negative or equivocal studies. We feel by taking this path, you have a book in which you can have confidence.

About Doses and When to Take Supplements

Each health condition covered in this book includes specific, useful information about nutritional, herbal, and homeopathic support for the condition. Keep in mind that unless the text specifies differently, the suggested amounts of vitamins, minerals, amino acids, herbs, or homeopathic ingredients apply only to an average-size male or female adult. Children's doses should be determined in consultation with a nutritionally oriented physician.

Unless otherwise specified in the text, nutritional supplements and herbs should be taken with meals.

PART ONE

CONDITIONS

ACNE

ACNE (also called *acne vulgaris*) is a skin condition characterized by reddened, inflamed lesions (sometimes called pustules or "whiteheads") on the face, neck, shoulders, and elsewhere. Acne occurs most commonly in teenagers and to a lesser extent in young adults. The condition results in part from excessive stimulation of the skin by androgens (male hormones). Bacterial infection of the skin also appears to play a role.

Dietary Changes That May Be Helpful

Food allergy appears to play a role in adult acne, but it is less important for teenage acne.

Nutrients That May Be Helpful

Several studies indicate that **zinc** (page 224) supplements reduce the severity of acne.[1] In one study, zinc was found to be as effective as oral antibiotic therapy.[2] Many people with acne take 30 mg of zinc two or three times per day for a few months, then 30 mg per day thereafter. It often takes twelve weeks before any improvement is seen.

Large quantities of **vitamin A** (page 209)—such as 300,000 IU per day for females and 400–500,000 IU per day for males—have been used successfully to treat a severe type of acne known as cystic acne.[3] However, those quantities of vitamin A are toxic and should be taken only under the supervision of a health professional.

Vitamin B6 (page 214) at 50 mg per day may alleviate premenstrual flare-ups of acne experienced by some women.[4]

Are There Any Side Effects or Interactions?

Individuals who take 30 mg or more of zinc per day for more than a few months should balance the zinc with **copper** (page 151) in order to prevent copper deficiency. For 30 mg per day of zinc, 2 mg per day of copper is usually taken. For 60–90 mg per day of zinc, 3–4 mg per day of copper is a reasonable amount.

Studies suggest that vitamin A in amounts greater than 10,000 IU per day may cause birth defects if taken by a pregnant woman. Large doses of vitamin A (more than 25,000 IU per day for an adult) can also be toxic and should be monitored by a nutritionally oriented doctor.

Herbs That May Be Helpful

A large study compared the topical use of 5% **tea tree** (page 313) oil to 5% benzoyl peroxide for common acne. Although the tea tree oil was slower and less potent in its action, it had far fewer side effects and was thus considered more effective overall.[5] For topical treatment of acne, many people use the oil at a dilution of 5–15%.

Historically, tonic or alterative herbs, such as **burdock** (page 239), have been used in the treatment of skin conditions. These herbs are believed to have a cleansing effect when taken internally.[6] Many people take 2–4 ml of burdock root tincture per day. Dried root preparations in a capsule or tablet can be used at 1–2 grams three times per day. Many herbal preparations combine burdock root with other alterative herbs, such as yellow dock, **red clover** (page 301), or cleavers.

Are There Any Side Effects or Interactions?

Tea tree oil should not be applied to broken skin or to areas affected by rashes not due to fungus. The oil may burn if it gets into the eyes, nose, mouth, or other tender areas. Some people have allergic reactions, including rashes and itching, when applying tea tree oil. For this reason, only a small amount should be applied when first using it. The oil should never be taken internally.

Use of burdock root at the dosages listed above is generally safe. However, burdock root in large quantities may stimulate the uterus, and it should be used with caution during pregnancy.

Checklist for Acne

Nutritional Supplements	Herbs	Homeopathic Remedies
Zinc, Vitamin A, Vitamin B6	Tea tree oil, Burdock	Sulfur 6c, Hepar sulfuris 6c

ALZHEIMER'S DISEASE

ALZHEIMER'S DISEASE is a brain disorder that occurs in the later years of life. Individuals with Alzheimer's disease develop progressive loss of memory and gradually lose the ability to function in the world and to take care of themselves.

The cause of this disorder is not known. However, some, but not all, studies suggest that it may be related to an accumulation of aluminum in the brain.[1]

Dietary Changes That May Be Helpful

Although the connection between Alzheimer's disease and aluminum exposure has not been proven, it seems prudent to take steps to minimize exposure to this metal. Avoid foods cooked in aluminum pots, foods that come into direct contact with aluminum foil, and beverages stored in aluminum cans. Some water authorities add aluminum to the water supply to prevent the accumulation of particulate matter in the water. In such areas, bottled water may be preferable.

Nutrients That May Be Helpful

Phosphatidylserine (page 196), which is related to **lecithin** (page 176), is a naturally occurring compound present in the brain. Phosphatidylserine (100 mg three times per day) has been shown to improve mental function in individuals with Alzheimer's disease.[2] However, the phosphatidylserine used in these studies was obtained from the brains of cows, which may not be the safest source for this nutrient. Fortunately, a plant source of phosphatidylserine is also available—however, this is a slightly different form of phosphatidylserine, and its effectiveness needs documentation.[3]

Acetyl-L-carnitine is a molecule that occurs naturally in the brain and other tissues. Acetyl-L-carnitine improves memory and enhances overall performance in some individuals with Alzheimer's disease.[4] Most research involving acetyl-L-carnitine uses 500 mg three times per day.

Large amounts of **vitamin E** (page 220) may slow the progression of Alzheimer's disease, according to researchers from the Alzheimer's Disease Co-operative Study. A two-year study of 341 individuals with Alzheimer's disease of moderate severity found that 2,000 IU per day of vitamin E extended the time patients were able to care for themselves, such as bathing, dressing, and other necessary daily functions, compared to those taking a placebo.[5]

Preliminary findings indicate a beneficial effect of **tyrosine** (page 207), along with other amino acids, in people affected by dementia including Alzheimer's disease.[6]

Are There Any Side Effects or Interactions?

There are no known contraindications to the use of these nutrients in the amounts mentioned. Although the preliminary research is contradictory, patients with Alzheimer's disease should avoid zinc supplements until further studies clarify the role of zinc in this disease. [7,8]

Herbs That May Be Helpful

An extract made from the leaves of the *Ginkgo biloba* tree is a leading treatment for early-stage Alzheimer's disease in Europe. While not a cure for this serious condition, **Ginkgo biloba** (page 268) extract (GBE) may improve memory and quality of life and slow progression in the early stages. Research shows that 240 mg per day of GBE can improve memory, attention, and mood. Improvements were noted as early as after one month of supplementation and became progressively better over the course of two studies.[9,10]

This is very exciting information, considering that the only drug currently approved in the United States for early-stage Alzheimer's disease is Cognex. This medication is extremely toxic to the liver and has not proven useful for long-term treatment of Alzheimer's disease. GBE offers a safer and more successful alternative. Many people use 60 mg of GBE three times per day.

A class of herbs often used for elderly persons experiencing mental decline is the tonic, or adaptogenic, herbs. Examples include **Asian ginseng** (page 232) (100–200 mg per day of the standardized herbal extract), **eleuthero** (Siberian ginseng) (page 257) (2–3 grams per day of the dried root or 300–400 mg per day of the concentrated solid extract standardized on eleutherosides B and E), **astragalus** (page 233) (two to three 500 mg capsules three times per day), and ashwagandha.

Asian ginseng has the longest history of use in traditional Chinese medicine and is commonly used for older individuals showing signs of memory loss. Asian ginseng improves and sharpens mental concentration and performance, including attention and memory.[11,12] While not as thoroughly researched as GBE for this condition, studies show that ginseng is effective at improving memory and also countering depression in the elderly. Some herbal supplements combine GBE with Asian ginseng.

Are There Any Side Effects or Interactions?

Ginkgo is essentially devoid of any serious side effects. Mild headaches lasting for a day or two and mild upset stomach have been reported in a very small percentage of people using ginkgo. There are no known contraindications to the use of ginkgo by pregnant and lactating women.

Used as recommended, Asian ginseng and eleuthero are generally safe. In rare instances, Asian ginseng may cause overstimulation and possibly insomnia. Consuming caffeine with ginseng increases the risk of overstimulation and gastrointestinal upset. Persons with uncontrolled high blood pressure should not use ginseng. Long-term use of ginseng may cause menstrual abnormalities and breast tenderness in some women. Ginseng is not recommended for pregnant or lactating women.

Astragalus has no known side effects when used as recommended.

Checklist for Alzheimer's Disease

Nutritional Supplements	Herbs	Homeopathic Remedies
Phosphatidylserine, Acetyl-L-carnitine, Vitamin E, Tyrosine	Ginkgo biloba, Asian ginseng, Eleuthero, Astragalus, Ashwagandha	No homeopathy commonly used for this condition

ANTIOXIDANTS AND FREE RADICALS

OXYGEN IS essential to life, since humans need to breathe air containing oxygen in order to sustain life. Yet oxygen is very active and combines readily with many compounds in our body. Some of these compounds can cause damage.

During cellular respiration (the process that creates energy), some oxygen molecules are converted into oxidizing agents (also called "free radicals"), such as superoxides or hydrogen peroxide.

These molecules are unstable and react with other compounds in an effort to become stabilized. This quest for stability can be quite damaging to normal body tissues, but fortunately the body is equipped with an "antioxidant" defense system.

Environmental Sources of Free Radicals

The environment is a source of free radicals. Such oxidizing agents include: ionizing radiation (from industry, sun exposure, cosmic rays, and medical X rays); ozone and nitrous oxide (primarily from automobile exhaust); heavy metals (such as mercury, cadmium, and lead); cigarette smoke (both active and passive); alcohol; unsaturated fat (may create a strain on the natural antioxidants of the body); and other chemicals and compounds from food, water, and air.

When these free radicals enter the body, they can react with healthy tissue, setting off potentially damaging reactions. Free radicals are believed to play a role in more than sixty different health conditions, including the aging process, cancer, and atherosclerosis.[1] Reducing exposure to free radicals and increasing intake of antioxidant nutrients can reduce the risk of free radical–related health problems.

Natural Antioxidants

Free radicals are inherently unstable, since they contain "extra" energy. To reduce their energy load, free radicals react with certain cells in the body, interfering with the cells' ability to function normally. Fortunately there are many natural antioxidants that interfere with free radicals before they can damage the body. Antioxidants work in several ways: they may reduce the energy of the free radical, stop the free radical from forming in the first place, or interrupt an oxidizing chain reaction to minimize the damage of free radicals.

Superoxide dismutase (SOD), catalase, and glutathione peroxidase are enzymes produced by the body itself to defuse many types of free radicals. Supplements of these compounds are also available to augment the body's supply. However, these anti-

oxidant enzymes may not absorb well. It may be more effective to take the "building blocks" the body requires to make SOD, catalase, and glutathione peroxidase. These building block nutrients include the minerals **manganese** (page 183), **zinc** (page 224), and **copper** (page 151) for SOD and **selenium** (page 203) for glutathione peroxidase.

In addition to enzymes, many vitamins and minerals act as antioxidants in their own right, such as **vitamin C** (page 217), **vitamin E** (page 220), **beta-carotene** (page 209), **lutein** (page 179), **lycopene** (page 180), **vitamin B3** (page 213) in the form of niacin, **vitamin B2** (page 212), **vitamin B6** (page 214), **coenzyme Q10** (page 152), and **cysteine** (page 154) (an amino acid). Herbs, such as **bilberry** (page 234), **turmeric** (page 314) (curcumin), **grape seed** or **pine bark extracts** (proanthocyanidins, page 199), and **ginkgo biloba** (page 268), can also provide powerful antioxidant protection for the body.

A wide variety of antioxidant enzymes, vitamins, minerals, and herbs may be the best way to provide the body with the most complete protection against free radical damage. See the individual nutrient or herb entries in this book for more information on a particular antioxidant.

ASTHMA

ASTHMA is a lung disorder in which spasms of the bronchial passages restrict the flow of air in and out of the lungs. The number of people with asthma and the death rate from this condition have been increasing since the late 1980s. Environmental pollution appears to be one of the causes of this growing epidemic.

Dietary Changes That May Be Helpful

Unrecognized food allergy is a contributing factor in at least 75% of childhood asthmatics and about 40% of adult asthmatics.[1] A medically supervised "allergy elimination diet" often helps identify problematic foods. A health care professional should supervise this allergy test, since there is a chance of triggering an asthma attack during the elimination-and-rechallenge.

Some asthmatics react to food additives, such as sulfites and tartrazine (yellow dye #5). A naturally occurring class of chemicals known as salicylates may also provoke asthma in sensitive individuals. A nutritionally oriented doctor or an allergist can help determine whether chemical sensitivities are present.

Nutrients That May Be Helpful

Vitamin B6 (page 214) deficiency is common in asthmatics.[2] This deficiency may relate to the asthma itself or to certain antiasthma drugs (such as theophylline and aminophylline) that deplete vitamin B6.[3] In a study of asthmatic children, 200 mg per day of vitamin B6 for two months reduced the severity of their illness and reduced the amount of asthma medication needed.[4] In another study, asthmatic adults experienced a dramatic decrease in the frequency and severity of asthma attacks while taking 50 mg of vitamin B6 twice a day.[5]

Magnesium (page 182) levels are frequently low in asthmatics.[6] Magnesium supplements might help prevent asthma attacks, since magnesium can prevent spasms of the bronchial passages. Intravenous injections of magnesium can stop an acute asthma attack within minutes.[7] Although the effect of oral magnesium has not been well studied, many doctors recommend magnesium supplements for their asthma patients. The usual amount of magnesium taken by an adult is 200–400 mg per day (children take proportionately less, based on their body weight).

Supplementation with 1 gram of **vitamin C** (page 217) per day reduces the tendency of the bronchial passages to go into spasm.[8] Some individuals with asthma have shown considerable improvement after taking 1–2 grams of vitamin C per day. A buffered form of vitamin C (such as sodium ascorbate or calcium ascorbate) may work better for some asthmatics than regular vitamin C (ascorbic acid).[9]

Very high amounts of **vitamin B12** (page 216) supplements (1,500 mcg per day) have been found to reduce the tendency for asthmatics to react to sulfites.[10] The trace mineral molybdenum also helps the body detoxify sulfites.[11] However, a nutritionally oriented physician should be involved in the evaluation and treatment of sulfite sensitivity.

Betaine hydrochloride, or HCl, (page 139) may be helpful to some individuals with asthma.[12] **Ionized air** (page 172) may also play a role in allergies.

Research suggests that some allergy-provoking substances, such as dust and pollen, have a positive electrical charge. Meanwhile, negative ions appear to counteract the allergenic effects of these positively charged ions on respiratory tissues. Negative ions generally lead to favorable effects, and many individuals experience relief from their respiratory allergies.[13] Other allergy sufferers report considerable relief, with a few allergy reactions resolving completely, after negative ion therapy. The majority of allergy sufferers can reduce reliance on other treatments (nutritional, biochemical, or prescription) during negative ion therapy.

Are There Any Side Effects or Interactions?

Individuals undergoing dialysis should not take vitamin C or magnesium without medical supervision. Ingestion of large amounts of vitamin B6 (more than 200 mg per day for adults, proportionately less for children) can cause nerve damage. Large amounts of vitamin B6 should therefore be monitored by a health care professional. Magnesium in larger amounts can cause diarrhea. Vitamin B12 supplements are not associated with side effects.

The normal stomach produces about the same amount of HCl as is found in twenty 10-grain tablets or capsules. However, people should not take more than 10 grains (650 mg) of HCl without the recommendation of a nutritionally oriented physician. No side effects are associated with the use of ionized air.

Herbs That May Be Helpful

Ephedrine, an alkaloid extracted from **ephedra** (page 259), is an approved over-the-counter treatment for bronchial tightness associated with asthma.[14] Over-the-counter drugs containing ephedrine can be safely used by adults in the amount of 12.5–25 mg every four hours. Adults should take a total dose of no more than 150 mg every twenty-four hours. Refer to labels for children's dosages. Ephedrine has largely been replaced by other bronchodilating drugs, such as alupent and albuterol. Ephedra, also known as ma huang, continues to be an important component of traditional herbal preparations for asthma. Some people use 1–2 grams of the herb per day.

Traditionally, herbs that have a soothing effect on bronchioles are also used for asthma. These would include **marshmallow root** (page 289), **mullein** (page 291), and **licorice** (page 286).

Are There Any Side Effects or Interactions?

Ephedra and ephedrine should be used with caution, since they may increase the heart rate and elevate blood pressure. Anyone with high blood pressure, heart conditions, diabetes, glaucoma, thyroid disease, and those taking MAO-inhibiting antidepressants should consult with a physician before using any type of product with ephedra. Ephedra-based products should be avoided during pregnancy and lactation and used with caution in children under the age of six years.

Marshmallow root is very safe. There have been extremely rare reports of allergic reactions. Mullein is generally safe, and there are no known contraindications to its use during pregnancy or lactation, except for rare reports of skin irritation.

Licorice products without the glycyrrhizin removed may increase blood pressure and cause water retention. Some people are more sensitive to this effect than are others. Deglycyrrhizinated licorice extracts do not cause these side effects.

Checklist for Asthma

Nutritional Supplements	Herbs	Homeopathic Remedies
Vitamin B6, Magnesium, Vitamin C, Vitamin B12, Betaine hydrochloride, Ionized air	Ephedra, Marshmallow root, Mullein, Licorice	No homeopathy commonly used for this condition

ATHEROSCLEROSIS

ATHEROSCLEROSIS, or hardening of the arteries, is a very common disease of the major blood vessels. It is characterized by fatty streaks along the vessel walls and deposits of cholesterol and calcium.

Atherosclerosis of arteries supplying the heart is called coronary artery disease. It can restrict the flow of blood to the heart, which often triggers heart attacks—the leading cause of death in Americans and Europeans. Atherosclerosis of the arteries supplying the legs causes a condition called intermittent claudication.

People with elevated cholesterol levels are much more likely to have atherosclerosis than people with low cholesterol levels. Many important nutritional approaches to protecting against atherosclerosis are aimed at lowering serum cholesterol levels. People concerned about atherosclerosis should also read the section on **high cholesterol** (page 62).

People with diabetes are also at very high risk for atherosclerosis. Those with diabetes who are concerned about atherosclerosis should also read the section on **diabetes** (page 39).

People with elevated triglycerides may be at high risk for atherosclerosis. For a discussion about fish, fish oil, and other natural substances that lower triglycerides and may also reduce the risk of atherosclerosis, see the section on **hypertriglyceridemia** (page 69).

Lifestyle Changes That May Be Helpful

Virtually all doctors acknowledge that smoking is directly linked to atherosclerosis and heart disease. Quitting smoking protects many people from atherosclerosis and heart disease and is a critical step in the process of disease prevention.

Obesity and type A behavior are both associated with an increased risk of atherosclerosis, while exercise is linked to protection from this condition. These are discussed in more detail in the section on cholesterol.

Dietary Changes That May Be Helpful

The most important dietary changes in protecting arteries from atherosclerosis include avoiding meat and dairy fat, increasing fiber, and possibly avoiding foods that contain trans fatty acids (margarine and other processed foods).

Independent of their effect on serum cholesterol, foods that contain high amounts of cholesterol—mostly egg yolks—can induce atherosclerosis.[1] It makes sense to reduce the intake of egg yolks. However, eating eggs does not increase serum cholesterol as much as eating saturated fat, and eggs may not increase serum cholesterol at all if the overall diet is low in fat. A decrease in atherosclerosis resulting from a pure vegetarian diet—meaning no meat, poultry, dairy, or eggs—combined with exercise and stress reduction has been proven by medical research.[2]

Garlic (page 265) acts as a blood thinner[3] and may reduce other risk factors for atherosclerosis.[4] Doctors of natural medicine generally view garlic as an antiatherogenic agent, and many recommend eating garlic or taking 900 mg of garlic powder per day from capsules. Garlic may also be taken as a tincture in the amount of 2–4 ml, three times daily.

Nutrients That May Be Helpful

Many cardiologists agree that LDL—low density lipoproteins, or "bad" cholesterol—triggers atherosclerosis only when it has been damaged by reactive molecules called free radicals. Several **antioxidant** (page 8) supplements protect LDL cholesterol.

Vitamin E (page 220) is an antioxidant that serves to protect LDL from oxidative damage[5] and has been linked to prevention of heart disease in double-blinded research.[6] **Vitamin C** (page 217) also protects LDL,[7] although it is less clear whether vitamin C protects against atherosclerosis. Virtually all nutritionally oriented doctors recommend 400–800 IU of vitamin E per day to lower the risk of atherosclerosis and heart attacks. Many such doctors also suggest that people take vitamin C—often 1 gram per day. See the section on cholesterol for more details.

In some studies, people who consume more **selenium** (page 203) in their diet have a lower risk of heart disease.[8][9] In one double-blinded report, individuals who already had one heart attack were given 100 mcg of selenium per day or placebo for six months.[10] At the end of the trial, there were four deaths from heart disease in the placebo group but none in the selenium group (although the numbers were too small for this difference to be statistically significant). Some nutritionally oriented doctors recommend that people with atherosclerosis supplement with 100–200 mcg of selenium per day.

Quercetin (page 201), a **bioflavonoid** (page 140), also protects LDL cholesterol from damage.[11] Several studies have found eating foods high in quercetin lowers the risk of heart disease,[12][13][14] but the research on this subject is not consistent.[15] Quercetin is found in apples, onions, black tea, and as a supplement. Dietary amounts linked to protection from heart disease are as low as 35 mg per day.

Blood levels of an amino acid called homocysteine are strongly linked to both atherosclerosis and heart disease in general.[16] Researchers believe that even slight elevations of homocysteine trigger atherosclerosis at its early stages and significantly increase the risk of heart disease.

Higher blood levels of **vitamins B6** (page 214), **B12** (page 216), and **folic acid** (page 163) are associated with low levels of homocysteine,[17] and supplementing with these vitamins lowers homocysteine levels.[18] [19] For the few cases in which B6, B12, and folic acid fail to normalize homocysteine, adding 6 grams per day of betaine may be effective.[20] Of these four supplements, folic acid appears to be the most important.[21] Attempts to lower homocysteine by simply changing the diet rather than using vitamin supplements have not been successful.[22] While several trials have consistently shown that B6, B12, and folic acid are helpful, the amounts used vary from study to study. Many nutritionally oriented doctors recommend 50 mg of vitamin B6, 100–300 mcg of vitamin B12, and 800 mcg of folic acid.

Chondroitin sulfate (page 149) is another nutrient that may prove to be important for healthy blood vessels. Preliminary research shows that chondroitin sulfate may prevent atherosclerosis in animals and humans and may also prevent heart attacks in people who already have atherosclerosis.[23] [24] However, further research is needed to determine the value of chondroitin sulfate supplements for preventing or treating atherosclerosis.

Resveratrol (page 202), found primarily in red wine, is a naturally occurring antioxidant that decreases the "stickiness" of blood platelets and helps blood vessels remain open and flexible.[25] [26] [27]

Are There Any Side Effects or Interactions?

Vitamin E side effects are very rare, as are side effects from vitamin C. However, some individuals experience diarrhea when taking a few thousand milligrams of vitamin C per day. Selenium in excess of 1,000 mcg per day can cause the loss of fingernails, skin rash, and changes to the nervous system. No clear toxicity has been identified with quercetin.

Folic acid, although safe, can mask the symptoms of vitamin B12 deficiency, which is why these vitamins should always be taken together. Vitamin B12 supplements are not associated with side effects. Vitamin B6 side effects are rare, but nervous system changes can occur with dosages above 200 mg per day.

At intakes of chondroitin sulfate greater than 10 grams per day, nausea may occur. No other adverse effects have been reported. Care should be taken if using a form of chondroitin sulfate that contains sodium, as this may worsen high blood pressure.

Herbs That May Be Helpful

As is the case with nutritional supplements and foods that protect the cardiovascular system, herbs that help prevent atherosclerosis are those that provide one of the following actions:

- Reduce the levels of **cholesterol** (page 62) and **triglycerides** (page 69) in the bloodstream
- Reduce the stickiness of platelets in the blood
- Improve the strength of blood vessel walls
- Improve the flow of blood through the body
- Provide **antioxidant** (page 8) protection to the cardiovascular system—particularly with regard to blocking oxidation of LDL cholesterol

For more detailed information on lowering serum cholesterol and triglycerides using herbs, please refer to the respective herb entries from the checklist.

Checklist for Atherosclerosis

Nutritional Supplements	Herbs	Homeopathic Remedies
Vitamin E, Vitamin C, Selenium, Quercetin, Vitamin B6, Vitamin B12, Folic acid, Betaine, Chondroitin sulfate, Resveratrol	Asian ginseng, Bilberry, Butcher's broom, Fenugreek, Fo-ti, Garlic, Ginger, Ginkgo biloba, Guggul, Hawthorn, Psyllium, Turmeric	No homeopathy commonly used for this condition

ATHLETIC PERFORMANCE

ASIDE FROM training, nutrition may be the most important influence on athletic performance. An adequate number of calories, carbohydrates, protein, and even dietary fat and water are necessary for a healthy body and especially for an athlete's body. Nutrient needs often increase faster than calorie needs for the athlete, yet many athletes do not always eat an optimal diet. Meanwhile, even marginal deficiencies of essential nutrients can reduce endurance, shorten the time to fatigue, or make it more difficult to improve performance.

Nutrients That May Be Helpful

Strenuous exercise increases the production of harmful substances called free radicals, which can damage muscle tissue and result in inflammation and aching muscles. Exercising in cities or smoggy areas also increases exposure to free radicals. **Antioxidants** (page 8), including **vitamin C** (page 217) and **vitamin E** (page 220), neutralize free radicals before they can damage the body; although antioxidants do not improve athletic performance, they may aid in exercise recovery. Regular exercise increases the efficiency of the antioxidant defense system, but an extra boost of antioxidant vitamins may be needed in older or untrained individuals or athletes who are undertaking an especially vigorous training protocol or athletic event.[1]

The **B-complex vitamins** (page 210) are also important for athletes because they are needed to unlock the energy from carbohydrates. Exercisers may have slightly increased requirements for some of the B vitamins, such as **vitamin B2** (page 212), **vitamin B6** (page 214), and **pantothenic acid** (page 193).[2] Athletic performance could suffer if these increased needs are not met.

Intense exercise alters the body's use of and requirements for several minerals. For example, exercise can decrease blood levels and increase urinary losses of **chromium** (page 150) and **zinc** (page 224). Low levels of these minerals interfere with blood sugar regulation, energy production, tissue repair, and resistance to colds and infections.[3] Chromium, in a form called chromium picolinate, has been studied for its potential role in altering body composition. Although preliminary research in animals[4] and humans[5][6] suggested that chromium picolinate increases fat loss and lean muscle tissue gain, follow-up research in people has not confirmed chromium picolinate to have a significant effect in altering body composition.[7]

Iron (page 173) is crucial for the athlete because it transports oxygen to and within the muscle cells. However, some athletes do not get enough of this mineral. In fact, up to 80% of exercising women are iron deficient, which can result in reduced endurance, muscle soreness, fatigue, lethargy, irritability, and poor concentration.[8] Nonetheless, it is unwise to supplement with iron unless a deficiency has been diagnosed. Athletes who experience undue fatigue (an early warning sign of iron deficiency) should have their iron status evaluated by a nutritionally oriented physician.

Magnesium (page 182) plays many roles in the athlete's body. This mineral aids in muscle contraction and relaxation, facilitates nerve function, maintains the heartbeat and blood pressure, and helps build muscle. Strenuous exercise may increase magnesium requirements while increasing urinary losses of magnesium, thus placing an extra drain on magnesium status.[9]

Certain amino acids, the building blocks for protein, might be ergogenic aids (performance enhancers). However, while it is now established that athletes have an increased need for protein compared with other adults, the maximum amount of protein suggested by researchers—1.5 grams for every 2.2 pounds of body weight—is already in the diet of most athletes. Eating larger amounts of protein may be linked to osteoporosis and kidney disease.

For those few athletes who consume less than optimal amounts of protein from their diets, branched-chain amino acids (page 138), or BCAAs, which include the amino acids leucine, isoleucine, and valine, are needed for the maintenance of muscle tissue and for intense exercise. BCAA supplements may reduce muscle loss and speed muscle gain.[10]

Research shows that individuals who supplement with carnitine (page 146) while engaging in an exercise regimen are less likely to experience muscle soreness.[11]

A small number of clinical trials also indicate that supplements of pyruvate (page 200), an altered form of sugar, enhance exercise endurance.[12][13] However, the research with pyruvate is preliminary and further trials are needed to determine if the effect on performance is significant.

Whey protein (page 223) is a dairy-based source of amino acids. Whey protein provides the body with the BCAAs that are needed for the maintenance of muscle tissue.

Other amino acids also influence athletic performance. Leucine (page 177) supplements or protein powders that contain leucine are used by some bodybuilders and other athletes to promote muscle recovery.[14] Some, but not all, studies indicate that inosine (page 169) can benefit athletes by improving aerobic performance.[15]

Some experts have claimed that ornithine (page 190) promotes muscle-building activity in the body, but subsequent research has not supported these claims.[16] A similar compound, ornithine alpha-ketoglutarate (page 191), or OKG, is formed from the amino acids ornithine and glutamine (page 166); OKG is believed to enhance the body's release of muscle-building hormones, such as growth hormone and insulin, and increase arginine and glutamine levels in muscle. OKG also encourages synthesis of polyamine and helps prevent the breakdown of muscle while increasing muscle growth.[17][18]

Creatine (page 153) assists in the production of energy and muscle-building processes. Most of the creatine in the body is stored in the muscles as creatine or in a form called phosphocreatine.[19] Creatine is a quickly available energy source for muscle contraction.[20] It also increases the synthesis of muscle protein and assists in the formation of polyamines (powerful growth promoters).[21] Creatine also promotes protein synthesis by causing the muscles to swell, which is called "cell volumizing."

Gamma oryzanol (page 164) is a mixture of sterols and ferulic acid esters. Preliminary evidence suggests that it increases testosterone levels, the release of endorphins, and the growth of lean muscle tissue.[22]

Medium chain triglycerides (page 184) are a class of fatty acids, but unlike other fats, the medium chain triglycerides are more rapidly absorbed and burned as energy.[23] However, most people consume an adequate, if not excessive, amount of fat in their diets, so extra fat intake as medium chain triglycerides is probably unnecessary.

Are There Any Side Effects or Interactions?

Vitamin E side effects are very rare, as are side effects from vitamin C. However, some individuals experience diarrhea when taking a few thousand milligrams of vitamin C per day. Vitamin B2 is non-toxic, even in high amounts. Vitamin B6 side effects are rare, but nervous system changes can occur with dosages above 200 mg per day. Toxicity has not been reported for pantothenic acid at supplemental doses; very large amounts (several grams per day) can cause diarrhea.

In supplemental doses (typically 50–300 mcg per day), chromium has not been linked consistently with any toxicity in humans. Zinc intake in excess of 300 mg per day may impair immune function. In addition, it is important to balance zinc and **copper** (page 151) intake.

Huge overdoses of iron (as when a child swallows many iron pills) can be fatal. Keep iron-containing supplements out of a child's reach. Hemochromatosis, hemosiderosis, polycythemia, and iron-loading anemias (such as thalassemia and sickle cell anemia) are conditions that involve excessive storage of iron. Supplementing iron can be quite dangerous for people with these diseases.

Taking too much magnesium often leads to diarrhea. Occasionally, this can happen at doses as low as 350–500 mg per day. Excessive magnesium intake is more serious, but it is rarely caused by magnesium supplements. People with kidney disease should not take magnesium supplements without consulting a physician.

Side effects have not been reported with the use of BCAAs. Carnitine has not been consistently linked with any toxicity symptoms. People who are allergic to dairy products could react to whey protein and should therefore avoid it. As with protein in general, long-term excessive intake is associated with deteriorating kidney function and possibly osteoporosis. However, neither kidney nor bone problems have been directly associated with whey protein; the other dietary sources of protein probably contribute more protein to the diet than whey protein.

There are no reported side effects with the use of inosine, ornithine, or ornithine alpha-ketoglutarate. Little is known about creatine side effects, but no consistent toxicity has been reported to date.

No side effects have been reported with the use of gamma oryzanol. Consuming medium chain triglycerides on an empty stomach can lead to gastrointestinal upset. Anyone with cirrhosis or other liver problems or lung problems, such as chronic pulmonary obstructive disease, should not use medium chain triglycerides.

Herbs That May Be Helpful

Some athletes during their training utilize energizing herbs, such as **Asian ginseng** (page 232), **eleuthero** (Siberian ginseng) (page 257), and **guaraná** (page 273).

Are There Any Side Effects or Interactions?

Guaraná may cause insomnia, trembling, anxiety, palpitations, urinary frequency, and hyperactivity. Its use should be avoided during pregnancy and lactation. Long-term use may cause decreased fertility, cardiovascular disease, and several forms of cancer, according to epidemiological studies of caffeine use.

Checklist for Athletic Performance

Nutritional Supplements	Herbs	Homeopathic Remedies
Vitamin C, Vitamin E, Vitamin B-complex (B2, B6, pantothenic acid), Chromium, Zinc, Iron, Magnesium, Branched-chain amino acids (BCAAs), Carnitine, Pyruvate, Whey protein, Leucine, Inosine, Ornithine, Ornithine alpha-ketoglutarate (OKG), Creatine monohydrate, Gamma oryzanol, Medium chain triglycerides	Asian ginseng, Eleuthero, Guaraná	No homeopathy commonly used for this condition

AUTISM

AUTISM is a severe psychiatric disorder that begins in childhood. Autistic individuals generally have only weak contact with reality.

Nutrients That May Be Helpful

Vitamin B6 (page 214) has helped to normalize the function of nerve cells in autistic children.[1] Uncontrolled and double-blinded research shows that vitamin B6 can be helpful for autistic children.[2][3] In these trials, children typically took between 3.5 mg and almost 100 mg of B6 for every 2.2 pounds of body weight, with some researchers recommending 30 mg per 2.2 pounds of body weight. Although toxicity was not reported, such amounts are widely considered to have potential toxicity, can damage the nervous system, and should only be administered by a nutritionally oriented doctor. At least one prominent researcher has suggested that vitamin B6 may be better supported by research than drug treatment in dealing with autism.[4]

Some researchers have added **magnesium** (page 182) to vitamin B6, reporting that taking both nutrients may work better than taking B6 alone.[5] The amount of magnesium—10–15 mg per 2.2 pounds of body weight—is high enough to cause diarrhea in some people and should be administered by a nutritionally oriented doctor. Doctors of natural medicine will often try vitamin B6 or the combination of B6 and magnesium for at least three months to see if these nutrients help autistic children.

Are There Any Side Effects or Interactions?

As mentioned above, the amounts of vitamin B6 and magnesium often used for autism are very high and have the potential for toxicity. A health care physician should be consulted during treatment.

Checklist for Autism

Nutritional Supplements	Herbs	Homeopathic Remedies
Vitamin B6, Magnesium	No herbs commonly used for this condition	No homeopathy commonly used for this condition

BENIGN PROSTATIC HYPERPLASIA

THE PROSTATE is a small gland that surrounds the neck of the bladder and urethra. Its major function is to contribute to seminal fluid. If it enlarges or swells, it can put pressure on the urethra, acting a bit like a clamp—this condition is known as benign prostatic hyperplasia (BPH). Half of all fifty-year-old men have BPH. A man with BPH has to urinate more often and experiences less force and caliber while urinating, often dribbling. If the prostate enlarges too much, urination is difficult or impossible and there is an increased risk of **urinary tract infection** (page 120) and kidney damage.

Most medical textbooks and doctors will advise surgery for men with BPH serious enough to cause obstruction. The prognosis for these surgeries is quite good.

Nutrients That May Be Helpful

In 1941, Dr. William Cooper and James Hart wrote about using **flaxseed oil** (page 162) in the treatment of BPH.[1] In this study, nineteen men were given 2,000 mg of flaxseed oil per day. The dose was given for three days and then reduced to 1,300 mg per day for several weeks. After that time, a maintenance dose of less then 1,000 mg was used. All patients began retaining less urine; 63% had no residual urine at the conclusion of the testing. Nighttime urination problems stopped in 68%. All patients noted less fatigue and leg pain along with an increase in sexual libido. Dribbling was eliminated in 95% of the cases. Urine stream was more forceful and the size of the prostate was reduced. Unfortunately, there has been no recent follow-up to this preliminary research.

Other researchers have noticed that the portion of the seminal fluid for which the prostate is responsible is high in the mineral **zinc** (page 224). In a study of nineteen males, those with BPH had normal levels of zinc in the blood, which did not increase when zinc supplements were given. However, the semen zinc levels increased.

This group was given 150 mg of zinc for two months, which was then dropped to 50–100 mg. In fourteen of the nineteen men (74%), the prostate shrunk in size. Unfortunately, this study was never published, and there is no other study using men as subjects. This was verified by rectal palpation, X ray, and endoscopy.[2] Animal studies have confirmed this finding but only using locally injected zinc. While the research supporting zinc is therefore very weak, some doctors of natural medicine nonetheless recommend its use.[3]

Because zinc competes with copper for absorption, when recommending this amount of zinc most nutritionally oriented doctors suggest also taking at least 2 or 3 mg of **copper** (page 151).

Another group of researchers looked at the amino acid content (the building blocks of protein) of prostate fluid. The group determined that the fluid contained high amounts of three key amino acids: glycine, alanine, and glutamic acid; a controlled study of forty-five men with BPH was then done. After three months, 66% of the patients treated with this amino acid mixture showed reduced urinary urgency, 50% had less delay in starting urine flow, 46% had less difficulty in maintaining flow, and 43% had reduced frequency. No side effects were observed.[4]

Beta-sitosterol is another nutrient that may benefit men with BPH. One double-blind study of 100 men showed that beta-sitosterol, taken either as 20 mg of beta-sitosterol three times per day or a placebo for six months, improved urine flow, reduced the size of the prostate, and led to subjective feelings of improvement of BPH.[5]

Are There Any Side Effects or Interactions?

Toxicity has not been reported with regard to flaxseed. Zinc intake in excess of 300 mg per day may impair immune function.[6] Although the preliminary research is contradictory, patients with Alzheimer's disease should avoid zinc supplements until further studies clarify the role of zinc in this disease.[7][8]

Zinc inhibits copper absorption, which can lead to anemia and lower levels of HDL cholesterol ("good" cholesterol).[9][10][11] Copper intake should be increased if zinc supplementation continues for more than a few days (except for individuals with Wilson's disease).[12] Many zinc supplements, to prevent copper inhibition, include copper in the formulation.

Zinc competes for absorption with **iron** (page 173),[13][14] **calcium** (page 144),[15] and **magnesium** (page 182).[16] A **multimineral** (page 187) supplement will prevent mineral imbalances that can result from taking high doses of zinc for extended periods of time.

Herbs That May Be Helpful

In Europe, herbal supplements have become one of the leading methods for managing early stages of BPH. Successful treatment of BPH is an ongoing process. Men with BPH will probably need to take one or a combination of these herbs indefinitely. Any nutritional support for BPH should be done after consulting a doctor.

The fat-soluble extract of the **saw palmetto** (page 306) berry has become the leading natural treatment for BPH. This extract, when used regularly, has been shown to help keep symptoms in check.[17] Saw palmetto may inhibit 5-alpha-reductase, the enzyme that converts testosterone to its more active form, dihydrotestosterone (DHT). Saw palmetto also blocks DHT from binding in the prostate.[18] Studies have used 320 mg of the standardized (85% liposterolic acids) herbal extract, capsules, or tablets per day.

In a recent study, a group of 305 patients with mild to moderate symptoms of BPH was given 160 mg of saw palmetto twice a day for three months; the study reported an 88% success rate.[19]

Since saw palmetto reduces levels of 5-alpha-reductase, an additional benefit of this herb may be reduced risk of developing prostate cancer. While no tests have been done to show that reducing this enzyme's activity will reduce prostate cancer risk, lower levels of this enzyme are detected in men in countries with lower incidence of prostate cancer.[20]

An extract from the bark of the African tree *Pygeum africanum* has also been used for BPH. Approved for use in Germany, France, and Italy, **pygeum** (page 300) has anti-inflammatory and decongesting properties that help with early-stage BPH.[21] Studies have used 50–100 mg of pygeum (standardized to 13% sterols) herbal extract, capsules, or tablets twice per day. *Pygeum africanum* contains three compounds that help the prostate: pentacyclic triterpenoids have a diuretic action; phytosterols act as an anti-inflammatory; ferulic esters help rid the prostate of any cholesterol deposits that accompany BPH.

Another herb for BPH is a concentrated extract made from the roots of the **nettle** (page 293) plant *Urtica dioica*. The root extract may increase the volume and maximum flow of urine in men with early-stage BPH.[22] It has been successfully combined with both saw palmetto and pygeum for treatment of BPH. An appropriate amount appears to be 120 mg nettle root extract, capsules, or tablets twice per day or a 2–4 ml tincture three times daily.

Are There Any Side Effects or Interactions?

No significant side effects have been noted in clinical studies with saw palmetto extracts. Please note that BPH can only be diagnosed by a physician; use of saw palmetto extract for this condition should only occur after a thorough work-up and diagnosis by a doctor.

Side effects from pygeum are very rare, but they include mild gastrointestinal irritation in some patients. Allergic reactions to nettle are rare. However, when contact is made with the skin, fresh nettles can cause a rash.

Checklist for Benign Prostatic Hyperplasia

Nutritional Supplements	Herbs	Homeopathic Remedies
Flaxseed oil, Zinc, Amino acids (glycine, alanine, glutamic acid), Beta-sitosterol	Saw palmetto, Pygeum, Nettle	Lycopodium 6c, Apis mellifica 6c, Sabal serrulata 6c

BURSITIS

BURSITIS is an inflammation of a fluid-filled sac (bursa), which the body situates in places where movement would otherwise cause friction. The most common bursa to become inflamed is in the shoulder. The cause of bursitis is mostly unknown, but trauma or arthritis may be involved.

Nutrients That May Be Helpful

Intramuscular or subcutaneous injections of **vitamin B12** (page 216)[1] or the combination of B12 and **B3** (page 213) in niacin form[2] have not only relieved symptoms but have also decreased calcifications in chronically inflamed bursae. The mechanism is not understood. Oral B vitamins are unlikely to have the same effect, since absorption of vitamin B12 is quite limited. A nutritionally oriented doctor should be consulted regarding B12 or B12/niacin injections.

Are There Any Side Effects or Interactions?

Vitamin B3 as niacin, at intakes as low as 50–100 mg, can cause flushing, headache, and stomachache in some people. The niacinamide form does not cause these side effects. Vitamin B12 is not associated with the side effects of vitamin B3.

Herbs That May Be Helpful

While there have been few studies on herbal therapy for bursitis, most practitioners of natural medicine would consider using anti-inflammatory herbs that have proven useful in conditions such as rheumatoid arthritis. These would include **boswellia** (page 238), **turmeric** (page 314), **white willow** (page 318), and topical **cayenne** (page 246) ointment. Refer to **rheumatoid arthritis** (page 115) for specific recommendations for these herbs.

Are There Any Side Effects or Interactions?

Boswellia is generally safe when used as directed. Rare side effects can include diarrhea, skin rash, and nausea. Turmeric is extremely safe. It has been used in large quantities as a food with no adverse reactions. However, persons with symptoms from gallstones should avoid turmeric.

Long-term use of willow is not advisable, as it may cause some of the same problems that aspirin does—primarily stomach ulcers. However, willow is much safer than aspirin. As is the case with aspirin, willow should not be used to lower fevers in children. People who are allergic to aspirin should avoid white willow.

Besides causing a mild burning for the first few applications (or severe burning if accidentally placed in sensitive areas, such as the eyes), there are no side effects from use of cayenne. As with anything applied to the skin, some people may have an allergic reaction, so the first application should be to a very small area of skin.

Checklist for Bursitis

Nutritional Supplements	Herbs	Homeopathic Remedies
Vitamin B12, Vitamin B3	Boswellia, Turmeric, White willow, Cayenne	Rhus toxicodendron 6c, Ruta graveolens 6c, Belladonna 6c

CANKER SORES

CANKER SORES, or mouth ulcers, are small ulcerations within the mouth. Doctors call this common condition aphthous stomatitis.

Lifestyle Changes That May Be Helpful

Minor trauma from poor-fitting dentures, rough fillings, or braces can aggravate mouth ulcers and should be remedied by a dentist.

Dietary Changes That May Be Helpful

Food sensitivities or allergies can make mouth ulcers worse.[1][2][3] While a double-blind study found allergies to play only a minor role,[4] people with recurrent mouth ulcers should discuss the diagnosis and treatment of food sensitivities with a nutritionally oriented doctor. For some people, treating allergies may be a key component to restoring health.

Nutrients That May Be Helpful

Several reports have found a surprisingly high incidence of **iron** (page 173) and B vitamin deficiency among people with recurrent mouth ulcers.[5][6][7] Supplementing with B vitamins—300 mg **vitamin B1** (page 211), 20 mg **vitamin B2** (page 212), and 150 mg **vitamin B6** (page 214)—can provide some people with relief.[8] Thiamin (B1) deficiency specifically has been linked to an increased risk.[9]

Some people with recurrent mouth ulcers respond to **Lactobacillus acidophilus** (page 135)[10] and Lactobacillus bulgaricus.[11] Chewing four lactobacillus tablets three times per day may reduce soreness in some people with recurrent mouth ulcers.[12]

Are There Any Side Effects or Interactions?

Iron should not be supplemented unless a deficiency is diagnosed with blood tests. Vitamins B1 and B2 are nontoxic, even in very high amounts. Although side effects with vitamin B6 are rare, very high levels of this vitamin can damage sensory nerves. Pregnant and lactating women should not take more than 100 mg per day of vitamin B6. There are no reported side effects with even large intakes of acidophilus.

Herbs That May Be Helpful

Licorice (page 286) that has had the glycyrrhizic acid removed is called deglycyrrhizinated licorice (DGL). Glycyrrhizic acid is the portion of licorice root that can increase blood pressure and cause water retention in some people. The wound-healing and soothing components of the root remain in DGL.

A mixture of DGL and warm water, applied to the inside of the mouth, may shorten the healing time for mouth ulcers.[13] This DGL mixture is made by combining 200 mg of powdered DGL and 200 ml of warm water. It can then be swished in the mouth for two to three minutes and spit out. This can be continued each morning and evening for one week.

The antiviral, immune-enhancing, and wound-healing properties of **echinacea** (page 255) make this herb a reasonable choice for mouth ulcers. Many people try 4 ml of liquid echinacea swished in the mouth for two to three minutes, then swallowed. This can be repeated three times per day. Tablets and capsules containing echinacea may also be helpful.

Because of its soothing effect on mucous membranes (including the lining of the mouth) and healing properties, **chamomile** (page 247) can be tried for mouth ulcers and other mouth irritations.[14] Many people with mouth ulcers make a strong tea or tincture three to four times per day and then swish it in the mouth before swallowing.

Myrrh (page 292), another traditional remedy with good wound-healing properties, has a long history of use for mouth and gum irritations. Many people have tried mixing 200–300 mg of herbal extract or 4 ml of myrrh tincture with warm water two to three times per day and swishing it in the mouth before swallowing.

Are There Any Side Effects or Interactions?

Licorice products without the glycyrrhizin removed may increase blood pressure and cause water retention; deglycyrrhizinated licorice (DGL) extracts do not cause these side effects.

People should not take echinacea without consulting a physician if they have an autoimmune illness, such as lupus, or other progressive diseases, such as tuberculosis or multiple sclerosis. Those who are allergic to flowers of the daisy family should take echinacea with caution.

Although rare, allergic reactions to chamomile have been reported. These reactions have included bronchial constriction with internal use and allergic skin reactions with topical use. While such side effects are extremely uncommon, persons with allergies to plants of the *Asteraceae* family (ragweed, asters, and chrysanthemums) should avoid use of chamomile.

Myrrh is not associated with any side effects.

Checklist for Canker Sores

Nutritional Supplements	Herbs	Homeopathic Remedies
Iron, Vitamin B-complex (B1, B2, B6), Acidophilus	Licorice (DGL), Echinacea, Chamomile, Myrrh	Natrum muriaticum 6c, Mercurius sol 6c, Arsenicum album 6c, Rhus toxicodendron 6c, Borax 6c

CARPAL TUNNEL SYNDROME

IN MANY CASES, carpal tunnel syndrome (CTS) is thought to result from long-term repetitive motions of the hands and wrists, such as from typing. Although repetitive motion is often a culprit, it does not explain the frequent occurrence of CTS with non-motion-related conditions, such as pregnancy. Conventional treatment includes splinting, rest, anti-inflammatory drugs, and, frequently, surgery—which relieves pressure and eliminates the symptoms.

Nutrients That May Be Helpful

Vitamin B6 (page 214) is the most frequently used and well-known nutritional treatment for CTS. It appears that many people with CTS have vitamin B6 deficiencies.[1] Some studies show that people with CTS are helped when given 100 mg of vitamin B6 three times per day.[2][3] Although some researchers have found benefits with lesser amounts,[4][5][6] the results have not been consistent.[7][8][9] Often, CTS will improve in two to three months with vitamin B6 supplementation.

In order to be effective, vitamin B6 must be transformed in the body to pyridoxal-5'-phosphate. Some doctors of natural medicine suggest that people who do not respond well to the vitamin B6 supplements try 50 mg of pyridoxal-5'-phosphate three times per day.

Are There Any Side Effects or Interactions?

Although side effects from vitamin B6 supplements are rare, at very high levels this vitamin can damage sensory nerves, leading to numbness in the hands and feet as well as difficulty walking. Vitamin B6 supplementation should be stopped if these symptoms develop.

Pregnant and lactating women should not take more than 100 mg of vitamin B6 per day. For other adults, vitamin B6 is usually safe in amounts of 200–500 mg per day,[10] although occasional problems have been reported in this range.[11] Any adult taking more than 100–200 mg of vitamin B6 per day for more than a few months should consult a doctor. Side effects from vitamin B6 become more common when intake exceeds 2,000 mg per day; consequently, this supplement level should be avoided.[12]

Checklist for Autism

Nutritional Supplements	Herbs	Homeopathic Remedies
Vitamin B6	No herbs commonly used for this condition	Ruta graveolens 6c, Rhus toxicodendron 6c

CATARACTS

CATARACTS develop when damage to the protein of the lens of the eyes clouds the lens and impairs vision.

Most people, if they live long enough, will develop cataracts.[1] Cataracts are more likely to occur in those who smoke, have diabetes, or are exposed to excessive sunlight. All of these factors create what scientists call oxidative damage. Oxidative damage to the lens of the eye appears to cause cataracts in animals[2] and people.[3]

Nutrients That May Be Helpful

People with low blood levels of **antioxidants** (page 8) and those who eat few antioxidant-rich fruits and vegetables are at high risk for cataracts.[4] [5] The major antioxidants in the lens of the eye are **vitamin C** (page 217)[6] and glutathione (an antioxidant enzyme).[7] Vitamin C is needed to activate **vitamin E** (page 220),[8] which in turn activates glutathione. Both nutrients are important for healthy vision.

Vitamin C levels in the eye decrease with age;[9] however, supplementing with vitamin C prevents this decrease[10] and is linked to a lower risk of developing cataracts.[11] [12] Healthy people are more likely to take vitamin C and vitamin E supplements than those with cataracts,[13] and people who supplement with vitamin C develop far fewer cataracts.[14] [15]

Vitamin E supplements also protect against cataracts in animals[16] and people.[17] Many people take 400 IU of vitamin E per day as prevention.

Some studies find that eating more foods rich in **beta-carotene** (page 209) or supplementing with **vitamin A** (page 209) lowers the risk of cataracts.[18] It is still not clear whether beta-carotene per se protects the eye or if the beta-carotene is found in foods that contain other protective factors. People who eat a lot of spinach, which is high in **lutein** (page 179), a nutrient similar to beta-carotene, appear to be at low risk for cataracts.[19]

Vitamin **B2** (page 212) and vitamin **B3** (page 213) are needed to protect glutathione, an important antioxidant in the eye. Vitamin B2 deficiency is linked to cataracts.[20] [21] Older people taking 3 mg of vitamin B2 and 40 mg of vitamin B3 per day may be partly protected against cataracts.[22]

The flavonoid **quercetin** (page 201) may also help by blocking sorbitol accumulation in the eye.[23] This may be especially helpful for those with diabetes.

Are There Any Side Effects or Interactions?

Some individuals develop diarrhea after as little as a few thousand milligrams of vitamin C per day, while others are not bothered by ten times this amount. However, high levels of vitamin C can deplete the body of copper,[24] an essential nutrient. It is prudent to ensure adequate copper intake at higher intakes of vitamin C (copper is found in many multivitamin/mineral supplements).

One form of vitamin B3, called niacinamide or nicotinamide, is almost always safe to take, although rare liver problems have occurred at doses in excess of 1,000 mg per day. Another form of vitamin B3, called niacin or nicotinic acid, at doses as low as 50–100 mg may cause flushing, headache, and stomachache in some people. However, very high doses (above 1 gram) of this form of vitamin B3 can also cause a variety of serious health problems.

Herbs That May Be Helpful

Bilberry (page 234), a close relative of blueberry, is high in the **bioflavonoid** (page 140) complex anthocyanosides.[25] Anthocyanosides protect both the lens and the retina from oxidative damage. This bioflavonoid also helps with adaptation to bright light and improves night vision. The potent antioxidant activity of anthocyanosides makes it useful for reducing the risk of cataracts.[26] [27]

Many people take 240–480 mg per day of bilberry extract, capsules, or tablets standardized to contain 25% anthocyanosides. In recommended amounts, there are no known side effects with bilberry extract.

Checklist for Cataracts

Nutritional Supplements	Herbs	Homeopathic Remedies
Vitamin C, Vitamin E, Vitamin A/Beta-Carotene, Lutein, B-Complex (B2, B3), Quercetin	Bilberry	No homeopathy commonly used for this condition

CHEMOTHERAPY SUPPORT

CHEMOTHERAPY SUPPORT, the systemic use of anticancer drugs, is a common treatment for many cancers.

Unfortunately, during the process of eliminating cancerous cells, healthy cells are also damaged, and many side effects can develop. Several nutritional approaches show promise for alleviating side effects and/or increasing the effectiveness of chemotherapy treatment.

Malabsorption and Weight Loss

Chemotherapy often causes nausea, malabsorption, and weight loss. The best way to combat these problems may involve working with a nutritionally oriented doctor or dietitian on an individual basis. A **multiple vitamin/mineral** (page 187) can be a first step in counteracting the decreased absorption of nutrients caused by chemotherapy.

Nausea

At least one trial suggests that **N-acetyl cysteine** (page 189), or NAC, at 1,800 mg per day may reduce nausea and vomiting caused by chemotherapy.[1] NAC is an amino acid–like supplement that produces **antioxidant** (page 8) activity. **Ginger** (page 267) can also be helpful in alleviating nausea and vomiting caused by chemotherapy.[2][3] A reasonable amount is 2–4 grams of the dried rhizome powder two to three times per day. Ginger in the form of tablets, capsules, and liquid herbal extracts is also available, which can be taken in 250 mg amounts every two or three hours, for a total of 1 gram per day.

Mouth Sores

Chemotherapy often causes painful mouth sores, a condition called mucositis. Applying 400 IU of **vitamin E** (page 220) topically twice per day to the sores can reduce the problem, according to double-blind research.[4] This can be achieved by breaking a vitamin E capsule and squeezing it onto the sores. It makes sense to use the d-alpha tocopherol form rather than tocopheryl forms of vitamin E, because the tocopheryls may not be active when applied to body surfaces.

Nutrients That May Help Chemotherapy Work

In animal and test-tube studies, individual nutrients—usually antioxidants such as **vitamin A** (page 209),[5] vitamin E (page 220),[6] and **vitamin C** (page 217)[7]—have increased the effectiveness of chemotherapy. Although more research is needed in cancer patients, a few human trials suggest similar effects, including increased survival.[8] Nutritional support for chemotherapy patients should be discussed with a nutritionally oriented doctor.

Nutrients and Specific Chemotherapy Drugs

Methotrexate, a chemotherapy drug, interferes with the metabolism of **folic acid** (page 163), a B vitamin. Cancer patients taking methotrexate should not supplement folic acid beyond the 400 mcg found in a multivitamin without first discussing it with their oncologist, because supplementation might interfere with the action of the drug. Sometimes oncologists supply leucovorin—a special form of folic acid—after methotrexate has done its work in the body. The leucovorin is used to protect against unnecessary side effects caused by methotrexate.

Adriamycin, also called doxorubicin, sometimes causes heart damage. A variety of antioxidants appear to reduce this toxicity. For example, **coenzyme Q10** (page 152) has been used successfully for this purpose.[9] Nutritionally oriented doctors sometimes recommend 90–120 mg of coenzyme Q10.

In animals, vitamin C protects against Adriamycin-induced heart damage.[10] For this reason, some nutritionally oriented doctors recommend several grams of vitamin C per day to people taking Adriamycin.

In test tubes, vitamin E has been found to enhance the ability of Adriamycin to kill cancer cells.[11] Anecdotes have appeared suggesting that hair loss caused by Adriamycin may be reduced by taking high amounts (1,600 IU per day) of vitamin E.[12] In animals, vitamin E protects against heart damage caused by Adriamycin.[13] Many nutritionally oriented doctors recommend at least 800 IU of vitamin E to people taking Adriamycin.

Under certain circumstances, **vitamin B2** (page 216), or riboflavin, can also have antioxidant activity. In rats, supplementation with vitamin B2 helps protect against Adriamycin-induced heart damage.[14]

Cisplatin, another chemotherapy drug, often leads to depletion of **magnesium** (page 182).[15] In some reports, this depletion happens in a majority of cases.[16] People taking cisplatin should have their magnesium status checked by a nutritionally oriented doctor, who will prescribe magnesium supplements when appropriate. Glutathione significantly reduces the toxicity caused by cisplatin and improves quality of life for these patients, but it must be given intravenously by a doctor.[17][18]

Fluorouracil sometimes causes problems on the skin of palms and soles. Reports have appeared showing that 100 mg per day of **vitamin B6** (page 214) can sometimes eliminate the pain associated with this condition.[19][20]

Are There Any Side Effects or Interactions?

No consistent adverse effects of NAC have been reported in humans. One small study found that daily amounts of 1.2 grams or more could lead to oxidative damage. Extremely large amounts of cysteine, the amino acid from which NAC is derived, may be toxic to nerve cells in rats.

Vitamin E toxicity is very rare; supplements are widely considered to be safe. Women who are or could become pregnant should take less than 10,000 IU per day of vitamin A to avoid the risk of birth defects. For other adults, intake above 25,000 IU per day can—in rare cases—cause headaches, dry skin, hair loss, fatigue, bone problems, and liver damage.

Some individuals develop diarrhea after as little as a few thousand milligrams of vitamin C per day, while others are not bothered by ten times this amount. However, high levels of vitamin C can deplete the body of copper, an essential nutrient. It is prudent to ensure adequate copper intake at higher intakes of vitamin C (copper is found in many multivitamin/mineral supplements).

Congestive heart failure patients taking coenzyme Q10 should not abruptly discontinue taking supplements without first consulting a physician. Vitamin B2 is nontoxic, even in very high amounts. Taking too much magnesium can lead to diarrhea. This can happen at doses as low as 350–500 mg per day. People with kidney disease should not take magnesium supplements without consulting a physician.

Although side effects from vitamin B6 supplements are rare, at very high levels this vitamin can damage sensory nerves, leading to numbness in the hands and feet as well as difficulty walking. Vitamin B6 supplementation should be stopped if these symptoms develop. Pregnant and lactating women

should not take more than 100 mg of vitamin B6. For other adults, vitamin B6 is safe in amounts of 200–500 mg per day, although occasional problems have been reported in this range.

Herbs That May Be Helpful

Using herbal adaptogens following chemotherapy can help the bone marrow in the production of white blood cells and help optimize immune function. Three herbs that have proven particularly useful following chemotherapy are **astragalus** (page 233) (two to three 500 mg capsules three times per day), **eleuthero** (Siberian ginseng) (page 257) (2–3 grams per day of the dried root or 300–400 mg per day of the concentrated solid extract standardized on eleutherosides B and E), and **Asian ginseng** (page 232) (100–200 mg per day of the standardized herbal extract).[21][22][23] Astragalus is often used in combination with another Chinese herb, *Ligustrum lucidum*.

Other herbal adaptogens that may also prove helpful include **maitake** (page 288), **shiitake** (page 310), **reishi** (page 303), and **schisandra** (page 307).

Are There Any Side Effects or Interactions?

Astragalus, eleuthero, and Asian ginseng are generally safe. Astragalus has no known side effects when used as recommended.

In rare instances, Asian ginseng may cause overstimulation and possibly insomnia. Consuming caffeine with ginseng increases the risk of overstimulation and gastrointestinal upset. Persons with uncontrolled high blood pressure should not use ginseng. Long-term use of ginseng may cause menstrual abnormalities and breast tenderness in some women. Ginseng is not recommended for pregnant or lactating women.

There have been no reports of any side effects with the use of maitake. Shiitake has an excellent record of safety but has been known to induce temporary diarrhea and abdominal bloating when used in high dosages. Its safety during pregnancy has not yet been established. Side effects from reishi can include dizziness, dry mouth and throat, nose bleeds, and abdominal upset; these rare effects may develop with continuous use over three to six months. As it may increase bleeding time, reishi is not recommended for those taking anticoagulant (blood-thinning) medications. Pregnant and lactating women should consult a physician before taking reishi. Side effects involving schisandra are uncommon, but they may include abdominal upset, decreased appetite, and skin rash.

Checklist for Chemotherapy Support

Nutritional Supplements	Herbs	Homeopathic Remedies
Multiple vitamin/mineral, N-acetyl cysteine, Vitamin E, Vitamin A, Vitamin C, Folic acid, Coenzyme Q10, Vitamin B2 (riboflavin), Magnesium, Vitamin B6	Ginger, Astragalus, Eleuthero, Asian ginseng, *Ligustrum lucidum*, Maitake, Shiitake, Reishi, Schisandra	Gelsemium 6c, Ipecac 30c, Nux vomica 6c, Cadmium sulfuricum 30c

COMMON COLD/SORE THROAT

THE COMMON COLD is an acute (short-term) viral infection of the upper respiratory tract, often causing runny nose, sore throat, and malaise.

Colds can be spread through the air, such as when a person sneezes, or by contact with contaminated objects.

Dietary Changes That May Be Helpful

Sugar has been found to interfere with immune functioning,[1] so it makes sense to avoid excess sweets.

Nutrients That May Be Helpful

A review of twenty-one placebo-controlled studies using 1–8 grams of **vitamin C** (page 217) found that "In each of the twenty-one studies, vitamin C reduced the duration of episodes and the severity of the symptoms of the common cold by an average of 23%."[2][3][4] The optimum amount of vitamin C to take for cold treatment is debatable, but 1–3 grams per day is commonly used.

Zinc (page 224) gluconate lozenges are helpful for cold sufferers.[5][6] A few reports claim that zinc is ineffective, but these trials have been found to use inactive forms of zinc.[7] Successful research uses zinc gluconate lozenges containing 15–25 mg of zinc per lozenge. They can be used at the first sign of a cold;

up to ten lozenges per day can be taken for several days during the cold. Long-term zinc supplementation in healthy individuals should be lower, about 15 mg per day, and must include **copper** (page 151) to avoid a copper deficiency.

Are There Any Side Effects or Interactions?

Some individuals develop diarrhea after as little as a few thousand milligrams of vitamin C per day, while others are not bothered by ten times this amount. However, high levels of vitamin C can deplete the body of copper,[8,9] an essential nutrient. It is prudent to ensure adequate copper intake at higher intakes of vitamin C (copper is found in many multiple vitamin/mineral supplements).

More is not necessarily better when it comes to zinc. Zinc intake in excess of 300 mg per day may impair immune function.[10] Some people report that zinc lozenges lead to mild problems, such as nausea, mouth irritation, and a bad taste.

Herbs That May Be Helpful

Echinacea (page 255) stimulates the immune system[11] and reduces the incidence of colds when taken as a preventive. It doubles as a useful treatment for a cold, because it helps speed the healing process.[12]

As an immune system stimulant, echinacea is best taken for a specific period of time. At the onset of a cold, it can be taken three to four times per day and continued for ten to fourteen days. To help prevent a cold, it can be taken three times per day for six to eight weeks. A "rest" period is recommended, since echinacea's effects may diminish if used continuously. Many people take up to 900 mg of echinacea in tablet or capsule form, or 4 ml three times per day of the liquid extract.

In traditional herbal medicine, **goldenseal** (page 270) root is often taken with echinacea. Two alkaloids in the root (berberine and canadensis) have an antimicrobial and mild immune-stimulating effect.[13] Goldenseal soothes irritated mucous membranes in the throat,[14] making it useful for those experiencing a sore throat with their cold.

Goldenseal root should only be used for short periods of time. Goldenseal root extract, capsules, or tablets are typically taken in amounts of 4–6

grams three times per day. Using goldenseal powder as a tea or tincture may soothe a sore throat.

Herbs high in mucilage, such as **slippery elm** (page 311) and **marshmallow root** (page 289), are often helpful for symptomatic relief of coughs and irritated throats.

Herbal supplements can play a role in long-term attempts to strengthen the immune system and fight infections. Adaptogens, which include **eleuthero** (Siberian ginseng) (page 257), **Asian ginseng** (page 232), **astragalus** (page 233), and **schisandra** (page 307), can help keep various body systems—including the immune system—functioning optimally. Astragalus is well regarded for boosting immune function. Schisandra may also be helpful for coughs.

Elderberry (page 256) has been shown in research to inhibit the influenza virus. **Horseradish** (page 280) has antibiotic properties, which may account for its easing of throat and upper respiratory tract infections. **Mullein** (page 291) has expectorant and demulcent properties, which accounts for this herb's historical use as a remedy for the respiratory tract, particularly in cases of irritating coughs with bronchial congestion.

The resin of the herb **myrrh** (page 292) has been shown to kill various microbes and to stimulate macrophages (a type of white blood cell). **Red raspberry** (page 302) may also help relieve some of the symptoms of the common cold, such as sore throat.

Are There Any Side Effects or Interactions?

People should not take echinacea without consulting a physician if they have an autoimmune illness, such as lupus, or other progressive diseases, such as tuberculosis or multiple sclerosis. Those who are allergic to flowers of the daisy family should take echinacea with caution. Taken as recommended, goldenseal is generally safe. However, as with all alkaloid-containing plants, high amounts may lead to gastrointestinal distress and possible nervous system effects. Goldenseal is not recommended for pregnant or lactating women.

Slippery elm is quite safe, with no known side effects. Marshmallow is also very safe. There have been extremely rare reports of allergic reactions.

Used as recommended, Asian ginseng is generally safe. In rare instances, it may cause overstimulation and possibly insomnia. Consuming caffeine with ginseng increases the risk of overstimulation and gastrointestinal upset. Persons with uncontrolled high blood pressure should not use ginseng. Long-term use of ginseng may cause menstrual abnormalities and breast tenderness in some women. Ginseng is not recommended for pregnant or lactating women.

Reported side effects have been minimal with use of eleuthero. Mild, transient diarrhea has been reported in a very small number of users. Eleuthero may cause insomnia in some people if taken too close to bedtime. Eleuthero is not recommended for individuals with uncontrolled high blood pressure. It can be used during pregnancy or lactation. However, pregnant or lactating women using eleuthero should avoid products that have been adulterated with *Panax ginseng* or other related species that are contraindicated.

Astragalus and elderberry have no known side effects when used as recommended. Side effects involving schisandra are uncommon but may include abdominal upset, decreased appetite, and skin rash. Very large amounts of horseradish can cause vomiting or excessive sweating. Horseradish should be avoided by patients with hypothyroidism. Mullein is generally safe, and there are no known contraindications to its use during pregnancy or lactation, except for rare reports of skin irritation. Myrrh is not associated with any side effects. Raspberry may cause mild loosening of stools and nausea.

Checklist for Common Cold/Sore Throat

Nutritional Supplements	Herbs	Homeopathic Remedies
Vitamin C, Zinc	Echinacea, Goldenseal, Slippery elm, Marshmallow root, Eleuthero, Asian ginseng, Astragalus, Schisandra, Elderberry, Horseradish, Mullein, Myrrh, Red raspberry	Aconite 30c, Kali bichromicum 6c, Rhus toxicodendron 6c. Natrum muriaticum 6c, Euphrasia 6c

CONGESTIVE HEART FAILURE

CONGESTIVE HEART FAILURE (CHF) is a chronic condition that results when the heart muscle is unable to pump blood as quickly as is needed. It leads to breathlessness, fatigue, and accumulation of fluid in the lungs or the veins (primarily in the legs), or both.

Hypertension (page 67), or high blood pressure, can cause congestive heart failure.

Cautions About Exercise

Too much exercise can be life-threatening for those with CHF. How much is "too much" varies from person to person. Therefore, any exercise program undertaken by someone with CHF requires professional supervision. Nevertheless, even with severe disease, appropriate exercise can benefit those with CHF.[1]

Nutrients That May Be Helpful

As is true for many heart conditions, **coenzyme Q10** (page 152) helps people with CHF[2]—an effect proven in double-blinded research.[3] Many people take 30 mg three times per day. Coenzyme Q10 may take several months to show beneficial results. People with CHF taking coenzyme Q10 should *not* stop taking it suddenly. Sudden withdrawal may exacerbate CHF.

Those with CHF have insufficient oxygenation of the heart, which can damage the heart muscle. Such damage may be reduced by taking **carnitine** (page 146) supplements.[4] Carnitine is a natural substance made from the amino acids **lysine** (page 181) and **methionine** (page 186). Levels of carnitine are low in people with CHF.[5] Therefore, many nutritionally oriented doctors recommend that those with CHF take 500 mg of carnitine two to three times per day.

Magnesium (page 182) deficiency frequently occurs with CHF, leading to heart arrhythmias. Magnesium supplements reduce the risk of these arrhythmias.[6] Those with CHF are often given drugs that deplete both magnesium and **potassium** (page 197). It is important to protect against the arrhythmias, which could result from a lack of either mineral.[7] Many nutritionally oriented doctors suggest magnesium supplements of 300 mg per day.

Whole fruit and fruit and vegetable juice, all of which are high in potassium, are also recommended by some doctors; however, this dietary change should be discussed with a health care provider, because several drugs given to those with CHF can actually cause *retention* of potassium, making dietary potassium, even from fruit, dangerous.

Taurine (page 206), an amino acid, helps the heart pump. Research repeatedly shows that taurine helps those with CHF.[8] [9] [10] [11] Most nutritionally oriented doctors suggest 6 grams per day.

The body needs **arginine** (page 137), another amino acid, to make nitric oxide, which increases blood flow. This process is impaired in those with CHF. Arginine has been used experimentally in amounts of 5.6–12.6 grams per day in the treatment of CHF.[12] A doctor should be consulted before taking arginine.

Are There Any Side Effects or Interactions?

Carnitine has not been consistently linked with any toxicity symptoms. Potassium and magnesium should not be taken by anyone taking "sparing" diuretic drugs. Excessive magnesium intake can cause diarrhea. People with kidney disease should not take magnesium supplements without consulting a doctor. High potassium intake can produce stomach irritation.

Taurine has not been consistently linked with any toxicity. Individuals with kidney or liver disease should consult their nutritionally oriented doctors before supplementing with arginine. Individuals with herpes (either cold sores or genital herpes) should not take arginine, because it can stimulate the virus.

Herbs That May Be Helpful

Studies have shown that standardized extracts made from the leaves and flowers of **hawthorn** (page 276), *Crataegus oxyacantha,* are effective in the support of early-stage congestive heart failure.[13] [14] Hawthorn extracts help early-stage CHF by increasing blood flow to the heart, increasing the strength of heart contractions, reducing resistance to blood flow in the extremities, and acting as an **antioxidant** (page 8).[15] [16] [17]

People often use hawthorn extract in capsules or tablets standardized to either total flavonoid content (usually 2.2%) or oligomeric procyanidins (usually 18.75%). Many people take 80–300 mg twice per day or a tincture in the amount of 4–5 ml three times daily. Hawthorn berry products that are not standardized are weaker, and the recommended amount is approximately 4–6 grams per day.

Those with early-stage CHF might consider other herbs that help improve circulation. **Ginkgo biloba** (page 268) and **garlic** (page 265) herbal extracts in capsules, tablets, or tinctures are two possible choices.

Checklist for Congestive Heart Failure

Nutritional Supplements	Herbs	Homeopathic Remedies
Coenzyme Q10, Carnitine, Magnesium, Potassium, Taurine, Arginine	Hawthorn, Ginkgo biloba, Garlic	No homeopathy commonly used for this condition

CONSTIPATION

CONSTIPATION results when food moves too slowly through the gastrointestinal (GI) tract.

Dietary Changes That May Be Helpful

Insoluble **fiber** (page 159) acts like a sponge. Adding water to the "sponge" makes it soft and easy to push through the GI tract. Insoluble fiber comes from vegetables, beans, brown rice, whole wheat, rye, and other whole grains. Switching from white bread and white rice to whole grain and brown rice may help relieve constipation. It is important to drink lots of fluid along with the fiber—at least 16 ounces of water per serving of fiber. Otherwise, a "dry sponge" is now in the system, which can worsen the constipation.

In addition, flaxseed or wheat bran can be added to the diet. Some doctors of natural medicine also recommend 15 ml per day of **flaxseed oil** (page 162) to help relieve constipation. Wheat bran helps constipation but is not by itself a cure,[1] although higher amounts are sometimes more successful.[2] **Psyllium** (page 299) seeds may also help.[3]

Food allergies in children or a lack of stomach acid or pancreatic enzymes in adults may make constipation worse. If other approaches do not help, these possibilities can be discussed with a nutritionally oriented physician.

Lifestyle Changes That May Be Helpful

Exercise may increase the muscular contractions of the intestine, which sometimes helps move the contents through the body.[4] Nonetheless, the effect of exercise on constipation remains controversial.[5]

Nutrients That May Be Helpful

Chlorophyll (page 148), the substance responsible for the green color in plants, is useful for many gastrointestinal problems, including constipation.

Are There Any Side Effects or Interactions?

No side effects have been reported with the use of chlorophyll.

Herbs That May Be Helpful

The most frequently sold laxatives worldwide come from plants. Herbal laxatives are either bulk-forming or stimulating.

Bulk-forming laxatives come from plants with a high fiber and mucilage content that expand when they come into contact with water; examples include psyllium, flaxseed, and fenugreek (page 262). As the volume in the bowel increases, a reflex contraction is stimulated. These mild laxatives are best suited for long-term treatment of constipation.

Many nutritional doctors recommend 7.5 grams of psyllium seeds or 5 grams of psyllium husks, mixed with water or juice, one to two times per day. Some doctors use a combination of senna (18%) and psyllium (82%) for the treatment of chronic constipation. This has been shown to work for people in nursing homes.[6]

Stimulant laxatives are high in anthraquinones, which stimulate bowel muscle contraction. The most frequently used stimulant laxatives are senna leaves, cascara bark, and aloe latex. While senna (page 309) is the most popular, cascara (page 243) has a somewhat milder action. Aloe (page 231) is very potent and should be used with caution.

The unprocessed roots of fo-ti (page 264) possess a mild laxative effect. The bitter compounds in dandelion (page 251) leaves and root are also mild laxatives.

Are There Any Side Effects or Interactions?

These natural stimulant laxatives are for short-term use; they are rarely recommended for long-term use, unless in very low amounts for chronic constipation. Overuse can lead to dehydration and dependency. They are not typically recommended for pregnant and lactating women (senna is an exception). Those with inflammatory bowel diseases, such as Crohn's disease (page 34) or ulcerative colitis, should not use laxatives.

Side effects from psyllium (such as allergic skin and respiratory reactions to psyllium dust) have largely been limited to workers in psyllium manufacturing plants.

Senna can cause the colon to become dependent on it to move properly. Therefore, senna must not be used for more than ten consecutive days. Chronic senna use (for more than ten days) can also cause loss of fluids, low potassium levels, and diarrhea, all of which can lead to dehydration and negative effects on the heart and muscles. Similarly, aloe laxative preparations, if used for more than ten consecutive days, can aggravate constipation and cause dependency. Those with an intestinal obstruction should not employ cascara.

Fo-ti may cause mild diarrhea. Some people who are sensitive to fo-ti may develop a skin rash, and very high doses may cause numbness in the arms or legs. Dandelion leaf and root should be used with caution by persons with gallstones. If there is an obstruction of the bile ducts, then dandelion should be avoided altogether. In cases of stomach ulcer or gastritis, dandelion should be used cautiously, as it may cause overproduction of stomach acid.

Checklist for Constipation

Nutritional Supplements	Herbs	Homeopathic Remedies
Fiber, Flaxseed oil, Chlorophyll	Psyllium, Flaxseed, Fenugreek, Senna, Cascara, Aloe, Fo-ti, Dandelion	Nux vomica 6c, Sepia 30c, Sulfur 6c

CROHN'S DISEASE

CROHN'S DISEASE is a poorly understood inflammatory disease that affects the final part of the small intestine and the beginning section of the colon. It often causes bloody stools and malabsorption problems.

Dietary Changes That May Be Helpful

People with Crohn's disease eat more sugar than others.[1] While details of how sugar injures the intestine are still being uncovered, many doctors suggest eliminating all sugar (including soft drinks and processed foods with added sugar) from the diets of those with Crohn's.

A high animal protein and high fat diet (other than fish) has also been linked to Crohn's disease.[2] As with many other health conditions, it may be beneficial to eat less meat and dairy fat and more fruits and vegetables.

When those with Crohn's disease avoid foods they are allergic to, they fare much better. One study reported that people with Crohn's are most likely to react to cereals, dairy, and yeast.[3] Yeast and some dairy (cheese) are both high in histamine, which is part of the allergenic response. Those with Crohn's lack the ability to break down histamine at a normal rate.[4] It would probably be helpful to identify potential allergies and avoid those foods with the help of a nutritionally oriented doctor.

Lifestyle Changes That May Be Helpful

People with Crohn's disease are more likely to smoke, and there is evidence that continuing to smoke aggravates disease progression.[5]

Nutrients That May Be Helpful

Crohn's disease often leads to malabsorption. For this reason, it may be helpful to take a high potency **multiple vitamin/mineral** (page 187) supplement. In particular, people with Crohn's tend to be deficient in **zinc** (page 224), **folic acid** (page 163), **vitamin B12** (page 216), and **iron** (page 173).[6] Zinc, folic acid, and vitamin B12 are needed to repair intestinal cells damaged by Crohn's disease. Some doctors recommend 25–50 mg of zinc (balanced with 2–4 mg of copper), 800 mcg of folic acid, and 800 mcg of vitamin B12. Iron status should be evaluated by a nutritionally oriented doctor before considering supplementation.

Vitamin A (page 209) is needed for the growth and repair of cells that line both the small and large intestine.[7] Over the years, reports of those with Crohn's responding to vitamin A have appeared in medical journals.[8][9] For adults with Crohn's disease, some nutritionally oriented doctors recommend 50,000 IU per day. A dose this high should never be taken without qualified guidance, nor should it be given to a woman who is or could become pregnant.

Vitamin D (page 219) malabsorption is common in Crohn's,[10] which can lead to a deficiency.[11] Successful treatment with vitamin D for osteomalacia (bone brittleness caused by vitamin D deficiency) triggered by Crohn's disease has been reported.[12] A nutritionally oriented doctor can evaluate vitamin D status and suggest the right level of vitamin D supplements.

Crohn's disease is considered one of the two major forms of inflammatory bowel disease. EPA and DHA, the omega-3 fatty acids found in **fish oil** (page 160), have anti-inflammatory activity. Supplementing with a combination of EPA and DHA at 2,700 mg per day may reduce the recurrence rate of Crohn's.[13] Using an enteric-coated, "free fatty acid" form of EPA/DHA may lead to better results.

Are There Any Side Effects or Interactions?

Women who are or could become pregnant should not take more than 10,000 IU (3,000 mcg) per day of vitamin A, to avoid the risk of birth defects. For other adults, intake above 25,000 IU (7,500 mcg) per day can—in rare cases—cause headaches, dry skin, hair loss, fatigue, bone problems, and liver damage.

Excessive vitamin D intake can cause several symptoms, including headaches, weight loss, and kidney stones. Patients with sarcoidosis or hyperparathyroidism should not take vitamin D without consulting a physician.

Side effects from EPA and DHA include nose bleeds (because of reduced blood clotting), gastrointestinal upset, and "fishy" burps.

Herbs That May Be Helpful

A combination of herbs has been used to help soothe inflammation throughout the digestive tract. The formula contains **marshmallow root** (page 289), **slippery elm** (page 311), wild indigo, **goldenseal** (page 270), **echinacea** (page 255), and cranesbill. Marshmallow and slippery elm are mucilaginous plants that help soothe inflamed tissues. Wild indigo and goldenseal help inhibit growth of abnormal gut bacteria and also have astringent effects. Cranesbill is another astringent. Echinacea promotes normal immune function.

Are There Any Side Effects or Interactions?

Goldenseal should not be used during pregnancy or lactation. Echinacea is essentially non-toxic when taken orally. People should not take echinacea without consulting a physician if they have an autoimmune illness, such as lupus, or other progressive diseases, such as tuberculosis or multiple sclerosis. Those who are allergic to flowers of the daisy family should take echinacea with caution. There are no known contraindications to the use of echinacea during pregnancy or lactation.

Checklist for Crohn's Disease

Nutritional Supplements	Herbs	Homeopathic Remedies
Multiple vitamin/mineral (zinc, folic acid, B12, iron), Vitamin A, Vitamin D, Fish oil (EPA/DHA), Zinc	Marshmallow root, Slippery elm, Wild indigo, Goldenseal, Echinacea, Cranesbill	No homeopathy commonly used for this condition

DEPRESSION

DEPRESSION, characterized by unhappy feelings of hopelessness, can be a response to stressful events, hormonal imbalances, biochemical abnormalities, or other causes. Mild depression that passes quickly may not require any diagnosis or treatment. However, when depression becomes recurrent, constant, or severe, it should be diagnosed by a licensed counselor, psychologist, or psychiatrist. Diagnosis may be crucial to determining appropriate treatment. For example, depression caused by low thyroid function can be successfully treated with prescription thyroid medication. Suicidal depression often requires prescription antidepressants. Persistent mild-to-moderate depression triggered by stressful events is often best treated with counseling and not necessarily with pills of any sort.

When depression is not a function of external events, it is called endogenous. Endogenous depression is often due to biochemical abnormalities. Lifestyle changes and herbs may be used with people who suffer from depression with a variety of causes, but dietary and nutrient interventions are usually best geared to endogenous depression.

Dietary Changes That May Be Helpful

Although some of the research has produced mixed results,[1] several double-blind studies have shown that food allergies can trigger mental symptoms, including depression.[2] [3] Individuals with depression who do not respond to other natural or conventional approaches should consult a nutritionally oriented doctor to diagnose possible food sensitivities and avoid offending foods.

Restricting sugar and caffeine in people with depression may elevate mood.[4] How much of this effect results from the sugar and how much from the caffeine remains unknown. People with depression may want to avoid sugar and caffeine for one week to see what happens.

Lifestyle Changes That May Be Helpful

Exercise increases the body's production of endorphins—chemical substances that can relieve depression. Scientific research shows that routine exercise can positively affect mood and help with depression.[5] As little as three hours per week of aerobic exercises can profoundly reduce the level of depression.[6]

Nutrients That May Be Helpful

Oral contraceptives can deplete the body of **vitamin B6** (page 214), a nutrient needed for maintenance of normal mental functioning. Double-blind research shows that women who are depressed and who have become depleted of vitamin B6 while taking oral contraceptives typically respond to vitamin B6 supplementation.[7] In one trial, 20 mg of vitamin B6 were taken twice per day. Some evidence suggests that people who are depressed—even when not taking the oral contraceptive—are still more likely to be B6 deficient than people who are not depressed.[8]

Several studies also indicate that vitamin B6 supplementation helps alleviate depression associated with **premenstrual syndrome** (page 109),[9] or PMS, although the research remains inconsistent.[10] Many nutritionally oriented doctors suggest that women who have depression associated with PMS take 100–300 mg of vitamin B6 per day.

Iron (page 173) deficiency is known to affect mood and can exacerbate depression—a problem that is easy to fix with iron supplements. Iron deficiency can be diagnosed and treated by any nutritionally oriented doctor.

Deficiency of **vitamin B12** (page 216) can create disturbances in mood that respond to B12 supplementation.[11] Depression caused by vitamin B12 deficiency can occur in the absence of anemia.[12] Diagnosis of deficiency requires a doctor knowledgeable in the field of nutrition.

Sometimes mood will improve with vitamin B12 injections even in the absence of a B12 deficiency.[13] Providing high amounts of vitamin B12 can only be done by injection. However, once a B12 deficiency has been successfully treated by injection, oral maintenance supplementation (1,000 mcg per day) is often possible.

A deficiency of the B vitamin **folic acid** (page 163) can also disturb mood. A large percentage of depressed people have low folic acid levels.[14] Folic acid supplements appear to improve the effects of lithium in treating manic-depressives.[15] Depressed alcoholics report feeling better with large amounts of a modified form of folic acid.[16] Anyone suffering from chronic depression should be evaluated for possible folic acid deficiency by a nutritionally oriented doctor. Those with abnormally low levels of folic acid are sometimes given short-term, high amounts of folic acid (10,000 mcg per day).

An amino acid called **tyrosine** (page 207) can convert into norepinephrine—a neurotransmitter that affects mood. Women taking oral contraceptives have lower levels of tyrosine, and some researchers think this might be related to depression caused by the pill.[17] Tyrosine metabolism may be abnormal in other depressed people as well,[18] and preliminary research suggests supplementation might help.[19] [20] Several nutritionally oriented doctors recommend a twelve-week trial of tyrosine supplementation for people who are depressed. Published research has used a high amount—100 mg per 2.2 pounds of body weight (or about 7 grams per day for an average adult).

L-phenylalanine (page 194) is another amino acid that converts to mood-affecting substances (including phenylethylamine). Preliminary research reported that L-phenylalanine improved mood for thirty-one out of forty depressed people.[21] DLPA is a mixture of the essential amino acid L-phenylalanine and its mirror image D-phenylalanine. DLPA (or the D- or L-form alone) may be effective in the treatment of depression.[22] Some doctors of natural medicine suggest a one-month trial with 3–4 grams per day of phenylalanine for people with depression, although some research finds that even very low amounts—75–200 mg per day—are helpful.[23]

Phosphatidylserine (page 196), or PS, is a natural substance derived from the amino acid serine. It affects neurotransmitter levels in the brain that affect mood. In a controlled trial, older women given 300 mg of PS had significantly less depression compared with placebo.[24] After forty-five days, the level of depression in the PS group was more than 60% less than the level achieved with placebo.

Niacinamide, a form of **vitamin B3** (page 213), has shown some success in the alleviation of depression.[25]

Dehydroepiandrosterone (DHEA, page 155), a hormone available over-the-counter in health food stores, may help some people with depression according to preliminary research.[26] People should not take DHEA to treat depression without the supervision of a nutritionally oriented doctor.

Are There Any Side Effects or Interactions?

Large amounts of vitamin B6 can cause side effects and should be used with caution or under the guidance of a nutritionally oriented physician. People who have not been diagnosed with iron deficiency should not supplement iron (see the section on iron for more details).

Before taking 1,000 mcg or more of folic acid per day, it's important to be assessed by a nutritionally oriented doctor for possible vitamin B12 deficiency. People who are B12 deficient and take large amounts of folic acid can run into potentially serious problems. Although the amounts of tyrosine used for depression have not been clearly linked to toxicity in humans, it is prudent to be monitored by a doctor who works with amino acid supplements.

The maximum amount of DLPA or L-phenylalanine that is safe is unknown, but nerve damage has not been reported with 1,500 mg per day or less of DLPA; DLPA has occasionally caused mild side effects, such as nausea, heartburn, and transient headaches, in smaller amounts. There are no side effects associated with phosphatidylserine. Niacinamide is almost always safe to take, although rare liver problems have occurred at doses in excess of 1,000 mg per day.

DHEA is a hormone, and as such there are serious concerns about its inappropriate use. See the section on DHEA (pages 155–156) for more information on its side effects.

Herbs That May Be Helpful

St. John's wort (page 312) extracts are among the leading medicines used in Germany for the treatment of mild to moderate depression. Using St. John's wort extract can significantly relieve the symptoms of depression. Patients receiving St. John's wort show a remarkable improvement in mood and ability to carry out their daily routine. Symptoms such as sadness, hopelessness, worthlessness, exhaustion, and poor sleep also decrease.[27][28] One study documented that St. John's wort is as effective as the prescription antidepressant imipramine for treating depression.[29] Best of all, compared to prescription antidepressants, side effects with St. John's wort are rare.

In modern herbal medicine, the amount of St. John's wort taken is typically based on hypericin concentration in the extract, which should be approximately 1 mg per day. For example, an extract standardized to contain 0.2% hypericin would require a daily intake of 500 mg (usually given in two divided dosages). Many European studies use higher intakes of 900 mg daily (supplying 2.7 mg of hypericin). As an antidepressant, St. John's wort should be monitored for four to six weeks to check effectiveness. If possible, St. John's wort should be taken near mealtime.

Ginkgo (page 268) and damiana (page 250) may also be supportive in the alleviation of depression. Yohimbe (page 323) inhibits monoamine oxidase (MAO) and therefore may be of benefit in depressive disorders.

Are There Any Side Effects or Interactions?

St. John's wort makes the skin more light-sensitive. Persons with fair skin should avoid exposure to strong sunlight and other sources of ultraviolet light, such as tanning beds. It is also advisable to avoid foods like red wine, cheese, yeast, and pickled herring. St. John's wort should not be used at the same time as prescription antidepressants. St. John's wort should not be used during pregnancy or lactation.

Ginkgo is essentially devoid of any serious side effects. Mild headaches lasting for a day or two and mild upset stomach have been reported in a very small percentage of people using ginkgo. There are no known contraindications to the use of ginkgo by pregnant and lactating women. Higher doses of damiana may induce a mild sense of euphoria. The leaves have a minor laxative effect, which is more pronounced at higher intakes, and may cause loosening of stools.

Patients with kidney disease or peptic ulcer and pregnant or lactating women should not use yohimbe. Standard doses may sometimes cause dizziness, nausea, insomnia, or anxiety. Using more than 40 mg of yohimbe per day can cause dangerous side effects, including loss of muscle function, chills, and vertigo. Some people will also experience hallucinations when taking higher amounts of yohimbe. Foods with high amounts of tyramine (such as cheese, red wine, and liver) should not be eaten while a person is taking yohimbe, as it may cause severe hypertension and other problems. Similarly, yohimbe should only be combined with other antidepressant drugs under the close supervision of a physician.

Checklist for Depression

Nutritional Supplements	Herbs	Homeopathic Remedies
Vitamin B6, Iron, Vitamin B12, Folic acid, Tyrosine, Phenylalanine/DLPA, Phosphatidylserine, Vitamin B3 (Niacinamide), DHEA	St. John's wort, Ginkgo biloba, Damiana, Yohimbe	No homeopathy commonly used for this condition

DIABETES

DIABETES here refers to diabetes mellitus. Other uncommon forms of diabetes are not covered in this discussion.

People with diabetes cannot properly process glucose, a sugar the body uses for energy. As a result, glucose stays in the blood, causing blood glucose to rise. At the same time, however, the cells of the body are starved for glucose. Diabetes can lead to poor wound healing, higher risk of infections, and many other problems involving the eyes, kidneys, nerves, and heart.

There are two types of diabetes mellitus. Adult-onset diabetes is also called type II or non-insulin-dependent diabetes (NIDDM). With NIDDM, the pancreas makes enough insulin, but the body has trouble using the insulin. NIDDM responds so well to natural medicine that even conventional medicine recommends starting treatment with dietary and lifestyle changes.

Childhood-onset diabetes is the other form of diabetes mellitus. It is also called type I or insulin-dependent diabetes (IDDM). In IDDM, the pancreas cannot make the insulin needed to process glucose. Natural medicine cannot cure IDDM, but by making the body more receptive to insulin supplied by injection, it may help.

People with diabetes have a high risk for heart disease. As a result, information in the section on **atherosclerosis** (page 11) is also important to read.

Dietary Changes That May Be Helpful

People with diabetes cannot properly process sugar. Although short-term high-sugar diets do not cause blood sugar problems for diabetics,[1][2][3] sugar is not necessarily innocent. Research shows that sugar causes diabetes in animals.[4]

The **fiber** (page 159) in carbohydrates helps protect against NIDDM. Most sugar comes from low-fiber foods, while high-fiber foods are often low in sugar. Therefore, eating more sugar usually means decreasing fiber—a mistake for diabetics. When whole foods, such as beans, whole raw fruit, and pasta, are compared with processed sugary foods, the high-sugar foods increase blood sugar more than the whole foods.[5]

Most doctors of natural medicine recommend that diabetics cut intake of sugar, such as snacks and processed foods. The best replacements for low-fiber, high-sugar foods (such as fruit juice) or starch (such as white bread) are high-fiber, whole foods.

High-fiber supplements, such as **psyllium** (page 299),[6] guar gum (found in beans),[7] pectin (from fruit),[8] oat bran,[9] and glucomannan,[10] improve glucose tolerance. Good results are seen with the consumption of 1–3 ounces of powdered **fenugreek** (page 262) seeds per day.[11][12] Most,[13][14][15] but not all, studies[16] find high-fiber diets help diabetics. Focus should be placed on fruits, vegetables, seeds, oats, and whole-grain products, although psyllium and glucomannan supplements also help.

Eating fish also affords some protection from diabetes.[17] Glucose tolerance improves in healthy people taking omega-3 **fish oil** (page 160) supplements.[18] Some studies find that omega-3 fish oil improves glucose tolerance,[19][20] **high triglycerides** (page 69),[21] and **cholesterol** (page 62) levels in diabetics.[22] However, others report that cholesterol increases[23] and diabetes worsens with fish oil supplements.[24][25][26] Until this issue is resolved, diabetics should feel free to increase their fish intake, but they should not take omega-3 fish oil supplements unless a nutritionally oriented physician has been consulted.

Vegetarians have a low risk of NIDDM.[27] When people with diabetic nerve damage switch to a vegan diet (no meat, dairy, or eggs), improvements can occur after several days.[28] In one study, pain completely disappeared in seventeen of twenty-one people.[29] Fats from meat and dairy also cause heart disease, the leading killer of people with diabetes.

Vegetarians eat less protein than meat eaters. Reducing protein intake lowers kidney damage caused by diabetes[30][31] and may also improve glucose tolerance.[32] Switching to a low-protein diet should be discussed with a nutritionally oriented doctor.

Monounsaturated oils may be good for diabetics.[33] The easiest way to incorporate monounsaturates into the diet is to use olive oil. However, those who are overweight need to be careful—olive oil is high in calories.

Should Children Avoid Milk to Avoid IDDM?

Countries with high milk consumption have a high risk of IDDM.[34] Animal research indicates that avoiding milk affords protection from IDDM.[35] Milk contains a protein that is related to a protein in the pancreas, the organ where insulin is made. Some researchers believe that children who are allergic to milk may develop antibodies that attack the pancreas, causing IDDM. Many, but not all, studies indicate that children with IDDM drink cow's milk at an earlier age than other children.[36] Children with IDDM may have high levels of antibodies that attack milk protein.[37]

Immune problems in people with IDDM have been tied to other allergies as well,[38] and the importance of avoidance of dairy remains unclear.[39] Until more is known, most doctors of natural medicine recommend abstaining from dairy in infancy and early childhood, particularly for children with a family history of IDDM. Recent research suggests a possible link between milk consumption in infancy and an increased risk of NIDDM.[40]

Lifestyle Changes That May Be Helpful

Most people with NIDDM are obese.[41] Excess abdominal weight does not stop insulin formation,[42] but it does make the body insensitive to insulin.[43] Excess weight even makes healthy people prediabetic.[44] Weight loss reverses this problem.[45] NIDDM improves with weight loss in most studies.[46][47][48]

Being overweight does not cause IDDM, but it does increase the need for more insulin. It makes sense for people with IDDM to achieve and maintain a healthy weight.

Exercise helps decrease body fat[49] and improves insulin sensitivity.[50] Exercisers are less likely to develop NIDDM.[51] People with IDDM who exercise require less insulin.[52] However, exercise can induce low blood sugar or even increased blood sugar.[53] Therefore, diabetics should never begin an exercise program without consulting a health care professional.

Moderate drinking in healthy people improves glucose tolerance.[54] [55] [56] [57] However, alcohol worsens glucose tolerance in the elderly[58] and in diabetics.[59] Diabetics who drink have a high risk for eye[60] and nerve damage.[61] Until more is known, people with diabetes should avoid alcohol. For healthy people, light drinking won't increase the risk of diabetes, but heavy drinking will, and should therefore be avoided.

Diabetics who smoke are at higher risk for kidney damage,[62] heart disease,[63] and other diabetes-linked problems. Smokers are more likely to become diabetic.[64] It is important to quit.

Nutrients That May Be Helpful

People with low blood levels of **vitamin E** (page 220) are more likely to develop NIDDM.[65] Double-blind studies show that vitamin E improves glucose tolerance in people with NIDDM.[66] [67] [68] Vitamin E even improves glucose tolerance in elderly nondiabetics.[69] [70] It may require three months or more of supplementation for benefits to become apparent. The most common amount used is 900 IU of vitamin E per day.

Vitamin E prevents blood from clotting too fast[71] and has other effects that protect diabetics' blood vessels from damage.[72] Vitamin E protects animals from diabetic cataracts.[73]

Glycosylation is an important index of diabetes. It refers to how much sugar attaches abnormally to proteins. Vitamin E reduces this problem in some,[74] [75] although not all, studies.[76]

People with IDDM have low **vitamin C** (page 217) levels.[77] As with vitamin E, vitamin C may reduce glycosylation.[78] Vitamin C also lowers sorbitol in diabetics;[79] sorbitol is a sugar that can accumulate and damage the eyes, nerves, and kidneys of diabetics. Vitamin C may improve glucose tolerance in NIDDM,[80] [81] although not every study confirms this benefit.[82] Most doctors of natural medicine suggest that diabetics supplement with 1–3 grams per day of vitamin C.

Many diabetics have low blood levels of **vitamin B6** (page 214).[83] [84] Levels are even lower in diabetics with nerve damage.[85] Vitamin B6 supplements improve glucose tolerance in women with diabetes caused by pregnancy.[86] [87] Vitamin B6 is also effective for glucose intolerance induced by the birth control pill.[88] For other people with diabetes, 1,800 mg per day of a special form of vitamin B6—pyridoxine alpha-ketoglutarate—improves glucose tolerance dramatically.[89] Standard vitamin B6 has helped in some,[90] but not all, studies.[91]

Vitamin B12 (page 216) is needed for normal functioning of nerve cells. Vitamin B12 taken orally, intravenously, or by injection reduces nerve damage caused by diabetes in most people.[92] Oral vitamin B12 up to 500 mcg three times per day has been used.

Biotin (page 141) is a B vitamin needed to process glucose. When people with IDDM were given 16 mg of biotin per day for just one week, their fasting glucose levels dropped by 50%.[93] Similar results have been reported using 9 mg per day for two months in people with NIDDM.[94] Biotin may also reduce pain from diabetic nerve damage.[95] Some doctors of natural medicine try 16 mg of biotin for a few weeks to see if blood sugar levels will fall.

High levels—several grams per day—of niacin, a form of **vitamin B3** (page 213), impair glucose tolerance and should not be taken by people with diabetes.[96] [97] Surprisingly, smaller amounts (500–750 mg per day for one month followed by 250 mg per day) may help some people with NIDDM.[98]

Preliminary studies suggested that niacinamide, the other form of vitamin B3, might be useful in the very early stages of IDDM,[99] but most research does not support this claim.[100] [101] [102]

Animal studies show that **chromium** (page 150) improves glucose tolerance.[103] Medical reports dating back to 1853 and including modern research indicate that chromium-containing **brewer's yeast** (page 143) can be useful in treating diabetes.[104] [105] Double-blind research shows that chromium supplements improve glucose tolerance in people with both NIDDM[106] and IDDM, apparently by increasing sensitivity to insulin.[107] Chromium improves the processing of glucose in people with prediabetic glucose intolerance[108] and in women with diabetes associated with pregnancy.[109] Chromium even helps healthy people,[110] although one such report found chromium useful only when accompanied by 100 mg of niacin.[111] Chromium may also lower triglycerides (a risk factor for heart disease) in diabetics.[112]

The typical amount of chromium used in research trials is 200 mcg per day. Some doctors of natural medicine recommend up to 1,000 mcg per day for diabetics.[113]

Diabetes patients tend to have low **magnesium** (page 182) levels.[114] Double-blind research indicates that supplementing with magnesium overcomes this problem.[115] Magnesium leads to improved insulin production in elderly people with NIDDM.[116] Elders without diabetes can also produce more insulin as a result of magnesium supplements, according to some,[117] but not all, studies.[118] Insulin requirements are lower in people with IDDM who supplement with magnesium.[119]

Diabetes-induced damage to the eyes is more likely to occur to magnesium-deficient people with IDDM.[120] In pregnant women with IDDM who are magnesium deficient, the lack of magnesium may even account for the high rate of spontaneous abortion and birth defects associated with IDDM.[121]

The American Diabetes Association admits "strong associations . . . between magnesium deficiency and insulin resistance" but will not say magnesium deficiency is a risk factor.[122] Many doctors of natural medicine, however, recommend that diabetics with normal kidney function supplement with 300–400 mg of magnesium per day.

People with IDDM tend to be **zinc** (page 224) deficient,[123] which may impair immune function.[124] Zinc supplements have lowered blood sugar levels in people with IDDM.[125] People with NIDDM also have low zinc levels, caused by excess loss of zinc in their urine.[126] Many doctors of natural medicine recommend that people with NIDDM supplement with moderate amounts of zinc (15–25 mg per day) as a way to correct for the deficit.

People with diabetes cannot adequately process carbohydrates. **Coenzyme Q10** (page 152), or coQ10, is needed for normal carbohydrate metabolism. Animals with diabetes are coQ10 deficient. In one trial, blood sugar levels fell substantially in 31% of people with diabetes after they supplemented with 120 mg of coQ10 per day.[127]

Inositol (page 170) is needed for normal nerve function. Diabetes can cause nerve damage, or diabetic neuropathy. Some of these abnormalities have been reversed by inositol supplementation (500 mg taken twice per day).[128]

Alpha-lipoic acid is a powerful natural antioxidant. It has been used to improve diabetic neuropathies (at an intake of 600 mg per day) and has reduced pain in several studies.[129]

Carnitine (page 146) is a substance needed for the body to properly use fat for energy. When diabetics are given carnitine (1 mg per 2.2 pounds of body weight), high blood levels of fats—both cholesterol and triglycerides—dropped 25–39% in just ten days.[130] In higher amounts (1 gram per day by injection), carnitine may reduce pain from diabetic nerve damage as well.[131]

Taurine (page 206) is an amino acid found in protein-rich food. People with IDDM have low taurine levels, which leads to "thickened" blood—a condition that increases the risk of heart disease. Supplementing taurine (1.5 grams per day) restores taurine levels to normal and corrects the problem of blood viscosity within three months.[132]

Supplementing with 4 grams of **evening primrose oil** (page 158) per day for six months has been found to reverse the cause of diabetic nerve damage and improve this painful condition. In double-blind research, 6 grams per day helps reduce nerve damage in people with both IDDM and NIDDM.[133] **Quercetin** (page 201) may also help reduce the risk of some diabetic complications, such as diabetic cataracts and retinopathy.

Vanadyl sulfate, a form of **vanadium** (page 208), may improve glucose control in individuals with NIDDM.[134] However, the long-term safety of the large amounts of vanadium required for this effect remain unknown. Furthermore, many doctors of natural medicine expect that amounts this high will turn out to be unsafe.

Are There Any Side Effects or Interactions?

Vitamin E toxicity is very rare; supplements are widely considered to be safe. Since vitamin C can interfere with lab tests assessing sugar levels in urine, diabetics supplementing with this vitamin should inform their doctor.[135] Vitamin B6 side effects are rare, but nervous system changes can occur above 200 mg per day. Vitamin B12 and biotin are not associated with side effects. Niacinamide is almost always safe to take, but niacin, in amounts as low as 50–100 mg, may cause flushing, headache, and stomachache in some people.

Side effects have not been reported from the use of brewer's yeast; it is not related to *Candida albicans,* which causes yeast infection.

Taking too much magnesium often leads to diarrhea. For some people this can happen at amounts as low as 350–500 mg per day. Excessive magnesium intake is more serious but is uncommon. People with kidney disease should not take magnesium supplements without consulting a doctor.

Zinc has been reported to increase glycosylation with IDDM—an indicator of trouble.[136] (This problem does not occur with NIDDM.[137]) While doctors of natural medicine believe this increase may be an error,[138] people with IDDM supplementing with zinc should consult a nutritionally oriented doctor. People supplementing with zinc should take 1–3 mg of **copper** (page 151) to protect against copper deficiency.

Congestive heart failure patients who are taking coenzyme Q10 should not discontinue taking coenzyme Q10 supplements without first consulting a doctor.

There is limited information about vanadium toxicity; however, workers exposed to vanadium dust can develop toxic effects. High blood levels have been linked to manic-depressive mental disorders, but the meaning of this remains uncertain. Vanadium sometimes inhibits but at other times stimulates cancer growth in animals. The effect in humans remains unknown.

Herbs That May Be Helpful

Gymnema (page 275) assists the pancreas in the production of insulin in NIDDM. Gymnema also improves the ability of insulin to lower blood sugar in both IDDM and NIDDM. This herb can be an excellent substitute for oral blood sugar–lowering drugs in NIDDM. Some people take 400 mg per day of gymnema extract.[139 140]

Asian ginseng (page 232) is commonly used in traditional Chinese medicine to treat diabetes. It has been shown to enhance the release of insulin from the pancreas and to increase the number of insulin

receptors.[141 142] It also has a direct blood sugar–lowering effect.[143] A recent study found that 200 mg of ginseng extract per day improved blood sugar control as well as energy levels in NIDDM.[144]

Bilberry (page 234) may lower the risk of some diabetic complications, such as diabetic cataracts and retinopathy. **Ginkgo biloba** (page 268) extract may prove useful for prevention and treatment of early-stage diabetic neuropathy. Other herbs that may help are fenugreek seeds (discussed earlier as a source of fiber), **bitter melon** (page 235), **aloe vera** (page 231) juice, and **eleuthero** (Siberian ginseng) (page 257).

Maitake (page 288) is being studied as a potential tool in the management of diabetes; however, further research is needed in this area.

Are There Any Side Effects or Interactions?

Use of more than 100 grams of fenugreek seeds daily can cause intestinal upset and nausea. Otherwise, fenugreek is extremely safe.

Used at the recommended amounts, gymnema is generally safe and without side effects. The safety of gymnema during pregnancy and lactation has not yet been determined. Persons with NIDDM should only use gymnema to lower blood sugar under the clinical supervision of a health care professional. Gymnema cannot be used in place of insulin to control blood sugar by persons with IDDM and NIDDM.

Used at the recommended dosage, Asian ginseng is generally safe. In rare instances, ginseng may cause overstimulation and possibly insomnia. Consuming caffeine with ginseng increases the risk of overstimulation and gastrointestinal upset. Persons with uncontrolled high blood pressure should not use ginseng. Long-term use of ginseng may cause menstrual abnormalities and breast tenderness in some women. Ginseng is not recommended for pregnant or lactating women.

In recommended amounts, there are no known side effects with bilberry extract. Bilberry does not interact with commonly prescribed drugs, and there are no known contraindications to its use during pregnancy or lactation.

Ginkgo biloba is essentially devoid of any serious side effects. Mild headaches lasting for a day or two and mild upset stomach have been reported in a very small percentage of people using ginkgo. There are no known contraindications to the use of ginkgo by pregnant and lactating women.

Excessively high doses of bitter melon juice can cause abdominal pain and diarrhea. Small children or anyone with hypoglycemia should not take bitter melon, since this herb could theoretically trigger or worsen low blood sugar, or hypoglycemia. Furthermore, diabetics taking hypoglycemic drugs (such as chlorpropamide, glyburide, or phenformin) or insulin should use bitter melon with caution, as it may potentiate the effectiveness of the drugs, leading to severe hypoglycemia.

Checklist for Diabetes

Nutritional Supplements	Herbs	Homeopathic Remedies
Fiber, Psyllium, Fish oil (EPA/DHA), Vitamin E, Vitamin C, B-complex (B6, B12, biotin, B3), Chromium, Brewer's yeast, Magnesium, Zinc, Coenzyme Q10, Inositol, Alpha-lipoic acid, Carnitine, Taurine, Evening primrose oil,	Fenugreek, Gymnema, Asian ginseng, Bilberry, Ginkgo biloba, Bitter melon, Aloe vera, Eleuthero, Maitake	No homeopathy commonly used for this condition

DIARRHEA

ANY ATTACK of frequent watery stools is called diarrhea. Many different conditions can trigger it. Acute diarrhea is often caused by an infection and may require medical management. The primary role of nutrition is to prevent depletions of fluid, sodium, potassium, and calories. Diarrhea can cause dehydration, low blood sugar, and chemical imbalances that can be serious or even life-threatening, particularly in children.

A health care provider should be consulted if diarrhea continues for more than a few days, since it may indicate a more serious health condition.

Dietary Changes That May Be Helpful

Some foods contain sugars that absorb slowly, such as fructose in fruit juice or sorbitol in dietetic confectionery, and can hold water in the intestines, leading to diarrhea.[1]

People who are lactose intolerant—meaning they lack the enzyme needed to digest milk sugar—often develop diarrhea after consuming dairy products.

Large amounts of vitamin C or magnesium can also cause diarrhea, although the amount varies considerably from person to person. Unlike infectious diarrhea, diarrhea caused by fructose, sorbitol, or high amounts of vitamin C or magnesium is not accompanied by other signs of illness, aside from cramping and occasional nausea.[2] Avoiding the offending food or supplement brings rapid relief.

While **fiber** (page 159) is often useful for constipation, it may also play a role in alleviating diarrhea. For example, 9–30 grams per day of **psyllium** (page 299) seed (an excellent source of fiber) makes the stools more solid and can help resolve symptoms of noninfectious diarrhea.[3] Drinking lots of coffee will cause diarrhea in some people.[4]

Allergies and food sensitivities can trigger diarrhea. For example, some infants suffer diarrhea when fed cow's milk–based formula but improve when switched to soy-based formula.[5]

Nutrients That May Be Helpful

Acute diarrhea can damage the lining of the intestine. **Folic acid** (page 163) helps repair this damage. Supplementing with large amounts of folic acid (5,000 mcg, three times per day for several days) has been shown to shorten the duration of acute infectious diarrhea by 42%.[6] These larger amounts are probably needed because diarrhea can cause malabsorption problems. However, folic acid should not routinely be taken in amounts greater than 800 mcg per day.

Brewer's yeast (page 143) has been shown to alter the immune system or the flora living in the intestine and may relieve infectious diarrhea.[7][8] Three capsules or tablets of brewer's yeast three times per day for two weeks has been found to be helpful.[9]

Beneficial bacteria, such as lactobacilli and bifidobacteria, normally live in a healthy colon, where they inhibit the overgrowth of disease-causing bacteria.[10] Diarrhea flushes intestinal microorganisms out of the digestive tract, leaving the body vulnerable to opportunistic infections. Replenishing with **acidophilus** (page 135) and other beneficial bacteria can help prevent new infections.

Supplementing with one hundred million to a billion bifidobacteria per day may provide protection for small children.[11] (Lactobacilli and bifidobacteria supplements often list the number of microorganisms on the label.) The combination of bifidobacteria and strep thermophilus (found in certain yogurts) dramatically reduces the incidence of acute diarrhea in hospitalized children.[12] Active-culture yogurt may prevent antibiotic-induced diarrhea.[13] Lactobacillus acidophilus, another microorganism found in both supplements and some yogurt, also inhibits disease-causing bacteria.[14]

Some doctors of natural medicine suggest that **betaine hydrochloride** (page 139) may be helpful to some individuals with diarrhea. If lactose intolerance is the cause of diarrhea, supplemental use of **lactase** (page 175) prior to consuming any dairy products can be helpful.[15]

The malabsorption problems that develop during diarrhea can lead to deficiencies of many vitamins and minerals.[16] For this reason, it makes sense for people with diarrhea to take a **multiple vitamin/mineral** (page 187) supplement.

Are There Any Side Effects or Interactions?

Folic acid supplements can mask a **vitamin B12** (page 216) deficiency in individuals lacking adequate vitamin B12. See the section on folic acid for more information on this vitamin interaction.

Side effects have not been reported from the use of brewer's yeast. It is not related to *Candida albicans*, which causes yeast infection.

There are no reported side effects with even large intakes of acidophilus and other probiotic bacteria. The normal stomach produces about the same amount of hydrochloride (HCl) as is found in twenty 10-grain tablets or capsules. However, people should not take more than 10 grains (650 mg) of HCl without the recommendation of a nutritionally oriented physician. Lactase is safe and does not produce side effects.

Herbs That May Be Helpful

The following recommendations are for milder forms of diarrhea. For more serious cases of diarrhea, proper medical evaluation and monitoring should occur before taking any herbal supplements.

Carob (page 242) is rich in tannins that have an astringent or binding effect on the mucous membranes of the intestinal tract. It is often used for young children and infants with diarrhea.[17] Commonly, 15 grams of carob powder are mixed with applesauce for children.

Chamomile (page 247) reduces intestinal cramping and eases the irritation and inflammation associated with diarrhea.[18] Chamomile is typically drunk as a tea. Many people dissolve 2–3 grams of powdered chamomile or add 3–5 ml of a chamomile liquid extract to hot water and drink it three times per day, between meals.

Herbs high in mucilage, such as **marshmallow root** (page 289), can help reduce the irritation to the walls of the intestinal tract that can occur with diarrhea. People often take 1,000 mg of marshmallow root extract, capsules, or tablets three times per day. Marshmallow root may also be taken as a tincture in the amount of 5–15 ml, three times daily.

Other astringent herbs traditionally used for diarrhea include blackberry leaves, blackberry root bark, blueberry leaves, and **red raspberry** (page 302) leaves.[19] Raspberry leaves are high in tannins and like their relative, blackberry, may relieve acute diarrhea.

Are There Any Side Effects or Interactions?

Carob and marshmallow are generally very safe; only rarely have allergic reactions been reported. Though rare, allergic reactions to chamomile have also been reported. These reactions have included bronchial constriction with internal use and allergic skin reactions with topical use. While such side effects are extremely uncommon, persons with allergies to plants of the *Asteraceae* family (ragweed, aster, and chrysanthemum) should avoid use of chamomile. Raspberry may cause mild loosening of stools and nausea.

Checklist for Diarrhea

Nutritional Supplements	Herbs	Homeopathic Remedies
Fiber, Folic acid, Brewer's yeast, Acidophilus, Betaine hydrochloride, Lactase, Multiple vitamin/mineral supplement	Psyllium, Carob, Chamomile, **Marshmallow root**, Blackberry, Blueberry, **Red raspberry**	Arsenicum album 6c, Argentum nitricum 6c, Podophyllum 30c, Pulsatilla 6c, Sulfur 6c

DUPUYTREN'S CONTRACTURE

IN DUPUYTREN'S CONTRACTURE, a poorly understood formation of fibers occurs in the palm of the hand. The fibrous tissue can cause the fingers of the hand to curl up.

Conventional treatments involve injection of steroids into the hand or removal of some of the diseased tissue with surgery. Even with surgery, however, recurrences are not uncommon.

Nutrients That May Be Helpful

Fifty years ago, researchers investigated the effects of taking **vitamin E** (page 220) to treat Dupuytren's contracture. Several studies reported that 200–2,000 IU of vitamin E per day for several months was helpful,[1] although others did not find it useful.[2] Overall, there are more positive trials than negative ones,[3] although the early research has not been followed up. Nonetheless, many doctors of natural medicine believe that a three-month trial using very high amounts of vitamin E (2,000 IU per day) is worth a try.

Are There Any Side Effects or Interactions?

Vitamin E toxicity is very rare.

Checklist for Dupuytren's Contracture

Nutritional Supplements	Herbs	Homeopathic Remedies
Vitamin E	No herbs commonly used for this condition	No homeopathy commonly used for this condition

EAR INFECTIONS (RECURRENT)

MANY CHILDREN suffer recurrent infections of the middle ear. Antibiotics are frequently used, but according to some research are not effective.[1] Likewise, inserting tubes surgically in the ear—another common conventional treatment—has not consistently provided any long-term benefit.[2]

Dietary Changes That May Be Helpful

The incidence of allergy among children with recurrent ear infections is much higher than among the general public.[3] In one study, more than half of all children with recurrent ear infections were found to be allergic to certain foods. Removing those foods led to significant improvement in 86% of the allergic children tested.[4] Other reports show similar results.[5][6] People with recurrent ear infections should discuss allergy diagnosis and elimination with a nutritionally oriented doctor.

Although sugar intake has not been studied in relation to recurrent ear infections, eating sugar is known to impair immune function.[7][8] Therefore, many nutritionally oriented doctors recommend that children with recurrent ear infections reduce or eliminate sugar from their diets.

Xylitol, a natural sugar found in some fruits, interferes with the growth of some bacteria that may cause ear infections. In a double-blind trial, children who chewed gum sweetened with xylitol had a reduced risk of ear infections.[9]

Lifestyle Changes That May Be Helpful

When parents smoke, their children are more likely to have recurrent ear infections.[10] It is important that children are not exposed to passive smoke.

Nutrients That May Be Helpful

Vitamin C (page 217) stimulates immune function in most studies.[11] [12] Vitamin C has not been studied in regard to ear infections specifically; nonetheless, some nutritionally oriented doctors recommend between 500 mg and 1,000 mg of vitamin C per day for ear infections.

Zinc (page 224) supplements increase immune function,[13] [14] although the studies showing this have not focused on ear infections. Some nutritionally oriented doctors recommend zinc supplements for anyone with recurrent infections, suggesting 25 mg per day for adults and lower amounts for children. For example, a 30-pound child could be given 5 mg of zinc.

Vitamin A (page 209) is needed by the immune system. Vitamin A supplements have helped vitamin A–deficient children with measles or infectious diarrhea in many studies.[15] Vitamin A supplements have not been studied as a treatment for ear infections in children who are not vitamin A deficient. Nonetheless, some nutritionally oriented doctors give children with ear infections 5,000–10,000 IU of vitamin A per day.

Are There Any Side Effects or Interactions?

People taking zinc for more than a few weeks should take copper as well. Taking too much zinc (several hundred milligrams per day for an adult) will actually depress immune function and must be avoided.[16] Women who could become pregnant should not take more than 10,000 IU of vitamin A per day.

Herbs That May Be Helpful

Some children with recurrent ear infections benefit from echinacea (page 255), which helps support healthy immune function.[17] Echinacea lowers the risk of colds and upper respiratory tract infections—which are common in children experiencing recurrent ear infections. Many people use 40 drops of the tincture two to three times per day for six to eight weeks. Children can be given half the adult dose.

Ear drops with mullein (page 291), St. John's wort (page 312), and garlic (page 265) in an oil base are traditional remedies used to alleviate the pressure in the middle ear during acute ear infections.

Because of its antimicrobial activity, goldenseal (page 270) has a long history of use for infections, including recurrent ear infection.

Are There Any Side Effects or Interactions?

Echinacea is essentially nontoxic when taken orally. People should not take echinacea without consulting a physician if they have an autoimmune illness, such as lupus, or other progressive diseases, such as tuberculosis or multiple sclerosis. Those who are allergic to flowers of the daisy family should take echinacea with caution. There are no known contraindications to the use of echinacea during pregnancy or lactation.

St. John's wort makes the skin more light-sensitive. Persons with fair skin should avoid exposure to strong sunlight and other sources of ultraviolet light, such as tanning beds. It is also advisable to avoid foods like red wine, cheese, yeast, and pickled herring. St. John's wort should not be used at the same time as prescription antidepressants. St. John's wort should not be used during pregnancy or lactation.

Most people enjoy garlic; however, some individuals who are sensitive to it may experience heartburn and flatulence. Because of garlic's anticlotting properties, persons taking anticoagulant drugs should check with their nutritionally oriented doctor before taking garlic. Those scheduled for surgery should inform their surgeon if they are taking garlic supplements. There are no known contraindications to the use of garlic during pregnancy and lactation.

Taken as recommended, goldenseal is generally safe. However, as with all alkaloid-containing plants, high amounts may lead to gastrointestinal distress and possible nervous system effects. Goldenseal is not recommended for pregnant or lactating women.

Checklist for Ear Infections

Nutritional Supplements	Herbs	Homeopathic Remedies
Vitamin C, Zinc, Vitamin A	Echinacea, Mullein, St. John's wort, Garlic, Goldenseal	Aconite 30c, Belladonna 30c, Pulsatilla 6c

ECZEMA

ECZEMA is a common skin condition characterized by an itchy, red rash. Many skin diseases cause similar rashes, so it is important to have the disease properly diagnosed before it can be treated.

Dietary Changes That May Be Helpful

Eczema can be triggered by allergies.[1] [2] A nutritionally oriented doctor should be consulted to determine if allergies are a factor. Once the trigger for the allergy has been identified, avoidance of the allergen can lead to significant improvement.[3]

When heavy coffee drinkers with eczema avoided coffee, eczema symptoms were reported to improve.[4] In this study, the reaction was to coffee—not caffeine, indicating that some people with eczema may be allergic to coffee. People with eczema who, with the guidance of a nutritionally oriented doctor, are using a hypoallergenic diet to investigate food allergies should avoid coffee as part of this trial.

Nutrients That May Be Helpful

People with eczema do not have the normal ability to process fatty acids, which can result in a deficiency of gamma-linolenic acid (GLA).[5] GLA is found in **evening primrose oil (page 158)** (EPO), borage oil, and black currant seed oil. Most double-blind research has shown that EPO overcomes this block and is useful in the treatment of eczema.[6] [7] [8] The effects for reduced itching are usually most striking.[9] Much of the research uses 12 pills per day; each pill containing 500 mg of EPO, of which 45 mg is GLA. One study questioned the effectiveness of evening primrose oil for eczema;[10] however, this negative study has been criticized.[11]

Older reports using large amounts of vegetable oil (containing precursors to GLA) claimed some success,[12] [13] but these studies were not controlled and do not meet modern standards of research. As a result, it makes more sense to use GLA-containing oils (such as EPO), rather than vegetable oil.

Ten grams of **fish oil** (page 160) providing 1.8 grams of EPA (eicosapentaenoic acid) per day were given to a group of eczema sufferers in a double-blind trial. After twelve weeks, those using the fish oil experienced significant improvement.[14] According to the researchers, fish oil may be effective because it reduces levels of leukotriene B4, a substance that has been linked to eczema.[15] The eczema-relieving effects of fish oil may require taking ten pills per day of fish oil.

Although **vitamin E** (page 220) at 400 IU per day has been reported in anecdotal accounts to alleviate eczema,[16] no formal study has investigated this effect.

In 1989, *Medical World News* reported that researchers from the University of Texas found that **vitamin C** (page 217), at 50–75 mg per 2.2 pounds of body weight, reduced symptoms of eczema in a double-blind trial.[17] Vitamin C may be beneficial in eczema by affecting the immune system.

Are There Any Side Effects or Interactions?

Consistent, reproducible problems from taking evening primrose oil have not been reported. A nutritionally oriented doctor should be consulted before long-term use of more than 3–4 grams of fish oil, since a high intake has been reported to elevate blood sugar levels. Side effects from EPA and DHA include nose bleeds (because of reduced blood clotting), gastrointestinal upset, and "fishy" burps.

Vitamin E toxicity is very rare; supplements are widely considered to be safe. Some individuals develop diarrhea after as little as a few thousand milligrams of vitamin C per day, while others are not bothered by ten times this amount. However, high levels of vitamin C can deplete the body of copper, an essential nutrient. It is prudent to ensure adequate copper intake at higher intakes of vitamin C (copper is found in many multivitamin/mineral supplements).

Herbs That May Be Useful

Licorice (page 286) root, used either internally or topically, may help alleviate symptoms of eczema. A traditional Chinese herbal preparation, which includes licorice, has been successful in treating childhood and adult eczema. The product, known as Zemaphyte, is currently under investigation in England. One or two packets of the combination is mixed in hot water and taken once per day.[18] [19] Topically, glycyrrhetinic acid, a constituent of licorice root, reduces the inflammation and itching associated with eczema.[20] Some people apply creams or ointments containing glycyrrhetinic acid three or four times per day. Licorice root may also be taken as a tincture in the amount of 2–5 ml, three times daily.

Numerous other herbal preparations are used topically to relieve the redness and itching of eczema. A cream prepared with **witch hazel** (page 321) and **phosphatidyl choline** (page 176) is as effective as 1% hydrocortisone in the topical management of eczema.[21] Other topical herbal preparations to consider are **chamomile** (page 247), **calendula** (page 241), and **chickweed** (page 248) ointments.

Although **burdock** (page 239) root is listed in traditional herbal books for the treatment of eczema, there is little evidence to support its use for this condition.

Sarsaparilla (page 305) may be beneficial as an anti-inflammatory. Capsules or tablets should provide at least 9 grams of the dried root per day, usually taken in divided doses. Tincture is used in the amount of 3 ml three times per day.

Red clover (page 301) is considered beneficial for all manner of chronic conditions, particularly those afflicting the skin, such as eczema. However, the mechanism of action and responsible constituents for its purported benefit in skin conditions is unknown. Wild **oat** (page 294) can be used to treat a variety of skin conditions, including eczema.

Are There Any Side Effects or Interactions?

Licorice products without the glycyrrhizin removed may increase blood pressure and cause water retention. Some people are more sensitive to this effect than others. Long-term intake of products containing more than 1 gram of glycyrrhizin (which is the amount in approximately 10 grams of root) per day is the usual amount required to cause these effects. As a result of these possible side effects, long-term intake of high levels of glycyrrhizin are discouraged and should only be undertaken if prescribed by a qualified health care professional. Deglycyrrhizinated licorice extracts do not cause these side effects.

Witch hazel may cause minor skin irritation in some people when applied topically; this herb is not typically recommended for internal use. Although rare, allergic reactions to chamomile have been reported. These reactions have included bronchial constriction with internal use and allergic skin reactions with topical use. While such side effects are extremely uncommon, persons with allergies to plants of the *Asteraceae* family (ragweed, aster, and chrysanthemum) should avoid use of chamomile. There are no contraindications to the use of chamomile during pregnancy or lactation.

Except for the very rare person who is allergic to calendula and therefore should not use it, there are no known side effects or interactions. No untoward effects have been reported with chickweed.

Sarsaparilla can cause nausea and kidney damage. Large doses for long periods of time are to be avoided. As sarsaparilla can increase absorption and/or elimination of digitalis and bismuth, such combinations are contraindicated.[22]

Nonfermented red clover is relatively safe; however, fermented red clover should be avoided altogether. Oats are not associated with any adverse effects.

Checklist for Eczema

Nutritional Supplements	Herbs	Homeopathic Remedies
Evening primrose oil, Fish oil (EPA/DHA), Vitamin E, Vitamin C, Phosphatidyl choline	Licorice, Witch hazel, Chamomile, Calendula, Chickweed, Sarsaparilla, Red clover, Oats	No homeopathy commonly used for this condition

FIBROCYSTIC BREAST DISEASE

FIBROCYSTIC BREAST DISEASE is a term colloquially given to a group of benign conditions affecting the breast. It is a very common benign condition in younger women. Both breasts become tender or painful and lumpy, and the symptoms vary at different times of the menstrual cycle.

Dietary Changes That May Be Helpful

Total caffeine elimination reduces symptoms of fibrocystic disease.[1] [2] Caffeine is found in coffee, black and green tea, cola drinks, chocolate, and a number of over-the-counter drugs. The decrease in breast tenderness can take six months or more to occur after caffeine is eliminated. Breast lumpiness may not go away, but the pain often decreases.

Many doctors misunderstand the effect of caffeine. When researchers tell women to cut back or to eliminate caffeine for less than six months, the results are unimpressive.[3] [4] Moreover, some doctors are under the impression that fibrocystic women do not drink much coffee. However, for every study that says fibrocystic disease patients do not drink more coffee than other women,[5][6] there is a study that says otherwise.[7][8] More important, the original research did not claim that fibrocystic patients drink much coffee—only that they are especially sensitive to it.

Twins with similar or identical genes should be affected the same by caffeine. For example, if one twin has fibrocystic symptoms and the other does not, the twin with symptoms will most likely be the coffee drinker, researchers have found.[9]

Fibrocystic disease has been linked to excess estrogen. When those with fibrocystic disease are put on a low-fat diet, their estrogen levels decrease.[10][11] After three to six months, the pain and lumpiness also decrease.[12][13] The link between fat and symptoms appears to be most strongly related to saturated fat.[14] Foods high in saturated fat include meat and dairy products. Fish, nonfat dairy, and tofu are possible replacements.

Lifestyle Changes That May Be Helpful

Exercise may decrease breast tenderness. In one study, women who ran 45 miles per menstrual cycle reported less breast tenderness as well as improvement in other symptoms, such as anxiety.[15]

Nutrients That May Be Helpful

Several studies report that 200–600 IU of **vitamin E** (page 220) per day, taken for several months, may reduce symptoms.[16][17] Most double-blind research has not found vitamin E to relieve fibrocystic breast disease symptoms.[18][19] Nonetheless, many women take 400 IU of vitamin E for three months to see if it helps.

As with vitamin E, the effectiveness of **vitamin B6** (page 214) remains unclear. Some,[20] but not all,[21] studies find that it reduces symptoms. Those with premenstrual syndrome in addition to breast tenderness should discuss the use of vitamin B6 with their nutritionally oriented doctor.

Some doctors of natural medicine use **iodine** (page 171) for fibrocystic symptoms. In animals, iodine deficiency can cause the equivalent of fibrocys-

tic disease.[22] What appears to be the most effective form—diatomic iodine[23]—is not readily available. Because some people are sensitive to iodine and high doses can alter thyroid function, it should not be taken without a doctor's involvement.

Research suggests that **evening primrose oil** (page 158), or EPO, may reduce symptoms of fibrocystic disease.[24][25] Many women take 3 grams per day of EPO for the alleviation of fibrocystic breast disease. It may take up to six months for optimal results.[26]

Are There Any Side Effects or Interactions?

Although side effects from vitamin B6 supplements are rare, at very high levels this vitamin can damage sensory nerves, leading to numbness in the hands and feet as well as difficulty walking. Vitamin B6 supplementation should be stopped if these symptoms develop. Pregnant and lactating women should not take more than 100 mg of vitamin B6. For other adults, vitamin B6 is usually safe in amounts of 200–500 mg per day,[27] although occasional problems have been reported in this range.[28] Side effects from vitamin B6 become more common when intake exceeds 2,000 mg per day; consequently, this supplement level should be avoided.[29]

High doses (several milligrams per day) of iodine can interfere with normal thyroid function and should not be taken without consulting a nutritionally oriented doctor.

Herbs That May Be Helpful

Since many women with fibrocystic breast disease and cyclical breast tenderness also suffer from **premenstrual syndrome** (page 109), or PMS, there is often an overlap in herbal recommendations.

Vitex (page 317) has been shown to help reestablish normal balance of estrogen and progesterone during a woman's menstrual cycle. This is important, because some women will suffer from PMS and other menstrual irregularities due to underproduction of the hormone progesterone during the second half of their cycle. Vitex stimulates the pituitary gland to produce more luteinizing hormone, and this leads to a greater production of progesterone.[30] Studies have shown that using vitex once in the morning over a period of several months will help normalize hormone balance and alleviate the symptoms of PMS.[31]

Use 40 drops of a liquid, concentrated vitex extract or one capsule of the equivalent dried, powdered extract once per day in the morning with some liquid. Vitex should be taken for at least four cycles to determine efficacy. Vitex should not be taken during pregnancy or with hormone therapy.

In traditional Chinese medicine, **dong quai** (page 254), or *Angelica sinensis,* is often referred to as the "female ginseng." Dong quai helps promote normal hormone balance and is particularly useful for women experiencing premenstrual cramping and pain.[32] Many women take 2–3 grams of dong quai capsules or tablets per day.

Are There Any Side Effects or Interactions?

Minor gastrointestinal upset and a mild skin rash with itching have been reported in less than 2% of the women monitored while taking vitex. Vitex is not recommended for use during pregnancy. It should not be taken together with hormone therapy.

Dong quai may cause some fair-skinned persons to become more sensitive to sunlight. Persons using it on a regular basis should limit prolonged exposure to the sun or other sources of ultraviolet radiation. Dong quai is not recommended for pregnant or lactating women.

Checklist for Fibrocystic Breast Disease

Nutritional Supplements	Herbs	Homeopathic Remedies
Vitamin E, Vitamin B6, Iodine, Evening primrose oil	Vitex, Dong quai	No homeopathy commonly used for this condition

FIBROMYALGIA

FIBROMYALGIA is a complex syndrome with no known cause or cure. Its predominant symptom is severe muscle pain, although other symptoms, such as fatigue, chest pain, low-grade fever, swollen lymph nodes, unrestful sleep or insomnia, frequent abdominal pain, irritable bowel syndrome, and depression, may be involved.[1]

Of the estimated three to six million people[2] afflicted with this disorder, the majority are women between twenty-five and forty-five years old.

Lifestyle Changes That May Be Helpful

Low-intensity exercise may improve fibromyalgia symptoms, and patients who exercise regularly suffer less severe symptoms than patients who remain sedentary.[3][4][5] Since stress can exacerbate symptoms, stress-reduction techniques, such as meditation, have also proved to be helpful.[6] Acupuncture may also improve symptoms.[7]

Nutrients That May Be Helpful

Some, but not all, clinical research suggests that a combination of **magnesium** (page 182) and malic acid might improve muscle pain.[8] [9] The amounts used in these studies were 300–600 mg of elemental magnesium and 1,200–2,400 mg of malic acid daily for eight weeks. This is available in combination as magnesium malate. However, the evidence remains very weak, since magnesium malate was effective in an uncontrolled study but not in a double-blind report. One study also found low red blood-cell magnesium in fibromyalgic patients.

Other studies have found fibromyalgic patients to have low **vitamin B1** (page 211) status and reduced activity of some thiamin-dependent enzymes.[10] [11] What, if any, role this marginal deficiency plays in this condition remains unknown.

One early study describes the use of **vitamin E** (page 220) supplements in the treatment of "fibrositis"—probably the rough equivalent of what is today called fibromyalgia. Several dozen individuals were treated with vitamin E in the range of 100–300 IU per day with positive and sometimes dramatic benefit.[12]

Are There Any Side Effects or Interactions?

Magnesium at high intakes can produce diarrhea in some people. For some people, this can happen at amounts as low as 350–500 mg per day. Excessive magnesium intake is more serious but is uncommon. People with kidney disease should not take magnesium supplements without consulting a doctor. Vitamin B1 is nontoxic, even at very high amounts.

Herbs That May Be Helpful

While no herbal supplements have been studied specifically for fibromyalgia, herbs used to relieve symptoms of chronic fatigue syndrome (CFS) should also be useful for fibromyalgia. These include the initial use of 2 grams of **licorice** (page 286) root three times per day for six to eight weeks, followed by the ongoing use of an adaptogenic herb, such as **Asian ginseng** (page 232), 1–2 grams per day, or **eleuthero** (Siberian ginseng) (page 257), 2–3 grams per day.

Are There Any Side Effects or Interactions?

Licorice products without the glycyrrhizin removed may increase blood pressure and cause water retention. Some people are more sensitive to this effect than others. Long-term intake of more than 1 gram of glycyrrhizin (which is the amount in approximately 10 grams of root) daily is the usual amount required to cause these effects. As a result of these possible side effects, long-term intake of high levels of glycyrrhizin are discouraged and should only be undertaken if prescribed by a qualified health care professional. Deglycyrrhizinated licorice extracts do not cause these side effects.

Used at the recommended dosage, Asian ginseng is generally safe. In rare instances, ginseng may cause overstimulation and possibly insomnia. Consuming caffeine with ginseng increases the risk of overstimulation and gastrointestinal upset. Persons with uncontrolled high blood pressure should not use ginseng. Long-term use of ginseng may cause menstrual abnormalities and breast tenderness in some women. Ginseng is not recommended for pregnant or lactating women.

Checklist for Fibromyalgia

Nutritional Supplements	Herbs	Homeopathic Remedies
Magnesium, Malic acid, Vitamin B1, Vitamin E	Licorice, Asian ginseng, Eleuthero	No homeopathy commonly used for this condition

GALLSTONES

GALLBLADDER ATTACKS

cause extreme pain in the upper-right quarter of the abdomen, often moving to the back, and can be accompanied by nausea and vomiting. The attacks frequently occur as a result of the bile duct being blocked by gallstones. Gallstones are found in the gallbladder and are made primarily of cholesterol. They are commonly associated with bile containing excessive cholesterol, a deficiency of bile acids and lecithin, or a combination of these factors.

Dietary Changes That May Be Helpful

As stated, **cholesterol** (page 62) is the primary ingredient in most gallstones. Some,[1] but not all,[2] research links dietary cholesterol to the risk of gallstones. Some doctors of natural medicine suggest avoiding eggs, either due to the cholesterol content or because eggs may be allergenic.

Vegetarians have half the risk of forming gallstones compared with meat eaters.[3] [4] Vegetarians often eat fewer calories and less cholesterol. They also tend to weigh less than meat eaters, which may reduce their risk.

Constipation (page 32) has been linked to gallstones.[5] When constipation is successfully resolved, it appears to reduce the risk of gallstone formation.[6]

Gallbladder attacks (though not the stones themselves) can result from food allergies. One study found that all sixty-nine of the subjects with gallbladder problems showed complete relief from gallbladder pain when allergy-provoking foods were identified[7] and eliminated from the diet. Pain returned when the problem foods were reintroduced into the diet. Nutritionally oriented doctors can help diagnose food allergies.

Lifestyle Changes That May Be Helpful

People with gallstones may eat too many calories[8] and are often overweight.[9] Obese women have seven times the risk compared to women who are not overweight.[10] Even slightly overweight women have significantly higher risks.[11] Losing weight may help,[12] but rapid weight loss might make matters worse.[13] Any weight-loss program should be reviewed by a doctor. **Weight loss** (page 124) plans generally entail reducing dietary fat, which itself correlates with protection against gallstone formation and attacks.[14] [15]

Nutrients That May Be Helpful

Those with gallstones are likely to have insufficient stomach acid.[16] It may be helpful to have a doctor assess adequacy of stomach acid and, if appropriate, supplement with **betaine hydrochloride** (page 139).

Phosphatidyl choline (page 176), or PC—a purified extract from lecithin—is one of the components of bile that helps protect against gallstone formation. Some studies suggest that 300–2,000 mg per day of PC is helpful.[17] [18] Although not every study reports success,[19] many doctors suggest PC supplements as part of gallstone treatment.

Are There Any Side Effects or Interactions?

Large amounts of HCl can burn the lining of the stomach. If a burning sensation is experienced, HCl should be immediately discontinued. People should not take more than 10 grains (650 mg) of HCl without the recommendation of a nutritionally oriented physician. All people with gastrointestinal symptoms—particularly heartburn—should see a nutritionally oriented doctor before taking HCl.

At intakes of several grams per day, phosphatidyl choline can cause abdominal discomfort, diarrhea, or nausea.

Herbs That May Be Helpful

Milk thistle (page 290) extracts in capsules or tablets may be beneficial in preventing gallstones. In one study, silymarin (the active component of milk thistle) reduced cholesterol levels in the bile,[20] which is one important way to avoid gallstone formation. The recommended dose is 600 mg of milk thistle extract (standardized to 70–80% silymarin) per day.

Are There Any Side Effects or Interactions?

Since milk thistle stimulates liver and gallbladder activity, it may have a mild, transient laxative effect in some individuals. This will usually cease within two to three days.

Checklist for Gallstones

Nutritional Supplements	Herbs	Homeopathic Remedies
Betaine hydrochloride, Phosphatidyl choline	Milk thistle	No homeopathy commonly used for this condition

GINGIVITIS

GINGIVITIS, also called periodontal disease, is an inflammation of the gums (gingiva).

This common problem is often progressive and can eventually result in loss of the underlying bone that supports the teeth. After age thirty, periodontal disease is responsible for more tooth loss than are dental cavities. Severe gingivitis sometimes requires surgery to repair damaged gum tissue.

Nutrients That May Be Helpful

Individuals with periodontal disease who take 1 gram of **calcium** (page 144) per day for six months show improvement in gum condition and tooth mobility.[1]

A 0.1% solution of **folic acid** (page 163) used as a mouth rinse (5 ml twice a day for 30–60 days) reduces gum inflammation and bleeding in people with gingivitis.[2] [3] Depending on the preparation, the folic acid solution is rinsed in the mouth for one to five minutes and then either swallowed or spat out. Folic acid may also be effective when taken in capsule or tablet form (4 mg per day).[4]

Coenzyme Q10 (page 152) (50 mg per day for three weeks) has been found to relieve the symptoms of gingivitis.[5] **Vitamin C** (page 217) deficiency is known to cause periodontal disease. In one study, administration of vitamin C plus **bioflavonoids** (page 140)—300 mg per day of each—improved gingival health in a group of individuals with gingivitis. The improvement was somewhat less when vitamin C was given without the bioflavonoids.[6]

Are There Any Side Effects or Interactions?

Folic acid is remarkably safe. However, folic acid supplements can mask a vitamin B12 deficiency in individuals lacking adequate vitamin B12, which could lead to permanent neurological damage. Although this problem is rare, folic acid and vitamin B12 should always be taken together, to prevent masked vitamin B12 deficiencies.

Some individuals develop diarrhea after as little as a few thousand milligrams of vitamin C per day, while others are not bothered by ten times this amount. However, high levels of vitamin C can deplete the body of copper, an essential nutrient. It is prudent to ensure adequate copper intake at higher intakes of vitamin C (copper is found in many multivitamin/mineral supplements).

Herbs That May Be Helpful

Herbs that may help treat gingivitis include **chamomile** (page 247), **echinacea** (page 255), **green tea** (page 272), **peppermint** (page 297), sage, clove, and **myrrh** (page 292). A mouthwash combination that includes sage oil, peppermint oil, mint oil, menthol, chamomile tincture, expressed juice from *Echinacea purpurea*, myrrh tincture, clove oil, and caraway oil has been used successfully to treat gingivitis.[7] In cases of acute gum inflammation, 0.5 ml of the herbal mixture in half a glass of water three times daily can be used. Rinse slowly in the mouth before spitting out. For daily hygiene, use slightly less of the mixture in half a glass of water and repeat only one or two times daily.

A toothpaste containing sage oil, peppermint oil, chamomile tincture, expressed juice from *Echinacea purpurea*, myrrh tincture, and rhatany tincture has been used to accompany this mouthwash in managing gingivitis.[8]

Of the many herbs listed above, chamomile, echinacea, and myrrh should be priorities, if only a few are to be used. These three herbs can provide anti-inflammatory and antimicrobial actions critical to successfully treating gingivitis.

Are There Any Side Effects or Interactions?

Although rare, allergic reactions to chamomile have been reported. These reactions have included bronchial constriction with internal use and allergic skin reactions with topical use. While such side effects are extremely uncommon, persons with allergies to plants of the *Asteraceae* family (ragweed, aster, and chrysanthemum) should avoid use of chamomile. There are no contraindications to the use of chamomile during pregnancy or lactation.

Echinacea is essentially nontoxic when taken orally. People should not take echinacea without consulting a physician if they have an autoimmune illness, such as lupus, or other progressive diseases, such as tuberculosis or multiple sclerosis. Those who are allergic to flowers of the daisy family should take echinacea with caution. There are no known contraindications to the use of echinacea during pregnancy or lactation.

Green tea is extremely safe. The most common adverse effect reported from consuming large amounts of green tea is insomnia, anxiety, and other symptoms caused by the caffeine content in the herb.

Peppermint tea is generally considered safe for regular consumption. Peppermint oil, in large amounts, can cause burning and gastrointestinal upset in some people. It should be avoided by persons with chronic heartburn. Rare allergic reactions have been reported with topical use of peppermint oil. Use peppermint tea with caution in infants and young children, as they may choke in reaction to the strong menthol; chamomile is usually a better choice for this group.

No adverse effects have been reported with myrrh.

Checklist for Gingivitis

Nutritional Supplements	Herbs	Homeopathic Remedies
Calcium, Folic acid, Coenzyme Q10, Vitamin C, Bioflavonoids	Chamomile, Echinacea, Green tea, Peppermint, Sage, Clove, Myrrh, Rhatany	Arnica 30c, Gelsemium 6c, Calendula MT, Mercurius sol 6c

GLAUCOMA

THE TERM GLAUCOMA describes a group of eye conditions involving increased pressure within the eyeball. This pressure can ultimately cause blindness if left untreated. In many cases, the cause is unknown. In some cases, however, glaucoma is caused by an underlying condition that should be treated with conventional medicine. Therefore, it is important for people with glaucoma to be diagnosed by and under the care of an ophthalmologist; regular eye exams are especially important after age forty.

Dietary Changes That Might Be Helpful

At least two older reports claim that allergy can exacerbate glaucoma.[1] [2] If other approaches are not successful, it makes sense to consult a nutritionally oriented physician to diagnose and treat possible allergies.

Nutrients That Might Be Helpful

Vitamin C (page 217), according to six out of seven reports studying people with glaucoma, significantly reduces elevated pressure within the eye.[3] These studies used at least several grams per day of vitamin C, but the intake varied widely. Doctors of natural medicine often suggest that people with glaucoma take the amount of vitamin C causing loose stools, and then reduce this amount slightly—an amount called bowel tolerance—as a way to help people with glaucoma.[4] The amount of vitamin C needed to reach bowel tolerance varies considerably from person to person, ranging from about 5 to 20 or more grams per day. Vitamin C does not cure glaucoma and must be used continually to reduce ocular pressure.

Many years ago, rutin, a **bioflavonoid** (page 140), was used to reduce pressure within the eyes of people with glaucoma.[5] The amount used—20 mg three times per day—was quite moderate. Seventeen of twenty-six people showed clear improvement. The effects of rutin or other bioflavonoids in people with glaucoma have apparently not been studied since.

Less than 1 mg of **melatonin** (page 185) has lowered pressure within the eyes of healthy people,[6] but studies have not yet been published on the effects of using melatonin with people who have glaucoma.

Magnesium (page 182) can act as a dilator of blood vessels. One study looked at whether magnesium might improve vision in people with glaucoma by enhancing blood flow to the eyes. In that trial, people were given 245 mg of magnesium per day. Improvement in vision was noted after four weeks, but the change did not quite reach statistical significance.[7]

Are There Any Side Effects or Interactions?

Some individuals develop diarrhea after as little as a few thousand milligrams of vitamin C per day, while others are not bothered by ten times this amount. However, high levels of vitamin C can deplete the body of copper, an essential nutrient. It is prudent to ensure adequate copper intake at higher intakes of vitamin C (copper is found in many multivitamin/ mineral supplements).

There are very few side effects with melatonin; however, there are reports of morning grogginess, undesired drowsiness, sleepwalking, and disorientation. There are certain individuals who should not use melatonin supplements. For example, melatonin should not be taken by pregnant or breast-feeding women, individuals with depression or schizophrenia, and those with autoimmune disease, including lupus.

Taking too much magnesium, even 350–500 mg for some people, can cause diarrhea. People with kidney disease should supplement with magnesium only after consulting a nutritionally oriented physician.

Checklist for Glaucoma

Nutritional Supplements	Herbs	Homeopathic Remedies
Vitamin C, Bioflavonoids, Melatonin, Magnesium	No herbs commonly used for this condition	No homeopathy commonly used for this condition

HAY FEVER

HAY FEVER is an allergic condition triggered by inhalant substances (frequently pollens) leading to sneezing and inflammation of the nose and conjunctiva of the eyes.

Nutrients That May Be Helpful

Vitamin C (page 217) acts as a natural antihistamine—an effect that has been reported to help in some,[1,2] but not all, studies.[3] Some hay fever sufferers take 1,000–3,000 mg of vitamin C per day.

Quercetin (page 201), a bioflavonoid, works well with vitamin C as an antihistamine[4] and may help reduce the severity of hay fever symptoms. Together, they can be taken at the beginning of hay fever season to help hay fever sufferers through the season. Doctors of natural medicine often suggest 400 mg of quercetin two to three times per day. Other **bioflavonoids** (page 140) that can be tried are hesperidin and rutin.

Ionized air (page 172) may also play a role in allergies. Research suggests that some allergy-provoking substances, such as dust and pollen, have a positive electrical charge. Meanwhile, negative ions appear to counteract the allergenic effects of these positively charged ions on respiratory tissues.[5]

Negative ions generally lead to favorable effects and many individuals experience relief from their respiratory allergies. Other allergy sufferers report considerable relief, with a few allergy reactions resolving completely after negative ion therapy. The majority of allergy sufferers can reduce reliance on other treatments (nutritional, biochemical, or prescription), during negative ion therapy.

Are There Any Side Effects or Interactions?

Some individuals develop diarrhea after as little as a few thousand milligrams of vitamin C per day, while others are not bothered by ten times this amount. However, high levels of vitamin C can deplete the body of copper, an essential nutrient. It is prudent to ensure adequate copper intake at higher intakes of vitamin C (copper is found in many multivitamin/mineral supplements).

Herbs That May Be Helpful

Nettle (page 293) leaf may reduce the symptoms of hay fever, including sneezing and itchy eyes.[6] For help with hay fever symptoms, some people take 450 mg of nettle leaf capsules or tablets two to three times per day or a 2–4 ml tincture three times per day.

Are There Any Side Effects or Interactions?

Allergic reactions to nettle are rare. However, when contact is made with the skin, fresh nettles can cause a rash.

Checklist for Hay Fever

Nutritional Supplements	Herbs	Homeopathic Remedies
Vitamin C, Quercetin, Bioflavonoids, Ionized air	Nettle	Euphrasia 6c, Allium cepa 6c, Sabadilla 6c

HEMORRHOIDS

HEMORRHOIDS are enlarged raised veins in the anus or rectum. They can bleed and become inflamed, often causing pain and itching.

Common hemorrhoids are often linked to **diarrhea** (page 44).[1]

Although the belief that hemorrhoids are caused by **constipation** (page 32) is questioned by researchers,[2] most doctors feel that many hemorrhoids are triggered by the straining that accompanies chronic constipation.[3] Therefore, natural approaches to hemorrhoids sometimes focus on overcoming constipation.

Dietary Changes That May Be Helpful

Countries with high **fiber** (page 159) intakes have a very low incidence of hemorrhoids. Double-blind research shows that increasing dietary fiber from **psyllium** (page 299) seed powder (7 grams taken three times per day) reduces bleeding and pain from hemorrhoids.[4]

Insoluble fiber—the kind found primarily in whole grains and vegetables—increases the bulk of stool. Drinking water with a high-fiber meal or supplement results in softer, bulkier stools that can move more easily. People with hemorrhoids accompanied by constipation should read about fiber in the section on constipation.

Psyllium husk has also been useful in the treatment of diarrhea.[5] People with hemorrhoids associated with chronic diarrhea should read the section on diarrhea.

Herbs That May Be Helpful

Topical use of astringent herbs is a mainstay treatment for hemorrhoids. A leading herb for topical use is **witch hazel** (page 321).[6] Witch hazel is typically applied to hemorrhoids three to four times daily in an ointment base. Poor venous circulation is a component of hemorrhoids—for this the internal use of **horse chestnut** (page 278) or **butcher's broom** (page 240) extracts can be helpful. Some people use horse chestnut seed extracts standardized for aescin content (16–21%) or isolated aescin preparations at an initial intake of 90–150 mg of aescin per day.

Butcher's broom products can also be used in the amount of 1,000 mg two or three times per day.

Constipation may worsen hemorrhoid symptoms. Bulk-forming laxatives to alleviate constipation are often recommended for those with hemorrhoids. An excellent herbal product is psyllium seeds.[7] Take 7.5 grams of the seeds (2 teaspoons) or 1 teaspoon of the husks one to two times per day mixed with water or juice. It is important to maintain adequate fluid intake while using psyllium.

Are There Any Side Effects or Interactions?

Using psyllium in recommended amounts is generally safe. People with chronic constipation should seek the advice of a health care professional. Side effects, such as allergic skin and respiratory reactions to psyllium dust, have largely been limited to people working in plants manufacturing psyllium products.

Witch hazel may cause minor skin irritation in some people when applied topically. This herb is typically not recommended for internal use. There are no significant side effects with butcher's broom.

Internal use of purified horse chestnut extracts standardized for aescin at the doses listed above is generally safe. There have been two reports of kidney damage in persons consuming very large quantities of aescin. Horse chestnut should be avoided by anyone with liver or kidney disease. Its internal use is also contraindicated during pregnancy and lactation. Topically, horse chestnut has been associated with rare cases of allergic skin reactions. Since circulation disorders and trauma associated with swelling may be the sign of a serious condition, a health care professional should be consulted before self-treating with horse chestnut.

Checklist for Hemorrhoids

Nutritional Supplements	Herbs	Homeopathic Remedies
Fiber	Psyllium, Witch hazel, Horse chestnut, Butcher's broom	Hamamelis 6c, Calcarea fluorica 6c, Arnica 30c, Aesculus hippocastanum 30c, Pulsatilla 6c

HIGH CHOLESTEROL

ELEVATED SERUM CHO-LESTEROL is associated with a high risk of heart disease. Most medical doctors suggest cholesterol levels should stay under 200 mg/dl (5.2 mmol/liter). Cholesterol levels lower than 200 are not without risk; many people with levels below 200 have heart attacks. But as a guideline, as levels fall below 200, heart disease risk declines. Many nutritionally oriented doctors consider cholesterol levels of no more than 180 to be optimal.

Medical labs also break down total cholesterol measurement into LDL cholesterol (which is directly linked to heart disease) and HDL cholesterol (the so-called "good" cholesterol). The relative amount of LDL to HDL is more important than total cholesterol. It is possible for someone with high HDL to be at low risk for heart disease even with total cholesterol above 200. Check with your doctor for details.

Because high cholesterol is linked to atherosclerosis and heart disease, it is important to also read the section on **atherosclerosis** (page 11).

Dietary Changes That May Be Helpful

There are many dietary interventions that may help lower serum cholesterol levels. For example, eating saturated fat from animal foods is linked to high serum cholesterol[1] and heart disease.[2] Avoiding dairy fat and meat reduces cholesterol and may reverse heart disease.[3] Skimmed milk and nonfat yogurt and cheese are essentially fat-free. "Low-fat" dairy is not: 25% of calories from 2% milk come from fat. Americans eat a little saturated fat from plant foods like coconut and palm oil. Palm oil may elevate cholesterol.[4][5]

Yogurt and other fermented milk products lower cholesterol.[6] Eating fish may increase HDL cholesterol[7] and is linked to a reduced risk of heart disease in most[8] but not all studies.[9] Fish contains little saturated fat, and **fish oil** (page 160) contains EPA and DHA, omega-3 oils that protect against heart disease.[10]

Vegetarians have low cholesterol[11] and less heart disease[12] in part because they avoid animal fat. Vegans (no meat, dairy, or eggs) have the lowest cholesterol levels,[13] and going on such a diet can reverse heart disease.[14]

Dietary Cholesterol

Most dietary cholesterol comes from egg yolks. Therefore, eating eggs increases serum cholesterol in most studies.[15] Yet, eating eggs does not increase serum cholesterol as much as eating saturated fat, and eating eggs may not increase serum cholesterol at all if the overall diet is low in fat.[16] Consequently, some doctors of natural medicine do not discourage egg consumption.

Eggs are not innocent, however. When cholesterol from eggs is cooked or exposed to air, it oxidizes. Eating oxidized cholesterol may increase heart disease.[17] Eating eggs also makes serum cholesterol susceptible to damage, which is linked to heart disease.[18] Egg eaters are more likely to die from heart disease even when serum cholesterol levels are not elevated.[19]

Fiber

Fiber (page 159) from beans,[20] **oats** (page 294),[21] **psyllium** (page 299) seed,[22] and fruit pectin lowers cholesterol levels in most studies.[23] Doctors of natural medicine often recommend that people with elevated cholesterol eat more of these high-fiber foods. However, even grain fiber (which does not lower cholesterol) protects against heart disease.[24] It makes sense to eat more of all types of fiber.

Soy

Tofu, tempeh, miso, and some protein powders in health food stores are derived from **soy** (page 204) beans. Soy protein reduces cholesterol.[25] Isoflavones from soy beans may also have this effect.[26]

Sugar

Eating sugar reduces HDL.[27] It also increases other risk factors linked to heart disease.[28] Although the exact relationship between sugar and heart disease is unclear, many nutritionally oriented doctors recommend that people with high cholesterol reduce their sugar intake.

Coffee

Drinking boiled or French press coffee increases cholesterol levels.[29] Modern paper coffee filters trap the offending chemicals and keep them from entering the cup. Therefore, paper-filtered coffee does not increase cholesterol levels in most studies.[30][31] However, paper-filtered coffee does appear to significantly increase homocysteine—a risk factor for heart disease.[32] The effects of decaffeinated coffee remain in debate.[33]

Alcohol

Moderate drinking (one to two drinks per day) increases HDL.[34] This effect happens equally for wine and other drinks.[35][36] Alcohol also "thins" blood.[37] However, alcohol causes liver disease, cancer, high blood pressure, alcoholism, and, at high intake, even *increased* risk of heart disease. As a result, many doctors of natural medicine do not recommend alcohol, even for people with high cholesterol. Nonetheless, those who have one to two drinks per day appear to live longer[38] and are less likely to have heart disease.[39] People with high cholesterol should consult a nutritionally oriented doctor before deciding whether light drinking might do more good than harm.

Olive Oil

Olive oil lowers LDL,[40] especially when it replaces saturated fat in the diet.[41] People from countries that use olive oil appear to be at low risk for heart disease.[42]

Trans Fatty Acids

Trans fatty acids are found in processed foods containing hydrogenated oils. The highest levels occur in margarine. Margarine consumption is linked to increased risk of heart disease.[43] Eating trans fatty acids increases the LDL-to-HDL ratio.[44] Margarine and other foods containing partially hydrogenated oils should be avoided.

Garlic

Garlic (page 265) is available as a whole food, in powder as a spice, and as a supplement. Eating garlic helps lower cholesterol.[45] Garlic also acts as a blood thinner[46] and may reduce other risk factors for heart disease.[47] Doctors of natural medicine typically recommend eating garlic, taking 900 mg of garlic powder from capsules, or a tincture of 2–4 ml three times daily.

Number and Size of Meals

The practice of eating many small meals rather than three large ones is called "grazing." When people eat more small meals, serum cholesterol levels fall.[48][49] It is probably best to avoid large meals and to eat more frequent but smaller meals.

Lifestyle Changes That May Be Helpful

Exercise increases HDL,[50] an effect that occurs even from walking.[51] Exercisers have a low risk of heart disease.[52] People over forty years of age or who have heart disease should talk with their doctor before starting an exercise program; overdoing it can actually trigger heart attacks.[53]

Obesity increases the risk of heart disease,[54] in part because weight gain lowers HDL.[55] **Weight loss** (page 124) increases HDL and reduces **triglycerides** (page 69), another risk factor for heart disease.[56]

Smoking is linked to a lowered level of HDL.[57] It also causes heart disease.[58] Quitting reduces the risk of having a heart attack.[59]

The combination of feelings of hostility, stress, and time urgency is called type A behavior. Men[60][61] (but not women[62]) with these traits are at high risk for heart disease in most, but not all, studies.[63] Stress[64] or type A behavior[65] may elevate cholesterol in men. Reducing stress and feelings of hostility reduces the risk of heart disease.[66]

Nutrients That May Be Helpful

High levels (several grams per day) of **vitamin B3** (page 213) in the form of niacin lowers cholesterol.[67] The other form of B3—niacinamide—does not. Some cardiologists and doctors of natural medicine recommend large amounts of niacin for people who have high cholesterol levels. Because of toxicity, high levels of niacin should only be taken under the supervision of a nutritionally oriented doctor or a cardiologist. To avoid the side effects of niacin, doctors of natural medicine increasingly use **inositol hexaniacinate** (page 170), recommending 500–1,000 mg be taken three times per day rather than niacin.[68][69] This form of niacin lowers serum cholesterol but unlike niacin appears safe.[70]

In some,[71] but not all, studies[72] **vitamin E** (page 220) increases HDL cholesterol. Vitamin E also protects LDL cholesterol from becoming damaged.[73] Most cardiologists believe that only damaged LDL cholesterol increases the risk of heart disease. People who take several hundred IU of vitamin E per day have a much lower risk of heart disease.[74][75] Double-blind research indicates that vitamin E significantly reduces the risk of heart disease.[76] Doctors of natural medicine generally recommend that everyone

supplement at least 400 IU of vitamin E per day to lessen the risk of having a heart attack.

Like vitamin E, **vitamin C** (page 217) protects LDL from damage.[77] In some studies, cholesterol levels fall when people with elevated cholesterol levels supplement with vitamin C.[78] The decrease is due to a drop in LDL.[79] An amount sometimes recommended by nutritionally oriented doctors is 1 gram per day.

Pantethine (page 193) is a special form of vitamin B5 (pantothenic acid). Pantethine may help reduce the amount of cholesterol made in the body. Several studies have found that pantethine (300 mg taken two to four times per day) significantly lowers serum cholesterol levels and increases HDL.[80][81][82] Common pantothenic acid does not appear to have this effect.

Vitamins **B6** (page 214), **B12** (page 216), and **folic acid** (page 163) lower homocysteine[83]—a substance linked to heart disease risk. Homocysteine may increase the rate at which LDL is damaged.[84] Therefore, limiting homocysteine levels should help protect against heart disease, an idea supported by preliminary research. See the section on atherosclerosis for more information about vitamins B6 and B12 and folic acid.

Quercetin (page 201) is a **bioflavonoid** (page 140) that protects LDL from damage.[85] Several studies have found that people who eat foods high in quercetin have a much lower risk of heart disease,[86][87][88] though the research is not consistent.[89] Quercetin is found in apples, onions, and black tea and as a supplement. Dietary amounts linked to protection from heart disease are as low as 35 mg per day.

Supplementation with the mineral **chromium** (page 150) has increased HDL levels in people.[90] Chromium supplementation has reduced LDL[91] and increased HDL[92] in humans. **Brewer's yeast** (page 143) containing chromium lowers serum cholesterol.[93] People with higher blood levels of chromium are at lower risk of heart disease.[94] A reasonable and safe amount is 200 mcg per day.

Several studies show that supplementing with **calcium** (page 144) reduces cholesterol levels.[95][96] Possibly the calcium is binding fat and preventing its absorption.[97] Reasonable supplemental levels are 800–1,000 mg per day.

Magnesium (page 182) is needed by the heart in order to beat. Although the mechanism is unclear, magnesium supplements (432 mg per day) lowered cholesterol in a South American study.[98] Intravenous magnesium reduces death following a heart attack in most, but not all, studies.[99] Disturbing research reports that magnesium supplements given to people with heart disease *increases* the number of heart attacks.[100] The benefits of taking magnesium supplements for people at risk for heart disease remains unclear despite the relative success of post–heart attack intravenous magnesium.

Carnitine (page 146) is needed by the heart muscle to utilize fat for energy. Some studies report that carnitine reduces serum cholesterol,[101] although other studies do not support such findings.[102] HDL cholesterol may increase with carnitine supplementation.[103] [104] People who do suffer a heart attack appear to have a reduced risk of dying if they supplement with carnitine.[105] Most studies use 1–4 grams of carnitine per day.

Soy (page 204) protein appears to lower cholesterol in people.[106] The saponins in soy bind to cholesterol to limit its absorption in the intestine, and soy's phytosterols also block the absorption of cholesterol.

Another nutrient that may be helpful in lowering high cholesterol levels is chondroitin sulfate (page 149). Preliminary research suggests that chondroitin sulfate may lower blood cholesterol levels.[107]

Are There Any Side Effects or Interactions?

Soy contains a compound called phytic acid, which can interfere with mineral absorption. In the amounts often used to affect cholesterol levels, niacin can be toxic.[108] Therefore, no one should take large amounts without the supervision of a cardiologist or nutritionally oriented doctor.

Although the inositol hexaniacinate form of niacin has not been linked with side effects, the amount of research remains quite limited. Therefore, it makes sense for people taking this supplement in large amounts (500 mg three times per day) to be followed by a nutritionally oriented doctor.

Vitamin B6, in large amounts, can damage sensory nerves, leading to numbness in the hands and feet. Folic acid is remarkably safe; however, folic acid

supplements can mask the symptoms of vitamin B12 deficiency, which could lead to permanent neurological damage. Although this problem is rare, folic acid and vitamin B12 should always be taken together.

Vitamin E toxicity is very rare, and supplements are widely considered to be safe. Some individuals may develop diarrhea after as little as a few thousand milligrams of vitamin C per day, while others are not bothered by ten times this amount. However, high levels of vitamin C deplete the body of copper. No clear toxicity from quercetin has been identified.

Supplemental intake (typically 50–300 mcg per day) of chromium has not been linked consistently with any toxicity in humans. Side effects other than allergic reactions have not been reported from the use of brewer's yeast. Individuals with sarcoidosis, hyperparathyroidism, or with chronic kidney disease should not supplement with calcium. In addition, individuals with a history of kidney stones should use calcium supplements cautiously. For other adults, 1,200–1,500 mg per day is safe. Magnesium at high intakes can produce diarrhea in some people.

Carnitine has not been consistently linked with any toxicity symptoms. At intakes of chondroitin sulfate greater than 10 grams per day, nausea may occur. No other adverse effects have been reported. Care should be taken if using a form of chondroitin sulfate that contains sodium, as this may worsen high blood pressure.

Herbs That May Be Helpful

More than thirty-two human studies have demonstrated the ability of garlic (page 265) to lower serum cholesterol levels. Common garlic intakes in these studies ranged from 600–900 mg for a duration of four to sixteen weeks. Reports that have analyzed the results of all studies performed to date on the cholesterol-lowering effect of garlic indicate that over a one-to-four-month period, the administration of garlic powder tablets reduces total serum cholesterol by 9–12%.[109] [110]

Persons with no aversion to the odor can chew one whole clove of raw garlic daily. Otherwise, odor-controlled, enteric-coated tablets standardized for allicin content can be taken in the amount of 900 mg daily (providing 5,000 mcg of allicin), divided into two daily doses. For health maintenance, half of the therapeutic regimen is adequate.

Guggul (page 274), the mixture of ketonic steroids from the gum oleoresin of *Commiphora mukul,* is an approved treatment of hyperlipidemia in India and has been a mainstay of Ayurvedic herbal approaches to preventing atherosclerosis. Clinical studies indicate that guggul is effective in the treatment of high cholesterol. One study found total serum cholesterol to drop by 17.5%.[111] Another study compared guggul to the drug clofibrate.[112] With guggul, the average fall in serum cholesterol was 11%. With clofibrate, the reduction averaged 10%. HDL rose in 60% of patients responding to guggul, while clofibrate had no effect.

Daily intakes of guggul are typically based on the amount of guggulsterones in the extract. The recommended amount of guggulsterones is 25 mg three times per day. Most extracts contain 5–10% guggulsterones, and nutritionally oriented doctors usually recommend taking it for twelve to twenty-four weeks.

Fo-ti (page 264) root has been shown to lower cholesterol levels, according to animal and human research, as well as to decrease hardening of the arteries.[113] [114] A tea can be made from processed roots by boiling 3–5 grams in 250 ml (1 cup) of water for ten to fifteen minutes. Three or more cups are drunk each day. Fo-ti tablets, each in the amount of 500 mg, are also available. Many people take five tablets three times per day.

Wild yam (page 320) has been shown to raise HDL.[115] Wild yam can be taken as 2–3 ml of tincture three to four times per day or one or two capsules or tablets of the dried root three times per day.

Alfalfa (page 230) leaves contain substances called saponins, which block absorption of cholesterol and prevent the formation of atherosclerotic plaques.

Other herbal supplements that may help lower serum cholesterol include **psyllium** (page 299), **fenugreek** (page 262), **green tea** (page 272), and **maitake** (page 288).

Are There Any Side Effects or Interactions?

Most people enjoy garlic; however, some individuals who are sensitive to it may experience heartburn and flatulence. Because of garlic's anticlotting properties, persons taking anticoagulant drugs should check with their doctor before taking garlic. Those scheduled for surgery should inform their surgeon if they are taking garlic supplements. There are no known contraindications to the use of garlic during pregnancy and lactation.

Early studies with the crude oleoresin of *Commiphora mukul* reported numerous side effects, including diarrhea, anorexia, abdominal pain, and skin rash. Modern extracts are more purified, and far fewer side effects (e.g., mild abdominal discomfort) have been reported with long-term use. Guggul should be used with caution by persons with liver disease and in cases of inflammatory bowel disease and diarrhea. A physician should be consulted for any case of elevated cholesterol and triglycerides.

The unprocessed fo-ti roots may cause mild diarrhea. Some people who are sensitive to fo-ti may develop a skin rash. Very high doses may cause numbness in the arms or legs.

Some people may experience nausea when taking large amounts of wild yam. Alfalfa is usually safe; however, there have been isolated reports of persons allergic to alfalfa. Persons with lupus or a history of lupus should avoid the use of alfalfa products.

Using psyllium in the suggested amounts is generally safe. Side effects, such as allergic skin and respiratory reactions to psyllium dust, have largely been limited to people working in plants manufacturing psyllium products.

Use of more than 100 grams of fenugreek seeds daily can cause intestinal upset and nausea; otherwise, it is extremely safe. Green tea is extremely safe. The most common adverse effect reported from consuming a large amount of green tea is insomnia, anxiety, and other symptoms caused by the caffeine content in the herb. Used as suggested, there have been no reports of any side effects with maitake.

Checklist for High Cholesterol

Nutritional Supplements	Herbs	Homeopathic Remedies
Fish oil (EPA/DHA), Fiber, Soy, B-complex (B3, pantethine, B6, B12, folic acid), Vitamin E, Vitamin C, Quercetin, Chromium, Calcium, Magnesium, Carnitine, Chondroitin sulfate	Garlic, Guggul, Fo-ti, Wild yam, Alfalfa, Psyllium, Fenugreek, Green tea, Maitake	No homeopathy commonly used for this condition

HYPERTENSION (HIGH BLOOD PRESSURE)

HYPERTENSION technically indicates high blood pressure, a condition with many causes. Approximately 90% is essential, or idiopathic, hypertension, a condition that is poorly understood but treatable nonetheless.

Dietary Changes That May Be Helpful

Essential hypertension is related to salt intake.[1] Eliminating salt from the diet lowers blood pressure in most people.[2] With the prevalence of processed and restaurant food, eliminating salt is difficult, but decreasing dietary salt intake by itself is often much less successful in treating hypertension.

Vegetarian diets lower blood pressure.[3] This occurs partly because fruits and vegetables contain **potassium** (page 197), a blood pressure–lowering mineral.[4] However, fruit contains so much potassium that people taking potassium-sparing drugs (as some hypertensives do) can end up with too much potassium. Those taking such medications should consult their doctor before increasing fruit intake. The **fiber** (page 159) provided by vegetarian diets may also help reduce high blood pressure.[5]

Sugar,[6] coffee, stress,[7] and alcohol[8] can increase blood pressure, although it is unknown if eliminating these factors will help lower blood pressure. **Garlic** (page 265) lowers blood pressure[9] and can be added to food and/or taken as a supplement.

Food allergy can contribute to hypertension in some people.[10] Exposure to lead and other heavy metals has been linked to high blood pressure.[11]

Those suspecting a food allergy or heavy metal exposure should check with a nutritionally oriented doctor.

Lifestyle Changes That May Be Helpful

Smoking is particularly bad for people with high blood pressure.[12] Daily exercise can lower blood pressure significantly.[13] People over forty years of age should consult with their doctor before starting an exercise regimen.

Many people with high blood pressure are overweight. **Weight loss** (page 124) significantly lowers blood pressure in most people.[14]

Nutrients That May Be Helpful

Many studies have found that **calcium** (page 144) supplements—typically 800–1,500 mg per day—lower blood pressure. This effect is small unless the first (systolic) blood pressure number is high and the second (diastolic) number is normal.[15] This condition is called isolated systolic hypertension.

Some,[16] but not all,[17] studies show that **magnesium** (page 182) supplements—typically 350–500 mg per day—lower blood pressure. The results are particularly effective in people who are taking a form of medication called depleting diuretics.[18]

Vitamin C (page 217) has been reported to lower blood pressure.[19] Many people take 1–2 grams per day to help support healthy blood pressure levels.

Coenzyme Q10 (page 152) is frequently deficient in people with hypertension. When these people take supplements of coenzyme Q10—typically 50 mg twice per day—blood pressure goes down significantly.[20]

Omega-3 fatty acids, such as EPA and DHA, in **fish oil** (page 160) may lower blood pressure.[21] Most studies use at least 3 grams per day of EPA and DHA combined. Most fish oil supplements contain 30% EPA plus DHA, requiring 10 grams of fish oil to deliver 3 grams of EPA plus DHA.

Taurine (page 206), an amino acid, has been used to lower blood pressure in animals[22] and people (at 6 grams per day),[23] probably by reducing levels of the hormone epinephrine.

Are There Any Side Effects or Interactions?

Individuals with sarcoidosis, hyperparathyroidism, or chronic kidney disease should not supplement with calcium. In addition, individuals with a history of kidney stones should talk with a nutritionally oriented doctor before using calcium supplements. Taking too much magnesium can lead to diarrhea. People with kidney disease should not take magnesium supplements without consulting a doctor.

Some individuals develop diarrhea after as little as a few thousand milligrams of vitamin C per day, while others are not bothered by ten times this amount. However, high levels of vitamin C can deplete the body of copper, an essential nutrient. It is prudent to ensure adequate copper intake at higher intakes of vitamin C (copper is found in many multivitamin/mineral supplements).

Congestive heart failure patients who are taking coenzyme Q10 should not abruptly discontinue taking supplements without first consulting a doctor. Side effects from the EPA and DHA in fish oil include nose bleeds (because of reduced blood clotting),[24] gastrointestinal upset, and "fishy" burps.

Herbs That May Be Helpful

Herbs should not be considered the primary tool in reducing high blood pressure, but herbal supplements can be used to support healthy heart function and circulation.

Garlic has a mild blood pressure–lowering effect.[25] Garlic's positive effect on the heart includes reduction of platelet stickiness and lowering of cholesterol and triglyceride levels. **Hawthorn** (page 276) may also exert a very mild blood pressure–lowering effect.[26]

Blood pressure is lower in individuals who regularly drink **green tea** (page 272), suggesting that this herb helps lower high blood pressure. **Reishi** (page 303), a type of mushroom, contains several constituents that seem to help lower blood pressure. **Kudzu** (page 284) has also been suggested to help lower high blood pressure. In traditional Asian use, **maitake** (page 288) has been used to manage high blood pressure.

Are There Any Side Effects or Interactions?

Most people enjoy garlic; however, some individuals who are sensitive to it may experience heartburn and flatulence. Because of garlic's anti-clotting properties, persons taking anticoagulant drugs should check with a doctor before taking garlic. Those scheduled for surgery should inform their surgeon if they are taking garlic supplements.

Green tea is extremely safe. The most common adverse effects reported from consuming large amounts of green tea are insomnia, anxiety, and other symptoms caused by the caffeine content in the herb. Side effects from reishi can include dizziness, dry mouth and throat, nose bleeds, and abdominal upset; these rare effects may develop with continuous use over three to six months. As it may increase bleeding time, reishi is not recommended for those taking anticoagulant (e.g., blood-thinning) medications. Pregnant or lactating women should consult a physician before taking reishi. There have been no reports of toxicity in humans from the use of kudzu or maitake.

Checklist for Hypertension (High Blood Pressure)

Nutritional Supplements	Herbs	Homeopathic Remedies
Potassium, Fiber, Calcium, Magnesium, Vitamin C, Coenzyme Q10, Fish oil (EPA/DHA), Taurine	Garlic, Hawthorn, Green tea, Reishi, Kudzu, Maitake	No homeopathy commonly used for this condition

HYPERTRIGLYCERIDEMIA (HIGH TRIGLYCERIDES)

MANY PEOPLE have elevated blood levels of triglycerides (TGs). TGs are composed of three fatty chains linked together. This is the way most fat exists in both food and the human body.

People with diabetes often have elevated TG levels; see the section on **diabetes** (page 39) for further information. Successfully dealing with diabetes will, in some cases, lead to normalization of TG levels. Most, although not all, studies indicate that people with elevated triglycerides are at higher risk of heart disease; see the sections on **high cholesterol** (page 62) and **atherosclerosis** (page 11).

Dietary Changes That May Be Helpful

While moderate drinking does not affect TG levels, heavy drinking is believed to be the second most prevalent cause (after diabetes) of hypertriglyceridemia.[1] Alcoholics with elevated TG levels should deal with the disease of alcoholism first.

Sugar increases TG levels as well.[2] [3] It makes sense for people with elevated TGs to reduce intake of sugar, sweets, and other sugar-containing foods.

Diets high in **fiber** (page 159) have lowered TGs in several studies,[4] although many researchers have not seen this effect.[5] Water-soluble fibers, such as pectin found in fruit, guar gum and other gums found in beans, and beta-glucan found in **oats** (page 294), may be particularly helpful in lowering triglycerides.

Low-fat, high-carbohydrate diets have lowered TGs in some,[6] but not all, studies.[7] Suddenly switching to a high-carbohydrate, low-fat diet will generally increase TGs temporarily, but making the switch gradually protects against this short-term problem.[8] Cardiologists and most nutritionally oriented doctors recommend a diet low in saturated fat (meaning avoidance of red meat and all dairy except nonfat dairy) to reduce TGs and the risk of heart disease.[9]

Some,[10] [11] but not all, studies[12] report that fish eaters have a lower risk of heart disease. Significant amounts of TG-lowering omega-3 oils EPA and DHA can be found in the **fish oil** (page 160) of salmon, herring, mackerel, sardines, anchovies, albacore tuna, and black cod. Many doctors of natural medicine recommend that people with elevated TGs increase their intake of these fatty fish.

Lifestyle Changes That May Be Helpful

Exercise lowers TG levels.[13] People who have diabetes, heart disease, or are over the age of forty should talk with a doctor before beginning an exercise program.

Smoking has been linked to elevated TG levels.[14] As always, it makes sense for smokers to quit.

Obesity (page 124) increases TG levels.[15] Maintaining ideal body weight helps protect against elevated TG levels. Many nutritionally oriented doctors encourage people who have elevated TGs and who are overweight to lose the extra weight.

Nutrients That May Be Helpful

Many double-blind studies consistently demonstrate that the omega-3 fish oils EPA and DHA, mentioned above, lower TG levels.[16] The amount used in much of the research is 3,000 mg per day of omega-3 fatty acid. To calculate how much omega-3 fatty acid is in a supplement, add together the amounts of EPA and DHA. For example, if a given fish oil capsule contains 1,000 mg of fish oil, of which 180 mg is EPA and 120 mg is DHA, then the total omega-3 oil content is 300 mg. At this level, ten capsules per day would be required to reach 3,000 mg. Other forms of omega-3 oil, such as flaxseed oil, do not lower TGs; while they have other benefits, they should not be used for this purpose.

Cod liver oil will also lower TGs.[17] Cod liver oil is less expensive than omega-3 fish oil. However, most cod liver oil contains large amounts of **vitamin A** (page 209) and **vitamin D** (page 219). Too much of either can cause side effects. Doctors will often order blood work for people who take high doses of vitamins A or D, and the cost of the blood work may exceed the savings in using cod liver oil. Those wishing to use cod liver oil instead of omega-3 fish oil should consult a nutritionally oriented doctor.

Omega-3 oil from fish oil and cod liver oil has been reported to affect blood in many other ways that might lower the risk of heart disease.[18] However, it sometimes increases LDL—the bad form of cholesterol. A doctor can check to see if fish oil has this effect on an individual. Research shows that when 900 mg of **garlic** (page 265) extract is added to fish oil, the combination still dramatically lowers TG levels but no longer increases LDL.[19] Therefore, it appears that taking garlic supplements may be a way to avoid the increase in LDL cholesterol sometimes associated with taking fish oil. People who take omega-3 fish oil may also need to take **vitamin E** (page 220) to protect the oil from oxidative damage in the body.[20]

Carnitine (page 146) is another supplement that has lowered TGs in several studies.[21] [22] Some nutritionally oriented doctors recommend 1–3 grams of carnitine per day.

Pantethine is a special form of the B vitamin **pantothenic acid** (page 193). Several studies show that 300 mg of pantethine taken three times per day will lower TG levels.[23][24][25] The form found in most B vitamins—pantothenic acid—does not have this effect. Some nutritionally oriented doctors recommend supplementing with pantethine to reduce TG levels.

The niacin form of **vitamin B3** (page 213) is used by both cardiologists and nutritionally oriented doctors to lower cholesterol levels, but niacin also lowers TG levels.[26] The amount of niacin needed to lower cholesterol and TGs is several grams per day. Such quantities often have side effects and should not be taken without the supervision of a cardiologist or nutritionally oriented doctor. To avoid the side effects of niacin, doctors of natural medicine increasingly use **inositol hexaniacinate** (page 213) at 500 mg three times per day rather than niacin.[27][28]

Are There Any Side Effects or Interactions?

Since fish oil reduces blood clotting, people taking supplements may sometimes experience nose bleeds. Some people who supplement with several grams of fish oil will experience gastrointestinal upset and burp up a "fishy" smell.

Vitamin B3 comes in two basic forms—niacin (also called nicotinic acid) and niacinamide (also called nicotinamide). Niacinamide is almost always safe to take, although rare liver problems have occurred at doses in excess of 1,000 mg per day. Niacin, at amounts as low as 50–100 mg, may cause flushing, headache, and stomachache in some people.

Cardiologists, in treating specific health problems, sometimes prescribe very high amounts of niacin—often several 1,000 mg per day. These doses can cause liver damage, diabetes, gastritis, eye damage, and elevated blood levels of uric acid (which can cause gout) and should never be taken without the supervision of a cardiologist or nutritionally oriented doctor.

Although the inositol hexaniacinate form of niacin has not been linked with side effects, the amount of research remains quite limited. Therefore, it makes sense for people taking this supplement in large amounts (500 mg three times per day) to be followed by a nutritionally oriented doctor.

Herbs That May Be Helpful

More than thirty-two human studies have demonstrated the ability of garlic to lower serum triglyceride levels. Common **garlic** (page 265) intakes in these studies range from 600–900 mg for a duration of four to sixteen weeks. Reports that have analyzed the results of all studies performed to date on the TG-lowering effect indicate that over a one-to-four-month period, garlic supplements reduce triglyceride levels by 8–27%.[29][30]

Persons with no aversion to the odor can chew one whole clove of raw garlic daily. Otherwise, odor-controlled, enteric-coated tablets standardized for allicin content can be taken in the amount of 900 mg daily (providing 5,000 mcg of allicin), divided into two daily doses. For health maintenance, half of the therapeutic regimen is adequate.

Guggul (page 274), the mixture of ketonic steroids from the gum oleoresin of *Commiphora mukul,* is an approved treatment of hyperlipidemia in India and has been a mainstay of Ayurvedic herbal approaches to preventing atherosclerosis. Clinical studies indicate that guggul is effective in the treatment of high triglycerides. One study found total serum triglycerides to drop by 30.3%.[31]

Daily intakes of guggul are typically based on the amount of guggulsterones in the extract. The recommended amount of guggulsterones is 25 mg three times per day. Most extracts contain 5–10% guggulsterones, and nutritionally oriented doctors often recommend taking it for twelve to twenty-four weeks.

Wild yam (page 320)—2–3 ml of tincture three to four times per day or one or two capsules or tablets of the dried root can be taken three times each day—has been shown to lower blood triglycerides.[32]

Reishi (page 303), a type of mushroom, contains several constituents that seem to help decrease triglyceride levels.

Other herbal supplements that may help lower serum triglycerides include **psyllium** (page 299), fenugreek (page 262), **green tea** (page 272), and **maitake** (page 288).

Are There Any Side Effects or Interactions?

Most people enjoy garlic; however, some individuals who are sensitive to it may experience heartburn and flatulence. Because of garlic's anticlotting properties, persons taking anticoagulant drugs should check with their doctor before taking garlic. Those scheduled for surgery should inform their surgeon if they are taking garlic supplements. There are no known contraindications to the use of garlic during pregnancy and lactation.

Early studies with the crude guggul reported numerous side effects, including diarrhea, anorexia, abdominal pain, and skin rash. Modern extracts are more purified, and far fewer side effects (e.g., mild abdominal discomfort) have been reported with long-term use. Guggul should be used with caution by persons with liver disease and in cases of inflammatory bowel disease and diarrhea. A physician should be consulted for any case of elevated cholesterol and triglycerides.

Some people may experience nausea when taking large amounts of wild yam. Side effects from reishi can include dizziness, dry mouth and throat, nose bleeds, and abdominal upset; these rare effects may develop with continuous use over three to six months. As it may increase bleeding time, reishi is not recommended for those taking anticoagulant (e.g., blood-thinning) medications. Pregnant or lactating women should consult a physician before taking reishi.

Using psyllium as suggested is generally safe. People with chronic constipation should seek the advice of a health care professional. Side effects, such as allergic skin and respiratory reactions to psyllium dust, have largely been limited to people working in plants manufacturing psyllium products.

Use of more than 100 grams of fenugreek seeds daily can cause intestinal upset and nausea; otherwise, it is extremely safe. Green tea is extremely safe. The most common adverse effects reported from consuming large amount of green tea are insomnia, anxiety, and other symptoms caused by the caffeine content in the herb. Used as suggested, there have been no reports of any side effects with maitake.

Checklist for Hypertriglyceridemia

Nutritional Supplements	Herbs	Homeopathic Remedies
Fiber, Fish oil (EPA/DHA), Carnitine, Pantethine, Vitamin B3 (niacin)	Oats, Garlic, Guggul, Wild yam, Reishi, Psyllium, Fenugreek, Green tea, Maitake	No homeopathy commonly used for this condition

IMMUNE FUNCTION

THE IMMUNE SYSTEM is an intricate network of specialized tissues, organs, cells, and chemicals.

The lymph nodes, spleen, bone marrow, thymus gland, and tonsils all play a role, as do lymphocytes (specialized white blood cells), antibodies, and interferon.

There are two types of immunity: innate and adaptive. Innate immunity, which is present at birth, is the first barrier against microorganisms. For example, the skin, mucus secretions, and acidity of the stomach act as barriers to keep unwanted germs away from more vulnerable tissues.

The second immune system barrier to infection, adaptive immunity, is acquired later in life, for example after an immunization or successfully fighting off an infection. The adaptive immune system retains a memory of all the invaders it has faced. This is why people usually get the measles only once although they may be repeatedly exposed. Unfortunately, some bugs, such as the viruses that cause the common cold, "disguise" themselves and must be fought off time and again by the immune system.

Dietary Changes That May Be Helpful

All forms of sugar (including honey) interfere with the ability of white blood cells to destroy bacteria.[1 2] Alcohol (a common ingredient in drugstore cold and cough remedies) interferes with a wide variety of immune defenses.[3] Excessive dietary fat reduces natural killer cell activity.[4]

When the **common cold/sore throat** (page 28) and **ear infections** (page 47) continually recur, many nutritionally oriented physicians consider whether allergies may be a contributing factor. Many medical doctors treat ear infections with antibiotics or surgery and drainage tubes. Neither approach appears to work.[5 6] The link between allergy and ear infection has been well documented.[7] Frequently these infections disappear when the food (often milk) causing a reaction is avoided.

Lifestyle Changes That May Be Helpful

The immune system is suppressed during times of stress, while optimal nutrition helps maintain a strong immune system and combat the harmful effects of stress. Other challenges to a healthy immune system include chronic **insomnia** (page 79), overwork, and the aging process. Immunity gradually declines over the years, increasing susceptibility to infection. Exercise increases natural killer cell activity, which may help prevent infections.[8 9]

Nutrients That May Be Helpful

Zinc (page 224) supplements may increase immune function.[10 11] Some nutritionally oriented doctors recommend zinc supplements for anyone with recurrent infections, suggesting 25 mg per day for adults and lower amounts for children (depending on body weight).

A double-blind study of 100 men and women with colds provided half of the group with lemon-flavored zinc gluconate lozenges containing 13.3 mg of zinc to dissolve in the mouth, every two waking hours for the duration of their cold symptoms. The other half of the group unknowingly received a supply of dummy lozenges developed to have a medicinal taste similar to the zinc lozenges.[12]

The zinc lozenge takers reported fewer days of coughing, headaches, hoarse voice, stuffy nose, nasal drainage, or a sore throat. In fact, while the average cold sufferer reports symptoms lasting for 7.6 days, zinc lozenge users stopped experiencing cold symptoms after just 4.4 days. Because the effects of zinc gluconate on the cold happen only with lozenges, it may be that the zinc helps not by stimulating immunity but by killing viruses topically in the throat.

Vitamin A (page 209) is needed by a healthy immune system. Vitamin A supplements have helped vitamin A–deficient children with measles or infectious diarrhea in many studies.[13] Without enough vitamin A, microorganisms can penetrate skin and mucous membranes (including the lungs). Infections may cause a reduction in the body's ability to store vitamin A; without normal storage, extra vitamin A may be necessary.

Vitamin C (page 217) stimulates the immune system in part by elevating interferon levels, which accounts for this vitamin's antiviral activity.[14] In a Japanese study, surgical patients receiving transfusions were given 2 grams per day of vitamin C and did not contract hepatitis, a common problem in postoperative patients.[15] A second study claiming to show that patients receiving vitamin C had not benefited actually demonstrated a 29% lower risk of contracting hepatitis, though these results were not statistically significant.[16]

Harri Hemilä at the University of Helsinki, Finland, after reviewing twenty double-blind studies, reports that while vitamin C has only a small effect in preventing a cold, it does reduce a cold's duration and severity. In fact, vitamin C given in therapeutic doses (1 to 8 grams per day) at the onset of a cold reduces the duration of cold episodes by as much as 48%. This effect appears to be dose-dependent—that is, the greater the dose of vitamin C taken, the stronger the effect.[17]

Lactobacillus acidophilus (page 135), the friendly bacteria found in yogurt, produces acids that kill invading bacteria.[18]

Are There Any Side Effects or Interactions?

Some people report that zinc lozenges lead to mild problems, such as nausea, mouth irritation, and a bad taste. People taking zinc for more than a few weeks should take copper as well. Taking too much zinc (several hundred milligrams per day for an adult) will actually depress immune function and must be avoided.[19] Women who could become pregnant should not take more than 10,000 IU of vitamin A per day.

Some individuals develop diarrhea after as little as a few thousand milligrams of vitamin C per day, while others are not bothered by ten times this amount. However, high levels of vitamin C can deplete the body of copper, an essential nutrient. It is prudent to ensure adequate copper intake at higher intakes of vitamin C (copper is found in many multivitamin/mineral supplements). There are no reported side effects with even large intakes of acidophilus.

Herbs That May Be Helpful

Echinacea (page 255) helps support healthy immune function.[20] Echinacea lowers the risk of colds and upper respiratory tract infections. Many people use 40 drops of the tincture two to three times per day for six to eight weeks; echinacea in capsule form is also commonly available.

Garlic (page 265) has natural antibiotic abilities. Supplementing with garlic increases natural killer cell activity in AIDS patients.[21][22]

Complex polysaccharides present in astragalus (page 233) and the maitake (page 288) mushroom have the unique ability to act as immunomodulators and, as such, are researched for their potential role in AIDS. The primary polysaccharide, beta-D-glucan, is well absorbed when taken orally and is currently under review as a supportive tool for HIV infection.

Oxyindole alkaloids help cat's claw (page 245) stimulate the immune system.[23]

Green tea (page 272) has been shown to stimulate production of immune cells and has antibacterial properties.[24][25][26]

Research has investigated fo-ti's (page 264) role in strong immune function, red blood cell formation, and antibacterial action.[27]

Are There Any Side Effects or Interactions?

Echinacea is essentially nontoxic when taken orally. People should not take echinacea without consulting a physician if they have an autoimmune illness, such as lupus, or other progressive diseases, such as tuberculosis or multiple sclerosis. Those who are allergic to flowers of the daisy family should take echinacea with caution. There are no known contraindications to the use of echinacea during pregnancy or lactation.

Most people enjoy garlic; however, some individuals who are sensitive to it may experience heartburn and flatulence. Because of garlic's anticlotting properties, persons taking anticoagulant drugs should check with their doctor before taking garlic. Those scheduled for surgery should inform their surgeon if they are taking garlic supplements. There are no known contraindications to the use of garlic during pregnancy and lactation.

No serious adverse effects have yet been reported with cat's claw, although those with an autoimmune illness, multiple sclerosis, or tuberculosis should first consult a physician. European practitioners avoid combining this herb with hormonal drugs, insulin, or vaccines. Cat's claw, until proven safe, should be taken only with great caution by pregnant or lactating women.

The unprocessed roots of fo-ti may cause mild diarrhea. Some people who are sensitive to fo-ti may develop a skin rash. Very high doses may cause numbness in the arms or legs.

Checklist for Immune Function

Nutritional Supplements	Herbs	Homeopathic Remedies
Zinc, Vitamin A, Vitamin C, Acidophilus	Echinacea, Garlic, Astragalus, Maitake, Cat's claw, Green tea, Fo-ti	No homeopathy commonly used for this condition

INFERTILITY (FEMALE)

INFERTILITY is defined by doctors as the failure to become pregnant after a year of unprotected intercourse. It can be caused by sex-hormone abnormalities, low thyroid function, endometriosis, scarring of the tubes connecting the ovaries with the uterus, or a host of other causes. Some of the causes of infertility readily respond to natural medicine, while others do not. The specific cause of infertility should always be diagnosed by a physician before considering possible solutions.

Dietary Changes That May Be Helpful

Caffeine consumption equivalent to more than two cups of coffee per day has been linked to tubal disease and endometriosis—both of which can cause female infertility.[1] As little as one to one and a half cups of coffee per day appear to delay conception in women trying to get pregnant.[2] Some studies find one cup of coffee per day cuts fertility in half,[3] although others report that it takes two[4] or three[5] cups to have detrimental effects.

Caffeine is found in regular coffee, black and green tea, some soft drinks, chocolate, cocoa, and many over-the-counter pharmaceuticals. While not every study finds that caffeine reduces female fertility,[6] most doctors of natural medicine recommend that women trying to get pregnant avoid caffeine.

Decaffeinated coffee has been linked to spontaneous abortion.[7] Some researchers suspect that the tannic acid found in any kind of coffee and black tea may contribute to infertility.[8]

Lifestyle Changes That May Be Helpful

The more women smoke, the less likely they are to conceive.[9] In fact, women whose mothers smoked during *their* pregnancy are only half as likely to conceive as those whose mothers were nonsmokers.[10] It is important to quit smoking.

Even moderate drinking in women is linked to an increased risk of infertility in some,[11] although not all, research.[12] Until more is known, women wishing to conceive should probably avoid alcohol.

Excessive or insufficient weight can also be causes of female infertility.[13] Infertile women who are overweight or underweight should consult a nutritionally oriented physician.

Some conventional medications can interfere with fertility. If in doubt, individuals taking prescription drugs should consult their physician.

Nutrients That May Be Helpful

Gross deficiencies of many nutrients, including **iron** (page 173) and the **B-complex vitamins** (page 210), reduce female fertility, but not much is known about the specific role most nutrients play.[14] Nonetheless, double-blind research has shown that taking a **multiple vitamin/mineral** (page 187) supplement increases female fertility.[15]

Vitamin E (page 220) deficiency in animals leads to infertility.[16] In a preliminary human trial, 100–200 IU of vitamin E given to each man and woman of infertile couples led to a significant increase in fertility.[17]

Women who are infertile should rule out the possibility of iron deficiency with the help of a doctor. A preliminary report found women sometimes regain their fertility when given iron supplements.[18]

PABA (page 192) appears to enhance the effects of cortisone,[19] estrogen, and possibly other hormones by delaying their breakdown in the liver. Some infertile women have increased their ability to become pregnant after taking PABA.[20]

Are There Any Side Effects or Interactions?

Iron supplements should only be taken by women who are deficient in this mineral. No serious side effects have been reported with 300–400 mg per day of PABA. Larger amounts of PABA (such as 8 grams per day or more) can cause low blood sugar, rash, fever, and (on rare occasions) liver damage.

Herbs That May Be Helpful

Vitex (page 317) is sometimes used as an herbal treatment for infertility—particularly in cases with established luteal phase defect (shortened second half of the menstrual cycle) and high prolactin levels. In one study, forty-eight women diagnosed with infertility (ages twenty-three to thirty-nine) took vitex once daily for three months.[21] Forty-five women completed the study, with successful treatment reported in thirty-nine women. Seven women became pregnant during the study, while in twenty-five of the women, progesterone levels normalized—which increases the chances for pregnancy. Many women take 40 drops of a liquid extract of vitex each morning with some liquid. Encapsulated powdered vitex provides a similar amount of the product, with one capsule taken in the morning.

Are There Any Side Effects or Interactions?

Side effects are rare using vitex. Minor gastrointestinal upset and a mild skin rash with itching has been reported in less than 2% of the women monitored while taking vitex. Vitex is not recommended for use during pregnancy. It should not be taken together with hormone therapy.

Checklist for Infertility (Female)

Nutritional Supplements	Herbs	Homeopathic Remedies
Iron, B-complex vitamins, Multiple vitamin/mineral, Vitamin E, PABA	Vitex	No homeopathy commonly used for this condition

INFERTILITY (MALE)

INFERTILITY is defined by doctors as the failure of a couple to achieve pregnancy after a year of unprotected intercourse. In men, infertility is usually associated with a decrease in the number or quality of sperm. There are multiple possible underlying causes for this. Some of the causes of infertility readily respond to natural medicine, while others do not. The specific cause of infertility should always be diagnosed by a physician before considering possible solutions.

Lifestyle Changes That May Be Helpful

Some conventional medications can interfere with fertility. If in doubt, individuals taking prescription drugs should consult their physician.

Nutrients That May Be Helpful

Vitamin C (page 217) protects sperm from oxidative damage.[1] Supplementing vitamin C improves the quality of sperm in smokers.[2] When sperm stick together (a condition called agglutination), fertility is reduced. Vitamin C reduces sperm agglutination,[3] increasing the fertility of men with this condition.[4] Many doctors of natural medicine recommend 1 gram of vitamin C per day for infertile men, particularly those diagnosed with sperm agglutination.

A lack of **zinc** (page 224) can reduce testosterone levels.[5] For men with low testosterone levels, zinc supplementation raises testosterone and also increases fertility.[6] For men with low semen zinc levels, zinc supplements may increase both sperm counts and fertility.[7] Most studies have infertile men take zinc supplements for at least several months. The ideal amount of supplemental zinc remains unknown, but some doctors of natural medicine recommend 25 mg three times per day.

Arginine (page 137) is an amino acid found in many foods. It is needed to produce sperm. Most research shows that several months of arginine supplementation increases sperm count and quality[8][9] and also fertility.[10][11] However, some studies have reported that arginine helps few,[12] if any, infertile men.[13] Nonetheless, many doctors of natural medicine suggest 4 grams of arginine per day for several months to see if it will help infertile men.

Coenzyme Q10 (page 152) is a nutrient used by the body in the production of energy. While its exact role in the formation of sperm is unknown, there is evidence that as little as 10 mg per day (over a two-week period) will increase sperm count and motility.[14]

Vitamin E (page 220) deficiency in animals leads to infertility.[15] In a preliminary human trial, 100–200 IU of vitamin E given to each man and woman of infertile couples led to a significant increase in fertility.[16]

Vitamin B12 (page 216) is needed to maintain fertility. Vitamin B12 injections have increased sperm counts for men with low numbers of sperm.[17] These results have been duplicated in double-blind research.[18] Men seeking B12 injections should consult a nutritionally oriented physician.

Carnitine (page 146) is a substance made in the body and also found in supplements. It appears to be necessary for normal functioning of sperm cells. Supplementing with 3 grams per day for four months has helped to normalize sperm in men with low sperm quality in several studies.[19 20]

Are There Any Side Effects or Interactions?

Some individuals develop diarrhea after as little as a few thousand milligrams of vitamin C per day, while others are not bothered by ten times this amount. However, high levels of vitamin C can deplete the body of copper, an essential nutrient. It is prudent to ensure adequate copper intake at higher intakes of vitamin C (copper is found in many multivitamin/ mineral supplements).

People taking zinc for more than a few weeks should take copper as well. Taking too much zinc (several hundred milligrams per day for an adult) will actually depress immune function and must be avoided.[21]

Arginine is remarkably free of side effects for the vast majority of people who take it, although some doctors are concerned that increases in growth hormone triggered by arginine could overwork the pancreas. Individuals with kidney or liver disease should consult their nutritionally oriented physician before supplementing with arginine. Individuals with herpes (either cold sores or genital herpes) should not take arginine, since it can stimulate the virus. Large amounts of arginine in animals can both promote and interfere with cancer growth; the meaning of this for humans remains unknown.

Congestive heart failure patients who are taking coenzyme Q10 should not abruptly discontinue taking supplements without first consulting a physician. Vitamin E, vitamin B12, and carnitine are not associated with side effects.

Herbs That May Be Helpful

Yohimbe (page 323) dilates blood vessels, making this herb useful for treating male impotence, which can be a cause of infertility. A tincture of yohimbe bark is often used in the amount of 5–10 drops three times per day. There are also standardized yohimbe products available for the treatment of impotence. The alkaloid known as yohimbine is the primary active constituent in yohimbe. A typical daily amount of yohimbine is 15–30 mg. It is best to use yohimbine under the supervision of a nutritionally oriented doctor.

Damiana (page 250) is sometimes helpful for men with impotence. Damiana is not usually used alone; it is believed to be more effective when combined with other herbs of similar or complementary activity. **Ginkgo biloba** (page 268), by increasing circulation to the capillaries, may help some impotent men.

Are There Any Side Effects or Interactions?

Men with kidney disease or peptic ulcer should not use yohimbe. Yohimbe may sometimes cause dizziness, nausea, insomnia, or anxiety. Using more than 40 mg of yohimbine per day can cause dangerous side effects, including loss of muscle function, chills, and vertigo. Some people will also experience hallucinations when taking higher amounts of yohimbine.

Foods with high amounts of tyramine (such as cheese, red wine, and liver) should not be eaten while a person is taking yohimbe, as it may cause severe hypertension and other problems. Similarly, yohimbe should only be combined with other antidepressant drugs under the close supervision of a physician.

Higher doses of damiana may induce a mild sense of euphoria. The leaves have a minor laxative effect, which is more pronounced at higher intakes, and may cause loosening of stools.

Ginkgo biloba is essentially devoid of any serious side effects. Mild headaches lasting for a day or two and mild upset stomach have been reported in a very small percentage of people using ginkgo. There are no known contraindications to the use of ginkgo by pregnant and lactating women.

Checklist for Infertility (Male)

Nutritional Supplements	Herbs	Homeopathic Remedies
Vitamin C, Zinc, Arginine, Coenzyme Q10, Vitamin E, Vitamin B12, Carnitine	Yohimbe, Damiana, Ginkgo biloba	Lycopodium 30c, Argentum nitricum 30c, Selenium metallicum 30c

INSOMNIA

THE INABILITY to get a good night's sleep can result from waking up in the middle of the night and having trouble getting back to sleep. It also occurs when people have a hard time getting to sleep in the first place. Insomnia can be a temporary, occasional, or chronic problem.

Dietary Changes That May Be Helpful

Caffeine is a stimulant.[1] The effects of caffeine can last up to twenty hours,[2] so some people will have disturbed sleep patterns even when their last cup of coffee was in the morning. Besides regular coffee, black and green tea, cocoa, chocolate, some soft drinks, and many over-the-counter pharmaceuticals also contain caffeine.

Doctors of natural medicine will sometimes recommend eating a high-carbohydrate food before bedtime, such as a slice of bread or some crackers. Eating carbohydrates can significantly increase serotonin levels in the body;[3] the hormone serotonin is known to reduce anxiety and promote sleep.

Lifestyle Changes That May Be Helpful

Insomnia can be triggered by psychological stress. Dealing with that stress, through counseling or other techniques, may be the key to a better night's rest. Psychological intervention has helped in many studies.[4]

A steady sleeping and eating schedule combined with caffeine avoidance and counseling sessions using behavioral therapy has reduced insomnia for some people, as has listening to relaxation tapes.[5]

Only scanty research explores the effect of exercise on sleep, yet some doctors of natural medicine recommend daily exercise as a way to reduce stress, which in turn can help with insomnia.

A naturopathic therapy for insomnia is to precede sleep with a fifteen- to twenty-minute, hot Epsom-salts bath. One or two cups of Epsom salts (magnesium sulfate) in a hot bath acts as a muscle relaxant.

Smokers are more likely to have insomnia than nonsmokers.[6] As with many other health conditions, it is important for people with insomnia to quit smoking.

Nutrients That May Be Helpful

Melatonin (page 185) is a natural hormone that regulates the human biological clock. The body produces less melatonin with advancing age, which may explain why elderly people often have difficulty sleeping[7] and why melatonin supplements improve sleep in the elderly.[8]

Other adults with insomnia also have lower melatonin levels.[9] Double-blinded research with young adults shows that melatonin facilitates sleep.[10]

Normally, the body makes melatonin for several hours per night—an effect best duplicated with time-release supplements. Studies using time-release melatonin have reported good results.[11] Many doctors of natural medicine suggest 1–3 mg of melatonin taken one and a half to two hours before bedtime.

Are There Any Side Effects or Interactions?

There are few known side effects with melatonin; however, there are reports of morning grogginess, undesired drowsiness, sleepwalking, and disorientation. There are certain individuals who should not use melatonin supplements. For example, melatonin should probably not be taken by pregnant or breast-feeding women, individuals with depression or schizophrenia, and those with autoimmune disease, including lupus, at least until more is known about melatonin's effects.

Herbs That May Be Helpful

Herbal remedies have been used safely for centuries for insomnia. In modern herbal medicine, the leading herb for insomnia is valerian (page 316). Valerian root makes getting to sleep easier and increases deep sleep and dreaming. Valerian does not cause a morning "hangover," a side effect common to prescription sleep drugs and melatonin in some individuals.[12] [13] Many people use 300–400 mg of a concentrated valerian root supplement thirty minutes before bedtime.

One German study compared the effect of a combination product containing an extract of valerian root (320 mg at bedtime) and extract of lemon balm (page 285), *Melissa officinalis*, with the sleeping drug Halcion.[14] After monitored sleep for nine nights, the herbal duo matched Halcion in boosting the ability to get to sleep as well as in the quality of sleep. However, the Halcion group felt hung over and had trouble concentrating the next day, while those taking the valerian/lemon balm combination reported no negative effect.

Combining valerian root with other mildly sedating herbs is common both in Europe and the U.S. Chamomile (page 247), hops (page 277), passion flower (page 295), lemon balm, scullcap (page 308), and catnip (page 244) are popular choices.[15] These herbs can also be used alone as mild sedatives for those suffering from insomnia or nervous exhaustion. Chamomile is a particularly good choice for younger children whose insomnia may be related to gastrointestinal upset.

Historically, wild oats (page 294) have been used to ease insomnia; oat alkaloids are believed to account for this herb's relaxing effect. However, some European experts do not endorse this herb as a sedative.

Are There Any Side Effects or Interactions?

Valerian should not be taken with alcohol. Recent research indicates that valerian does not impair the ability to drive or to operate machinery. Valerian does not lead to addiction or dependence. There are no known contraindications to using valerian during pregnancy or lactation.

No significant adverse effects have been reported with lemon balm. Unlike sedative drugs, lemon balm has been shown to be safe even while driving or operating machinery. Lemon balm's sedating effects are not intensified by alcohol. Persons with glaucoma should avoid lemon balm essential oil, as animal studies show that it may raise pressure in the eye.

Although rare, allergic reactions to chamomile have been reported. These reactions have included bronchial constriction with internal use and allergic skin reactions with topical use. While such side effects are extremely uncommon, persons with allergies to plants of the *Asteraceae* family (ragweed, aster, and chrysanthemum) should avoid use of chamomile. There are no contraindications to the use of chamomile during pregnancy or lactation.

Use of hops is generally safe, and there are no known contraindications or potential interactions with other medications. There are some reports of persons experiencing an allergic skin rash after handling the dried fruit; this is most likely due to a pollen sensitivity.

Used in the recommended amounts, passion flower is generally safe and has not been found to negatively interact with other sedative drugs; however, some experts suggest not using passion flower with MAO-inhibiting antidepressant drugs. Passion flower has not been proven to be safe during pregnancy and lactation.

Use of scullcap in the recommended amounts is generally safe. Due to limited information on the safety of scullcap during pregnancy and lactation, it should be avoided by pregnant and lactating women. Recently, cases of liver damage were reportedly associated with intake of scullcap. On closer examination, it appears that these scullcap products actually contained germander, an herb known to cause liver toxicity.

Using reasonable doses, no side effects with catnip have been noted. Oats are not associated with any adverse effects, although those with gluten sensitivity (celiac disease) should use oats with caution.

Checklist for Insomnia

Nutritional Supplements	Herbs	Homeopathic Remedies
Melatonin	Valerian, Lemon balm, Chamomile, Hops, Passion flower, Scullcap, Catnip, Oats	Kali phosphoricum 6c, Arsenicum album 30c, Ignatia 30c, Coffea cruda 6c, Nux vomica 30c

IRRITABLE BOWEL SYNDROME

IRRITABLE BOWEL SYNDROME (IBS) may be the most common gastrointestinal disorder. The common symptoms are bloating, abdominal discomfort, gas, and alternating diarrhea and constipation.

IBS patients are also likely to have backaches, fatigue, and other seemingly unrelated problems. The exact cause of IBS remains unknown.

Dietary Changes That May Be Helpful

Although increased **fiber** (page 159) intake can be helpful in IBS, many IBS sufferers are sensitive to wheat in any form, including wheat bran.[1][2][3] Rye, brown rice, oatmeal, and barley are high in hypoallergenic fiber, as are vegetables and **psyllium** (page 299) husk.

Some,[4] and perhaps most[5] people with IBS are sensitive to certain foods. However, these food sensitivities vary from person to person. It is beneficial to work with a nutritionally oriented doctor to find which foods cause an IBS flare-up.

Lifestyle Changes That May Be Helpful

At one time, IBS was thought to be "all in the head." Nonetheless, those with IBS are not psychologically different from other people. However, stress aggravates IBS, and reducing stress or practicing stress management skills can be beneficial. Hypnosis for relaxation may also be helpful for those with IBS.[6][7]

Nutrients That May Be Helpful

Some young women with IBS experience worsening symptoms before and during their menstrual periods. Such women may be helped by taking **evening primrose oil** (page 158) capsules or tablets containing 350–400 mg of gamma linolenic acid (GLA), the active ingredient.[8]

If lactose intolerance is the cause of diarrhea in individuals with irritable bowel syndrome, then supplemental use of the **lactase** (page 175) enzyme prior to consuming any dairy products can be helpful.

Some nutritionally oriented doctors believe that **acidophilus** (page 135) and other probiotic bacteria promote healthy digestion; use of these bacteria may lessen symptoms of irritable bowel syndrome.

Are There Any Side Effects or Interactions?

Consistent, reproducible problems from taking evening primrose oil have not been reported. Lactase is safe and does not produce side effects. There are no reported side effects with even large intakes of acidophilus and other probiotic bacteria.

Herbs That May Be Helpful

Enteric-coated **peppermint** (page 297) oil capsules, providing 0.2 ml of peppermint oil, have been shown in some, but not all, studies to be an effective symptomatic treatment for IBS.[9] Many people take one to two capsules three times per day, between meals. The enteric coating protects the peppermint oil while it passes through the acidic environment of the stomach. In the intestinal tract, peppermint oil acts as a carminative (it reduces gas production), eases intestinal cramping, and soothes irritation. Peppermint may also be taken as a tincture in the amount of 2–3 ml, three times daily.

Chamomile (page 247) acts as a carminative as well as soothing and toning the digestive tract. Chamomile's essential oils also ease intestinal cramping and irritation.[10] It is often used for those with IBS experiencing alternating bouts of diarrhea and constipation.

Chamomile is typically taken in a tea form by dissolving 2–3 grams of powdered chamomile or by adding 3–5 ml of herb extract tincture to hot water, three times per day, between meals.

Supplements that combine an assortment of carminative herbs are often useful for IBS. A combination of peppermint leaves, **fennel** (page 261) seeds, caraway seeds, and **wormwood** (page 322) may be an effective treatment for upper abdominal complaints, including IBS.[11]

Some persons with IBS benefit from bulk-forming laxatives. Psyllium, mentioned above, helps regulate normal bowel activity and reduces the alternating constipation and diarrhea suffered by some people who have IBS.

Are There Any Side Effects or Interactions?

People with chronic constipation should seek the advice of a health care professional. Side effects to psyllium, such as allergic skin and respiratory reactions to psyllium dust, have largely been limited to people working in plants manufacturing psyllium products.

Peppermint tea is generally considered safe for regular consumption. Peppermint oil, in large amounts, can cause burning and gastrointestinal upset in some people. It should be avoided by persons with chronic heartburn. Some persons using the enteric-coated peppermint capsules may experience a burning sensation in the rectum. Use peppermint tea with caution in infants and young children as they may choke in reaction to the strong menthol; chamomile is usually a better choice for this group.

Although rare, allergic reactions to chamomile have been reported. These reactions have included bronchial constriction with internal use and allergic skin reactions with topical use. While such side effects are extremely uncommon, persons with allergies to plants of the *Asteraceae* family (rag-

weed, aster, and chrysanthemum) should avoid use of chamomile.

Pregnant or lactating women, as well as anyone with an estrogen-dependent cancer, should avoid fennel in large quantities until the importance of its estrogen-like activity is clarified.

Short-term use of wormwood tea or tincture has not resulted in any reports of significant side effects. Longer-term use can cause nausea, vomiting, insomnia, restlessness, vertigo, tremors, and seizures. Wormwood is contraindicated during pregnancy and lactation.

Checklist for Irritable Bowel Syndrome

Nutritional Supplements	Herbs	Homeopathic Remedies
Fiber, Evening primrose oil, Lactase, Acidophilus	Psyllium, Peppermint, Chamomile, Fennel, Wormwood	No homeopathy commonly used for this condition

KIDNEY STONES

MOST KIDNEY STONES are made of calcium oxalate. The information included in this section pertains only to calcium oxalate kidney stones, and the term "kidney stone" refers here only to this form of stone. People who have had kidney stones should talk with their doctor to find out what type of stones they have formed—approximately one stone in five is made of something other than calcium oxalate.

Calcium oxalate stone formation is rare in primitive societies, suggesting that this condition is preventable.[1] People who have formed a calcium oxalate stone are at high risk of forming another stone.

Dietary Changes That May Be Helpful

Most doctors agree that kidney stone formers should reduce their intake of oxalate from food as a way to reduce urinary oxalate.[2] Many foods contain oxalate. But only a few—spinach, rhubarb, beet greens, nuts, chocolate, tea, bran, almonds, peanuts, and strawberries—appear to increase urinary oxalate significantly.[3][4]

Drinking coffee or other caffeine-containing beverages increases urinary calcium.[5] Long-term caffeine consumers are reported to have an increased risk of **osteoporosis (page 100)**,[6] suggesting that people who regularly consume caffeine are chronically increasing urinary calcium loss. While consumption of caffeine has not yet been directly linked to kidney stones, it makes sense for stone formers to restrict caffeine until more is known.

Eating animal protein from meat, dairy, poultry, or fish increases urinary calcium. Perhaps for this reason, animal protein is linked to an increased risk of forming stones;[7] vegetarians are at lower risk.[8]

Salt increases urinary calcium excretion in stone formers.[9] [10] [11] In theory, this should increase the risk of forming a stone. Most nutritionally oriented doctors recommend that people with a history of kidney stones reduce salt intake.

Potassium (page 197) reduces urinary calcium excretion,[12] and people who eat high amounts of potassium appear to have a low risk of kidney stones.[13] The best way to increase potassium is to eat fruits and vegetables. The level of potassium in food is much higher than the small amounts found in supplements.

Bran (see **fiber,** page 159) reduces the absorption of calcium, which in turn causes urinary calcium to fall.[14] Many kidney stones can be prevented simply by incorporating 0.5 ounce of bran per day into the diet.[15] Oat and wheat bran are available in natural food stores. Before supplementing with bran, people should check with a nutritionally oriented doctor, because some—even a few with kidney stones—do not absorb enough calcium. For those people, supplementing with bran might deprive them of much-needed calcium.

Lifestyle Changes That May Be Helpful

Drinking water increases the volume of urine. In the process, substances that form kidney stones are diluted, reducing the risk that they will form into a stone. For this reason, people with a history of kidney stones should drink plenty of water—often two quarts per day. It is particularly important for people in hot climates to increase their fluid intake, to help prevent kidney stones.[16]

While an overall increase in fluids is helpful, some research has linked soft drinks (especially cola beverages) that contain phosphoric acid with a higher risk of stone formation.[17] For this reason, anyone with a tendency to form kidney stones should probably avoid soft drinks.

Nutrients That May Be Helpful

Taking **calcium** (page 144) supplements increases urinary calcium that in theory should increase the risk of forming kidney stones. However, calcium binds to oxalate in the gut, reducing absorption of oxalate. This causes a drop in urinary oxalate, which should reduce the risk of stone formation.[18] The question is, which counts more—the increase in urinary calcium, which might increase the risk, or the reduction in urinary oxalate, which might reduce it? According to the *New England Journal of Medicine*, people who eat more calcium have a lower risk of forming kidney stones than people who consume less calcium.[19] Therefore, it appears that calcium supplements are safe and possibly beneficial for many stone formers.

Kidney stone formers whose doctors suggest calcium supplementation should take the calcium with meals so that the calcium can reduce the absorption of oxalate. They should also avoid taking **vitamin D** (page 219) supplements without consulting a nutritionally oriented doctor. At least in theory, vitamin D might increase the risk of forming stones.[20]

When nutritionally oriented doctors recommend calcium supplements to stone formers, they often suggest 800 mg per day in the form of calcium citrate. Citrate may help reduce the risk of forming a stone.[21] [22]

Both **magnesium** (page 182) and **vitamin B6** (page 214) are used by the body to convert oxalate into other substances. A lack of either nutrient can increase urinary oxalate and increase the risk of forming a stone. Individuals with elevated urinary oxalate may lower their levels by supplementing with 50–100 mg of vitamin B6. Magnesium supplements of 200–300 mg taken with meals reduce both urinary calcium and oxalate.[23] Most, but not all, studies show that supplementing magnesium and vitamin B6 significantly lowers the risk of forming kidney stones.[24] [25] [26] [27]

Glucosamine sulfate (page 165) and **chondroitin sulfate** (page 149) may play a role in reducing the risk of kidney stone formation. One study indicates that

60 mg per day of such supplements significantly lowers urinary oxalate levels in stone formers.[28] Such a decrease should reduce the risk of stone formation.

Are There Any Side Effects or Interactions?

When people take calcium supplements, the increase in urinary calcium varies enormously from person to person. A few stone formers have such a large increase in urinary calcium when they take calcium supplements that their risk of forming a kidney stone may increase.[29] Therefore, before supplementing with calcium, people with a history of kidney stones should consult with a nutritionally oriented physician and evaluate their urinary calcium levels during supplementation.

It has been suggested that people who form kidney stones should avoid vitamin C supplements, because vitamin C can convert into oxalate and increase urinary oxalate.[30] [31] Recent research shows, however, that vitamin C conversion to oxalate takes place primarily after vitamin C in urine has left the body—which strongly suggests that taking vitamin C supplements is not a problem for most stone formers.[32] [33]

Magnesium at high intakes can produce diarrhea in some people. Although side effects from vitamin B6 supplements are rare, at very high levels this vitamin can damage sensory nerves, leading to numbness in the hands and feet as well as difficulty walking. Vitamin B6 supplementation should be stopped if these symptoms develop. Pregnant and lactating women should not take more than 100 mg of vitamin B6. For other adults, vitamin B6 is safe in amounts of 200–500 mg per day, although occasional problems have been reported in this range.

Checklist for Kidney Stones

Nutritional Supplements	Herbs	Homeopathic Remedies
Bran (Fiber), **Potassium, Calcium, Magnesium, Vitamin B6, Glucosamine sulfate, Chondroitin sulfate**	No herbs commonly used for this condition	No homeopathy commonly used for this condition

MACULAR DEGENERATION

THE MACULA is a portion of the retina in the back of the eye. Degeneration of the macula is the leading cause of blindness in elderly Americans.[1]

Lifestyle Changes That May Be Helpful

Smoking has been linked to macular degeneration. Quitting smoking may reduce the risk of developing macular degeneration.

Nutrients That May Be Helpful

Sunlight triggers oxidative damage in the eye, which in turn can cause macular degeneration.[2] Animals given **antioxidants** (page 8)—which protect against oxidative damage—have a lower risk of this vision problem.[3] People with high blood levels of antioxidants also have a lower risk.[4] Those with the highest levels of the antioxidants **selenium** (page 203), **vitamin C** (page 217), and **vitamin E** (page 220) may have a 70% lower risk of developing macular degeneration.[5] People who eat fruits and vegetables high in **beta-carotene** (page 209), another antioxidant, are also at low risk.[6] Consequently, many people who want to lower their risk for macular degeneration will supplement with antioxidants. Reasonable adult levels include 200 mcg of selenium, 1,000 mg of vitamin C, 400 IU of vitamin E, and 25,000 IU of natural beta-carotene per day.

Lutein (page 179) and zeaxanthin are antioxidants, much like beta-carotene; they are called carotenoids. These carotenoids, found in high concentrations in spinach and kale, concentrate in the part of the retina where macular degeneration strikes. Once there, they protect the retina from damage caused by sunlight.[7] As expected, spinach and kale eaters have a lower risk of macular degeneration, although blood levels of lutein have not correlated with risk of macular degeneration in one trial.[8 9]

Harvard researchers report that people eating the most lutein and zeaxanthin—a total of 5.8 mg per day—have a 57% decreased risk of macular degeneration compared with people eating the least.[10] Lutein and zeaxanthin can be taken as supplements; 6 mg or more per day of lutein may be a useful amount.

Two important enzymes needed for vision in the retina require **zinc** (page 224). Double-blind research using 80 mg of zinc or placebo for two years found that zinc prevented vision loss by 42% in those with macular degeneration;[11] although other double-blind research did not confirm these results.[12]

Are There Any Side Effects or Interactions?

Some individuals develop diarrhea after as little as a few thousand milligrams of vitamin C per day, while others are not bothered by ten times this amount.

Zinc intake in excess of 300 mg per day may impair immune function. **Copper** (page 151) should be taken along with zinc to prevent mineral imbalances.

Herbs That May Be Helpful

Ginkgo biloba (page 268) may help reduce the risk of developing macular degeneration.[13] Many people take 120–240 mg of standardized extract in capsules or tablets per day or a tincture of 0.5 ml three times daily for support of healthy vision.

Bilberry's (page 234) active bioflavonoid compounds, anthocyanosides, act as an antioxidant in the retina of the eye. This makes it a potential preventive measure against macular degeneration.[14] Bilberry has also been shown to strengthen capillaries and reduce hemorrhaging in the retina.[15] Many people take 240–480 mg per day of bilberry extract in capsules or tablets standardized to 25% anthocyanosides.

Are There Any Side Effects or Interactions?

Ginkgo biloba is essentially devoid of any serious side effects. Mild headaches lasting for a day or two and mild upset stomach have been reported in a very small percentage of people using ginkgo.

Checklist for Macular Degeneration

Nutritional Supplements	Herbs	Homeopathic Remedies
Selenium, Vitamin C, Vitamin E, Beta-carotene, Lutein, Zeaxanthin, Zinc	Ginkgo biloba, Bilberry	No homeopathy commonly used for this condition

MENOPAUSE

MENOPAUSE is the cessation of the monthly female menstrual cycle. Women who have not had a menstrual cycle for a year are considered postmenopausal. Most commonly, menopause takes place when a woman is in her late forties or early fifties. Women who have gone through menopause are no longer fertile. Menopause is not a disease and cannot be prevented.

Many hormonal changes occur as women go through menopause. Primarily as a result of decreases in estrogen, postmenopausal women are at higher risk of heart disease and osteoporosis. For a discussion of these conditions, see the sections on **osteoporosis** (page 100), **high cholesterol** (page 62), and **atherosclerosis** (page 11) sections. A number of unpleasant symptoms may also accompany menopause. Some, such as vaginal dryness, result from the lack of estrogen. Others, such as hot flashes, are caused by more complex hormonal changes.

Dietary Changes That May Be Helpful

Soybeans contain compounds called phytoestrogens, which are related in structure to estrogen. **Soy** (page 204) is known to affect the menstrual cycle in premenopausal women. Researchers have linked countries where people eat substantial amounts of soy products with a low incidence of hot flashes in women going through menopause.[1] As a result, some doctors of natural medicine recommend that women going through menopause eat tofu, soy milk, tempeh, roasted soy nuts, and other soy products. Supplements containing isoflavones extracted from soy are also available.

Nutrients That May Be Helpful

Many years ago, researchers looked at the effects of **vitamin E** (page 220) in reducing symptoms of menopause. Some,[2][3] but not all,[4] studies found vitamin E to be helpful. Many nutritionally oriented doctors suggest that women going through menopause take 800–1,000 IU per day of vitamin E for a trial period of at least three months to see if symptoms are reduced. If helpful, this amount can be continued.

1,200 mg of **vitamin C** (page 217) and 1,200 mg of the **bioflavonoid** (page 140) hesperidin, taken over the course of the day, was shown in one study to help relieve hot flashes.[5]

Are There Any Side Effects or Interactions?

Some individuals develop diarrhea after as little as a few thousand milligrams of vitamin C per day, while others are not bothered by ten times this amount. However, high levels of vitamin C can deplete the body of **copper** (page 151), an essential nutrient. It is prudent to ensure adequate copper intake at higher intakes of vitamin C; copper is found in many **multiple vitamin/mineral** (page 187) supplements.

No consistent toxicity has been linked to the bioflavonoids. The exception is for a bioflavonoid called cianidanol, which is not found in supplements.

Herbs That May Be Helpful

The leading herbal treatment for women suffering from hot flashes associated with menopause is **black cohosh** (page 236).[6] Black cohosh has weak estrogen-like activity, which may reduce hot flashes. Many women use a highly concentrated extract in the amount of 40 mg of black cohosh two times per day.

Vitex (page 317) does not contain hormones. Its benefits stem from its actions upon the pituitary gland—specifically on the production of estrogen and progesterone. Vitex increases the production of the hormones that help regulate a woman's cycle. Many people take 40 drops (in a glass of water) of the concentrated liquid herbal extract in the morning. Vitex is also available in powdered form in tablets and capsules, again to be taken in the morning.

Traditional uses of **dong quai** (page 254) include treatment for hot flashes associated with menopause. Dong quai is believed to have a balancing or adaptogenic effect on the female hormonal system. The powdered root can be used as an herbal extract, capsules or tablets, or as a tea. Many people take 3–4 grams per day.

Contrary to popular belief, **wild yam** (page 320) is not a natural source of progesterone. Although a pharmaceutical conversion process can produce progesterone from wild yam, the body cannot duplicate this conversion. Women who require progesterone should consult their nutritionally oriented physician and not rely solely on wild yam or other herbs.

Are There Any Side Effects or Interactions?

As black cohosh has an estrogen-like effect, women who are pregnant or lactating should not use the herb. Large doses of this herb may cause abdominal pain, nausea, headaches, and dizziness. Women taking estrogen therapy should consult a physician before using black cohosh.

Side effects are rare using vitex. Minor gastrointestinal upset and a mild skin rash with itching has been reported in less than 2% of the women monitored while taking vitex. Vitex is not recommended for use during pregnancy. It should not be taken during hormone therapy.

Dong quai is generally considered to be of extremely low toxicity. It may cause some fair-skinned persons to become more sensitive to sunlight. Persons using it on a regular basis should limit prolonged exposure to the sun or other sources of ultraviolet radiation. Dong quai is not recommended for pregnant or lactating women.

Checklist for Menopause

Nutritional Supplements	Herbs	Homeopathic Remedies
Soy, Vitamin E, Vitamin C, Bioflavonoids (hesperidin)	Black cohosh, Vitex, Dong quai, Wild yam	Calcarea carbonica 6c, Pulsatilla 6c, Ignatia 30c, Lachesis 6c, Sepia 30c

MENORRHAGIA (HEAVY MENSTRUATION)

DOCTORS CALL heavy menstrual blood loss menorrhagia. It needs to be diagnosed by a doctor to rule out a variety of potentially serious underlying conditions that sometimes cause increased menstrual bleeding.

Nutrients That May Be Helpful

Once women with menorrhagia have had serious underlying causes ruled out, they need to be tested for **iron** (page 173) deficiency—a condition diagnosed with simple blood tests. Since blood is rich in iron, blood loss can lead to iron depletion. If an iron deficiency is diagnosed, many doctors will recommend 100–200 mg of iron per day, although recommendations vary widely.

The relationship between iron deficiency and menorrhagia is complicated. Not only can the condition lead to iron deficiency, but iron deficiency can lead to menorrhagia. Supplementing with iron decreases excess menstrual blood loss in women who have no other underlying cause for their condition.[1][2] Iron supplements should only be taken by individuals with iron deficiency.

Women with menorrhagia may be deficient in **vitamin A** (page 209). Many women taking 25,000 IU of vitamin A twice per day for fifteen days have been reported to show significant improvements and a complete normalization of menstrual blood loss.[3] However, women who are or could become pregnant should not supplement with more than 10,000 IU (3,000 mcg) per day of vitamin A.

Years ago, when some women used intrauterine devices (IUD) for birth control, **vitamin E** (page 220) at 100 IU per day for two weeks was found to help relieve menorrhagia caused by the IUD.[4] The cause of IUD-induced menstrual blood loss is different from other menorrhagia; therefore, it is possible that vitamin E supplements might not help with menorrhagia not associated with IUD use.

Both **vitamin C** (page 217) and **bioflavonoids** (page 140) protect capillaries (small blood vessels) from damage. In so doing, they might protect against the blood loss of menorrhagia. In one report, fourteen of sixteen women with menorrhagia improved when given 200 mg vitamin C and 200 mg bioflavonoids three times per day.[5]

Are There Any Side Effects or Interactions?

Hemochromatosis, hemosiderosis, polycythemia, and iron-loading anemias (such as thalassemia and sickle cell anemia) are conditions that involve excessive storage of iron. Supplementing iron can be quite dangerous for people with these diseases. Only individuals who have been diagnosed with iron deficiency should take iron supplements. Supplemental doses required to overcome iron deficiency can cause constipation.

Women who are or could become pregnant should take less than 10,000 IU per day of vitamin A to avoid the risk of birth defects. For other adults, intake above 25,000 IU per day can—in rare cases—cause headaches, dry skin, hair loss, fatigue, bone problems, and liver damage.

Some individuals develop diarrhea after as little as a few thousand milligrams of vitamin C per day, while others are not bothered by ten times this amount. However, high levels of vitamin C can deplete the body of **copper** (page 151), an essential nutrient. It is prudent to ensure adequate copper intake at higher intakes of vitamin C; copper is found in many **multiple vitamin/mineral** (page 187) supplements.

Herbs That May Be Helpful

With its emphasis on long-term balancing of a woman's hormonal system, **vitex** (page 317) is not a fast-acting herb. For **premenstrual syndrome** (page 109) or frequent or heavy periods, vitex can be used continuously for four to six months. Women with amenorrhea and infertility can remain on vitex for twelve to eighteen months, unless pregnancy occurs during treatment.

Many people take 40 drops (in a glass of water) of the concentrated liquid herbal extract in the morning. Vitex is also available in powdered form in tablets and capsules, again to be taken in the morning.

Are There Any Side Effects or Interactions?

Side effects are rare using vitex. Minor gastrointestinal upset and a mild skin rash with itching have been reported in less than 2% of the women monitored while taking vitex. Vitex is not recommended for use during pregnancy. It should not be taken together with hormone therapy.

Checklist for Menorrhagia

Nutritional Supplements	Herbs	Homeopathic Remedies
Iron, Vitamin A, Vitamin E, Vitamin C, Bioflavonoids	Vitex	Sepia 30c, Pulsatilla 30c, Cimicifuga 6c

MIGRAINE HEADACHES

MIGRAINES are very painful headaches sometimes involving nausea, vomiting, and changes in vision. They usually begin on only one side of the head and may become worse with exposure to light.

Dietary Changes That May Be Helpful

Migraines can be triggered by allergies and may be relieved by identifying and avoiding the problem foods.[1][2][3][4] Uncovering these foods with the help of a nutritionally oriented doctor is often a useful way to treat migraines. In children suffering migraines who also have epilepsy, there is evidence that eliminating offending foods will also reduce seizures.[5]

Some who suffer from migraines also react to salt, and eliminating salt is helpful for some of these people.[6] Lactose-intolerant individuals may benefit from avoiding milk and ice cream.[7] In addition, some migraine sufferers are unable to break down tyramine, a substance found in many foods.[8] This can lead to the absorption of intact tyramine,[9] which in turn may trigger a migraine.[10]

Tryptophan, an amino acid found in protein-rich foods, is converted to serotonin, a substance that might worsen some migraines. As a result, low-protein diets have been used with some success to reduce migraine attacks.[11][12] Some doctors have found reactions to smoking and birth control pills to be additional contributing factors in migraines.

Nutrients That May Be Helpful

Fish oil (page 160) containing EPA and DHA may reduce the symptoms of migraine headaches.[13][14] One study used 1 gram of fish oil per 10 pounds of body weight. Fish oil probably helps because of its effects in modifying prostaglandins, hormone-like substances made by the body.

On average, migraine patients have lower levels of magnesium (page 182) than other people.[15] Preliminary research shows that premenopausal women with migraines benefit from magnesium supplements.[16] Intravenous magnesium can relieve some migraines in a matter of minutes.[17] Double-blind research shows that 360 mg of magnesium per day decreases premenstrual migraines.[18] Most of the benefit of supplemental magnesium seems to be with younger women.

High doses of **calcium** (page 144) and **vitamin D** (page 219) have also been useful in treating several cases of migraines.[19] [20] Some nutritionally oriented doctors may recommend that people take 800 mg of calcium and 400 IU of vitamin D per day.

One group of researchers using high (400 mg per day) amounts of **vitamin B2** (page 212) in treating forty-nine migraine patients found beneficial results in most of the migraine sufferers.[21]

Individuals who develop migraines may be more likely to be lactose intolerant, in which case the supplemental use of the **lactase** (page 175) enzyme prior to consuming any dairy products can be helpful.

Are There Any Side Effects or Interactions?

Side effects from the EPA and DHA in fish oil include nose bleeds (because of reduced blood clotting), gastrointestinal upset, and "fishy" burps.

Taking too much magnesium can lead to diarrhea. People with kidney disease should not take magnesium supplements without consulting a nutritionally oriented doctor.

Individuals with sarcoidosis, hyperparathyroidism, or with chronic kidney disease should not supplement with calcium or vitamin D. In addition, individuals with a history of kidney stones should consult a nutritionally oriented physician before taking calcium supplements.

Vitamin B2 is nontoxic even in high amounts. Lactase is safe and does not produce side effects.

Herbs That May Be Helpful

The most frequently used herb for the long-term treatment and prevention of migraines is **feverfew** (page 263). Feverfew inhibits hyperaggregation of platelets and the release of serotonin and some inflammatory mediators.[22] Studies have shown that continuous use of feverfew leads to a reduction in the severity, duration, and frequency of migraine headaches.[23] [24]

Many people take standardized feverfew leaf extracts that supply a minimum of 250 mcg of parthenolide (the active constituent) per day. Results may not be evident for at least four to six weeks.

Clinical reports suggest success using 4–6 grams per day of powdered **ginger** (page 267) for migraines and the nausea that accompanies them.[25] Ginger may also be taken as a tincture in the amount of 1.5–3 ml, three times daily. **Ginkgo biloba** (page 268) extract may also help, because it reduces the formation of a substance known as platelet-activating factor,[26] which may contribute to migraines.

Are There Any Side Effects or Interactions?

Taken as recommended, standardized feverfew causes minimal side effects. Minor side effects from feverfew can include gastrointestinal upset and nervousness. Feverfew is not recommended during pregnancy or lactation.

Checklist for Migraine Headaches

Nutritional Supplements	Herbs	Homeopathic Remedies
Fish oil (EPA/DHA), Magnesium, Calcium, Vitamin D, Vitamin B2, Lactase	Feverfew, Ginger, Ginkgo biloba	Belladonna 6c, Bryonia 6c, Gelsemium 30c, Kali bichromicum 6c

MORNING SICKNESS

MORNING SICKNESS is the common but poorly understood nausea that frequently accompanies early pregnancy. It is generally not serious though it can be quite unpleasant.

Dietary Changes That May Be Helpful

Some obstetricians recommend that women with morning sickness eat dry crackers upon arising and drink liquids and eat solid foods separately from each other.

Women with a high intake of saturated fat (from meat and dairy) may have a much higher risk of severe morning sickness than women eating less saturated fat. A Harvard study found that the equivalent of one cheeseburger or three cups of milk more than tripled risk of developing morning sickness.[1]

Nutrients That May Be Helpful

Vitamin K (page 222) and **vitamin C** (page 217), taken together, may provide remarkable relief of symptoms for some women. In one study, women who took 5 mg of vitamin K and 25 mg of vitamin C per day reported the complete disappearance of morning sickness within three days;[2] however, most nutritionally oriented doctors use higher amounts of vitamin C (500–1,000 mg).

Vitamin B6 (page 210), at an intake of 10–25 mg taken three times per day, may also help relieve morning sickness.[3] [4]

Are There Any Side Effects or Interactions?

Vitamin K interferes with the action of prescription blood thinners. People taking these drugs should never supplement vitamin K without consulting a doctor.

Some individuals develop diarrhea after as little as a few thousand milligrams of vitamin C per day, while others are not bothered by ten times this amount. However, high levels of vitamin C can deplete the body of **copper** (page 151), an essential nutrient. It is prudent to ensure adequate copper intake at higher intakes of vitamin C; copper is found in many **multiple vitamin/mineral** (page 187) supplements.

Although side effects from vitamin B6 supplements are rare, at very high levels this vitamin can damage sensory nerves, leading to numbness in the hands and feet as well as difficulty walking. Vitamin B6 supplementation should be stopped if these symptoms develop. During pregnancy or lactation a maximum daily amount of 100 mg should not be exceeded without first consulting a nutritionally oriented doctor.

Herbs That May Be Helpful

Ginger (page 267) is well known for alleviating nausea and improving digestion. It has also been used to reduce vomiting in a more severe form of nausea associated with pregnancy known as hyperemesis gravidarum.[5] Women with hyperemesis gravidarum should consult their doctor before pursuing any course of treatment.

Many people take 250 mg of ginger capsules, tablets, or as a tea four times per day to reduce nausea.[6] It may also be taken as a tincture in the amount of 1.5–3 ml, three times daily. Ginger should only be used for short periods of time, and the amount taken daily should not exceed 1 gram per day.

Are There Any Side Effects or Interactions?

Side effects of ginger are rare when used as recommended. However, some people may be sensitive to the taste or experience heartburn. Persons with a history of gallstones should consult a doctor before using ginger. Short-term use of ginger for nausea and vomiting of pregnancy appears to pose no safety problems; however, long-term use during pregnancy is not recommended.

Checklist for Morning Sickness

Nutritional Supplements	Herbs	Homeopathic Remedies
Vitamin K, Vitamin C, Vitamin B6	Ginger	Sepia 30c, Ipecac 6c, Phosphorus 6c

MSG SENSITIVITY

MSG SENSITIVITY, also known as Chinese restaurant syndrome, is a group of symptoms that occur in some people after consuming monosodium glutamate (MSG).

Although some Chinese (and other) restaurants now avoid the use of MSG, many still use significant amounts of this flavor enhancer. The symptoms of Chinese restaurant syndrome commonly include headache, flushing, tingling, weakness, and stomachache.

Dietary Changes That May Be Helpful

Simply avoiding MSG will prevent the symptoms caused by its exposure in sensitive individuals. MSG is found in some Chinese and Japanese food (as Aji no Moto) and is also used as a meat tenderizer (as Accent). Often MSG is difficult to avoid, as it also occurs in hydrolyzed vegetable protein, textured vegetable protein, gelatin, yeast extracts, calcium and sodium caseinate, vegetable broth, whey, smoke flavoring, malt extracts, and several other food ingredients—without appearing on the label.

Nutrients That May Be Helpful

Years ago, researchers discovered that animals who were deficient in **vitamin B6** (page 214) could not properly process MSG.[1] Typical reactions to MSG have also been linked to vitamin B6 deficiency in people.[2] In one study, eight out of nine such people stopped reacting to MSG when given 50 mg of vitamin B6 per day for at least twelve weeks. The actual percentage of people with MSG sensitivity who are vitamin B6 deficient and who respond to B6 supplementation remains unknown. Nonetheless, many doctors of natural medicine suggest that people who have these symptoms try supplementing with vitamin B6 for three months as a trial.

Are There Any Side Effects or Interactions?

Vitamin B6 in large amounts can damage sensory nerves, leading to numbness in the hands and feet as well as difficulty walking. Vitamin B6 supplementation should be stopped if these symptoms develop. Pregnant and lactating women should not take more than 100 mg of vitamin B6; for other adults, 200–500 mg per day is probably safe.

Checklist for MSG Sensitivity

Nutritional Supplements	Herbs	Homeopathic Remedies
Vitamin B6	No herbs commonly used for this condition	No homeopathy commonly used for this condition

NIGHT BLINDNESS

PEOPLE WITH NIGHT BLINDNESS see poorly at night but see normally during the day. The condition does not actually involve true blindness, even at night.

Nutrients That May Be Helpful

Night blindness can be an early sign of **vitamin A** (page 209) deficiency, often the result of a diet lacking in vegetables containing beta-carotene, which the body can make into vitamin A.

A lack of **zinc** (page 224) can reduce retinol dehydrogenase, an enzyme needed to help vitamin A work in the eye. Zinc helps night blindness in those who are zinc deficient.[1] Most people do not get enough zinc in their diets. Therefore, many nutritionally oriented physicians suggest 15–30 mg of zinc per day to support healthy vision. Because long-term zinc supplementation reduces **copper** (page 151) levels, 1–3 mg of copper should accompany zinc supplementation lasting more than a few weeks.

Are There Any Side Effects or Interactions?

Women who are, or could become, pregnant should take less than 10,000 IU (3,000 mcg) per day of vitamin A to avoid the risk of birth defects. For other adults, intake above 25,000 IU (7,500 mcg) per day can—in rare cases—cause headaches, dry skin, hair loss, fatigue, bone problems, and liver damage. Zinc intake in excess of 300 mg per day may impair immune function.

Herbs That May Be Helpful

Bilberries (page 234), a close relative of blueberries, are high in a bioflavonoid complex known as anthocyanosides. Anthocyanosides speed the regeneration of rhodopsin, the purple pigment that is used by the rods in the eye for night vision.[2] This makes bilberry a possible first line of defense for those with poor night vision.[3] Bilberry extract standardized to 25% anthocyanosides can be taken at 240–480 mg per day in capsules or tablets.

Checklist for Night Blindness

Nutritional Supplements	Herbs	Homeopathic Remedies
Vitamin A, Zinc	Bilberry	No homeopathy commonly used for this condition

OSGOOD-SCHLATTER DISEASE

OSGOOD-SCHLATTER DISEASE (a form of osteochondrosis) occurs in adolescence and is often the result of a combination of rapid growth and competitive sports that overstress the knee joint. The patellar tendon, which normally attaches to the tibial tuberosity, is sometimes strained by the powerful quadriceps muscles.

This tearing or avulsion can be extremely painful and is sometimes disabling. It may occur in both knees. The knee is usually sore to pressure at the point where the large tendon from the kneecap attaches to the prominence below.

Nutrients That May Be Helpful

Based on the personal experience of a doctor who reported his findings,[1] some nutritionally oriented physicians recommend **vitamin E** (page 220) at 400 IU per day and **selenium** (page 203) at 50 mcg three times per day. Jonathan Wright, M.D., reports anecdotally that he has had considerable success with this regimen and often sees results in two to six weeks.[2]

Are There Any Side Effects or Interactions?

Vitamin E toxicity is very rare. Selenium is very safe, although taking more than 1,000 mcg per day may cause loss of fingernails, skin rash, and changes in the nervous system.

Checklist for Osgood-Schlatter Disease

Nutritional Supplements	Herbs	Homeopathic Remedies
Vitamin E, Selenium	No herbs commonly used for this condition	No homeopathy commonly used for this condition

OSTEOARTHRITIS

OSTEOARTHRITIS, a degenerative type of arthritis, develops when the linings of the joints wear down. Although it is associated with aging and injury (it used to be called "wear-and-tear arthritis"), its true cause remains unknown.

Dietary Changes That May Be Helpful

In the 1950s through the 1970s, a naturopathic doctor named Max Warmbrand used with some success a diet free of meat, dairy, chemicals, sugar, eggs, and processed foods for those with rheumatoid arthritis and osteoarthritis.[1]

Solanine is a substance found in nightshade plants, which include tomatoes, white potatoes, all peppers (except black pepper), and eggplant. If not destroyed in the intestine, solanine can be toxic. Eliminating solanine from the diet may give relief to some arthritis sufferers.[2] A survey of people avoiding nightshade plants revealed that 28% had a "marked positive response" and another 44% had a "positive response." Unfortunately, researchers have never put this diet to a strict clinical test, although the treatment continues to be used by many doctors to help patients with both rheumatoid and osteoarthritis. It can take up to six months for this diet to bring relief. It is very difficult for some people to eliminate tomatoes and peppers, and many people are simply not helped. Therefore, this diet is often attempted in only severe cases of arthritis that do not respond to other natural treatments.

Most of the studies linking allergies to joint disease have focused on rheumatoid arthritis, although mention of what was called rheumatism (some of which was probably osteoarthritis) in older reports suggests a possible link.[3] If other therapies are unsuccessful in relieving symptoms of osteoarthritis, food allergy identification with the help of a nutritionally oriented physician could be considered.

Nutrients That May Be Helpful

Glucosamine sulfate (page 165), a nutrient derived from seashells, contains a building block needed for the repair of joint cartilage. Osteoarthritis symptoms are lessened and damaged joints may be repaired in people taking 500 mg of glucosamine sulfate three times per day.[4][5][6][7] It may take three to eight weeks before benefits from glucosamine sulfate become evident, and continued supplementation is needed in order to maintain benefits.

It has been reported that people who have osteoarthritis and eat high levels of antioxidants (page 8) in their diets exhibit a much slower rate of joint deterioration, particularly in the knees, than do people eating low levels of antioxidants.[8] The antioxidant vitamin E (page 220), for example, has been shown to reduce symptoms of osteoarthritis.[9][10] A reasonable amount is 400–600 IU of vitamin E per day.

Boron (page 142) affects calcium metabolism, and a link between boron deficiency and arthritis has been suggested.[11] Double-blind research has found that 6 mg of boron per day, taken for two months, may relieve symptoms of osteoarthritis.[12]

The omega-3 fatty acids, EPA and DHA, in fish oil (page 160) have been used extensively for rheumatoid arthritis because of their anti-inflammatory effects, but they may also play a role in the inflammatory component of osteoarthritis.[13]

Some people with osteoarthritis taking high doses of niacinamide (also called nicotinamide), a form of vitamin B3 (page 213), find relief from symptoms such as increased joint mobility, improved muscle strength, and decreased fatigue.[14][15][16] A therapeutic amount is 250 mg of niacinamide or nicotinamide in capsules or tablets four to sixteen times per day (with higher doses reserved for people with more advanced disease). Improvement may take three to four months of supplementation, and continued supplement use is needed to maintain symptom relief. A double-blind study has confirmed that niacinamide begins to improve osteoarthritis within twelve weeks.[17]

D-phenylalanine, the D-form of phenylalanine (page 194), has been used to treat chronic pain—including osteoarthritis—with mixed effectiveness.[18] A few studies suggest that individuals with arthritis may benefit from cartilage (page 147); however, well-designed research is lacking, and many experts question the use of cartilage in this regard.

Other supplements, such as chondroitin sulfate (page 149) and green lipped mussel, have occasionally been reported to help joint conditions. Levels of chondroitin sulfate may be reduced in joint cartilage affected by osteoarthritis and possibly other forms of arthritis; therefore, chondroitin sulfate may help restore joint function in people with osteoarthritis.[19] However, most doctors of natural medicine believe that chondroitin sulfate may simply duplicate the effects of glucosamine sulfate.

Are There Any Side Effects or Interactions?

Boron is rarely implicated in side effects, although one study found that 3 mg per day resulted in increased estrogen levels.[20] This is a concern, since estrogen may increase the risk of several cancers. Until more is known, it makes sense for supplemental boron intake to be limited to 1 mg per day.

Side effects from EPA and DHA in fish oil may include nose bleeds (because of reduced blood clotting), gastrointestinal upset, and "fishy" burps.

Niacinamide or nicotinamide is almost always safe to take, although rare liver problems have occurred at doses in excess of 1,000 mg per day.

The maximum amount of D-phenylalanine that is safe is unknown, but nerve damage has not been reported with 1,500 mg per day or less of D-phenylalanine. D-phenylalanine has occasionally caused mild side effects, such as nausea, heartburn, or transient headaches, in smaller amounts.

It has been suggested that some people should not use cartilage supplement. These would include individuals with circulation problems, hypertension, or other cardiovascular diseases, as well as women who want to be or are pregnant, nursing mothers, anyone having or having had surgery within thirty days, and athletes training intensely.

At intakes of chondroitin sulfate greater than 10 grams per day, nausea may occur. No other adverse effects have been reported.

Herbs That May Be Helpful

Boswellia (page 238) has unique anti-inflammatory action, much like the conventional nonsteroidal anti-inflammatory drugs (NSAIDs) used by many for inflammatory conditions. But unlike NSAIDs, long-term use of boswellia does not lead to irritation or ulceration of the stomach.

The silicon content of horsetail (page 281) is believed to exert a connective tissue strengthening and antiarthritic action. White willow (page 318) has anti-inflammatory and pain-relieving effects. Although the analgesic actions of willow are typically slow-acting, they last longer than standard aspirin

products. Cayenne (page 246) has been used topically. The authors of a study looking at patients with osteoarthritis and rheumatoid arthritis speculate that yucca saponins (page 324) block release of toxins from the intestines that inhibit normal formation of cartilage.

Are There Any Side Effects or Interactions?

Boswellia is generally safe when used as directed. Rare side effects can include diarrhea, skin rash, and nausea. Any inflammatory joint condition should be closely monitored by a nutritionally oriented physician.

Horsetail is generally considered safe for nonpregnant adults. The only concern would be that the correct species of horsetail is used; *Equisetum palustre* is another species of horsetail that contains toxic alkaloids and is a well-known livestock poison.

Long-term use of white willow may possibly cause gastrointestinal irritation. As is the case with aspirin, willow should not be used to lower fevers in children. People who are allergic to aspirin should avoid white willow.

Checklist for Osteoarthritis

Nutritional Supplements	Herbs	Homeopathic Remedies
Glucosamine sulfate, Antioxidants (vitamin E), Boron, Fish oil (EPA/DHA), Vitamin B3 (Niacinamide), D-phenylalanine, Cartilage, Chondroitin sulfate	Boswellia, Horsetail, White willow, Cayenne, Yucca	Rhus toxicodendron 6c, Ledum 6c, Belladonna 6c, Apis mellifica 6c, Bryonia 6c, Pulsatilla 6c, Ruta graveolens 6c

OSTEOPOROSIS

OSTEOPOROSIS is a very common condition that increases with age. It is more common in women than in men and more common in white and Asian people than in black people. The bones of people with this disease lack normal density, which increases the risk of fractures.

Dietary Changes That May Be Helpful

A diet high in animal protein—meat, poultry, and dairy—increases the risk of bone fractures.[1][2] Salt and caffeine have also been linked to bone loss.[3][4] Soft drinks, which have high levels of phosphoric acid, may be harmful to bones according to some,[5] though not all, studies.[6] But there is certainly no harm in decreasing drinks filled with sugar and chemicals. All of these changes are likely to reduce urinary loss of calcium.

Lifestyle Changes That May Be Helpful

Smoking leads to increased bone loss.[7] For this and many other health reasons, it should be avoided. Exercise protects against bone loss.[8] The more weight-bearing exercise done by men and post-menopausal women, the greater their bone mass and the lower their risk of osteoporosis. Walking is a good weight-bearing exercise. For premenopausal women, exercise is also important, but it can be overdone. Excessive exercise that leads to a cessation of the menstrual cycle can actually contribute to osteoporosis.[9]

Nutrients That May Be Helpful

Calcium (page 144) supplements help prevent and treat osteoporosis.[10] Many adults take 800–1,200 mg of calcium per day. Vitamin D (page 219) increases calcium absorption, but it is unclear whether vitamin D affects the risk of osteoporosis.[11][12] Since calcium may reduce absorption of magnesium (page 182) and zinc (page 224), which are important nutrients for preventing osteoporosis, it may be prudent to also supplement these minerals;[13][14] 25 mg of zinc and 200–400 mg of magnesium per day are reasonable amounts. **Copper** (page 151) helps in bone synthesis; a recent study found that 3 mg of copper per day may help prevent bone loss.[15] Often, all of these minerals are available in multimineral supplements.

Some research suggests that the minerals **boron** (page 142),[16] **manganese** (page 183),[17] silicon,[18] and strontium[19] may be helpful. One double-blind study with postmenopausal women added zinc (15 mg), copper (2.5 mg), and manganese (5 mg) to calcium (1,000 mg).[20] As expected, the calcium group lost less bone than the placebo group did. But the group receiving the additional trace minerals actually increased their bone mass significantly. Some osteoporosis supplement formulas include small amounts of all these minerals.

Folic acid (page 163), **vitamin B6** (page 214), and **vitamin B12** (page 216) are known to reduce blood levels of homocysteine in the body, while high homocysteine levels may contribute to osteoporosis. Some doctors of natural medicine suggest these B vitamins to help treat and prevent osteoporosis.[21] Doses found in **vitamin B-complex** (page 210) supplements and **multivitamins** (page 187) should be adequate, though the optimal amounts needed to affect bone mass are unknown.

Vitamin K (page 222) is needed for bone formation. Those with osteoporosis have low levels of this vitamin.[22] One study found that postmenopausal women with osteoporosis stop losing excessive calcium in their urine after taking 1 mg per day of vitamin K supplements.[23]

Are There Any Side Effects or Interactions?

Individuals with sarcoidosis, hyperparathyroidism, or with chronic kidney disease should not supplement with calcium. Individuals with a history of kidney stones should consult a nutritionally oriented physician before taking calcium supplements.

Boron may slightly increase estrogen levels. This is a concern since estrogen may increase the risk of several cancers. Until more is known, supplemental boron intake should be limited to 1 mg per day.

Preliminary research suggests that individuals with cirrhosis may not be able to properly excrete manganese; until more is known, these people should not supplement with manganese.

Folic acid, although safe, can mask the symptoms of vitamin B12 deficiency. Although side effects from vitamin B6 supplements are rare, at very high levels this vitamin can damage sensory nerves, leading to numbness in the hands and feet as well as difficulty walking. Vitamin B6 supplementation should be stopped if these symptoms develop.

Vitamin K interferes with the action of prescription blood thinners. People taking these drugs should never supplement vitamin K without consulting a doctor.

Herbs That May Be Helpful

Horsetail (page 281) is rich in silicon, and some experts have suggested that silicon is a vital component for bone and cartilage formation. This would indicate that horsetail may be beneficial in preventing osteoporosis.

Are There Any Side Effects or Interactions?

Horsetail is generally considered safe for nonpregnant adults. The only concern would be that the correct species of horsetail is used; *Equisetum palustre* is another species of horsetail that contains toxic alkaloids and is a well-known livestock poison.

Checklist for Osteoporosis

Nutritional Supplements	Herbs	Homeopathic Remedies
Calcium, Magnesium, Vitamin D, Boron, Multiple vitamin/mineral (B6, B12, silicon, strontium, zinc, copper, manganese), Folic acid, Vitamin K	Horsetail	Calcarea phosphorica 6c, Calcarea carbonica 6c, Strontium carb 6c

PAP SMEAR (ABNORMAL)

WOMEN ARE advised to have periodic Pap smears because cancer of the cervix is a fairly common and sometimes fatal disease. A Pap smear checks cells from the cervix for any evidence of precancerous or cancerous changes. If an abnormality is detected early, the doctor can prescribe effective treatment before the problem becomes more serious. Cervical dysplasia is a term used to describe abnormal cervical cells. Cervical dysplasia is usually graded according to its severity, which can range from mild inflammation to precancerous changes to localized cancer.

Nutrients That May Be Helpful

Women with cervical dysplasia may have lower blood levels of **beta-carotene** (page 209) and **vitamin E** (page 220) compared to healthy women.[1] Low levels of **selenium** (page 203)[2] and low dietary intake of **vitamin C** (page 217)[3] have also been observed in women with cervical dysplasia. Women with a low intake of **vitamin A** (page 209) have an increased risk of abnormal Pap smear.[4]

Large amounts of **folic acid** (page 163)—10 mg per day—have been shown to improve the abnormal Pap smears of women who are taking birth control pills.[5] Folic acid does not improve the Pap smears of women who are not taking oral contraceptives.[6][7] High blood levels of folic acid have been linked to protecting against the development of cervical dysplasia.[8]

Are There Any Side Effects or Interactions?

Taking more than 1,000 mcg of selenium per day may cause loss of fingernails, skin rash, and changes in the nervous system.

Some individuals develop diarrhea after as little as a few thousand milligrams of vitamin C per day, while others are not bothered by ten times this amount. However, high levels of vitamin C can deplete the body of **copper** (page 151), an essential nutrient. It is prudent to ensure adequate copper intake at higher intakes of vitamin C; copper is found in many **multiple vitamin/mineral** (page 187) supplements. Women who are or could become pregnant should take less than 10,000 IU per day of vitamin A to avoid the risk of birth defects. For other adults, intake above 25,000 IU per day can in rare cases cause headaches, dry skin, hair loss, fatigue, bone problems, and liver damage.

Folic acid is remarkably safe; however, folic acid supplements can mask the symptoms of vitamin B12 deficiency, which could lead to permanent neurological damage. Although this problem is rare, folic acid and **vitamin B12** (page 216) should always be taken together.

Checklist for Abnormal Pap Smear

Nutritional Supplements	Herbs	Homeopathic Remedies
Beta-carotene, Vitamin E, Selenium, Vitamin C, Vitamin A, Folic acid	No herbs commonly used for this condition	No homeopathy commonly used for this condition

PEPTIC ULCER

WHAT WE CALL an ulcer doctors call a peptic ulcer, to distinguish it from other forms of ulcer that can affect many parts of the body. Peptic ulcers are erosions in the stomach or duodenum (the first part of the small intestine); these ulcers often bleed and have many causes.

Many peptic ulcers are caused by an infection. The responsible bug is *Helicobacter pylori*. While at least one herb (licorice root, see below) may help kill these bacteria, until more is known, if your ulcer is due to infection it is wise to discuss treatment—a combination of antibiotics and bismuth—with a medical doctor.

Ulcers can also be caused or exacerbated by stress, alcohol, smoking, and dietary factors.

Dietary Changes That May Be Helpful

Those with ulcers appear to eat more sugar,[1] and sugar increases stomach acid.[2] Salt is a stomach and intestinal irritant. The higher the intake of salt, the higher the risk of stomach (though not duodenal) ulcer.[3] It is best to restrict the use of both sugar and salt.

Many years ago, researchers found that cabbage juice accelerated healing of peptic ulcers.[4 5] Drinking a quart per day is necessary, but pain relief may occur in just a few days. Carrot juice can be added to improve the flavor.

Fiber (page 159) slows the movement of food and acidic fluid from the stomach to the intestines, which should help those with duodenal ulcer.[6] When people with recently healed duodenal ulcers were put on a long-term (six months) high-fiber diet, the rate of ulcer recurrence was dramatically reduced.[7]

Ayurvedic doctors in India have traditionally used dried banana powder to treat ulcers. A research trial studying those with ulcers confirmed that it helps.[8] Bananas and unsweetened banana chips are probably good substitutes, although ideal intake remains unknown.

Years ago, food allergies were linked to peptic ulcer.[9] Exposure to allergic foods can actually cause stomach bleeding.[10] If an ulcer is not from an infection and does not respond to natural treatment, ask a nutritionally oriented doctor about the possibility of an allergy-triggered ulcer.

Lifestyle Changes That May Be Helpful

Aspirin and related drugs,[11] alcohol,[12] coffee[13] (even decaf),[14] and tea[15] increase stomach acidity, which can interfere with the healing of an ulcer. Smoking also slows ulcer healing.[16] Whether or not an ulcer was caused by infection, all of the above should be avoided.

Nutrients That May Be Helpful

Vitamin A (page 209) and zinc (page 224), both needed in the healing process, may help people with peptic ulcers.[17] [18] While the zinc research used 150 mg per day in adults (a very high amount), many people take 15–40 mg per day. Even at these doses, it is necessary to take 1–3 mg of copper (page 151) per day to avoid a copper deficiency. Very high amounts of vitamin A (100,000 IU per day) have also been used successfully, but such amounts can be quite toxic and require the supervision of a nutritionally oriented doctor. A safe dose for women of childbearing age is 10,000 IU (3,000 mcg) per day and probably 25,000 IU (7,500 mcg) for other adults.

Glutamine (page 166), an amino acid, is the principal source of energy for the cells that line the small intestine and stomach and helps them heal. Glutamine may help treat ulcers.[19] Some nutritionally oriented doctors suggest 500–1,000 mg of glutamine two to three times per day.

Research has shown that some bioflavonoids (page 140)—such as quercetin (page 201), catechin, and apigenin, which is found in chamomile (page 247)—inhibit the growth of H. pylori bacteria.[20] Bioflavonoids have also been used for ulcers because of their anti-inflammatory activity.[21] A reasonable amount is 500–1,000 mg of the bioflavonoid quercetin two to three times per day.

Are There Any Side Effects or Interactions?

Women who are or could become pregnant should take less than 10,000 IU per day of vitamin A to avoid the risk of birth defects. For other adults, intake above 25,000 IU per day can—uncommonly—cause headaches, dry skin, hair loss, fatigue, bone problems, and liver damage. Zinc intake in excess of 300 mg per day may impair immune function; seek guidance from a nutritionally oriented doctor.

No consistent toxicity has been linked to the bioflavonoids; the exception is for a bioflavonoid called cianidanol, which is not found in supplements.

Herbs That May Be Helpful

Licorice (page 286) root has a long history of use for soothing inflamed and injured mucous membranes in the digestive tract. Licorice may protect the stomach and duodenum (two areas where ulcers most commonly occur) by increasing production of mucin, a substance that protects the lining of these organs against stomach acid and other harmful substances.[22] Licorice also appears to inhibit Helicobacter pylori.[23]

For ulcers, many physicians use licorice root in its deglycyrrhizinated form (DGL). This removes the portion of licorice root associated with increasing blood pressure and causing water retention in some people, while retaining the mucous membrane–healing part of the root. In studies, DGL has compared favorably to the popular drug Tagamet for treatment of peptic ulcer disease.[24]

Doctors often suggest taking one to two chewable tablets of DGL (250–500 mg) fifteen minutes before meals and one to two hours before bedtime.

Chamomile (page 247) has a soothing effect on inflamed and irritated mucous membranes. It is also high in the bioflavonoid apigenin. Many people drink two to three cups of strong chamomile tea each day, which can be made by combining 3–5 ml of chamomile tincture with hot water. Chamomile is also available in capsules.

Marshmallow root (page 289) is high in mucilage. High-mucilage-containing herbs have a long history of use for irritated or inflamed mucous membranes in the digestive system.

Are There Any Side Effects or Interactions?

Licorice products without the glycyrrhizin removed may increase blood pressure and cause water retention. Some people are more sensitive to this effect that others. Long-term intake of products containing more than 1 gram of glycyrrhizin (which is the amount in approximately 10 grams of root) daily is the usual amount required to cause these effects. As a result of these possible side effects, long-term intake of high levels of glycyrrhizin are discouraged and should only be undertaken if prescribed by a qualified health care professional. Deglycyrrhizinated licorice extracts do not cause these side effects, because there is no glycyrrhizin in them.

Though rare, allergic reactions to chamomile have been reported. These reactions have included bronchial constriction with internal use and allergic skin reactions with topical use. While such side effects are extremely uncommon, persons with allergies to plants of the *Asteraceae* family (ragweed, aster, and chrysanthemum) should avoid use of chamomile.

Checklist for Peptic Ulcer

Nutritional Supplements	Herbs	Homeopathic Remedies
Fiber, Vitamin A, Zinc, Glutamine, Bioflavonoids (quercetin, catechin, apigenin)	Deglycyrrhizinated licorice, Chamomile, Marshmallow root	No homeopathy commonly used for this condition

PHOTOSENSITIVITY

SEVERAL CONDITIONS, such as erythropoietic protoporphyria and polymorphous light eruption, share the common symptom of hypersensitivity to light—typically sunlight. People taking certain prescription drugs (sulfonamides, tetracycline, and thiazide diuretics) and those diagnosed with systemic lupus erythematosis are more likely to overreact to sun exposure.

People with photosensitivities typically break out in a rash when exposed to sunlight; how much exposure causes a reaction varies from person to person.

Dietary Changes That May Be Helpful

One of the conditions that can trigger photosensitivity—porphyria cutanea tarda—has been linked to alcohol consumption.[1] People with this form of porphyria should avoid alcohol.

Lifestyle Changes That May Be Helpful

People with photosensitivities need to protect themselves from the sun by using sunscreen, wearing protective clothing (such as long-sleeved shirts), and avoiding excess exposure to the sun.

Nutrients That May Be Helpful

Beta-carotene (page 209) collects primarily in the skin. Years ago, researchers theorized that beta-carotene in skin might help protect against sensitivity to ultraviolet light from the sun. Large amounts of beta-carotene (up to 150,000 IU per day for at least several months) have allowed people with photosensitivities to stay out in the sun several times longer than they otherwise could tolerate.[2][3][4] The protective effect appears to result from beta-carotene's ability to protect against free radical damage caused by sunlight.[5]

Less is known about the effects of other antioxidants (page 8). Research with vitamin E (page 220) has been limited and has not yielded consistent results.[6][7]

Cases have been reported of people with photosensitivities who respond to vitamin B6 (page 214) supplements.[8][9] Amounts of vitamin B6 used to successfully reduce reactions to sunlight have varied considerably. Some nutritionally oriented doctors suggest a trial of 100–200 mg per day for three months.

Niacinamide, a form of vitamin B3 (page 213), can reduce the formation of a kynurenic acid—a substance that has been linked to photosensitivities. One trial studied the effects of niacinamide in people who had polymorphous light eruption, one of the photosensitivity diseases.[10] Taking one gram three times per day, most people remained free of problems despite exposure to the sun.

Adenosine monophosphate (AMP) is a substance made in the body and is also found as a supplement, although it is not widely available. Nineteen out of twenty-one people with porphyria cutanea tarda responded well to 160–200 mg of AMP per day taken for at least one month, reports one group of researchers.[11] Partial and even complete alleviation of photosensitivity associated with this condition occurred in several people.

Are There Any Side Effects or Interactions?

Beta-carotene does not cause any side effects, aside from excessive intake (more than 100,000 IU per day) sometimes giving the skin a yellow-orange hue. It is this very collection of beta-carotene in the skin, however, that is responsible for its ability to help people with photosensitivities.

Vitamin B6, in large amounts, can damage sensory nerves, leading to numbness in the hands and feet. Pregnant and lactating women should not take more than 100 mg of vitamin B6. For other adults, vitamin B6 is safe in amounts of 200–500 mg per day, although occasional problems have been reported in this range. Unlike niacin, the form of vitamin B3 called niacinamide is generally considered quite safe in moderate amounts, but such high levels are uncommon and need to be monitored by a nutritionally oriented doctor.

Checklist for Photosensitivity

Nutritional Supplements	Herbs	Homeopathic Remedies
Beta-carotene, Vitamin E, Vitamin B6, Vitamin B3 (Niacinamide), Adenosine monophosphate	No herbs commonly used for this condition	No homeopathy commonly used for this condition

PREGNANCY SUPPORT

<table>
<tr><td>

PREGNANCY lasts an average of forty weeks from the date of the last menstrual period to delivery. In the first trimester, many pregnant women experience nausea. Usually these women report that they feel best during the second trimester. During the third and final trimester, the increasing size of the fetus begins to pose mechanical strains on a woman, often causing back pain, sciatica, leg swelling, and other health problems.

</td></tr>
</table>

Dietary Changes That May Be Helpful

Nearly all pregnant women benefit from good nutritional habits prior to and during pregnancy. The increased number of birth defects during times of famine attest to the effects of poor nutrition during pregnancy.[1] A standard Western diet (high in fat, salt, sugar, and low in complex carbohydrates) often lacks essential vitamins and minerals needed during pregnancy and breast-feeding, which can result in compromised health of the newborn.[2]

Pregnant women should choose a well-balanced and varied diet that includes fresh fruits and vegetables, whole grains, legumes, beans, and fish. Foods such as refined sugars, processed foods, saturated fats, and other animal proteins should be limited. Organically grown produce is preferable to foods containing pesticides and preservatives.

Lifestyle Changes That May Be Helpful

A woman can reduce her risk of complications during pregnancy and delivery by avoiding harmful substances, such as alcohol, caffeine, nicotine, and recreational or prescription drugs.

Even minimal alcohol ingestion during pregnancy can increase the risk of hyperactivity, short attention span, and emotional problems in a woman's child.[3] Pregnant women should not drink alcohol.

Cigarette smoking causes lower birth weights and smaller-sized newborns. The rate of miscarriage in smokers is twice as high compared to non-smokers,[4] and babies born to mothers who smoke have more than twice the risk of dying from sudden infant death syndrome.[5]

Research also links caffeine to growth-retarded or low-birth-weight infants.[6] Women should limit caffeine intake to approximately 300 mg per day during pregnancy; this is equivalent to three small cups of coffee.

Nutrients That May Be Helpful

The requirement for the B vitamin **folic acid** (page 163) doubles during pregnancy.[7] Deficiencies of folic acid have been linked in studies to low-birth-weight infants as well as an increased incidence of neural tube defects. Women at high risk for giving birth to babies with neural tube defects have been reported to lower their risk by 72% if they take folate supplements prior to and during pregnancy.[8] In another study, folate supplements in pregnant women improved birth weight and Apgar scores and decreased the incidence of fetal growth retardation and maternal infections.[9] The recommended daily dose of folic acid during pregnancy is 800 mcg per day.

Supplementation of the niacin form of **vitamin B3** (page 213) taken during the first trimester has been positively correlated with higher birth weights, longer length, and larger head circumference (all signs of healthier infants).[10]

Calcium (page 144) needs are double during pregnancy.[11] Low dietary intake of this mineral is associated with pre-eclampsia, a potentially dangerous (but preventable) condition characterized by high blood pressure and swelling. Supplementation with calcium may reduce the risk of preterm delivery, which is often associated with pre-eclampsia. Calcium may also reduce the risk of hypertensive disorders of pregnancy.[12] Pregnant women should consume 1,500 mg of calcium per day. Food sources of calcium include milk products, dark leafy vegetables, tofu, sardines, and canned salmon.

Are There Any Side Effects or Interactions?

All vitamins and minerals have an optimal and safe recommended dose and in some cases have stricter parameters during pregnancy. Consult your health practitioner about proper prenatal supplements and their dosage.

Folic acid is remarkably safe. However, if someone is deficient in **vitamin B12** (page 216) and takes 1,000 mcg of folic acid per day or more, the folic acid can improve anemia caused by the B12 deficiency but not affect neurological symptoms. This is not a toxicity but rather a partial solution to one of the problems caused by B12 deficiency. Anyone supplementing with more than 1,000 mcg per day of folic acid needs to be initially evaluated by a doctor of natural medicine to avoid this potential problem.

The form of niacin called niacinamide is almost always safe to take, although rare liver problems have occurred at doses of several thousand milligrams per day. Niacin may cause flushing, headache, and stomachache in some people. These problems occasionally occur with doses as low as 50–100 mg. Vitamin B1 is nontoxic even in very high amounts.

People with sarcoidosis, hyperparathyroidism, or with chronic kidney disease should not supplement calcium. For other adults, 1,500 mg per day is considered quite safe.

Herbs That May Be Helpful

Tonic herbs, which nourish and tone the system, can be taken safely every day during pregnancy. Examples of these tonic herbs include **dandelion** (page 251) leaf and root, **red raspberry** (page 302) leaf, and **nettle** (page 293). Dandelion leaf and root are a rich source of vitamins and minerals, including **vitamin A** (page 209), calcium, **potassium** (page 197), and **iron** (page 173). Dandelion leaf is mildly diuretic and stimulating to bile flow and helps with the common digestive complaints of pregnancy. Dandelion root tones the liver.[13]

Red raspberry leaf is the most-often mentioned traditional herbal tonic for general support of pregnancy and breast-feeding. Rich in vitamins and minerals (especially iron), it tones the uterus, increases milk flow, and restores the system after childbirth.[14]

Nettle leaf provides the minerals calcium and iron, is mildly diuretic, and aids in elimination of excess water from tissues. Nettle enriches and increases the flow of breast milk and restores the mother's energy following childbirth.[15]

Are There Any Side Effects or Interactions?

Many herbs are considered safe during pregnancy, but there are also herbs that are potentially toxic during pregnancy. Some herbs may have the potential to cause birth defects, while others may cause health problems in the woman or the fetus or act as abortifacients (substances that induce abortion). All herbs should be reviewed with a reliable source before taking during pregnancy.

Dandelion leaf and root should be used with caution by persons with gallstones. In cases of stomach ulcer or gastritis, dandelion should be used cau-tiously, as it may cause overproduction of stomach acid. The milky latex in the stem and leaves of fresh dandelion may cause an allergic rash in some individuals. Raspberry may cause mild loosening of stools and nausea. Allergic reactions to nettle are rare; however, when contact is made with the skin, fresh nettles can cause a rash.

Checklist for Pregnancy Support

Nutritional Supplements	Herbs	Homeopathic Remedies
Folic acid, Vitamin B3, Calcium	Dandelion, Red raspberry, Nettle	Sepia 30c, Ipecac 6c, Phosphorus 6c, Ferrum phosphoricum 6c, Nux vomica 6c, Arnica 30c, Ignatia 30c, Pulsatilla 30c, Natrum muriaticum 30c

PREMENSTRUAL SYNDROME

MANY PREMENOPAUSAL women suffer from symptoms of premenstrual syndrome (PMS) at the end of a monthly cycle and are frequently relieved when the next menstrual cycle begins. Specific problems—cramping, bloating, mood changes, and breast tenderness—may vary from woman to woman. Women with breast tenderness should see the section on **fibrocystic breast disease** (page 51).

Dietary Changes That May Be Helpful

Women who eat more sugary foods appear to have an increased risk of PMS.[1] Alcohol can affect hormone metabolism, and alcoholic women are more likely to suffer PMS.[2] Tea consumption in China is strongly related to PMS.[3] The same is true for coffee and other caffeine-containing beverages in the U.S.[4] The more coffee women drink, the higher their risk.[5] Therefore, many nutritionally oriented doctors recommend that women with PMS avoid sugar, alcohol, and caffeine.

Several studies suggest that diets low in fat or high in **fiber** (page 159) may help to reduce symptoms.[6] Many nutritionally oriented doctors suggest diets very low in meat and dairy fat and high in fruit, vegetables, and whole grains.

Lifestyle Changes That May Be Helpful

Six months of jogging (averaging less than two miles per day) was reported to lower breast tenderness, fluid retention, depression, and stress in a group of women with PMS.[7] Nutritionally oriented doctors frequently recommend regular exercise as a way to reduce symptoms.

Nutrients That May Be Helpful

Vitamin B6 (page 214) can reduce effects of estrogen in animals, and excess estrogen may be responsible for PMS symptoms. A number of studies show that 200–400 mg of vitamin B6 per day for several months can relieve symptoms of PMS.[8 9 10 11 12] Although the amount of vitamin B6 is sometimes too low,[13] or the length of the trial too short,[14] some studies have not found vitamin B6 helpful.[15 16] Most nutritionally oriented doctors feel that vitamin B6 is worth a try and suggest 200–400 mg per day for at least three months. This amount can cause side effects. See the side effects section below.

Many years ago, research linked B vitamin deficiencies to PMS.[17 18] This work has only rarely been followed up, but some nutritionally oriented doctors still recommend the **B-complex vitamin** (page 210).[19]

Women with PMS show abnormalities in the processing of fatty acids.[20] In theory, these problems should resolve with **evening primrose oil** (page 158), or EPO. Of the double-blind trials, some report that EPO is quite helpful,[21 22 23 24] while others find it no better than placebo.[25 26] While the issue remains unresolved, many nutritionally oriented doctors consider EPO to be worth a try, suggesting 3–4 grams of EPO per day. EPO seems to work best when used over several cycles and may be more helpful in women with PMS who also experience breast tenderness or fibrocystic breast disease.[27]

Women with PMS are often deficient in **magnesium** (page 182).[28 29] Supplementing with magnesium may help reduce symptoms.[30 31] While the ideal amount of magnesium has yet to be determined, some doctors recommend 400 mg per day.[32]

Women who consume more **calcium** (page 144) from their diets are less likely to suffer severe PMS.[33] Double-blind research has shown that supplementing 1,000 mg of calcium per day relieves symptoms in women with PMS.[34 35]

Progesterone may relieve some symptoms of PMS, and **vitamin A** (page 209) appears to increase progesterone levels.[36] Very high doses of vitamin A—100,000 IU per day or more—have reduced symptoms of PMS,[37 38] but such an amount is dangerous. Women who are or who could become pregnant should not supplement with more than 10,000 IU (3,000 mcg) per day of vitamin A. Other people should not take 100,000 IU without the supervision of their nutritionally oriented doctor.

Although women with PMS do not appear to be **vitamin E** (page 220) deficient,[39] double-blind research shows that 300 IU of vitamin E per day may decrease symptoms of PMS.[40]

Some of the nutrients mentioned above appear together in **multiple vitamin/mineral** (page 187) supplements. One double-blind trial used multivitamin/mineral supplements containing vitamin B6 (600 mg per day), magnesium (500 mg per day), vitamin E (200 IU per day), vitamin A (25,000 IU per day), B-complex vitamins, plus other vitamins and minerals.[41] In the trial, all four groups of women with PMS benefited more from supplements than from placebo. These results have been independently confirmed.[42]

Are There Any Side Effects or Interactions?

Although side effects from vitamin B6 supplements are rare, at very high levels this vitamin can damage sensory nerves, leading to numbness in the hands and feet as well as difficulty walking. Vitamin B6 supplementation should be stopped if these symptoms develop.

Taking too much magnesium often leads to diarrhea. This can happen at doses as low as 350–500 mg per day. Excessive magnesium intake is more serious but is rarely caused by magnesium supplements. People with kidney disease should not take calcium or magnesium supplements without consulting a physician. Individuals with sarcoidosis, hyperparathyroidism, or with chronic kidney disease should not supplement with calcium.

Women who are or could become pregnant should take less than 10,000 IU per day of vitamin A to avoid the risk of birth defects. For other adults, intake above 25,000 IU per day can in rare cases cause headaches, dry skin, hair loss, fatigue, bone problems, and liver damage.

Herbs That May Be Helpful

Vitex (page 317) has been shown to help reestablish normal balance of estrogen and progesterone during a woman's menstrual cycle. This is important, because some women will suffer from PMS and other menstrual irregularities due to underproduction of the hormone progesterone during the second half of their cycle. Vitex stimulates the pituitary gland to produce more luteinizing hormone, and this leads to greater production of progesterone.[43] Studies have shown that using vitex once in the morning over a period of several months will help normalize hormone balance and alleviate the symptoms of PMS.[44]

Use 40 drops of a liquid, concentrated vitex extract or one capsule of the equivalent dried, powdered extract once per day in the morning with some liquid. Vitex should be taken for at least four cycles to determine efficacy.

In traditional Chinese medicine, **dong quai** (page 254), *Angelica sinensis,* is often referred to as the "female ginseng." Dong quai helps promote normal hormone balance and is particularly useful for women experiencing premenstrual cramping and pain.[45] Many women take 2–3 grams of dong quai capsules or tablets per day.

Are There Any Side Effects or Interactions?

Minor gastrointestinal upset and a mild skin rash with itching has been reported in less than 2% of the women monitored while taking vitex. Vitex is not recommended for use during pregnancy. It should not be taken together with hormone therapy.

Dong quai may cause some fair-skinned persons to become more sensitive to sunlight. Persons using it on a regular basis should limit prolonged exposure to the sun or other sources of ultraviolet radiation. Dong quai is not recommended for pregnant or lactating women.

Checklist for Premenstrual Syndrome

Nutritional Supplements	Herbs	Homeopathic Remedies
Fiber, Vitamin B6, Vitamin B-complex, Evening primrose oil, Magnesium, Calcium, Vitamin A, Vitamin E, Multiple vitamin/mineral	Vitex, Dong quai	Sepia 30c, Pulsatilla 30c, Cimicifuga 6c

PRITIKIN DIET PROGRAM

THE PRITIKIN DIET is a famous diet and philosophy of health developed by Nathan Pritikin.

In the minds of many people, the Pritikin Program is imagined to be a spartan, no-frills, uninteresting, and—worst of all—unpalatable diet. The Pritikin Program is also thought of as a "last resort" program that participants join because they have no other choices left.

It is true that for people living and eating the way most Westerners do, the Pritikin Program might seem to be the hardest thing they have ever done. But this is because most Westerners live and eat in a way that is far from natural.

The Diet

The Pritikin Program preceded and is remarkably similar to the Ornish program, developed by Dean Ornish, M.D., and is similar to any healthful diet—being low in refined carbohydrates (sugar) but high in unrefined carbohydrates, whole grains, vegetables, and fruits. These diets also exclude almost all processed grains, animal protein, eggs, and fat.

There are two reasons why Pritikin believed that the diet should be limited in the amounts of animal protein, fat, and refined carbohydrates it contains. First, these foods contain components that can be harmful, such as saturated fat. Second, eating these foods takes the place of more healthful foods.

For decades, doctors and researchers have warned that the diets common to Western countries are more likely to contribute to **atherosclerosis** (page 11), **diabetes** (page 39), and cancer compared to the diets of indigenous peoples. Native diets are naturally rich in complex or unrefined carbohydrates and typically lower in animal protein, fat, and sugar.

The Pritikin Program is not necessarily a **weight loss** (page 124) diet; however, most people involved in the program tend to lose weight (the average is 13 pounds during the first month). In addition, the Pritikin Program lowers **cholesterol** (page 62) and **triglyceride** (page 69) levels. For example, in the first month of the program, cholesterol levels often drop dramatically, such as from 235 to 175 mg/dl (from 6.1 to 4.5 mmol/liter). Similarly, triglyceride levels can drop from 174 to 130 mg/dl (2.0 to 1.5 mmol/liter).

The Pritikin Program is not a fad diet; it is a lifestyle modification program with the goal of reversing a lifetime of bad habits. The Pritikin Program is outlined in many books, including *The Pritikin Program for Diet & Exercise* and *The Pritikin Permanent Weight-Loss Manual*. Both of these books contain comprehensive explanations about the program for both the layman and professional. Both books also contain simple yet effective programs for daily exercise. The books also have the weight-loss program tiered for those who want to lose weight more or less rapidly. Finally, both books contain dozens of recipes that prove that the Pritikin Program does not always need to be dull, uninteresting, or unpalatable.

Numerous studies in the past few years have proven the safety and effectiveness of the Pritikin approach. Hundreds of other studies demonstrate the correlation between high-fat diets and degenerative disease, as well as the correlation between high-fiber diets and good health. Many colon problems have been treated with high-fiber diets, including **Crohn's disease** (page 34). In one study, thirty-two patients were fed a fiber-rich, unrefined carbohydrate diet for a period of four years. Another group of thirty-two did not eat the fiber-rich diet. The fiber-rich group spent only 20% as many days in the hospital and required surgery only 20% as often as the control group.[1]

The correlation between high cholesterol and the risk of heart disease is well documented. Also well documented is the use of high-fiber diets to lower cholesterol. Other sections in this book deal more extensively with the use of **fiber** (page 159) to help resolve specific health problems, including high cholesterol and diabetes.

PSORIASIS

PSORIASIS is a common disease that produces silvery, scaly plaques on the skin. A dermatologist should be consulted to confirm the diagnosis of psoriasis.

Dietary Changes That May Be Helpful

Alcohol appears to be a risk factor for psoriasis in men but not women.[1] [2] It would be prudent for men with psoriasis to drink moderately, if at all.

Anecdotal evidence suggests that people with psoriasis may improve on a hypoallergenic diet.[3]

One study reported that eliminating gluten (found in wheat, oats, rye, and barley) improved psoriasis for some people.[4] If other treatments are unsuccessful, a nutritionally oriented doctor can be consulted to investigate food allergies or a sensitivity to gluten.

Nutrients That May Be Helpful

Fish oil (page 160), which contains eicosapentaenoic acid (EPA), has been reported to improve psoriasis in double-blind research.[5] Typically, results require 1.8 grams of EPA per day taken for at least eight weeks. For many supplements, 10 grams of fish oil need to be taken in order to achieve the necessary 1.8 grams of EPA. Some researchers report that improvement of psoriasis symptoms takes two to three months to become evident.[6]

A higher amount—3.6 grams of EPA per day—was found to reduce psoriasis symptoms by 50% after five months of supplementation.[7] Limited research suggests that it may be possible to apply fish oil topically and still get significant results.[8] Some studies with oral fish oil do not report significant improvement,[9] although this apparent failure might result from using oils containing other essential fatty acids as a placebo.

Fish oil may serve another benefit. Some of the drugs used to treat psoriasis (etretinate and acetretin) raise blood levels of triglycerides, which might increase the risk of heart disease. Fish oil supplements help overcome this problem in people with psoriasis taking these medications.[10]

Activated **vitamin D** (page 219) is a prescription drug found in several forms. In one of these forms—1,25 dihydroxycholecalciferol—it is identical to the form of vitamin D produced by the liver and kidneys. Activated vitamin D is much more powerful than the nonprescription vitamin D. Several forms of activated vitamin D appear to be useful for people with psoriasis.[11] Topical application has worked well in some,[12] [13] [14] [15] but not all, studies.[16] [17] Activated vitamin D may work by helping skin cells replicate normally. It makes sense to discuss the use of activated vitamin D with a dermatologist, preferably in topical form. Oral activated vitamin D is considerably more toxic than the form of vitamin D available without prescription. Nonprescription vitamin D is unlikely to help treat psoriasis.

Fumaric acid is occasionally available in supplement form. In what chemists call an "esterified" form, fumaric acid has been used successfully with psoriasis in some studies.[18] [19] People interested in this treatment should talk with a dermatologist.

Are There Any Side Effects or Interactions?

A nutritionally oriented doctor should be consulted before long-term use of more than 3–4 grams of fish oil daily, since a high intake has been reported to elevate blood sugar levels. Side effects from EPA and DHA include nose bleeds (because of reduced blood clotting), gastrointestinal upset, and "fishy" burps.

Patients with sarcoidosis or hyperparathyroidism should not take vitamin D without consulting a physician. People taking cod liver oil can take too much, particularly if they also add vitamin D supplements. For most people, there is little reason to take more than 400 IU per day—a very safe adult dose. Too much vitamin D—significantly more than 1,000 IU per day for long periods of time—can ultimately lead to headaches, weight loss, kidney stones, and in rare cases deafness, blindness, and even death.

Herbs That May Be Helpful

Cayenne (page 246) contains a resinous and pungent substance known as capsaicin. This chemical relieves pain and itching by acting on sensory nerves. Capsaicin temporarily stimulates release of various neurotransmitters from these nerves, leading to their depletion. Creams containing 0.025–0.075% capsaicin are generally used. There may be a burning sensation for the first several times the cream is applied, but this should gradually decrease with each use. The hands must be carefully and thoroughly washed after use, or gloves should be worn, to prevent the cream from accidentally reaching the eyes, nose, or mouth and causing a burning sensation. Do not apply the cream to areas of broken skin. A tincture of cayenne can be used in the amount of 0.3–1 ml three times daily.

In traditional herbal texts, **burdock** (page 239) root is described as a blood purifier or alterative.[20] Burdock root was believed to clear the bloodstream of toxins. It was used both internally and externally for psoriasis. Traditional herbalists recommend 2–4 ml of burdock root tincture per day. For the dried root preparation in tablet or capsule form, the common amount to take is 1–2 grams three times per day. Many herbal preparations will combine burdock root with other alterative herbs, such as yellow dock, red clover, or cleavers.

"Sluggish" liver function can be a contributing factor in psoriasis, which is why **milk thistle** (page 290) seeds, which promote normal liver function, can be beneficial. Milk thistle can be taken in the amount of 420 mg of silymarin per day from capsules, tablets, or an herbal extract of milk thistle extract standardized to 70–80% silymarin content. According to research and clinical experience, improvement should be noted in about eight weeks. Once that occurs, intake is often reduced to 280 mg of silymarin per day. This lower amount may also be used for preventive purposes. For those who prefer, 12–15 grams of milk thistle seeds can be ground and eaten or made into a tea.

Psyllium (page 299) husk powder is sometimes used by psoriasis sufferers, since maintaining normal bowel health is important for managing psoriasis. Psyllium acts as a bulk-forming laxative to cleanse the bowel and encourage normal elimination. Many people take 7.5 grams of the seeds or 5 mg of the husks one to two times per day, with water or juice. It is important to maintain adequate fluid intake when using psyllium.

Sarsaparilla (page 305) may be beneficial as an anti-inflammatory. Capsules or tablets should provide at least 9 grams of the dried root per day, usually taken in divided doses. Tincture is used in the amount of 3 ml three times per day.

Bitter melon (page 235) inhibits the enzyme guanylate cyclase, which may benefit people with psoriasis.

Are There Any Side Effects or Interactions?

Besides causing a mild burning for the first few applications (or severe burning if accidentally placed in sensitive areas such as the eyes), there are no side effects from use of cayenne cream. As with anything applied to the skin, some people may have an allergic reaction to it, so the first application should be to a very small area of skin.

Use of burdock root is generally safe; however, burdock root in large quantities may stimulate the uterus and should be used with caution during pregnancy.

Milk thistle extract is virtually devoid of any side effects and may be used by a wide range of persons, including pregnant and lactating women. Since silymarin stimulates liver and gallbladder activity, it may have a mild, transient laxative effect in some individuals. This will usually cease within two to three days.

Using psyllium in recommended amounts is generally safe. People with chronic constipation should seek the advise of a health care professional. Side effects, such as allergic skin and respiratory reactions to psyllium dust, have largely been limited to people working in plants manufacturing psyllium products.

Sarsaparilla can cause nausea and kidney damage. Large doses for long periods of time are to be avoided. Since sarsaparilla can increase absorption and/or elimination of digitalis and bismuth, such combinations are contraindicated.[21]

Excessively high doses of bitter melon juice can cause abdominal pain and diarrhea. Small children or anyone with hypoglycemia should not take bitter melon, since this herb could theoretically trigger or worsen low blood sugar (hypoglycemia). Furthermore, diabetics taking hypoglycemic drugs (such as chlorpropamide, glyburide, or phenformin) or insulin should use bitter melon only under medical supervision, as it may potentiate the effectiveness of the drugs, leading to severe hypoglycemia.

Checklist for Psoriasis

Nutritional Supplements	Herbs	Homeopathic Remedies
Fish oil (EPA/DHA), Vitamin D, Fumaric acid	Cayenne, Burdock, Milk thistle, Psyllium, Sarsaparilla, Bitter melon	No homeopathy commonly used for this condition

RHEUMATOID ARTHRITIS

RHEUMATOID ARTHRITIS (RA) is a chronic inflammatory condition of the joints believed to be caused by autoimmunity (wherein the immune system attacks the body itself).

Dietary Changes That May Be Helpful

Fat can trigger autoimmune reactions.[1] People with RA may eat more fat, particularly animal fat.[2] Extremely low-fat diets have been reported to help people with RA,[3] and very low-fat, pure vegetarian diets have also proved helpful.[4][5] In one trial, fourteen weeks of a gluten-free (no wheat, rye, or barley) pure vegetarian diet, gradually changed to a lactovegetarian diet (permitting dairy), led to significant improvement in symptoms and objective laboratory measures of disease.[6]

In the 1950s through the 1970s, Max Warmbrand, a naturopathic doctor, used a very low-fat diet for those with both rheumatoid arthritis and osteoarthritis. He recommended a diet free of meat, dairy, chemicals, sugar, eggs, and processed foods.[7] Dr. Warmbrand claimed that his diet took at least six months to achieve noticeable results; a short-term (ten week) study with a similar approach failed.[8]

Solanine is a substance found in so-called nightshade plants: tomatoes, white potatoes, all peppers except black pepper, and eggplant. If not destroyed in the intestine, solanine can be toxic. A survey of people eliminating nightshade plants from their diets revealed that 28% had a "marked positive response" and another 44% had a "positive response."[9] Results often take six months, the elimination of tomatoes and peppers can be very difficult, and many people are simply not helped. Therefore, this diet is often reserved for severe cases of arthritis which do not respond to other natural treatments.

Rheumatoid arthritis may be linked to food allergies and sensitivities.[10] In many people, RA is made worse when they eat foods to which they are allergic or sensitive, and they are made better by avoiding these foods.[11][12][13][14] English researchers suggest that one-third of people with RA can control the disease completely through allergy elimination.[15] Finding and eliminating foods that trigger symptoms should be done with the help of a nutritionally oriented physician.

Lifestyle Changes That May Be Helpful

Although exercise may increase pain initially, gentle exercises help people with RA.[16] [17] Many doctors recommend swimming, stretching, or walking.

Nutrients That May Be Helpful

Rheumatoid arthritis causes inflamed joints, which in turn depletes the joints of **vitamin E** (page 220).[18] A double-blind report (using approximately 800 IU of vitamin E per day) found that vitamin E may relieve many symptoms of rheumatoid arthritis.[19]

Research suggests that people with RA may be partially deficient in **pantothenic acid** (page 193), or vitamin B5.[20] Those with RA have less morning stiffness, disability, and pain when they take 2,000 mg of pantothenic acid per day.[21] Many nutritionally oriented doctors suggest vitamin B5 (sometimes in lower amounts such as 1,000 mg) to people with RA.

Zinc (page 224) metabolism is altered in RA. Some studies have found zinc helpful,[22] although most have not.[23] [24] It has been suggested that zinc might help only those who are deficient.[25] Although there is no universally accepted test for zinc deficiency, some doctors check white blood cell zinc RA levels.

The relationship of **copper** (page 151) to RA is complex. Copper acts as an anti-inflammatory, because it is needed to activate superoxide dismutase, an enzyme that protects joints from inflammation. People with RA tend toward copper deficiency.[26] The *Journal of the American Medical Association* quoted one researcher as saying that while "regular aspirin had 6% the anti-inflammatory activity of [cortisone] . . . copper [added to aspirin] had 130% the activity."[27]

Several copper compounds have been used successfully with RA,[28] and a single-blind trial using "copper bracelets" reported surprisingly effective results.[29] However, under certain circumstances, copper might actually increase inflammation in rheumatoid joints.[30] Moreover, the most consis-

tently effective form of copper, copper aspirinate (a combination of copper and aspirin), is not readily available. A reasonable amount of copper might be 1–3 mg per day.

Many double-blind trials have shown that omega-3 fatty acids in **fish oil** (page 160), called EPA and DHA, help relieve symptoms of RA.[31] [32] [33] [34] [35] [36] The effect results from the anti-inflammatory activity of fish oil.[37] Many doctors recommend 3 grams per day of EPA and DHA. This amount is commonly found in 10 grams of fish oil. Positive results can take three months to become evident.

Evening primrose oil (page 158), or EPO, may help in RA because it partially converts to prostaglandin E1, which is known to have an anti-inflammatory effect. Double-blind research has reported significant improvement in morning stiffness using 6 grams of EPO per day.[38] Borage oil and black currant seed oil are thought to have similar benefits.[39] [40] However, some trials have not found EPO helpful.[41] Double-blind research has shown that fish oil and EPO can be successfully combined to help people with RA.[42]

Preliminary research suggests that **boron** (page 142) supplementation at 3–9 mg per day may be beneficial, particularly in juvenile RA.[43] However, more research on this is needed.

The DL-form of **phenylalanine** (page 194), or DLPA, has been used to treat chronic pain, including rheumatoid arthritis, with mixed effectiveness.[44] Some doctors of natural medicine suggest that individuals with arthritis may benefit from **cartilage** (page 147); however, well-designed research is lacking, and many experts question the use of cartilage in this regard.

Many individuals with rheumatoid arthritis have low levels of **histidine** (page 167); taking histidine supplements improves arthritis symptoms in some of these individuals.

Are There Any Side Effects or Interactions?

Very large amounts of pantothenic acid (several grams per day) can cause diarrhea.

Zinc intake in excess of 300 mg per day may impair immune function. People with Wilson's disease should never take copper. The level at which copper causes problems is unclear, but in combination with zinc, up to 3 mg per day is considered quite safe. Side effects from EPA and DHA in fish oil include nose bleeds (because of reduced blood clotting), gastrointestinal upset, and "fishy" burps.

Amounts of boron found in supplements have not been linked with toxicity. However, one study found that 3 mg per day resulted in small increases of estrogen levels. This is a concern, since estrogen may increase the risk of several cancers. Until more is known, supplemental boron intake should be limited to 1 mg per day.

The maximum amount of D-phenylalanine that is safe is unknown, but nerve damage has not been reported with 1,500 mg per day or less of D-phenylalanine. D-phenylalanine has occasionally caused mild side effects, such as nausea, heartburn, or transient headaches in smaller amounts.

There are no side effects reported with the use of histidine.

Herbs That May Be Helpful

Boswellia (page 238), a traditional herbal remedy from the Indian system of Ayurvedic medicine, has been investigated for its effects on arthritis. A study using boswellia found a beneficial effect on pain, stiffness, and improved joint function.[45] Boswellia is safe and showed no negative effects in the study. The herb has a unique anti-inflammatory action, much like the conventional nonsteroidal anti-inflammatory drugs (NSAIDs) used by many for inflammatory conditions. But unlike NSAIDs, long-term use of boswellia does not lead to irritation or ulceration of the stomach. Many people take 400–800 mg of gum resin extract in capsules or tablets three times per day.

Turmeric (page 314) is a yellow spice that is often used to make brightly colored curry dishes. The active principle is curcumin, a potent anti-inflammatory, which protects the body against the ravages of **free radicals** (page 8).[46] Many people take 400 mg of curcumin in capsules or tablets three times per day.

Ginger (page 267) has been used in Ayurvedic medicine as an anti-inflammatory.

A cream made from small amounts of hot **cayenne** (page 246) peppers, when rubbed onto arthritic joints, can help relieve pain.[47] It does this by depleting the nerves of certain neurotransmitters.

Although this may initially cause a burning feeling, it will lessen with each application and soon disappear for most people. A topically applied cream containing 0.025–0.075% of capsaicin (the active agent) is applied to the affected joints three to five times a day. A tincture of cayenne can be used in the amount of 0.3–1 ml three times daily.

Yucca (page 324), a popular traditional remedy, is a desert plant that contains soap-like components known as saponins. Yucca tea (7 or 8 grams of the root boiled in a pint of water for fifteen minutes) is often drunk for symptom relief three to five times per day.

Burdock (page 239) root has been used historically both internally and externally to treat painful joints. **Devil's claw** (page 253) has anti-inflammatory and analgesic actions. However, it is important to note that recent studies do not support devil's claw as a treatment for arthritis. The silicon content of **horsetail** (page 281) is said to exert a connective tissue strengthening and antiarthritic action.

Sarsaparilla (page 305) has anti-inflammatory properties, which may be helpful for rheumatoid arthritis. **White willow** (page 318) has anti-inflammatory and pain-relieving effects. Although the analgesic actions of willow are typically slow-acting, they last longer than standard aspirin products.

Are There Any Side Effects or Interactions?

Boswellia is generally safe when used as directed; rare side effects can include diarrhea, skin rash, and nausea. Persons with symptoms from gallstones should avoid turmeric.

There may be a short-lived burning sensation following initial application of cayenne cream. The hands should be washed after applying the cream, to avoid getting any in the eyes or mouth, where it can cause burning. Yucca tea can cause loose stools in some people; if it does, simply reduce the amount.

Use of burdock root is generally safe; however, burdock root in large quantities may stimulate the uterus and should be used with caution during pregnancy. Since devil's claw promotes stomach acid, anyone with gastric or duodenal ulcers should not use the herb.

Horsetail is generally considered safe for nonpregnant adults. The only concern would be that the correct species of horsetail is used; *Equisetum palustre* is another species of horsetail that contains toxic alkaloids and is a well-known livestock poison.

Sarsaparilla can cause nausea and kidney damage. Large doses for long periods of time are to be avoided. Since sarsaparilla can increase absorption and/or elimination of digitalis and bismuth, such combinations are contraindicated.

Long-term use of white willow may possibly cause gastrointestinal irritation. As is the case with aspirin, willow should not be used to lower fevers in children. People who are allergic to aspirin should avoid white willow.

Any inflammatory joint condition should be closely monitored by a nutritionally oriented physician.

Checklist for Rheumatoid Arthritis

Nutritional Supplements	Herbs	Homeopathic Remedies
Vitamin E, Pantothenic acid (vitamin B5), Zinc, Copper, Fish oil (EPA/DHA), Evening primrose oil, Boron, DL-phenylalanine (DLPA), Cartilage, Histidine	Boswellia, Turmeric, Ginger, Cayenne, Yucca, Burdock, Devil's claw, Horsetail, Sarsaparilla, White willow	Rhus toxicodendron 30c, Bryonia 6c, Ruta graveolens 6c, Pulsatilla 30c, Arnica gel

RICKETS

CHILDREN WITH RICKETS have abnormal bone formation resulting from inadequate **calcium** (page 144) in bones. This lack of calcium can result from inadequate exposure to sunshine (needed to make vitamin D) or from not eating enough **vitamin D** (page 219)—a nutrient needed for calcium absorption. Rickets is worsened by a lack of dietary calcium.

Rickets can also be caused by conditions that impair absorption of vitamin D and/or calcium, even when these nutrients are consumed in appropriate amounts. Activation of vitamin D in the body requires normal liver and kidney function. Damage to either organ can cause rickets. Some variations of rickets do not respond well to supplementation with vitamin D and calcium. Proper diagnosis must be made by a health care professional.

Dietary Changes That May Be Helpful

Dietary changes should only be considered if a medical professional has diagnosed rickets and determined that the cause is a simple nutritional deficiency. Rickets caused by a simple deficiency is more likely in a child who follows a pure vegetarian diet that does not include vitamin D and who has dark skin and/or lack of sunlight exposure (which reduces the amount of vitamin D made in the skin).

The few foods that contain vitamin D include egg yolks, butter, vitamin D-fortified milk, fish liver oil, breast milk, and infant formula. In addition to breast milk and formula, calcium is found in dairy products, sardines, canned salmon, green leafy vegetables, and tofu. Pure vegetarians may use supplements instead of eggs and dairy as sources for both calcium and vitamin D.

Lifestyle Changes That May Be Helpful

Sun exposure, required by the body to make vitamin D, must involve at least some direct exposure to skin (hands, face, arms, etc.). The ultraviolet light that triggers vitamin D formation is blocked by clothing. Depending on latitude, sunlight during the winter may not provide enough ultraviolet light to help the body make vitamin D. At other times during the year, even 30 minutes of exposure per day will usually lead to large increases in the amount of vitamin D made. If it is difficult to get sunlight exposure, full-spectrum lighting can be used to stimulate vitamin D production.

Nutrients That May Be Helpful

Vitamin D and calcium supplements should be used to treat rickets only if a medical professional has diagnosed rickets and has also determined that the cause is a nutritional deficiency. Amounts needed to treat rickets should be determined by a nutritionally oriented doctor, depending on the age, weight, and condition of the child. For prevention of rickets, 400 IU of vitamin D per day is considered reasonable. Doctors often suggest 1,600 IU for treating rickets caused by a lack of dietary vitamin D.

The National Institutes of Health in the United States has recommended that useful amounts of total calcium intake per day to prevent rickets are the following:

- 400 mg until six months of age
- 600 mg from six to twelve months
- 800 mg from one year through age five
- 800–1,200 mg from age six until age ten

Are There Any Side Effects or Interactions?

Individuals with sarcoidosis, hyperparathyroidism, or with chronic kidney disease should not supplement with calcium. In addition, individuals with a history of kidney stones should use calcium supplements cautiously. For other adults, 1,200–1,500 mg per day of calcium is safe.

Patients with sarcoidosis or hyperparathyroidism should not take vitamin D without consulting a physician. For most people, there is little reason to take more than 400 IU per day—a very safe adult dose. Excessive vitamin D intake—significantly more than 1,000 IU per day for long periods of time—can ultimately lead to headaches, weight loss, and kidney stones; and in rare cases deafness, blindness, and death.

Checklist for Rickets

Nutritional Supplements	Herbs	Homeopathic Remedies
Calcium, Vitamin D	No herbs commonly used for this condition	No homeopathy commonly used for this condition

URINARY TRACT INFECTION

**URINARY TRACT INFEC-
TIONS** (UTIs) are infections of the
kidney, bladder, and urethra. They
are generally triggered by bacteria
and are more common with any partial blockage of the urinary tract. In
some people, UTIs tend to recur.

Dietary Changes That May Be Helpful

Drinking **cranberry** (page 249) juice can be helpful in
the prevention of urinary tract infections.[1] Cranberry inhibits *E. coli* (the bacteria that causes most
urinary tract infections) from attaching to the walls
of the bladder.[2] However, cranberry is not a substitute for antibiotics in the treatment of acute urinary
tract infections.

Many people have trouble tolerating the large
amounts of unsweetened cranberry juice (50 ml or
more per day) needed to treat UTIs. Concentrated
cranberry extracts in capsules are now available.
Many people take 400 mg of these supplements
twice per day.

Sugar impairs the ability of white blood cells to
destroy bacteria.[3] Alcohol also suppresses the immune system,[4] while reducing dietary fat stimulates
immunity.[5] For these reasons, many doctors recommend a reduced intake of sugar, alcohol, and fat
during times of infection.

People who have recurrent or chronic infections
should discuss with a nutritionally oriented doctor
the possible role of allergies. Chronic infections have
been linked to allergies in many reports.[6][7][8][9] Identifying and eliminating the foods that trigger problems may help reduce the number of infections.

Nutrients That May Be Helpful

Vitamin C (page 217) stimulates the immune system
by helping to fight viruses[10] and increasing interferon.[11] Vitamin C can be particularly helpful for infections affecting the urinary tract. A high intake of
vitamin C tends to increase the acidity of the urine;
acidic urine is not well tolerated by the bacteria responsible for UTIs.[12] Consequently, some doctors of
natural medicine suggest that people with UTIs take
at least 5,000 mg of vitamin C per day. Lower
amounts are unlikely to significantly acidify urine.

Vitamin A (page 209) deficiency increases the risk of many infections. Although much of the promising research with vitamin A supplements and infections has focused on measles,[13] vitamin A is also thought to be helpful in other infections. Some doctors of natural medicine recommend that people with urinary tract infections take vitamin A.

Proteolytic enzymes (page 156), primarily bromelain, may alleviate symptoms of UTI.[14] One double-blind study reported that reduction of symptoms was excellent in 22% and good in 78% of the subjects—meaning that every patient had at least good results after taking this nutrient.

Since the immune system requires many nutrients to function properly, many people take a multiple vitamin/mineral (page 187) supplement to ensure that the immune system has the building blocks it needs. Research shows that healthy elderly people using such supplements for one year strengthen their immune systems and have an overall drop in the number of infections.[15]

Are There Any Side Effects or Interactions?

Some individuals develop diarrhea after as little as a few thousand milligrams of vitamin C per day. If large amounts of vitamin C (greater than 1,000 mg) are taken for more than a few weeks, copper (page 151) should also be supplemented, in order to prevent copper deficiency. Women who are, or could become, pregnant should not supplement with more than 10,000 IU (3,500 mcg) per day of vitamin A. Other adults can safely take as much as 25,000 IU (7,500 mcg) per day of vitamin A.

Herbs That May Be Helpful

Goldenseal (page 270) is reputed to help treat many types of infections. It contains berberine, an alka-

loid that prevents UTIs by inhibiting bacteria from adhering to the wall of the urinary bladder.[16] Goldenseal and other plants containing berberine (such as Oregon grape) may help in the treatment of recurrent urinary tract infections.

Many people take 250–500 mg of standardized goldenseal root extracts in capsules or tablets containing 10% berberine three times per day. The goldenseal root capsules, tablets, or tinctures that are not standardized can be used in amounts of 3–4 grams each day. Goldenseal is not a substitute for antibiotic treatment during an acute urinary tract infection.

The active constituent in uva ursi (page 315) is arbutin. In the alkaline environment of the urine, arbutin is converted into another chemical, called hydroquinone, which in turn kills bacteria. It is widely accepted in Europe as treatment for UTIs.[17] Many people take 5 ml of tincture three times per day or 100–250 mg of arbutin in herbal extract capsules or tablets three times per day.

Juniper (page 282) increases urine volume. Some evidence suggests it may lower uric acid levels, which may account for why juniper helps cases of urinary tract infection.

Are There Any Side Effects or Interactions?

Goldenseal is not recommended for use in pregnant or lactating women. Long-term use of uva ursi is not recommended, and some people may experience mild nausea after taking it. Uva ursi should not be used by pregnant or lactating women.

Due to potential damage to the kidneys, juniper should never be taken for more than six weeks continuously. Anyone with serious kidney diseases or taking diuretic drugs should not take juniper. Pregnant women should avoid juniper, as it may cause uterine contractions.

Checklist for Urinary Tract Infection

Nutritional Supplements	Herbs	Homeopathic Remedies
Vitamin C, Vitamin A, Proteolytic enzymes, Multiple vitamin/mineral	Cranberry, Goldenseal, Oregon grape, Uva ursi, Juniper	Cantharis 30c, Sepia 30c, Belladonna 6c, Staphysagria 12c, Nux vomica 6c

VITILIGO

VITILIGO is a disorder of skin pigmentation characterized by progressively widening areas of depigmented (very white) skin. The phenomenon is associated with the local destruction of melanocytes, the cells that produce melanin pigment to darken the skin. It affects 1–4% of the world's population.[1]

Nutrients That May Be Helpful

A clinical report describes the use of vitamin supplements in the treatment of vitiligo.[2] **Folic acid** (page 163) and/or **vitamin B12** (page 216) and **vitamin C** (page 217) were abnormally low in most of the fifteen people studied. Supplementation with high levels of folic acid (1–10 mg per day), along with vitamin C (1 gram per day) and intramuscular vitamin B12 injections (1,000 mcg every two weeks), produced marked repigmentation in eight people, occurring gradually over a period of many months.

Supplementation with the amino acid **L-phenylalanine** (page 194) may have value when combined with ultraviolet (UVA) radiation therapy. Several clinical trials, including one double-blind clinical trial, indicate that L-phenylalanine at or lower than about 50 mg per kilogram body weight per day (about 3,500 mg per day for a 150-pound person) increases the effectiveness of UVA radiation in promoting repigmentation. L-phenylalanine alone also produced a more modest repigmentation in some people.[3] Another study of vitiligo in children reported that L-phenylalanine plus UVA was effective treatment in the majority of children.[4]

One early report describes the presence of achlorhydria (lack of stomach digestive acid) in the stomachs of vitiligo sufferers and the use of dilute hydrochloric acid (HCl), or **betaine hydrochloride** (page 139), with success in treatment. HCl was given with meals over prolonged periods; repigmentation took a year or more.[5]

Another early report describes the use of **PABA** (page 192), or para-aminobenzoic acid—a factor that is commonly associated with the vitamins of the **B-complex** (page 210) family. Persistent use of 100 mg of PABA three or four times per day along with an injectable form of PABA and a variety of hormones tailored to the individual patients resulted in repigmentation of areas affected by vitiligo in many cases.[6]

Are There Any Side Effects or Interactions?

Folic acid is remarkably safe; however, folic acid supplements can mask the symptoms of vitamin B12 deficiency, which could lead to permanent neurological damage. Although this problem is rare, folic acid and vitamin B12 should always be taken together. Vitamin B12 supplements are not associated with side effects. Some individuals develop diarrhea after as little as a few thousand milligrams of vitamin C per day. High levels of vitamin C can deplete the body of **copper** (page 151).

Ingestion of very large quantities of individual amino acids can cause nerve damage. The maximum amount of L-phenylalanine that is safe is unknown, but nerve damage has not been reported with 1,500 mg per day or less of L-phenylalanine, although lesser amounts are occasionally associated with mild side effects, such as nausea, heartburn, or transient headaches.

Large amounts of betaine hydrochloride (HCl) can burn the lining of the stomach. If a burning sensation is experienced, HCl should be immediately discontinued. The normal stomach produces about the same amount of HCl as is found in twenty 10-grain tablets or capsules. However, people should not take more than 10 grains (650 mg) of HCl without the recommendation of a nutritionally oriented physician. All people with gastrointestinal symptoms—particularly heartburn—should see a nutritionally oriented doctor before taking HCl.

No serious side effects have been reported with 300–400 mg of PABA per day. Larger amounts (such as 8 grams per day or more) can cause low blood sugar, rash, fever, and (on rare occasions) liver damage. A nutritionally oriented physician should be consulted if taking more than 400 mg of PABA per day.

Herbs That May Be Helpful

An extract from khella (*Ammi visnaga*) is so far the only herb found to be useful in vitiligo.[7] Khellin, the active constituent, appears to work like psoralen drugs—it stimulates repigmentation of the skin by increasing sensitivity of remaining pigment-containing cells (melanocytes) to sunlight. Studies have used 120–160 mg of khellin per day.

Another herb that may prove useful for vitiligo is **St. John's wort** (page 312).[8] As with khella, it increases the response of the skin to sunlight. No studies have confirmed the use of St. John's wort for this condition to date.

Are There Any Side Effects or Interactions?

Khellin must be used with caution, as it can cause side effects such as nausea and insomnia. St. John's wort makes the skin more light-sensitive. Persons with fair skin should avoid exposure to strong sunlight and other sources of ultraviolet light, such as tanning beds. It is also advisable to avoid foods like red wine, cheese, yeast, and pickled herring. St. John's wort should not be used at the same time as prescription antidepressants. St. John's wort should not be used during pregnancy or lactation.

Checklist for Vitiligo

Nutritional Supplements	Herbs	Homeopathic Remedies
Folic acid, Vitamin B12, Vitamin C, L-phenylalanine, Betaine hydrochloride, PABA, Vitamin B-complex	Khella, St. John's wort	No homeopathy commonly used for this condition

WEIGHT LOSS AND OBESITY

ABOUT ONE-THIRD of the U.S. population is overweight. Because excess body weight is implicated in many different diseases, including heart disease, **diabetes** (page 39), several cancers, and **gallstones** (page 55), it seems prudent to maintain a healthy body weight. Unfortunately, losing weight—and keeping it off—is very difficult for most people.

Dietary Changes That May Be Helpful

Societies that eat very little fat have virtually no obesity. Reducing fat in the diet is an important component of weight loss efforts. Foods with a high proportion of calories from fat, which should be eliminated or limited in the diet, include red meat, poultry skins and dark meat, fried food, butter, margarine, cheese, milk (except skim milk), junk food, and most processed food. Vegetable oils should also be restricted. So should nuts, seeds, and avocados (although these foods are healthy for people who have no weight problem). Instead, the diet should be based on fruits, vegetables, whole grains, and nonfat dairy (and low-fat fish for non-vegetarians).

Eating more **fiber** (page 159) can be an important component to weight maintenance. Fiber fills people up, so they eat less; some studies find that soluble fibers work best. While soluble fiber can be found in beans and fruit, it is also available as a supplement. Glucomannan[1] and **psyllium** (page 299) contain soluble fiber and have been reported to help weight loss efforts in some studies. Some researchers add 10 or more grams per day to the diet.

Watch Out for Yo-Yo Dieting

People who go on and off diets frequently complain that the number of calories that result in weight gain gets less and less with each weight fluctuation. There is now clear evidence that the body gets stingier in its use of calories after each diet.[2] This means it becomes easier to gain weight and harder to lose it the next time. Therefore, a person should not make changes until they are ready to stick with them. Otherwise, they are better off not dieting in the first place.

Lifestyle Changes That May Be Helpful

Although exercise alone may not result in significant weight loss, when combined with dietary approaches, it usually helps. It remains unclear whether exercise merely increases the burning of calories or whether the exerciser continues to burn more calories after the exercise is completed.[3]

Nutrients That May Be Helpful

When people diet, their caloric intake drops sharply. When this happens, it becomes increasingly difficult to eat the recommended amounts of many vitamins and minerals. Therefore, proponents of most weight-loss programs advocate taking a **multiple vitamin/mineral** (page 187) supplement.

The mineral **chromium** (page 150) plays an essential role in the metabolism of carbohydrates and fats as well as in the production of insulin. Chromium, in a form called chromium picolinate, has been studied for its potential role in altering body composition. Although preliminary research in animals[4] and humans[5][6] suggested that chromium picolinate increases fat loss and lean muscle tissue gain, follow-up research in people has not confirmed chromium picolinate to have a significant effect in altering body composition.[7]

(-)**Hydroxycitric acid (HCA)** (page 168), a fruit extract taken from the rind of the *Garcinia cambogia* fruit grown in Southeast Asia, has a chemical composition similar to citric acid (the primary acid in oranges and other citrus fruits). Preliminary research, based on laboratory experiments and animal research, suggests that HCA may be a useful weight-loss aid.[8][9] HCA has been demonstrated in the laboratory (but not yet in clinical trials with people) to reduce the conversion of carbohydrates into stored fat by inhibiting certain enzyme processes.[10][11] Animal research indicates that HCA suppresses appetite and induces weight loss.[12][13][14][15] One case report found that eating 1 gram of the fruit containing HCA before each meal resulted in the loss of 1 pound per day.[16] However, much more research in human populations is needed to determine the effectiveness of HCA as a weight loss aid.

An altered form of the sugar molecule, **pyruvate** (page 200) might aid weight loss efforts.[17] A clinical trial found that pyruvate supplements, compared to placebo, enhance weight loss and also result in a greater reduction of body fat in overweight adults consuming a low-fat diet.[18] Animal studies suggest that pyruvate leads to weight loss by increasing the resting metabolic rate.[19]

Spirulina (page 205), or blue-green algae, is a rich source of protein, vitamins, minerals, and essential fatty acids. One double-blind trial of sixteen overweight individuals reports that 2.8 grams of spirulina taken three times per day for a four-week period results in a small, but statistically significant weight loss.[20]

Are There Any Side Effects or Interactions?

Supplemental intake (typically 50–300 mcg per day) of chromium has not been linked consistently with any toxicity in humans. One study suggested that chromium could cause mutagenic damage,[21] based on very high doses of chromium in ovarian cells of hamsters.[22] This risk, however, has not been demonstrated in humans. The potential side effects of HCA are not known; more research is needed in this area.

There are no side effects reported with spirulina. However, since spirulina can accumulate heavy metals from contaminated water, consuming spirulina from such areas can increase the body's load of lead, mercury, and cadmium.[23] There are a few reports of allergic reactions to spirulina.

Herbs That May Be Helpful

The herb **guaraná** (page 273) contains guaranine (which is nearly identical to caffeine) and the closely related alkaloids theobromine and theophylline; these compounds may curb appetite and increase weight loss. Caffeine's effects (and hence those of guaranine) are well known and include stimulating the central nervous system, increasing metabolic rate, and producing a mild diuretic effect.[24] Many doctors of natural medicine do not advocate using caffeine or caffeine-like substances to reduce weight.

Ephedra (page 259), commonly known as ma huang, is a diuretic and central nervous system stimulant. Studies show that ephedra, particularly when combined with caffeine, promotes weight loss. However, many nutritionally oriented doctors discourage the use of ephedra as a weight loss aid because of the many side effects that can occur with its use, especially since many of the side effects are intensified when ephedra is combined with caffeine.[25][26]

Are There Any Side Effects or Interactions?

As with any caffeinated product, guaraná may cause insomnia, trembling, anxiety, palpitations, urinary frequency, and hyperactivity. Guaraná should be avoided during pregnancy and lactation. Long-term use may cause decreased fertility, cardiovascular disease, and several forms of cancer according to epidemiological studies of caffeine use.

Ephedra has a long history of safe use at the recommended amount. However, abuse of the drug—especially for weight loss—can lead to amphetamine-like side effects, including elevated blood pressure, muscle disturbances, insomnia, dry mouth, heart palpitations, nervousness, and even death due to heart failure.

Anyone with high blood pressure, heart conditions, diabetes, glaucoma, or thyroid disease and those taking MAO-inhibiting antidepressants should consult with a physician before using any type of product with ephedra. Ephedra-based products should be avoided during pregnancy and lactation and used with caution in children under the age of six years.

Checklist for Weight Loss and Obesity

Nutritional Supplements	Herbs	Homeopathic Remedies
Fiber, Multiple vitamin/mineral, Chromium, Hydroxycitric acid (HCA), Pyruvate, Spirulina	Psyllium, Guaraná, Ephedra	No homeopathy commonly used for this condition

WILSON'S DISEASE

WILSON'S DISEASE is a genetic disorder that results in excessive accumulation of **copper** (page 151) in many parts of the body. If left untreated, this condition can be fatal, but fortunately it is readily treatable.

Dietary Changes That May Be Helpful

Most foods contain at least some copper, so it is not possible to avoid the metal completely. Foods high in copper, such as organ meats and oysters, should be eliminated from the diet. Some foods are relatively high in copper but are quite nutritious (e.g., nuts and legumes)—these foods should be eaten in moderation by people with Wilson's disease. Grains contain significant amounts of copper but are important components of a healthful diet, and dietary restriction may be neither wise nor necessary, particularly if zinc is supplemented.

Nutrients That May Be Helpful

Zinc (page 224) is known for its ability to reduce copper absorption and has been used successfully in patients with Wilson's disease,[1] with some trials lasting up to seven years.[2] Researchers have called zinc a "remarkably effective and nontoxic therapy for Wilson's disease."[3]

Zinc has also been used to keep normal copper levels from rising in people with Wilson's disease who had been successfully treated with prescription drugs.[4] Zinc in the amount of 50 mg taken three times per day has been used for this type of maintenance therapy,[5] although some researchers use the same level successfully with people who have untreated Wilson's disease.[6]

Zinc is so effective in lessening the body's burden of copper that a copper deficiency was reported in someone with Wilson's disease who took too much (480 mg) zinc.[7] Nonetheless, zinc does not help everyone with Wilson's disease. Sometimes increased copper in the liver has been reported after zinc supplementation;[8] however, leading researchers believe this increase is temporary and not harmful.[9]

Are There Any Side Effects or Interactions?

Zinc intake in excess of 300 mg per day may impair immune function. Although the preliminary research is contradictory, patients with Alzheimer's disease should avoid zinc supplementation until further studies clarify the role of zinc in this disease.

Checklist for Wilson's Disease

Nutritional Supplements	Herbs	Homeopathic Remedies
Zinc	No herbs commonly used for this condition	No homeopathy commonly used for this condition

YEAST INFECTION

YEAST INFECTIONS are one of the most common reasons that women consult health care professionals. Yeast infections result from an overgrowth of a species of fungus called *Candida albicans*.

The hallmark symptom of vaginitis caused by a yeast infection is itching of the external and internal genitalia, which is often associated with a white discharge that can be thick, curdy, or like cottage cheese. Severe infections lead to inflammation of the tissue and subsequent redness, swelling, and even pinpoint bleeding.

Dietary Changes That May Be Helpful

A well-balanced diet low in fats, sugars, simple carbohydrates, and refined foods is important for preventing vaginal infections caused by candida. A high-sugar diet encourages the overgrowth of the candida organisms.[1] Women who have a yeast infection (or are predisposed to such infections) should limit their intake of refined sugar, fruits, fruit juices, refined carbohydrates, and alcohol.

Lifestyle Changes That May Be Helpful

Yeast infections are three times more common in women who wear nylon underwear or tights than those wearing cotton underwear.[2] Additional predisposing factors for candida infection include the use of antibiotics, oral contraceptives, and steroids.

Underlying health conditions that may predispose someone to candida overgrowth include **pregnancy** (page 107), **diabetes** (page 39) mellitus, and HIV infection. Allergies have been reported to cause recurrent yeast vaginitis. When the allergens are avoided and the allergies treated, often the chronic recurring yeast infections are resolved.[3] In most cases, sexual transmission between partners is not considered an issue in yeast infection. However, in extremely persistent cases, sexual transmission should be considered, with the partner being examined and treated.

Nutrients That May Be Helpful

Lactobacillus **acidophilus** (page 135) are friendly bacteria that are an integral part of normal vaginal flora. Lactobacilli help to maintain the vaginal ecosystem by preventing the overgrowth of unfriendly bacteria and candida. Lactobacilli produce lactic acid, which acts like a natural antibiotic and competes with other organisms for the utilization of glucose.

Lactobacillus acidophilus can be taken orally in the form of acidophilus yogurt,[4] oral capsules, powder, or intravaginally. Many women find relief using an acidophilus yogurt douche daily for a few days or several weeks, depending on the severity of the infection.[5] Three capsules of acidophilus or one-quarter teaspoon of the powder can be taken one to three times daily. Lactobacillus can also be taken preventively during antibiotic use to reduce the risk of candida vaginitis.[6][7]

Boric acid capsules inserted in the vagina have been used to treat yeast vaginitis with great success. In one study of 100 women with chronic yeast vaginitis who were not successfully treated with any over-the-counter or prescription antifungal medicines, 98% of the women successfully treated their infections with boric acid capsules inserted into the vagina twice per day for two to four weeks.[8]

Are There Any Side Effects or Interactions?

There are no known contraindications to the use of Lactobacillus acidophilus. Boric acid capsules should not be used intravaginally during pregnancy.

Herbs That May Be Helpful

Topical use of diluted **tea tree** (page 313) oil may be useful for some women with vaginal yeast infections. It can be used as a diluted douche or as part of a coconut oil–based suppository (with 2% tea tree oil).[9] For more serious or persistent infections of the cervix or vagina, however, a health care professional should be consulted. Concentrations of tea tree oil as strong as 40% may be used with caution as a vaginal douche.

Internal use of **garlic** (page 265) may inhibit the growth of yeast organisms and increase resistance to yeast infections. Garlic exerts antibacterial, antiviral, and antifungal/antiyeast activity.[10] Garlic inhibits the growth of *Candida albicans,* the organism most widely responsible for intestinal, vaginal, and oral yeast infections. Garlic also shows long-term benefit in the treatment of recurrent yeast infections. For women with no aversion to the odor, one whole clove of raw garlic can be chewed daily. Otherwise, odor-controlled, enteric-coated tablets standardized for allicin content can be taken in the amount of 900 mg per day (providing 5,000 mcg of allicin). It is preferable to divide this into two equal doses. A tincture of 2–4 ml may be taken three times daily. For health maintenance, one-half of the therapeutic dose is adequate.

Another herb recommended for yeast infections is **pau d'arco** (page 296). This South American herb's active constituents have powerful antiyeast actions.[11] However, they are also somewhat toxic, and the amounts needed to kill off yeast and other microorganisms are not available in most herbal supplements.

Support of the immune system is also important with recurrent yeast infections. While **echinacea** (page 255) is not a substitute for antimicrobial medications, it is an excellent supportive tool for persons with recurring infections. Its ability to stimulate a "sluggish" immune system makes it an excellent choice for women with recurrent vaginal yeast infections. One study showed a 43% drop in recurrence rate in yeast infections with women using echinacea.[12]

Are There Any Side Effects or Interactions?

Tea tree oil should not be applied to broken skin or to areas affected by rashes. The oil can cause a burning sensation if it gets into eyes, nose, mouth, or other tender areas. Some women have allergic reactions, including rashes and itching, when applying tea tree oil. For this reason, only a small amount should be applied when first using it. The oil should never be taken internally.

Most people enjoy garlic; however, some individuals who are sensitive to it may experience heartburn and flatulence. Because of garlic's anticlotting properties, persons taking anticoagulant drugs should check with their doctor before taking garlic. Those scheduled for surgery should inform their surgeon if they are taking garlic supplements. There are no known contraindications to the use of garlic during pregnancy and lactation.

High doses of lapachol, the active ingredient in pau d'arco, can cause uncontrolled bleeding, nausea, and vomiting.[13] Use of the whole bark is much safer than isolated lapachol; the whole bark has no known serious side effects. Pregnant or lactating women should avoid use of pau d'arco.

Echinacea is essentially nontoxic when taken orally. People should not take echinacea without consulting a physician if they have an autoimmune illness, such as lupus, or other progressive diseases, such as tuberculosis or multiple sclerosis. Those who are allergic to flowers of the daisy family should take echinacea with caution. There are no known contraindications to the use of echinacea during pregnancy or lactation.

Checklist for Yeast Infection

Nutritional Supplements	Herbs	Homeopathic Remedies
Acidophilus, Boric acid	Tea tree oil, Garlic, Pau d'arco, Echinacea	Pulsatilla 6c, Kali bichromicum 6c, Sulfur 6c

YELLOW NAIL SYNDROME

PEOPLE WITH yellow nail syndrome have thickened nails with yellow or greenish discoloration, often accompanied by stunted growth and swelling of the ankles and sometimes other parts of the body.

Nutrients That May Be Helpful

Vitamin E (page 220) has been used successfully with people who have yellow nail syndrome.[1] [2] [3] Although topical use of the vitamin is helpful,[4] taking vitamin E supplements is much easier and less messy. A typical amount is 800 IU per day, with results beginning to appear after several months.

Are There Any Side Effects or Interactions?

Vitamin E toxicity is very rare. Supplements are widely considered to be safe.

Checklist for Yellow Nail Syndrome

Nutritional Supplements	Herbs	Homeopathic Remedies
Vitamin E	No herbs commonly used for this condition	No homeopathy commonly used for this condition

NUTRITIONAL SUPPLEMENTS

According to nutrition experts, the average Western diet contains too much fat and too little **fiber** (page 159). The combination of low fiber and high refined carbohydrates and fat contributes to an increased risk of heart disease, cancer, and **diabetes** (page 39). Even conventional medical authorities believe that the average Western diet is not ideal, since it is linked to poor health. A good diet should consist of fresh fruits and vegetables, whole grains, legumes, nuts and seeds, and (for nonvegetarians) nonfat dairy products and fish.

People do not eat the same foods their great-grandparents ate, and these dietary changes might affect nutrient requirements. Some foods were not available in Europe or Asia until the discovery of the New World. Before 1492, there were no potatoes in Ireland, no tomatoes in Italy, and no eggplant or green peppers in England. All these foods are New World crops. Other foods, such as rice and **soy** (page 204), are also relatively new to Europeans.

Another recent phenomena is that modern foods are generally picked before they are ripe. Ripening increases the nutrient content of the food, so diets based on unripened foods may be lacking in some nutrients.

Many of today's foods are processed with extra ingredients compared to food in the past. An example is a loaf of bread, which 100 years ago was prepared with only wheat, water, butter, baker's yeast, and a sweetener to help the yeast rise. Today, a modern loaf of bread may contain more than 100 ingredients, including preservatives, coloring agents, insecticides, herbicides, fungicides, and chemical residues from various packaging and cleaning procedures. These multiple ingredients may complicate digestion and increase the risk of allergic reaction.

Certain additives to the food chain have increased the need for certain vitamins and minerals. An example of this is the hydrazine residues in foods resulting from the fungicides used by farmers. The fungicides, along with nutrients from the soil, are absorbed by plants. Hydrazine compounds compete with and increase the body's need for **vitamin B6** (page 214).[1]

Plants do not always need the same nutrients as people. For example, plants do not require **selenium** (page 203), **iodine** (page 171), or **chromium** (page 150) to thrive. But if people are deprived of selenium, they can develop certain heart muscle problems and have an increased risk of cancer; if deprived of iodine, people can develop goiters; and if deprived of chromium, they can develop blood sugar problems.

People today do not eat the same quantities of quality food their ancestors ate (and in general, do not do as much work). For example, if people require the amount of **beta-carotene** (page 209) available in two pounds of carotene-containing food but now only eat two single carrots, then they are getting less than optimal amounts of beta-carotene.

Why Take Nutritional Supplements?

Some health experts claim that vitamin or mineral supplements are unnecessary if one eats a balanced, healthful diet. Furthermore, the experts making this argument often state that people who take extra vitamins or minerals are, at best, wasting their money and, at worst, endangering their health.

The few cases of vitamin toxicity—involving a handful of people taking extremely high dosages—do exist, but they are extremely rare. In most cases, any side effects caused by nutritional supplements are alleviated when the dosage of the supplement in question is reduced or discontinued. Please read specific supplement sections in this book for more details.

Supplement labels indicate what percentage of the recommended amount for each nutrient is provided in the supplement. These recommended amounts for nutrients continue to be debated by scientists. An example is vitamin C. While small amounts (such as 60 mg per day) prevent scurvy, it may not be the optimal amount for the body's functions.

Finally, it is important to remember that supplements should be used as additions to an already healthful diet—not as antidotes to years of poor eating habits. If used properly, there is strong scientific evidence that supplements optimize health. This book has numerous examples of this evidence.

This question of optimal nutrient levels, as opposed to "adequate" levels, is at the center of the controversy regarding the necessity of nutritional supplements.

ACIDOPHILUS (PROBIOTICS) AND FRUCTO-OLIGOSACCHARIDES

BENEFICIAL BACTERIA, such as *Lactobacillus acidophilus* and *Bifidobacterium bifidum*, are called probiotics. Probiotic bacteria favorably alter the intestinal microflora balance, inhibit the growth of harmful bacteria, promote good digestion, boost immune function, and increase resistance to infection.[1][2] Individuals with flourishing intestinal colonies of beneficial bacteria are better equipped to fight the growth of disease-causing bacteria.[3][4]

Acidophilus and bifidobacteria maintain a healthy balance of intestinal flora by producing organic compounds—such as lactic acid, hydrogen peroxide, and acetic acid—that increase the acidity of the intestine and inhibit the reproduction of many harmful bacteria.[5][6] Probiotic bacteria also produce substances called bacteriocins, which act as natural antibiotics to kill undesirable microorganisms.[7]

Regular ingestion of probiotic bacteria may help prevent vaginal **yeast infection** (page 127).[8][9] A review of the research concluded that both topical and oral use of acidophilus can prevent yeast infection caused by candida overgrowth.[10]

Diarrhea (page 44) flushes intestinal microorganisms out of the gastrointestinal tract, leaving the body vulnerable to opportunistic infections. Replenishing the beneficial bacteria with probiotic supplements can help prevent new infections. The incidence of "traveler's diarrhea," caused by pathogenic bacteria in drinking water or undercooked foods, can be reduced by the preventive use of probiotics.[11]

Probiotics are also important in recolonizing the intestine during and after antibiotic use. Probiotic supplements replace the beneficial bacteria, preventing up to 50% of infections occurring after antibiotic use.[12]

Probiotics also promote healthy digestion. Enzymes secreted by probiotic bacteria aid digestion. Acidophilus is a source of **lactase** (page 175), the enzyme needed to digest milk, which is lacking in lactose-intolerant individuals.[13] Symptoms of **irritable bowel syndrome** (page 81) may be alleviated by increased acidophilus intake.[14]

Fructo-oligosaccharides (FOS) are naturally occurring carbohydrates that cannot be digested or absorbed by humans but support the growth of beneficial bacteria.[15]

Where Are They Found?

Beneficial bacteria present in fermented dairy foods, namely live culture yogurt, have been used as a folk remedy for hundreds if not thousands of years. Yogurt is the traditional source of beneficial bacteria; however, different brands of yogurt can vary greatly in their bacteria strain and potency. Some (particularly frozen) yogurts do not contain any live bacteria. Supplements in powder, liquid extract, capsule, or tablet form containing beneficial bacteria are a source of probiotics.

FOS occur naturally in many foods, such as bananas, barley, garlic, honey, onions, wheat, and tomatoes; however, nutritional supplements containing FOS provide a more concentrated source of these compounds.

In What Conditions Might Acidophilus (Probiotics) Be Supportive?

- Canker sores (mouth ulcers) (page 21)
- Diarrhea (page 44)
- Immune strengthening (page 72)
- Indigestion
- Irritable bowel syndrome (page 81)
- Lactose intolerance
- Yeast infection (page 127)

Who Is Likely to Be Deficient?

Several groups of people are more likely to have depleted colonies of friendly bacteria. These include people using antibiotics, eating a poor diet, or suffering from diarrhea.

How Much Should I Take?

The amount of probiotics necessary to replenish the intestine varies by the extent of microbial depletion and presence of harmful bacteria. In general, many people find 1–2 billion colony forming units (CFUs) per day of acidophilus to be beneficial for the healthy maintenance of intestinal microflora. FOS is generally taken in the amount of 8 grams per day.

Are There Any Side Effects?

There are no reported side effects with even large intakes of probiotic bacteria.

Are There Any Interactions with Other Nutrients?

Acidophilus and bifidobacteria may produce B vitamins, including niacin, folic acid, biotin, and vitamin B6.

ARGININE

THE AMINO ACID ARGI-
NINE has several roles in the body,
such as assisting in wound healing,
ensuring that cells divide properly,
helping remove ammonium from the
body, facilitating immune function,
and promoting the secretion of several hormones including glucagon,
insulin, and growth hormone. Arginine is also a precursor to nitric
oxide, which the body uses to keep
blood vessels dilated, allowing the
heart to receive adequate oxygen.

Where Is It Found?

Dairy, meat, poultry, and fish are good sources of
arginine. Nuts and chocolate also contain significant
amounts of this amino acid.

In What Conditions Might Arginine Be Supportive?

- **Congestive heart failure** (page 30)
- **Infertility (male)** (page 77)

Who Is Likely to Be Deficient?

Normally, the body makes enough arginine, even
when the diet is lacking. However, during times of
unusual stress (including infection, burns, and injury), the body may not be able to keep up with increased requirements.

How Much Should I Take?

Most people do not need to take extra arginine.
While many of those with serious infections, burns,
or other trauma should take arginine, appropriate
doses must be determined by a doctor. Of those who
supplement with arginine, most take a few grams
per day.

Are There Any Side Effects?

Arginine is remarkably free of side effects for the
vast majority of people who take it, although some
doctors are concerned that increases in growth
hormone triggered by arginine could overwork the
pancreas.

Individuals with kidney or liver disease should
consult their nutritionally oriented doctor before

Arginine

supplementing with arginine. Individuals with herpes (either cold sores or genital herpes) should not take arginine, because it can stimulate replication of the virus. Large amounts of arginine in animals can both promote[1] and interfere with cancer growth;[2] the meaning of this for humans remains unknown.

Are There Any Interactions with Other Nutrients?

Arginine works with **ornithine** (page 190) in the synthesis of growth hormone.

BCAAs (BRANCHED-CHAIN AMINO ACIDS)

BRANCHED-CHAIN AMINO ACIDS (BCAAs) include **leucine** (page 177), isoleucine, and valine. BCAAs are needed for the maintenance of muscle tissue; they also are needed during times of physical stress and intense exercise. Research shows that BCAA supplements help those with amyotrophic lateral sclerosis (Lou Gehrig's disease) maintain muscle strength.[1] In addition, individuals with liver disease (hepatic encephalopathy) benefit from intravenous administration of BCAAs.[2]

Where Are They Found?

Dairy and red meat contain the greatest amount of BCAAs, although they are present in all protein-containing foods. **Whey protein** (page 223) and egg protein supplements are other sources of BCAAs. BCAA supplements provide the single amino acids leucine, isoleucine, and valine.

In What Conditions Might BCAAs Be Supportive?

- **Athletic performance** (page 14)
- Postsurgery recovery

Who Is Likely to Be Deficient?

Periods of physical stress, such as intense weight lifting and long-distance running, can create a catabolic state in which muscle tissue is broken down. In these situations, supplemental BCAAs—particularly leucine and its derivatives ketoisocaproate (KIC) and hydroxymethylbutyrate (HMB)—can be beneficial in reducing protein breakdown. Nonetheless, BCAA supplementation has not resulted in meaningful changes in body composition,[3] nor does it improve exercise performance.[4][5][6] During recovery from surgery, BCAA supplements may reduce muscle loss and speed muscle gain. BCAAs may also be useful to anyone wanting to prevent muscle breakdown.

How Much Should I Take?

A diet including animal protein provides an adequate amount of BCAA for most people. Athletes involved in intense training often take 5 grams of leucine, 4 grams of valine, and 2 grams of isoleucine per day to prevent muscle loss and increase muscle gain.

Are There Any Side Effects?

Side effects have not been reported with the use of BCAAs. A high intake of BCAAs is simply converted into other amino acids or used as energy.

Are There Any Interactions with Other Nutrients?

It is prudent to take BCAAs along with whole proteins, such as lean meat or poultry, and **multiple vitamin/minerals** (page 187), especially the **B-complex** (page 210) vitamins.

BETAINE HYDROCHLORIDE (HYDROCHLORIC ACID)

THE DIGESTIVE PROCESS takes place as food passes through the mouth, stomach, small intestine, and large intestine. One of the most important parts of digestion occurs in the stomach, where gastric (stomach) acid helps break down proteins for further digestion in the small intestine.

A low level of gastric acid increases the likelihood and severity of certain bacterial and parasitic intestinal infections.

A normal stomach's level of gastric acid is sufficient to destroy bacteria.[1] In one study, most fasting patients who had normal gastric acid in the stomach had virtually no bacteria in the small intestine. In those with low hydrochloric acid levels, there was some bacterial colonization of the stomach.[2]

Where Is It Found?

Gastric acid is produced by the parietal cells of the stomach. The acidity is quite strong in a normal stomach. In fact, the stomach can be between 100,000 and almost 1,000,000 times more acidic than water.

In What Conditions Might Betaine Hydrochloride Be Supportive?

- Allergy
- Anemia
- **Asthma** (page 9)

- **Atherosclerosis** (page 11)
- **Diarrhea** (page 44)
- **Gallstones** (page 55)
- Indigestion
- **Rheumatoid arthritis** (page 115)
- Thyroid conditions
- Tic douloureaux
- **Vitiligo** (page 122)
- **Yeast infection** (page 127)

Who Is Likely to Be Deficient?

Some nutritionally oriented physicians have found that most of their adult patients suffering from chronic health problems, such as allergies,[3] asthma,[4] and gallstones,[5] do not produce adequate amounts of stomach acid.

How Much Should I Take?

Betaine hydrochloride (HCl) is the most common hydrochloric acid-containing supplement. It normally comes in tablets or capsules measured in grains or milligrams. Some nutritionally oriented doctors recommend taking one or more tablets or capsules, each 5–10 grains (325–650 mg), with a meal that contains protein.

Occasionally, betaine is recommended to reduce blood levels of a substance called homocysteine, which is associated with heart disease. This form of betaine is different from betaine HCl.

Are There Any Side Effects?

Large amounts of HCl can burn the lining of the stomach. If a burning sensation is experienced, HCl should be immediately discontinued. The normal stomach produces about the same amount of HCl as is found in twenty 10-grain tablets or capsules. However, people should not take more than 10 grains (650 mg) of HCl without the recommendation of a nutritionally oriented physician. All people with gastrointestinal symptoms—particularly heartburn—should see a nutritionally oriented doctor before taking HCl.

Are There Any Interactions with Other Nutrients?

HCl helps make some minerals and other nutrients more absorbable.[6] [7] [8] Aspirin-containing compounds and other anti-inflammatory medicines, such as cortisone, can cause the stomach to bleed. People taking such medicines should discontinue taking HCl.

BIOFLAVONOIDS

BIOFLAVONOIDS are a class of water-soluble plant pigments. While they are not considered essential, they do support health as anti-inflammatory, antihistaminic, and antiviral agents.

Bioflavonoids block the "sorbitol pathway" that is linked to many symptoms of diabetes. Bioflavonoids also protect blood vessels and reduce platelet aggregation (acting as natural blood thinners).

As antioxidants, some bioflavonoids, such as **quercetin** (page 201), protect LDL cholesterol from oxidative damage. Others, such as the anthocyanidins from **bilberry** (page 234), may help protect the lens of the eye from cataracts. Preliminary evidence suggests that some bioflavonoids, such as naringenin, may have anticancer activity.

Where Are They Found?

Bioflavonoids are found in a wide range of foods. For example, citrus flavonoids are found in citrus fruits, rutin in buckwheat, epigallocatechin gallate (EGCG) in **green tea** (page 272), anthocyanidins in bilberry, and naringenin in grapefruit. In addition, OPCs, or oligomeric **proanthocyanidins** (page 199), are found in grape seeds and skins, and quercetin is found in many foods, including onions, tea, and apples.

In What Conditions Might Bioflavonoids Be Supportive?

- **Atherosclerosis** (page 11) (quercetin, bilberry)
- Bruising (bilberry)
- **Cataracts** (page 24) (quercetin, bilberry)
- Circulation (bilberry)
- **Diabetes** (page 39) (quercetin, bilberry)
- **Gingivitis** (page 56)
- **Glaucoma** (page 58) (rutin)
- **Hay fever** (page 59) (quercetin, hesperidin, rutin)
- **High cholesterol** (page 62) (quercetin)
- Injury (sprains, strains)
- **Macular degeneration** (page 85) (bilberry)
- **Menopause** (page 87) (hesperidin)
- **Menorrhagia (heavy menstruation)** (page 89)
- **Night blindness** (page 95) (bilberry)
- **Peptic ulcer** (page 103) (quercetin)
- Retinopathy (bilberry)
- Varicose veins (bilberry)

Who Is Likely to Be Deficient?

Bioflavonoid deficiencies have not been reported.

How Much Should I Take?

Although bioflavonoid supplements are not required to prevent deficiencies in individuals eating a healthy diet, doctors of natural medicine often recommend 1,000 mg of citrus bioflavonoids or 400 mg of quercetin, each taken three times per day.

Are There Any Side Effects?

No consistent toxicity has been linked to the bioflavonoids. The exception is for a bioflavonoid called cianidanol, which is not found in supplements.

Are There Any Interactions with Other Nutrients?

The bioflavonoids help protect vitamin C; the citrus bioflavonoids, in particular, improve the absorption of vitamin C.[1][2]

BIOTIN

BIOTIN, a water-soluble B vitamin, acts as a coenzyme during the metabolism of protein, fats, and carbohydrates.

Where Is It Found?

Good dietary sources of biotin include organ meats, oatmeal, egg yolk, **soy** (page 204), mushrooms, bananas, peanuts, and nutritional yeast. Bacteria in the intestine produce significant amounts of biotin, which is probably available for absorption and use by the body.

In What Conditions Might Biotin Be Supportive?

- Brittle nails
- Cradle cap
- **Diabetes** (page 39)

Who Is Likely to Be Deficient?

A biotin deficiency is very rare, even in those consuming a diet low in this B vitamin. However, if someone eats large quantities of raw egg whites, a biotin deficiency can develop, because a protein in the raw egg white inhibits the absorption of biotin. Cooked eggs do not present this problem. Long-term antibiotic use can interfere with biotin production in the intestine and increase the risk of deficiency symptoms, such as dermatitis, **depression** (page 36), hair loss, anemia, and nausea. Long-term use of antiseizure medications may also lead to biotin deficiency.[1]

How Much Should I Take?

The ideal intake of biotin is unknown; however the amount of biotin found in most diets, combined with intestinal production, appears to be adequate for preventing deficiency symptoms. The safe and adequate range of intake for biotin is 30–100 mcg for adults. Larger amounts of biotin (8–16 mg per day) may be supportive for diabetics by lowering blood glucose levels and preventing diabetic neuropathy.[2][3] Biotin in the amount of 2.5 mg per day strengthened the fingernails of two-thirds of the individuals with brittle nails, according to one clinical trial.[4]

Are There Any Side Effects?

As a water-soluble vitamin, excess intake of biotin is excreted in the urine; no toxicity symptoms have been reported.

Are There Any Interactions with Other Nutrients?

Biotin works with the other B vitamins, such as **folic acid** (page 163), **pantothenic acid,** also known as vitamin B5 (page 193), and **vitamin B12** (page 216). Symptoms of pantothenic acid or **zinc** (page 224) deficiency are lessened with biotin.[5]

BORON

BORON appears to increase absorption of **calcium** (page 144), **magnesium** (page 182), and phosphorus as well as control urinary loss of these minerals. The ability to use energy and to think may also depend somewhat on boron, but details are poorly understood.

Where Is It Found?

Raisins, prunes, and almonds are excellent sources. Fruit (other than citrus) and vegetables also contain boron.

In What Conditions Might Boron Be Supportive?

- **Osteoarthritis** (page 97)
- **Osteoporosis** (page 100)
- **Rheumatoid arthritis** (page 115)

Who Is Likely to Be Deficient?

This is unknown, but people who eat little fruit and few vegetables are likely to consume less than optimal amounts of boron.

How Much Should I Take?

Experts have suggested 1 mg per day of boron.[1]

Are There Any Side Effects?

Amounts found in supplements have not been linked with toxicity. However, one study found that 3 mg per day resulted in an increase of estrogen levels.[2] This is a concern, because estrogen may increase the risk of several cancers. Until more is known, some doctors of natural medicine recommend that supplemental boron intake should be limited to a maximum of 1 mg per day.

Are There Any Interactions with Other Nutrients?

Boron appears to conserve the body's use of calcium, magnesium, and phosphorus.

BREWER'S YEAST

BREWER'S YEAST is the dried, pulverized cells of *Saccharomyces cerevisiae,* a type of fungus. It is a rich source of the B-complex vitamins, protein (providing all the essential amino acids), and minerals, particularly chromium. Brewer's yeast should not be confused with baker's yeast, nutritional yeast, or torula yeast, which are low in chromium.

Where Is It Found?

Brewer's yeast, which has a very bitter taste, is recovered after being used in the beer-brewing process. Brewer's yeast can also be grown specifically for harvest as a nutritional supplement. "Debittered" yeast is also available, though most yeast sold in health food stores not tasting bitter is not real brewer's yeast—particularly if found in bulk.

In What Conditions Might Brewer's Yeast Be Supportive?

- Diabetes (page 39)
- Diarrhea (page 44)
- High cholesterol (page 62)

Who Is Likely to Be Deficient?

Brewer's yeast is not an essential nutrient, but it can be used as a source of **B-complex** (page 210) vitamins and protein. It is by far the best source of **chromium** (page 150), both in terms of quantity and bioavailability.

How Much Should I Take?

Brewer's yeast is often taken as a powder or as tablets or capsules, three times per day. High-quality brewer's yeast powder or flakes contain as much as 60 mcg of chromium per tablespoon. When doctors recommend brewer's yeast, they will often suggest 1–2 tablespoons of this high-potency bulk product. Remember, if it is not bitter, it is not likely to be real brewer's yeast and therefore will not contain chromium.

Are There Any Side Effects?

Side effects have not been reported from the use of brewer's yeast. It is not related to the *Candida albicans* fungus, which causes **yeast infection** (page 127). Some individuals have an allergy to brewer's yeast. People with severely impaired immune systems should not supplement with live or unsterilized brewer's yeast, because in such cases the brewer's yeast itself might lead to infection.[1]

CALCIUM

CALCIUM is the most abundant mineral in the human body. Of the two to three pounds of calcium contained in the average body, 99% is located in the bones and teeth. Calcium is needed to form bones and teeth and is also required for blood clotting, transmission of signals in nerve cells, and muscle contraction. The importance of calcium for preventing osteoporosis is probably its most well-known role.

Where Is It Found?

Most dietary calcium comes from dairy. Other good sources include sardines, canned salmon, green leafy vegetables, and tofu.

In What Conditions Might Calcium Be Supportive?

- **Gingivitis (periodontal disease)** (page 56)
- **High cholesterol** (page 62)
- **Hypertension (high blood pressure)** (page 67)
- **Kidney stones** (page 83)
- **Migraine headaches** (page 91)
- **Osteoporosis** (page 100)
- **Pregnancy** (page 107)
- **Premenstrual syndrome** (page 109)
- **Rickets** (page 118)

Who Is Likely to Be Deficient?

Severe deficiency of both calcium and **vitamin D** (page 219) is called **rickets** (page 118) in children and osteomalacia in adults. Vegans (pure vegetarians), people with dark skin, those who live in northern climates, and people who stay indoors almost all the time are likely to be vitamin D deficient. Vegans often eat less calcium and vitamin D than others. Most people eat well below the recommended amount of calcium. This lack of dietary calcium is thought to contribute to the risk of osteoporosis, particularly in white and Asian women.

How Much Should I Take?

The National Academy of Sciences has established new guidelines for calcium, which are 25–50% higher than previous recommendations. For ages nineteen to fifty, calcium intake is recommended to be 1,000 mg daily; for adults over age fifty-one, the recommendation is 1,200 mg daily. The most common supplemental amount for adults is 800–1,000 mg per day.[1] General recommendations for higher intakes (1,200–1,500 mg) usually include the several hundred milligrams of calcium most people consume from their diets.

Which Form of Calcium Is Best?

Dietary supplements may contain one of several different forms of calcium. One difference between the various calcium compounds is the percentage of elemental calcium present. A greater percentage of elemental calcium means that fewer tablets will be needed to achieve the desired calcium intake. For instance, in the calcium carbonate form, calcium accounts for 40% of the compound, while the calcium citrate form provides 24% elemental calcium.

Absorption of supplemental calcium also differs among calcium forms. Research shows that calcium in the form of calcium citrate/malate (CCM) has increased absorption compared to the calcium carbonate form.[2] However, calcium carbonate is at least as bioavailable as the calcium found in milk.[3] Other studies indicate that calcium absorption from several different supplement forms, including carbonate, acetate, lactate, gluconate, and citrate forms, is not significantly different from one to another.[4][5] Although the best form of calcium continues to be debated by researchers, they generally agree that it is best to take calcium supplements as part of a meal.

Are There Any Side Effects?

People with sarcoidosis, hyperparathyroidism, or with chronic kidney disease should not supplement with calcium without consulting a nutritionally oriented physician. People who have had kidney stones should read the section on **kidney stones** (page 83) before considering supplementation. For other adults, the highest dose ever suggested by nutritionally oriented doctors (1,200–1,500 mg per day) is considered quite safe.

Are There Any Interactions with Other Nutrients?

Vitamin D is needed for calcium to be absorbed. Therefore, many nutritionally oriented doctors recommend that those supplementing with calcium also supplement with 400 IU of vitamin D per day.

Calcium competes for absorption with a number of other minerals. Therefore, when taking calcium for more than a few weeks, it makes sense to take a multimineral supplement.

CARNITINE (L-CARNITINE)

L-CARNITINE is made in the body from the amino acids **lysine** (page 181) and **methionine** (page 186). It is needed to release energy from fat. When individuals supplement with carnitine while engaging in an exercise regimen, research shows that they are less likely to experience muscle soreness.[1]

Where Is It Found?

Dairy and red meat contain the greatest amounts of carnitine. Therefore, people who have a limited intake of meat and dairy products tend to have lower carnitine intakes.

In What Conditions Might Carnitine Be Supportive?

- Angina pectoris
- **Athletic performance** (page 14)
- **Congestive heart failure** (page 30)
- **Diabetes** (page 39)
- **High cholesterol** (page 62)
- **Hypertriglyceridemia (high triglycerides)** (page 69)
- **Infertility (male)** (page 77)

Who Is Likely to Be Deficient?

Carnitine deficiencies are rare, even in strict vegetarians, because the body produces carnitine relatively easily.

Rare genetic diseases can cause a carnitine deficiency. Also, deficiencies are occasionally associated with other diseases, such as **diabetes** (page 39) and cirrhosis.[2][3] A carnitine deficiency can also result from oxygen deprivation, as can occur in some heart conditions. In Italy, carnitine is prescribed for heart failure, heart arrhythmias, angina pectoris, and lack of oxygen to the heart.[4]

How Much Should I Take?

Most people do not need carnitine supplements. For therapeutic use, typical amounts are 1–3 grams per day.

Are There Any Side Effects?

L-carnitine has not been consistently linked with any toxicity symptoms.

Are There Any Interactions with Other Nutrients?

The body needs lysine, methionine, **vitamin C** (page 217), **iron** (page 173), **niacin** (page 213), and **vitamin B6** (page 214) to produce carnitine.

CARTILAGE

CARTILAGE, derived from shark and bovine (cow) sources, is a type of connective tissue comprised of mucopolysaccharides, protein substances, calcium, sulfur, and collagen. Early research in the 1950s and 1960s, using chips of bovine cartilage inserted into wounds, demonstrated that cartilage enhances wound healing.[1][2] Since then, cartilage has been investigated for its potential role in regulating **immune function** (page 72) and stopping the growth of tumors.[3] The role of shark cartilage in inhibiting angiogenesis (the growth of new blood vessels) is hypothesized to be beneficial in halting the growth and spread of cancer;[4] however, this remains to be proven by research.

Where Is It Found?

Cartilage is derived from either sharks or cows.

In What Conditions Might Cartilage Be Supportive?

- **Osteoarthritis** (page 97)
- **Rheumatoid arthritis** (page 115)
- Wound healing

Who Is Likely to Be Deficient?

Since it is not an essential nutrient, cartilage is not associated with deficiency states. A few studies suggest that individuals with cancer may benefit from cartilage supplements;[5][6] however, well-designed research is lacking, and many experts question the use of cartilage in this regard. A similar situation is seen with the use of cartilage in individuals with arthritis.

How Much Should I Take?

Anyone who is interested in taking bovine or shark cartilage supplements should consult a nutritionally oriented doctor for advice.

Are There Any Side Effects?

Researchers have suggested that there might be some people who should not use cartilage supplement, including those with cardiovascular disease, women who want to be or are pregnant, nursing mothers, anyone having or having had surgery within thirty days, and athletes training intensely. None of these contraindications has been proven, however.

CHLOROPHYLL

CHLOROPHYLL, the substance responsible for the green color in plants, has been used to ameliorate bad breath as well as to reduce the odors of urine, feces, and infected wounds. Chlorophyll has anti-inflammatory, antioxidant, and wound-healing properties.[1,2]

Historically, chlorophyll was used for gastrointestinal problems, such as constipation, and to stimulate blood cell formation in anemia. Some evidence suggests that chlorophyll helps detoxify cancer-promoting substances, suggesting that chlorophyll may reduce the risk of cancer.[3,4]

Where Is It Found?

Good dietary sources of chlorophyll include dark green leafy vegetables, algae, **spirulina** (page 205), chlorella, wheat grass, and barley grass. Supplements of chlorophyll as powder, capsule, tablet, and drinks are also available.

In What Conditions Might Chlorophyll Be Supportive?

- **Constipation** (page 32)
- Detoxification
- Halitosis (bad breath)
- Wound healing

Who Is Likely to Be Deficient?

Individuals who do not eat plenty of green foods lack chlorophyll in their diets.

How Much Should I Take?

Optimal levels remain unknown. Chlorophyll in the amount of 100 mg two or three times per day is used by many people for deodorization.

Are There Any Side Effects?

No side effects have been reported with the use of chlorophyll.

CHONDROITIN SULFATE

CHONDROITIN SULFATE consists of repeating chains of molecules called mucopolysaccharides. Chondroitin sulfate is classified as a type of glycosaminoglycan; it is rich in sulfur and is related to glucosamine. Chondroitin sulfate is a major constituent of cartilage, providing structure, holding water and nutrients, and allowing other molecules to move through cartilage—an important property, as there is no blood supply to cartilage.

Chondroitin and similar compounds are present in the lining of blood vessels and the urinary bladder. They help prevent abnormal movement of blood, urine, or components across the barrier of the vessel or bladder wall. Part of chondroitin's role in blood vessels is to prevent excessive blood clotting. However, it is unclear whether supplements of chondroitin are able to favorably affect blood clotting. In addition, chondroitin sulfate may lower blood cholesterol levels.[1]

Older preliminary research showed that chondroitin sulfate may prevent atherosclerosis in animals and humans and may also prevent heart attacks in people who already have atherosclerosis.[2][3][4]

Animal studies indicate that chondroitin sulfate may promote healing of bone, which is consistent with the fact that the majority of glycosaminoglycans found in bone consist of chondroitin sulfate.[5] Chondroitin sulfate also appears to help restore joint function in people with osteoarthritis.[6]

Where Is It Found?

The only significant food source of chondroitin sulfate is animal cartilage.

In What Conditions Might Chondroitin Sulfate Be Supportive?

- Atherosclerosis (page 11)
- High cholesterol (page 62)
- Kidney stones (page 83)
- Osteoarthritis (page 97)

Who Is Likely to Be Deficient?

Because the body makes chondroitin, the possibility of a dietary deficiency remains uncertain. Nevertheless, chondroitin sulfate may be reduced in joint cartilage affected by osteoarthritis and possibly other forms of arthritis.

How Much Should I Take?

For atherosclerosis, researchers have used very high amounts, such as 5 grams twice per day with meals, lowering the amount to 500 mg three times per day after a few months. Before taking such high amounts, people should consult a nutritionally oriented doctor. For osteoarthritis, a typical level is 400 mg three times per day. The ability for chondroitin to be absorbed orally is still under question.

Are There Any Side Effects?

Nausea may occur at intakes greater than 10 grams per day. No other adverse effects have been reported.

Are There Any Interactions with Other Nutrients?

The hypothesis that **glucosamine sulfate** (page 165) and chondroitin sulfate work synergistically in the support of osteoarthritis remains unproven. The fact that they are structurally similar suggests that they may act in similar ways.

CHROMIUM

CHROMIUM is an essential trace mineral that helps the body maintain normal blood sugar levels. It may also play a role in maintaining healthy levels of HDL (the "good" cholesterol). Chromium, in a form called chromium picolinate, has been studied for its potential role in altering body composition. Although preliminary research in animals[1] and humans[2][3] suggested that chromium picolinate increases fat loss and lean muscle tissue gain, follow-up research in people has not confirmed chromium picolinate to have a significant effect in altering body composition.[4]

Where Is It Found?

The best source of chromium is true **brewer's yeast** (page 143). Nutritional or torula yeast do not contain significant amounts and are not substitutes. Chromium is also found in grains and cereals, although it is lacking when these foods are refined. Stainless steel scrapings from pots and pans provides much of the chromium in many people's diets. Some brands of beer contain significant amounts.

In What Conditions Might Chromium Be Supportive?

- **Athletic performance** (page 14)
- **Diabetes** (page 39)
- **High cholesterol** (page 62)
- **Weight loss and obesity** (page 124)

Who Is Likely to Be Deficient?

Most people eat less than the U.S. National Academy of Science's recommended range of 50–200 mcg per day. The high incidence of adult-onset diabetes suggests to many doctors of nutritional medicine that most people should be supplementing small amounts of chromium.

How Much Should I Take?

A daily intake of 200 mcg is recommended by many doctors of nutritional medicine.

Are There Any Side Effects?

In supplemental doses (typically 50–300 mcg per day), chromium has not been linked consistently with any toxicity in humans. However, one research group has voiced possible concerns about mutagenic damage[5] based on their work with very high doses of chromium in cells from the ovaries of hamsters.[6] This work has not been repeated in humans, and chromium has not been linked to cancer in humans.[7]

Are There Any Interactions with Other Nutrients?

Preliminary research has found that vitamin C increases the absorption of chromium.[8]

COPPER

COPPER is needed to absorb and use **iron** (page 173). It is also part of the antioxidant enzyme superoxide dismutase (SOD). Copper is needed to make adenosine triphosphate (ATP), the energy the body runs on. Synthesis of some hormones requires copper, as does collagen (the "glue" that holds muscle tissue together) and tyrosinase (the enzyme that puts pigment into the skin).

Where Is It Found?

The best source of copper is oysters. Nuts, dried legumes, cereals, potatoes, vegetables, and meat also contain copper.

In What Conditions Might Copper Be Supportive?

- **Osteoporosis** (page 100)
- **Rheumatoid arthritis** (page 115)

Who Is Likely to Be Deficient?

Copper deficiency is uncommon. It can occur in people who supplement with zinc without also increasing copper intake. **Zinc** (page 224) and, to a lesser extent, **vitamin C** (page 217) interfere with copper absorption. Copper deficiency can cause anemia, a drop in HDL cholesterol (the "good" cholesterol), and several other health problems.

How Much Should I Take?

Most people consume less than the recommended amount of this mineral. Nonetheless, supplementing with 1–3 mg per day is important only for people who take zinc supplements, including the zinc found in **multiple vitamin/mineral** (page 187) supplements.

Are There Any Side Effects?

People with Wilson's disease should never take copper. People drinking tap water from new copper pipes should consult their nutritionally oriented doctor before supplementing, since they might be getting enough (or even too much) copper from their water.

The level at which copper causes problems is unclear. But in combination with zinc, up to 3 mg per day is considered quite safe.

Are There Any Interactions with Other Nutrients?

Zinc interferes with copper absorption. People taking zinc supplements for more than a few weeks should also take copper (unless they have Wilson's disease). Vitamin C may reduce copper absorption. Copper improves absorption and use of iron.

COENZYME Q10

COENZYME Q10 is a powerful **antioxidant** (page 8) that protects the body from free radicals. Coenzyme Q10 is also called ubiquinone, a name that signifies its widespread (ubiquitous) distribution in the human body. As a coenzyme, this nutrient aids metabolic reactions, such as the complex process of transforming food into ATP, the energy the body runs on.

Virtually every cell of the human body contains coenzyme Q10. The mitochondria, the area of cells where energy is produced, contain the most coenzyme Q10. The heart and liver, because they contain the most mitochondria per cell, have the greatest amount of coenzyme Q10.

Where Is It Found?

Coenzyme Q10 is found in spinach, broccoli, nuts, meat, and fish.

In What Conditions Might Coenzyme Q10 Be Supportive?

- Angina pectoris
- **Chemotherapy support** (page 25)
- **Congestive heart failure** (page 30)
- **Diabetes** (page 39)
- **Gingivitis (periodontal disease)** (page 56)
- **Hypertension (high blood pressure)** (page 67)
- **Infertility (male)** (page 77)

Who Is Likely to Be Deficient?

Deficiency is poorly understood, but it may be caused by synthesis problems in the body rather than an insufficiency in the diet. Low blood levels have been reported in those with heart failure, cardiomyopathy (another heart condition), gingivitis (inflammation of the gums), and AIDS. Coenzyme Q10 levels are generally lower in older individuals. The test used to assess coenzyme Q10 status is not routinely available from medical laboratories.

How Much Should I Take?

Adult levels of supplementation are usually 30–90 mg per day, although individuals with specific health conditions (with the involvement of a nutritionally oriented physician) may supplement with higher levels. Taking coenzyme Q10 supplements with a little fat, such as olive oil or peanut butter, will improve absorption of this nutrient.

Are There Any Side Effects?

Congestive heart failure patients who are taking coenzyme Q10 should not discontinue taking coenzyme Q10 supplements without first consulting a doctor.

CREATINE (CREATINE MONOHYDRATE)

CREATINE assists in the production of energy and muscle-building processes. Most of the creatine in the body is stored in the muscles as creatine or in a form called phosphocreatine.[1] Creatine is a quickly available energy source for muscle contraction.[2] It also increases the synthesis of muscle protein and assists in the formation of polyamines (powerful growth promoters).[3] Creatine also promotes protein synthesis.

Where Is It Found?

Animal proteins are the main dietary source of creatine. Supplements in the form of creatine monohydrate are well absorbed and tolerated by the stomach.

In What Conditions Might Creatine Be Supportive?

- **Athletic performance** (page 14)
- Postsurgery recovery

Who Is Likely to Be Deficient?

Individuals involved in intense physical activity or experiencing physical stress, especially those limiting their intake of red meat, may have low muscle stores of creatine.

How Much Should I Take?

There are two variations for supplementing with creatine. In the loading method, 20–30 grams of creatine per day (in divided doses) are taken for three to four days.[4] Muscle creatine levels increase rapidly, which is beneficial if a short-term rise in force is needed, such as during a weight-lifting competition, football game, or sprinting.

In the other method, 3–5 grams of creatine monohydrate per day are taken over an extended training period. Muscle creatine levels rise more slowly. This method is useful for athletes undergoing long-term training, such as bodybuilders and weight lifters during precompetition phases. Endurance athletes may also benefit from the improved recovery provided by this method of taking creatine.

Small amounts of creatine (3–5 grams) are best taken within thirty minutes after training.

Are There Any Side Effects?

Little is known about creatine side effects, but no consistent toxicity has been reported to date.

Are There Any Interactions with Other Nutrients?

Creatine may enhance the effects of other muscle-enhancing nutrients, such as **whey protein** (page 223), **glutamine** (page 166), and amino acids.

CYSTEINE

CYSTEINE is a nonessential amino acid (protein building block). Cysteine is one of the few amino acids that contains sulfur. This allows cysteine to bond in a special way and maintain the structure of proteins in the body. Cysteine is a component of the antioxidant glutathione. The body also uses cysteine to produce **taurine** (page 206), another amino acid.

Cysteine is occasionally converted into glucose and used as a source of energy. Cysteine strengthens the protective lining of the stomach and intestines, which may help prevent damage caused by aspirin and similar drugs.[1] In addition, cysteine may play an important role in the communication between immune system cells.[2]

Cysteine is rarely used as a dietary supplement. It is more common to supplement with **N-acetyl cysteine** (page 189), or NAC, which contains cysteine.

Where Is It Found?

The body can synthesize cysteine from **methionine** (page 186) and other building blocks. Cysteine, the amino acid from which NAC is derived, is found in most high-protein foods.

In What Conditions Might Cysteine Be Supportive?

• Refer to **N-acetyl cysteine** (page 189)

Who Is Likely to Be Deficient?

According to several studies, blood levels of cysteine and glutathione are low in individuals infected with HIV.[3][4][5] Cysteine has a role in the proper function of the immune system, so a deficiency of this amino acid may either contribute to or result from immune suppression of HIV.

How Much Should I Take?

When cysteine is used by itself, 200 mg two to four times per day is a typical amount. Refer to the section on N-acetyl cysteine (NAC) for further information. Unlike NAC, cysteine does not have an unpleasant odor or taste.

Are There Any Side Effects?

No consistent adverse effects of NAC have been reported in humans. One small study found that daily amounts of 1.2 grams or more could lead to oxidative damage. Extremely large amounts of cysteine, the amino acid NAC is derived from, may be toxic to nerve cells in rats.

Are There Any Interactions with Other Nutrients?

Adequate amounts of **methionine** (page 186) are needed in the diet, as the precursor to cysteine, to prevent cysteine deficiency.

DEHYDROEPIANDROSTERONE (DHEA)

DEHYDROEPIANDRO-STERONE (DHEA) is the most prevalent of the hormones produced by the adrenal glands. After being secreted by the adrenal glands, it circulates in the bloodstream as DHEA-sulfate (DHEAS) and is converted as needed into other hormones. As much as half of the testosterone in men and about three-quarters of the estrogen in women (and close to 100% after menopause) is derived from DHEA.[1]

Where Is It Found?

DHEA is produced by the adrenal glands. A synthetic form of this hormone is also available as a nutritional supplement in tablet, capsule, liquid, and sublingual form. Some products claim to contain "natural" DHEA precursors from **wild yam** (page 320); however, the body cannot convert any compounds in the yam to DHEA or other steroid hormones (although a series of reactions in a laboratory can make the conversion).

In What Conditions Might Dehydroepiandrosterone (DHEA) Be Supportive?

- **Depression** (page 36)
- Lupus
- Premature aging

Who Is Likely to Be Deficient?

DHEA levels peak early in life and start a lifelong descent in early adulthood. By the age of sixty, DHEA levels are only 5–15% of what they were at their peak at younger ages.[2] It remains unclear whether the lower level associated with age represents a deficiency. Women with asthma have been reported to have depressed levels of DHEA.[3]

Researchers from the University of California, San Francisco, report that DHEA and DHEAS levels are lower in depressed patients, and DHEA supplements of 30–90 mg per day for four weeks significantly improved depression in six depressed patients.[4] However, nutritional experts maintain that DHEA may be effective for only a minority of people with depression.[5]

How Much Should I Take?

DHEA supplementation is a controversial issue. Some experts believe that 2–10 mg of DHEA, depending on age, gender, and family history of disease, is a beneficial amount to take of this hormone. Other experts, however, do not feel that DHEA or other hormones should be taken as nutritional supplements. It would be prudent to consult a nutritionally oriented doctor to have DHEA levels monitored before and during supplementation.

Are There Any Side Effects?

DHEA is a hormone, and as such there are serious concerns about its inappropriate use. Excessive levels of DHEA may be of particular concern to women. For example, in one study, a woman taking 100 mg of DHEA per day for one year started to develop facial hair, presumably as a consequence of DHEA contributing to male hormones and triggering male secondary sex characteristics.[6]

Other concerns have been expressed that DHEA may contribute to liver damage or even liver cancer. Until more is known about DHEA, it would be prudent for individuals with a family history of hormone-related cancer (such as breast or prostate cancer) to avoid supplementing with DHEA, because DHEA is a precursor to estrogen and testosterone. While younger women with breast cancer may have low levels of DHEA, postmenopausal women with breast cancer appear to have high levels of DHEA, which has researchers concerned.[7]

ENZYMES, PROTEOLYTIC

PROTEOLYTIC ENZYMES help digest dietary protein. According to one theory, allergies are triggered by partially undigested protein, and these enzymes reduce allergy symptoms.[1] There is some scientific evidence to support this theory.[2]

Proteolytic enzymes such as trypsin, chymotrypsin, and bromelain are partially absorbed by the body.[3 4 5] Once absorbed, they have anti-inflammatory activity and may even demonstrate an antitumor effect.[6 7 8 9] Proteolytic enzymes may also improve immune system function, for example, in people with shingles (herpes zoster).[10] Bromelain is a natural blood thinner because it prevents excessive blood platelet stickiness.[11]

Where Are They Found?

The plant-based proteolytic enzyme bromelain comes from pineapples; papain comes from unripe papayas. Only small amounts of the animal-based proteolytic enzymes trypsin and chymotrypsin are found in the diet; however, the pancreas can synthesize these enzymes. Pancreatic enzymes, or pancreatin, contain several proteolytic enzymes along with enzymes that help digest fat and carbohydrates.

In What Conditions Might Enzymes Be Supportive?

- Indigestion and heartburn
- Injury (sprains, strains)
- **Urinary tract infection** (page 120)
- Pancreatic insufficiency
- Cystic fibrosis

Who Is Likely to Be Deficient?

Proteolytic enzymes belong to a broad class of enzymes called pancreatic enzymes. Consequently, people with pancreatic insufficiency and cystic fibrosis frequently require supplemental pancreatic enzymes. In addition, those with celiac disease, Crohn's disease, and perhaps indigestion may be deficient in pancreatic enzymes.[12] Since bromelain and papain are not essential, deficiencies do not exist.

How Much Should I Take?

Proteolytic enzymes taken to aid digestion are generally accompanied by other enzymes (called amylases and lipases) that help digest carbohydrates and fat. Pancreatin, which contains all three enzymes, is rated against a standard established by the U.S. Pharmacopeia (USP). For example, 9X pancreatin is nine times stronger than the government standard. Each X contains 25 USP units of amylase, 2 USP units of lipase, and 25 USP units of protease (or proteolytic enzymes). A dose of 1.5 grams of 9X pancreatin (or a higher dose at lower potencies) with each meal is likely to help digest food in people with pancreatic insufficiency.

The right dose of bromelain is complicated. Bromelain is measured in MCUs (milk clotting units) or GDUs (gelatin dissolving units). One GDU equals 1.5 MCU. Strong products contain at least 2,000 MCU (1,333 GDU) per gram (1,000 mg). A supplement containing 500 mg labeled "2,000 MCU per gram" would have 1,000 MCU of activity. Some doctors of natural medicine recommend 3,000 MCU taken three times per day for several days, followed by 2,000 MCU three times per day.[13] Much of the research, however uses smaller amounts, such as 2,000 MCU in divided amounts in the course of a day (500 MCU taken four times per day).

Supplemental enzymes that only state product weight but not activity units may lack potency.

Are There Any Side Effects?

The most important pancreatic enzymes in malabsorption diseases are usually fat-digesting enzymes called lipases. Since proteolytic enzymes can digest lipases, it may be prudent for people with enzyme deficiencies to avoid proteolytic enzymes in order to spare lipases.[14]

In theory, too much enzyme activity could be irritating, because it could start to "digest" parts of the body as the enzymes travel through the digestive system. Fortunately, that does not happen with supplemental amounts, though it is not clear at what level such problems might arise.

Are There Any Interactions with Other Nutrients?

Proteolytic enzymes should not be taken with **betaine hydrochloride** (page 139), or hydrochloric acid, which would destroy the enzymes.

EVENING PRIMROSE OIL (AND OTHER SOURCES OF GAMMA LINOLENIC ACID)

EVENING PRIMROSE OIL (EPO), black currant seed oil, and borage oil contain gamma linolenic acid (GLA), a fatty acid that the body converts to a hormone-like substance called prostaglandin E1 (PGE1). PGE1 has anti-inflammatory properties and may also act as a blood thinner and blood vessel dilator.

Linoleic acid, a common fatty acid found in nuts, seeds, and most vegetable oils (including EPO), should theoretically convert to PGE1. But many things can interfere with this conversion, including disease, the aging process, saturated fat, hydrogenated oils, blood sugar problems, and inadequate vitamin C, magnesium, zinc, and B vitamins. Supplements that provide GLA circumvent these conversion problems, leading to more predictable formation of PGE1.[1]

Where Is It Found?

Evening primrose oil is found primarily in supplements. The active ingredient, GLA, can also be found in black current seed oil and borage oil supplements.

In What Conditions Might Evening Primrose Oil Be Supportive?

- **Atherosclerosis** (page 11)
- **Bursitis** (page 20)
- **Diabetes** (page 39)
- **Eczema** (page 49)
- **Fibrocystic breast disease** (page 51)
- **Irritable bowel syndrome** (page 81)
- **Premenstrual syndrome** (page 109)
- **Rheumatoid arthritis** (page 115)

Who Is Likely to Be Deficient?

Those with premenstrual syndrome,[2] diabetes,[3] and eczema[4] can have a metabolic block that interferes with the body's ability to make GLA. Many people in Western societies may be at least partially GLA deficient as a result of aging, glucose intolerance, dietary fat intake, and other problems. Individuals with deficiencies benefit from supplemental GLA intake from evening primrose oil, black currant seed oil, or borage oil.

How Much Should I Take?

Although many people may have inadequate levels of GLA, the optimal intake for this nutrient remains unknown. Researchers often use 3,000–6,000 mg of evening primrose oil per day, which provides approximately 270–360 mg of GLA.

Are There Any Side Effects?

Consistent, reproducible problems from taking evening primrose oil have not been reported.

Are There Any Interactions with Other Nutrients?

Other nutrients are needed by the body, along with evening primrose oil, to make PGE1. Consequently, some experts suggest that **magnesium** (page 182), **zinc** (page 224), **vitamin C** (page 217), **niacin** (page 213), and **vitamin B6** (page 214) should be taken along with EPO.

FIBER

THERE ARE SEVERAL kinds of fiber. Water-soluble fiber helps control blood sugar levels and cholesterol. Insoluble fiber softens stool, which helps move it through the body in less time. Lignan, a fiber-like substance, has mild anti-estrogenic activity.

Where Is It Found?

Fruits (not fruit juice) and beans are high in water-soluble fiber. Vegetables and whole grains are high in insoluble fiber. **Oats** (page 294), barley, and **psyllium** (page 299) contain both soluble and insoluble fiber. The best source of lignan, by far, is flaxseed—not flaxseed oil, regardless of packaging claims to the contrary.

In What Conditions Might Fiber Be Supportive?

- Constipation (page 32)
- Diabetes (page 39)
- Diarrhea (page 44)
- Hemorrhoids (page 60)
- High cholesterol (page 62)
- Hypertension (high blood pressure) (page 67)
- Hypertriglyceridemia (high triglycerides) (page 69)
- Irritable bowel syndrome (page 81)
- Kidney stones (page 83)
- Peptic ulcer (page 103)
- Premenstrual syndrome (page 109)
- Weight loss and obesity (page 124)

Who Is Likely to Be Deficient?

Most people are fiber deficient. Eating white flour, white rice, and fruit juice (as opposed to real fruit) all contribute to this problem. Many so-called whole wheat products contain mostly white flour. Read labels and avoid "flour" and "unbleached flour," both of which are simply white flour. Junk food is also fiber depleted. The diseases listed on the previous page (plus colon and breast cancers) are much more likely to occur with low-fiber diets.

How Much Should I Take?

Western diets generally provide approximately 10 grams of fiber per day. So-called primitive societies consume 40–60 grams per day. Increasing fiber intake similar to the "primitive" diets is desirable.

Are There Any Side Effects?

While individuals can be allergic to certain high-fiber foods (most commonly wheat), high-fiber diets are more likely to improve health than cause any health problems. Beans, a good source of soluble fiber, also contain special sugars that are often poorly digested, leading to gas.

Are There Any Interactions with Other Nutrients?

Fiber reduces the absorption of most minerals. To minimize this effect, multimineral supplements should not be taken with high-fiber meals.

FISH OIL

FISH OIL contains EPA (eicosapentaenoic acid) and DHA (docosahexaenoic acid). Both are omega-3 oils. Most fish oil supplements are 18% EPA and 12% DHA, or a total of 30% omega-3. These special omega-3 oils, unlike other omega-3 oils, keep blood triglycerides in check (high triglycerides are linked with heart disease). EPA and DHA also keep blood from clotting too quickly. They also have anti-inflammatory activity.

DHA is essential for vision in infants. Fish oil may also help prevent some types of cancer in animals[1][2][3] and humans.[4]

Where Is It Found?

EPA and DHA are found in mackerel, salmon, herring, sardines, sable fish (black cod), anchovies, albacore tuna, and wild game. Cod liver oil contains large amounts of EPA and DHA.

In What Conditions Might Fish Oil Be Supportive?

- Crohn's disease (page 34)
- Diabetes (page 39)
- Eczema (page 49)
- Hypertension (high blood pressure) (page 67)
- Hypertriglyceridemia (high triglycerides) (page 69)
- Lupus

- **Migraine headaches** (page 91)
- **Osteoarthritis** (page 97)
- **Psoriasis** (page 112)
- **Rheumatoid arthritis** (page 115)
- Ulcerative colitis

Who Is Likely to Be Deficient?

To a limited extent, omega-3 oil from vegetable sources, such as **flaxseed oil** (page 162), can convert to EPA. Nonetheless, most nutritionally oriented doctors believe people do not ingest enough omega-3 oil. So-called primitive diets have much higher levels than modern diets.

How Much Should I Take?

Most healthy people do not supplement fish oil. Those who choose to supplement often take at least 3 grams of EPA plus DHA—an amount that may require 10 grams of fish oil to achieve because most fish oil contains only 18% EPA and 12% DHA (18% EPA + 12% DHA = 30% omega-3 oil x 10 grams = 3 grams EPA plus DHA).

Are There Any Side Effects?

While those with heart disease and diabetes often benefit from fish oil,[5] [6] both groups should check with their nutritionally oriented doctor before taking more than 3 or 4 grams of fish oil for several months. Elevations in blood sugar have sometimes been reported,[7] though this may simply be due to small increases in weight resulting from high dietary fish oil.[8] While EPA and DHA consistently lower triglycerides, they occasionally increase LDL cholesterol.[9] Also, because EPA and DHA reduce blood clotting, people taking them sometimes get nose bleeds.[10] Some people who supplement several grams of fish oil will experience gastrointestinal upset and burp up a "fishy" smell.

Due to its very high levels of vitamin A and vitamin D, cod liver oil should not be taken before consulting a nutritionally oriented doctor by women who are or who could become pregnant. Other adults should consult with a nutritionally oriented doctor before taking cod liver oil (plus other supplements) containing more than 25,000 IU (7,500 mcg) of vitamin A per day or 800 IU of vitamin D per day.

Are There Any Interactions with Other Nutrients?

Fish oil is easily damaged by oxygen, so a few milligrams or IUs of **vitamin E** (page 220) should be included in all fish oil supplements.[11] In addition, people who supplement with fish oil should take additional vitamin E supplements (several hundred IUs) to protect EPA and DHA within the body from oxidative damage.[12]

Some evidence suggests that adding vitamin E to EPA/DHA may prevent the fish oil-induced increase in serum glucose.[13] Similarly, the impairment of glucose tolerance sometimes caused by the omega-3 oil has been prevented by the addition of half an hour of moderate exercise three times a week.[14]

People who take fish oil containing EPA and DHA and who also take 15 grams of pectin per day have been reported to have reductions in LDL cholesterol.[15] This suggests that pectin may overcome the occasional problem of increased LDL cholesterol resulting from fish oil supplementation. The LDL cholesterol–raising effect of EPA and DHA may also be successfully prevented by taking garlic supplements (or presumably real garlic) along with EPA and DHA.[16]

FLAXSEED OIL

LIKE MOST vegetable oils, flaxseed oil contains linoleic acid, an essential fatty acid needed for survival. But unlike most oils, it also contains significant amounts of another essential fatty acid, alpha linolenic acid (ALA).

ALA is an omega-3 oil. To a limited extent, the body turns ALA into EPA—an omega-3 oil found in **fish oil** (page 160). EPA in turn converts to 3-series prostaglandins (prostaglandins are hormone-like substances made in many parts of the body rather than coming from one organ, as most hormones do). Indirectly, the 3-series prostaglandins have anti-inflammatory activity. Because the conversion from ALA to EPA is quite limited, some of the effects of fish oil (like controlling triglycerides) do not result when people supplement flaxseed oil.

In theory, flaxseed should be useful in the same conditions for which fish oil is used. However, it does not appear to lower triglycerides and may not protect against heart disease. Its anti-inflammatory activity also has yet to be proven, though researchers remain hopeful.

In 1994, a diet purportedly high in ALA was successful in preventing heart disease.[1] But this study altered many dietary factors, so it is possible that ALA was not responsible for the outcome.[2] In general, flaxseed oil does not appear to be a good replacement for fish oil for people with elevated triglycerides,[3][4] though it may help lower cholesterol.[5]

Even outside the realm of heart disease, most omega-3 oil research has been done with fish oil and not flaxseed oil. So why should anyone consider flaxseed oil?

Flaxseed oil appears to have anti-inflammatory activity[6] and may lower blood pressure.[7] Flaxseed oil will not cause a fishy-smelling burp (a possible side effect of fish oil). While it is best not to cook with flaxseed oil, unlike fish oil it can be used in salads. Some conversion to EPA does occur,[8] and this conversion can be increased by restricting the intake of other vegetable oils,[9] which should increase flaxseed oil's effectiveness.

Where Is It Found?

In addition to its presence in flaxseed oil, small amounts of ALA are found in canola, **soy** (page 204), black currant, and walnut oils.

In What Conditions Might Flaxseed Oil Be Supportive?

- **Benign prostatic hyperplasia** (page 18)
- **Constipation** (page 32)

Who Is Likely to Be Deficient?

ALA deficiencies are possible but believed to be rare, except in infants who are fed formula that is omega-3 deficient.

How Much Should I Take?

Some nutritionally oriented doctors recommend that people use 1 tablespoon, or five capsules, of flaxseed oil per day as a supplement in salads or on vegetables to ensure a supply of essential fatty acids.

For those who wish to replace fish oil with flaxseed oil, research suggests it takes ten times as much ALA to be the equivalent of EPA.[10] Typically, this means that 7.2 grams of flaxseed oil should equal 1 gram of fish oil.

Are There Any Side Effects?

Flaxseed oil toxicity has not been reported.

FOLIC ACID

FOLIC ACID is needed for DNA synthesis. DNA allows cells—including cells in the fetus when a woman is pregnant—to replicate normally. Adequate intake of folic acid early in pregnancy is important for preventing most neural tube birth defects[1] as well as some birth defects of the arms, legs, and heart.[2] It also appears to protect against cleft palate and cleft lip formation in most,[3,4] though not all,[5] studies.

Folic acid is needed to make SAM (S-adenosyl methionine), which affects (and may improve) mood. Folic acid is also needed to keep homocysteine (an amino acid) levels in blood from rising. Excess homocysteine dramatically increases the risk of heart disease and may be linked to osteoporosis and strokes.

Where Is It Found?

Beans, leafy green vegetables, citrus fruits, beets, wheat germ, and meat are good sources of folic acid.

In What Conditions Might Folic Acid Be Supportive?

- Abnormal Pap smear (page 102)
- Atherosclerosis (page 11)
- Chemotherapy support (page 25)
- Crohn's disease (page 34)
- Depression (page 36)
- Diarrhea (page 44)
- Gingivitis (periodontal disease) (page 56)
- High cholesterol (page 62)
- Osteoporosis (page 100)
- Pregnancy support (page 107)
- Vitiligo (page 122)

Who Is Likely to Be Deficient?

Most people do not consume the recommended amount of folic acid. Recently, scientists have found that many people with heart disease have elevated blood levels of homocysteine, which is often controllable with folic acid. This suggests that many people in Western societies have a mild folic acid deficiency. In fact, increasing folic acid intake could potentially prevent an estimated 13,500 deaths from cardiovascular diseases each year.[6] Folic acid deficiency is also common in alcoholics, people living at poverty level, those with malabsorption disorders, and women taking the birth control pill.

How Much Should I Take?

All women who are or who could become pregnant should take 400–800 mcg per day in order to reduce the risk of birth defects. Many nutritionally oriented doctors recommend 400 mcg to others.

Are There Any Side Effects?

Folic acid is remarkably safe.[7] However, if people are deficient in **vitamin B12** (page 216) and take 1,000 mcg of folic acid per day or more, then the folic acid can improve anemia caused by the B12 deficiency. This is not a toxicity but rather a partial solution to one of the problems caused by vitamin B12 deficiency.[8] The other problems caused by a lack of vitamin B12 (mostly neurological) do not improve with folic acid supplements.

Vitamin B12 deficiencies often occur without anemia (even in people who do not take folic acid supplements). Some doctors do not know that the absence of anemia does not rule out a B12 deficiency. If this confusion delays diagnosis of a vitamin B12 deficiency, the patient could be injured, sometimes permanently. This problem is rare and should not happen with doctors knowledgeable in this area using correct testing procedures.

Are There Any Interactions with Other Nutrients?

Folic acid is needed by the body to utilize vitamin B12. **Proteolytic enzymes** (page 156) and antacids[9] inhibit folic acid absorption;[10] people taking either are advised to supplement with folic acid.

GAMMA ORYZANOL

GAMMA ORYZANOL is a mixture of sterols and ferulic acid esters. Some evidence suggests that it increases testosterone levels, the release of endorphins, and the growth of lean muscle tissue.[1]

Where Is It Found?

Gamma oryzanol is a natural component of rice bran, corn, and barley oils.

In What Conditions Might Gamma Oryzanol Be Supportive?

- Athletic performance (page 14)
- Gastritis

Who Is Likely to Be Deficient?

Since gamma oryzanol is not an essential nutrient, it is not associated with a deficiency state. Athletes involved in competitive training or other physically active individuals may benefit from this compound.

How Much Should I Take?

Much of the human research with gamma oryzanol uses 300 mg per day.

Are There Any Side Effects?

No side effects have been reported in the amounts commonly used.

GLUCOSAMINE SULFATE

GLUCOSAMINE SULFATE provides the joints with the building blocks they need to repair damage caused by osteoarthritis or injuries. Specifically, glucosamine sulfate provides the raw material needed by the body to manufacture a mucopolysaccharide (called glycosaminoglycan) found in cartilage. Glucosamine sulfate may also play a role in wound healing.

Where Is It Found?

Glucosamine sulfate does not appear in significant amounts in most diets. Supplemental sources are derived from sea shells.

In What Conditions Might Glucosamine Sulfate Be Supportive?

- **Kidney stones** (page 83)
- **Osteoarthritis** (page 97)

Who Is Likely to Be Deficient?

A glucosamine sulfate deficiency in humans has not been reported.

How Much Should I Take?

There is no need for people other than those with osteoarthritis to routinely supplement with glucosamine sulfate. People with osteoarthritis should take 500 mg three times per day.

Are There Any Side Effects?

At the amount most frequently taken by adults—500 mg three times per day—toxicity has not been reported. Some glucosamine sulfate is processed with sodium chloride (table salt), which is restricted in some diets (particularly for people with high blood pressure).

Are There Any Interactions with Other Nutrients?

The hypothesis that glucosamine sulfate and **chondroitin sulfate** (page 149) work synergistically in the support of osteoarthritis remains unproven. The fact that they are structurally similar suggests that they may act in similar ways.

GLUTAMINE

GLUTAMINE is an amino acid (protein building block). It serves as a source of fuel for cells lining the intestines. Without it, these cells waste away. It is also used by white blood cells and is important for immune function. In animal research, glutamine has anti-inflammatory effects.

Where Is It Found?

Glutamine is found in many foods high in protein, such as fish, meat, beans, and dairy.

In What Conditions Might Glutamine Be Supportive?

- **Peptic ulcer** (page 103)
- Ulcerative colitis

Who Is Likely to Be Deficient?

Few people are glutamine deficient, in part because the body makes its own. During fasting, starvation, cirrhosis, and weight loss associated with AIDS and cancer, however, deficiencies often develop.

How Much Should I Take?

In the presence of good health, there is no need to supplement glutamine. A nutritionally oriented physician should be consulted for the supplemental use of glutamine for the support of serious health conditions.

Are There Any Side Effects?

No clear toxicity has emerged in glutamine studies.

HISTIDINE

HISTIDINE is called a semiessential amino acid (protein building block) because adults generally produce adequate amounts except during periods of growth. Histidine is also a precursor of histamine, a compound released by immune system cells during an allergic reaction.

Where Is It Found?

Dairy, meat, poultry, and fish are good sources of histidine and the other amino acids.

In What Conditions Might Histidine Be Supportive?

- Rheumatoid arthritis (page 115)

Who Is Likely to Be Deficient?

According to limited research, many individuals with rheumatoid arthritis have low levels of histidine. Taking histidine supplements might improve arthritis symptoms in some individuals.[1]

How Much Should I Take?

Most people do not need to supplement histidine. Optimal levels for others remain unknown. Human research has used between 1 gram and 8 grams per day.

Are There Any Side Effects?

There are no reported side effects with histidine.

HYDROXYCITRIC ACID

(-)**HYDROXYCITRIC ACID** (HCA) is a fruit extract with a chemical composition similar to citric acid (the primary acid in oranges and other citrus fruits). Preliminary research, based on laboratory experiments and animal research, suggests that HCA may be a useful weight loss aid.[1][2] HCA has been demonstrated in the laboratory (but not yet in clinical trials with people) to reduce the conversion of carbohydrates into stored fat by inhibiting certain enzyme processes.[3][4] Animal research indicates that HCA suppresses appetite and induces weight loss.[5][6][7][8] One case report found that eating 1 gram of the fruit containing HCA before each meal resulted in the loss of 1 pound per day.[9] However, much more research in human populations is needed to determine the effectiveness of HCA as a weight loss aid.

Where Is It Found?

HCA is found in only a few plants, with the richest source being the rind of a little pumpkin-shaped fruit called *Garcinia cambogia,* native to Southeast Asia. Thai and Indian cuisines use this fruit (also called the Malabar tamarind) as a condiment in dishes such as curry.

In What Conditions Might HCA Be Supportive?

- **Weight loss and obesity** (page 124)

Who Is Likely to Be Deficient?

Since it is not an essential nutrient, HCA is not associated with a deficiency state.

How Much Should I Take?

Optimal levels of HCA remain unknown. Dieters often take 250–500 mg of HCA three times per day (before each meal) as a weight loss aid, though these amounts are far below the levels used in animal research (figured on a per-pound body weight basis). The effectiveness of HCA is enhanced when used in conjuncture with a low-fat diet, because HCA does nothing to reduce the caloric effects of dietary fat. HCA supplements are available in many forms, including tablets, capsules, powders, snack bars, and chewing gum.

Are There Any Side Effects?

HCA has not been linked to any adverse effects.

INOSINE

INOSINE is a nucleoside, one of the basic compounds comprising cells. It plays many supportive roles in the body, including the release of insulin, use of carbohydrate by heart tissue, and contractions of the heart muscle. Inosine is also known as hypoxanthine riboside.

Where Is It Found?

Inosine is found in **brewer's yeast** (page 143) and organ meats.

In What Conditions Might Inosine Be Supportive?

- **Athletic performance** (page 14)

Who Is Likely to Be Deficient?

Inosine is not an essential nutrient, so deficiencies do not occur. Some, but not all, studies indicate that inosine can benefit athletes by improving aerobic performance.[1][2]

How Much Should I Take?

A common amount of inosine taken by athletes is 5,000–6,000 mg per day, though some of the limited research on inosine in athletes does not show any benefit.[3]

Are There Any Side Effects?

There are no reported side effects with the use of inosine.

INOSITOL

INOSITOL is required for proper formation of cell membranes. It affects nerve transmission and helps in transporting fats within the body.

Where Is It Found?

Nuts, beans, wheat and wheat bran, cantaloupe, and oranges are excellent sources of inositol. Most dietary inositol is in the form of phytate.

In What Conditions Might Inositol Be Supportive?

- **Depression** (page 36)
- **Diabetes** (page 39)

Who Is Likely to Be Deficient?

Clear deficiency of inositol has not been reported, although diabetics have increased excretion and may benefit from inositol supplementation.

How Much Should I Take?

Most people do not need to take inositol, and the small amounts commonly found in multivitamin supplements are probably unnecessary and ineffective. Nutritionally oriented doctors sometimes suggest 500 mg twice per day.

Are There Any Side Effects?

Toxicity has not been reported, although people with chronic renal failure show elevated levels.

Are There Any Interactions with Other Nutrients?

Large amounts of phytate, the common dietary form of inositol, reduces the absorption of **calcium** (page 144), **iron** (page 173), and **zinc** (page 224). However, supplemental inositol does not have this effect.

IODINE

IODINE is needed to make thyroid hormones, which are necessary for maintaining normal metabolism in all cells of the body.

Where Is It Found?

Seafood, iodized salt, and sea vegetables—for example, kelp (page 174)—are high in iodine. Processed food may contain added iodized salt. Iodine is frequently found in dairy products. Vegetables grown in iodine-rich soil also contain this mineral.

In What Conditions Might Iodine Be Supportive?

- Fibrocystic breast disease (page 51)
- Iodine deficiency–induced goiter

Who Is Likely to Be Deficient?

People who avoid dairy, seafood, processed food, and iodized salt can become deficient. Iodine deficiency can cause low thyroid function, goiter, and cretinism, but iodine deficiencies are now uncommon in Western societies.

How Much Should I Take?

Since the introduction of iodized salt, iodine supplements are unnecessary and not recommended for most people. For strict vegetarians who avoid salt and sea vegetables, 150 mcg per day is more than adequate.

Are There Any Side Effects?

High doses (several milligrams per day) can interfere with normal thyroid function and should not be taken without consulting a nutritionally oriented doctor.[1] The average diet provides about four times the recommended amount of iodine, which may result in health problems.[2] In fact, goiter, traditionally a disease of iodine deficiency, is now linked sometimes to high iodine intake.[3] There are also speculations of an iodine link to thyroid cancer.[4]

IONIZED AIR

IONS ARE charged particles— either positive or negative—found in the air. These ions are created naturally. For example, the action of ocean waves on a beach creates a large number of negatively charged ions, which may be why many people feel better at the seashore. Conversely, exposure to electrical equipment and other sources of positively charged ions is reported to cause poor health in many people. The percentage of the population who is sensitive to the ionization of the surrounding air is not currently known.

Positively charged ions, according to present knowledge, are detrimental to human health. The unfavorable interactions between humans and positive ions have occurred for millions of years. Folk knowledge has attributed evil effects to certain seasonal winds, which scientists now understand to be highly charged with positive ions.

Although nature produces negative ions, most people do not live in regions high in naturally occurring negative ions. For those who are bothered by positive ions, a negative ion generator might be a practical remedy for neutralizing the exposure to positive ions.

Ionized air may play a role in allergies. Research suggests that some allergy-provoking substances, such as dust and pollen, have a positive electrical charge. Negative ions appear to counteract the allergenic effects of these positively charged ions on respiratory tissues.[1][2] Negative ions also have other beneficial effects for the respiratory system.[3][4]

Jonathan Wright, M.D., reports anecdotally that although his patients note varying responses, negative ions generally lead to favorable effects, and many individuals experience relief from their respiratory allergies. Other allergy sufferers report considerable relief with a few allergy reactions resolving completely after negative ion therapy. According to Dr. Wright, the majority of allergy sufferers can reduce reliance on other treatments (nutritional, biochemical, or prescription) during negative ion therapy.[5]

In What Conditions Might Negative Ions Be Supportive?

- Allergic bronchitis
- Allergic sinusitis
- **Asthma** (page 9)
- Chronic respiratory tract allergies
- **Hay fever** (page 59)

IRON

IRON is part of hemoglobin, the oxygen-carrying component of the blood. Iron-deficient people tire easily, because their bodies are starved for oxygen. Iron is also part of myoglobin, which helps muscle cells store oxygen. Without enough iron, ATP (the fuel the body runs on) cannot be properly synthesized. As a result, some iron-deficient people become fatigued even when their hemoglobin levels are normal.

Although iron is part of the antioxidant enzyme catalase, iron is not generally considered an antioxidant, because too much iron can cause oxidative damage.

Where Is It Found?

The most absorbable form of iron, called heme iron, is found in oysters, meat, poultry, and fish. Non-heme iron is also found in these foods, as well as in dried fruit, molasses, leafy green vegetables, and wine. Acidic foods (such as tomato sauce) cooked in an iron pan can also be a source of dietary iron.

In What Conditions Might Iron Be Supportive?

If iron deficiency is the cause of the following health concerns, then iron may be helpful.

- **Athletic performance** (page 14)
- **Canker sores (mouth ulcers)** (page 21)
- **Crohn's disease** (page 34)
- **Depression** (page 36)
- **Infertility (female)** (page 75)
- Iron deficiency
- **Menorrhagia (heavy menstruation)** (page 89)

Who Is Likely to Be Deficient?

Vegetarians eat less iron than nonvegetarians, and the iron they eat is somewhat less absorbable. As a result, vegetarians are more likely to have reduced iron stores.[1] However, iron deficiency is not usually caused by a lack of iron in the diet alone; there is often an underlying cause, such as iron loss in menstrual blood.

Pregnant women, marathon runners, people who take aspirin, and those who have parasitic infections, hemorrhoids, ulcers, ulcerative colitis, Crohn's disease, or other conditions that cause blood loss or malabsorption are likely to become deficient.

Individuals who fit into one of these groups, even pregnant women, should not automatically take iron supplements. Fatigue, the first symptom of iron deficiency, can be caused by many other things. A nutritionally oriented doctor should assess the need for iron supplements, since taking iron when it is not needed does no good and may do some harm.

How Much Should I Take?

If a nutritionally oriented doctor diagnoses iron deficiency, iron supplementation is essential. A common adult dose is 100 mg per day. When iron deficiency is diagnosed, the doctor must also determine the cause. Usually it is not serious (such as normal menstrual blood loss or blood donation). Occasionally, however, iron deficiency signals ulcers or even colon cancer.

Many premenopausal women become marginally iron deficient unless they supplement with iron. Even so, the 18 mg of iron present in most multiple vitamin/mineral supplements is often adequate.

Are There Any Side Effects?

Huge overdoses (as when a child swallows an entire bottle of iron supplements) can be fatal. Keep iron-containing supplements out of a child's reach. Hemochromatosis, hemosiderosis, polycythemia, and iron-loading anemias (such as thalassemia and sickle cell anemia) are conditions involving excessive storage of iron. Supplementing iron can be quite dangerous for people with these diseases.

Supplemental doses required to overcome iron deficiency can cause **constipation** (page 32). Sometimes switching the form of iron, getting more exercise, or treating the constipation with **fiber** (page 159) and fluids is helpful. Sometimes it is necessary to reduce the amount of iron if constipation occurs.

Some researchers have potentially linked excess iron to **diabetes** (page 39),[2] cancer,[3] increased risk of infection,[4] lupus erythematosus (SLE),[5] and exacerbation of **rheumatoid arthritis** (page 115).[6] While none of these links has been proven, it is known that too much iron causes **free radical** (page 8) damage, which can cause or exacerbate most of these diseases. People who are not iron deficient should not supplement iron when potential risks might exist and no benefit can be found.

Are There Any Interactions with Other Nutrients?

Caffeine, high-fiber foods, and **calcium** (page 144) supplements reduce iron absorption. **Vitamin C** (page 217) slightly increases iron absorption.[7] Taking **vitamin A** (page 209) with iron helps treat iron deficiency, since vitamin A helps the body use iron stored in the liver.[8][9]

KELP

KELP is a sea vegetable that is a concentrated source of minerals, including **iodine** (page 171), **potassium** (page 197), **magnesium** (page 182), **calcium** (page 144), and **iron** (page 173).

Kelp as a source of iodine assists in making thyroid hormones, which are necessary for maintaining normal metabolism in all cells of the body.

Where Is It Found?

Kelp can be one of several brown-colored seaweed species called *Laminaria*.

In What Conditions Might Kelp Be Supportive?

- Iodine supplementation

Who Is Likely to Be Deficient?

People who avoid sea vegetables as well as dairy, seafood, processed food, and the salt shaker, can become deficient in iodine. Although rare in Western societies, iodine deficiency can cause low thyroid function, goiter, and cretinism.

How Much Should I Take?

Since the introduction of iodized salt, additional sources of iodine, such as kelp, are unnecessary. However, kelp can be consumed as a source of other minerals.

Are There Any Side Effects?

Extremely high intakes of kelp could provide too much iodine and interfere with normal thyroid function.

LACTASE

LACTASE is the enzyme in the small intestine that digests lactose (the naturally occurring sugar in milk). A few children and many people after childhood do not produce sufficient lactase, which impairs the body's ability to digest milk. These individuals are said to be lactose intolerant and suffer from symptoms including cramps, gas, and diarrhea.

A simple test for lactose intolerance is to drink at least two glasses of milk on an empty stomach and note any gastrointestinal symptoms that develop in the next four hours; repeat the test using several ounces of cheese (which does not contain much lactose). If symptoms result from milk but not cheese, then the person has lactose intolerance. If symptoms occur with both milk and cheese, the person may be allergic to dairy.

Where Is It Found?

Lactase is produced by the body. Dairy products have varying levels of lactose, which affects how much lactase is required for proper digestion. Milk, ice cream, and yogurt contain significant amounts of lactose—although for complex reasons yogurt often does not trigger symptoms in lactose-intolerant people.

In What Conditions Might Lactase Be Supportive?

If lactose intolerance is the cause of the following health concerns, then lactase may be helpful.

- **Diarrhea** (page 44)
- Gas
- Indigestion and heartburn
- **Irritable bowel syndrome** (page 81)
- **Migraine headaches** (page 91)

Who Is Likely to Be Deficient?

Only one-third of all people retain the ability to digest lactose into adulthood. Most individuals of Asian, African, and Native American descent are lactose intolerant. In addition, half of Hispanics and about 20 percent of Caucasians do not produce lactase as adults.[1] Individuals who develop migraines may be more likely to be lactose intolerant.[2]

How Much Should I Take?

Lactose-reduced milk is available and can be used in the same quantities as regular milk. Lactase drops can be added to regular milk twenty-four hours before drinking, to reduce lactose levels. Lactase drops, capsules, and tablets can also be taken directly, as needed, immediately before a meal containing dairy products. The degree of lactose intolerance varies by individual, so a greater or lesser amount of lactase may be needed to eliminate symptoms of lactose intolerance.

Are There Any Side Effects?

Lactase is safe and does not produce side effects.

Are There Any Interactions with Other Nutrients?

Some, but not all, studies suggest that lactose-intolerant individuals absorb less **calcium** (page 144).[3]

LECITHIN/PHOSPHATIDYL CHOLINE/CHOLINE

WHEN MEDICAL researchers use the term lecithin, they are referring to a purified substance called phosphatidyl choline (PC). Supplements labeled as lecithin usually contain 10–20% PC.

Relatively pure PC supplements are generally labeled as phosphatidyl choline. PC best duplicates supplements used in medical research.

Choline by itself (without the phosphatidyl group) is also available in food and supplements. In high doses, however, pure choline can make people smell like fish, so it is rarely used, except in the small doses found in **multiple vitamin** (page 187) supplements.

PC acts as a supplier of choline. Choline is needed for cell membrane integrity and to facilitate the movement of fats in and out of cells. It is also a component of the neurotransmitter acetylcholine. For this reason, PC has been used in a number of preliminary studies for a wide variety of neurological and psychiatric disorders.

Where Are They Found?

Choline, the major constituent of PC, is found in soybeans, liver, oatmeal, cabbage, and cauliflower. Egg yolks, meat, and some vegetables contain PC. Lecithin (containing 10–20% PC) is added to many processed foods in small amounts for the purpose of maintaining texture consistency.

In What Conditions Might PC Be Supportive?

- **Eczema** (page 49)
- **Gallstones** (page 55)
- Manic-depression
- Liver damage

Who Is Likely to Be Deficient?

Although choline deficiencies have been artificially induced in people, little is known about human deficiency in the real world.

How Much Should I Take?

Small amounts of choline are present in most **B-complex** (page 210) and multivitamin supplements.

Are There Any Side Effects?

At several grams per day, some people will experience abdominal discomfort, diarrhea, or nausea. Supplementing straight choline (as opposed to phosphatidyl choline) in large amounts (over 1,000 mg per day) can lead to a fishy odor; PC does not have this effect.

Are There Any Interactions with Other Nutrients?

The body uses both PC and **pantothenic acid** (page 193) to form acetylcholine.

Leucine

LEUCINE

LEUCINE is an essential amino acid. Leucine inhibits the breakdown of muscle proteins that may occur after trauma or severe stress.[1]

Leucine supplements or protein powders that contain leucine are used by some bodybuilders and other athletes to promote muscle recovery, although it has not produced significant changes in body composition.

Leucine and other amino acids may also be beneficial for individuals with phenylketonuria, a condition in which the body cannot metabolize the amino acid phenylalanine.[2] Phenylketonuria should only be treated under the care of a nutritionally oriented physician.

Where Is It Found?

Leucine is present in all protein foods, such as meat, fish, eggs, milk, and beans. It is also found in **soy** (page 204) protein, **whey protein** (page 223), and other protein supplements.

In What Conditions Might Leucine Be Supportive?

- **Athletic performance** (page 14)
- Phenylketonuria

Who Is Likely to Be Deficient?

Since all protein foods are good sources of leucine, only an individual deficient in protein would become deficient in leucine.[3] A strict vegetarian or vegan diet, without adequate soy or other protein sources, might be inadequate in its content of leucine, though most American vegan diets are not leucine deficient.

How Much Should I Take?

To influence protein metabolism and muscles, several grams of leucine are generally taken.

Are There Any Side Effects?

No consistent evidence of toxicity has been linked to leucine supplements.

LIPASE

LIPASE is any enzyme that helps to digest dietary fats.

Where Is It Found?

Lipase is produced by the pancreas and released into the small intestine, where it helps digest fat. Pancreatin contains lipase along with two other enzymes: proteases and amylase.

In What Conditions Might Lipase Be Supportive?

If inadequate fat digestion is the cause of the following health concern, then lipase may be helpful.

- Indigestion and heartburn

Who Is Likely to Be Deficient?

People with pancreatic insufficiency and cystic fibrosis frequently require supplemental lipase and other enzymes. Those with celiac disease, Crohn's disease, and perhaps some people suffering from indigestion may be deficient in pancreatic enzymes.

How Much Should I Take?

Lipase as a digestive aid is generally accompanied by other enzymes that help digest carbohydrates and protein. In the U.S., pancreatin, which contains the three enzymes (lipase, amylase, and proteases), is rated against a standard established by the United States Pharmacopeia (USP). For example, 9X pancreatin is nine times stronger than the USP standard. Each X contains 25 USP units of amylase, 2 USP units of lipase, and 25 USP units of proteolytic enzymes. A dose of 1.5 grams of 9X pancreatin (or a higher dose at lower potencies) with each meal can help digest food in people with pancreatic insufficiency.

Are There Any Side Effects?

Lipase does not generally cause any side effects at the amounts listed above.

Are There Any Interactions with Other Nutrients?

Lipase or other supplemental enzymes should not be taken with **betaine hydrochloride** (page 139), or hydrochloric acid, which could destroy the enzymes.

LUTEIN

LUTEIN is an antioxidant in the carotenoid family (naturally occurring fat-soluble pigments found in plants). One of its functions is to protect the retina of the eye from sunlight. Lutein is the primary carotenoid present in the central area of the retina called the macula. Lutein may act as a filter to protect the macula from potentially damaging forms of light. Consequently, lutein is associated with protection from age-related macular degeneration (the leading cause of blindness in older adults).

Where Is It Found?

Spinach, kale, collard greens, romaine lettuce, leeks, and peas are good sources of lutein.

In What Conditions Might Lutein Be Supportive?

- Cataracts (page 24)
- Macular degeneration (page 85)

Who Is Likely to Be Deficient?

While a deficiency has not been identified, people who eat more lutein-containing foods appear to be at lower risk of macular degeneration. In fact, it has been reported that adults with the highest dietary intake of lutein had a 57% decreased risk for macular degeneration compared to those with the lowest intake.

How Much Should I Take?

People showing protection from macular degeneration eat about 6 mg of lutein per day from food. Lutein, in supplemental form, should be taken with food to improve absorption.

Are There Any Side Effects?

No lutein toxicity has been identified.

Are There Any Interactions with Other Nutrients?

Lutein works together with zeaxanthin, another antioxidant found in the same foods and supplements as lutein.

LYCOPENE

LYCOPENE, found primarily in tomatoes, is a member of the carotenoid family—including **beta-carotene** (page 209) and similar compounds found naturally in food—and has potent **antioxidant** (page 8) capabilities.

A study conducted by Harvard researchers examined the relationship between carotenoids and the risk of prostate cancer.[1] Of the carotenoids, only lycopene was clearly linked to protection. The men who had the greatest amounts of lycopene (6.5 mg per day) in their diet showed a 21% decreased risk of prostate cancer compared with those eating the least.

This report suggests that lycopene may be an important tool in the prevention of prostate cancer.

This study also reported that those who ate more than ten servings per week of tomato-based foods had a 35% decreased risk of prostate cancer compared to those eating less than 1.5 weekly servings. When the researchers looked at only advanced (stage D) prostate cancer, the high lycopene eaters had a whopping 86% decreased risk (although this did not reach statistical significance due to the small number of cases).

Prior research has associated tomato intake with a reduced rate of prostate cancer.[2] Lycopene is the most abundant carotenoid in the prostate,[3] and high blood levels of lycopene have been linked to prostate cancer prevention.[4] Lycopene is also a more potent inhibitor of human cancer cells than other carotenoids—even beta-carotene.[5]

Another study found that, for the 25% of people with the greatest tomato intake, the risk for cancers of the gastrointestinal tract was 30–60% lower compared with those who ate fewer tomatoes. These reduced risks were statistically significant.[6] A study of women found that the 75% who ate the *least* amount of tomatoes had between 3.5 and 4.7 times the risk for cervical intra-epithelial neoplasia—precancerous changes of the cervix.[7]

Where Is It Found?

Tomatoes, tomato sauce, and pizza are high in lycopene. In the Harvard study, the only tomato-based food that did not correlate with protection was tomato juice. There is evidence that people inaccurately report their intake of juice; moreover, the lycopene in juice may not be well absorbed. Other plants, including watermelon and guava, also contain lycopene.

In What Conditions Might Lycopene Be Supportive?

- Cancer risk reduction

Who Is Likely to Be Deficient?

This is unknown, but people who do not eat diets high in tomatoes or tomato products are likely to consume less than optimal amounts.

How Much Should I Take?

The ideal intake of lycopene is currently unknown; however, the men in the Harvard study with the greatest protection against cancer consumed at least 6.5 mg per day.

Are There Any Side Effects?

There are no reports of adverse effects caused by high intakes of lycopene.

Are There Any Interactions with Other Nutrients?

A diverse intake of carotenoids, rather than single carotenoids, may increase the absorption of these nutrients. In particular, beta-carotene has been reported to increase levels of carotenoids in the body.[8]

LYSINE

LYSINE is an essential amino acid needed for growth and to help maintain nitrogen balance in the body. Essential amino acids cannot be made in the body and must be supplied by the diet or supplements. Lysine appears to help the body absorb and conserve calcium.[1] Linus Pauling believed that lysine helps maintain healthy blood vessels.[2]

Where Is It Found?

Brewer's yeast, legumes, dairy, wheat germ, fish, and meat all contain significant amounts of lysine.

In What Conditions Might Lysine Be Supportive?

- Herpes simplex

Who Is Likely to Be Deficient?

Most people, including vegans (vegetarians who also avoid dairy and eggs), consume adequate amounts of lysine. Athletes involved in frequent vigorous exercise have increased need for essential amino acids, although most diets, if they include meat, dairy, or eggs, meet these increased needs. The essential amino acid requirements of burn patients may exceed the amount of lysine in the diet.

How Much Should I Take?

Most people do not require lysine supplementation. Those who supplement often take 500–1,000 mg per day.

Are There Any Side Effects?

In animals, high doses of lysine have been linked to increased risk of gallstones[3] and elevated choles-terol.[4] At supplemental doses, problems have not been reported in humans.

Are There Any Interactions with Other Nutrients?

Lysine works with other essential amino acids to maintain growth, lean body mass, and maintenance of the body's store of nitrogen.

MAGNESIUM

MAGNESIUM is needed for bone, protein, and fatty acid formation, making new cells, activating B vitamins, relaxing muscles, clotting blood, and forming ATP— the energy the body runs on. Insulin secretion and function also require magnesium.

Where Is It Found?

Nuts and grains are good sources of magnesium. Beans, dark green vegetables, fish, and meat also contain significant amounts.

In What Conditions Might Magnesium Be Supportive?

- **Asthma** (page 9)
- **Athletic performance** (page 14)
- **Autism** (page 17)
- **Chemotherapy support** (page 25)
- **Congestive heart failure** (page 30)
- **Diabetes** (page 39)
- **Fibromyalgia** (page 53)
- **Glaucoma** (page 58)
- **High cholesterol** (page 62)
- **Hypertension (high blood pressure)** (page 67)
- **Kidney stones** (page 83)
- **Migraine headaches** (page 91)
- **Osteoporosis** (page 100)
- **Premenstrual syndrome** (page 109)

Who Is Likely to Be Deficient?

Magnesium deficiency is common in people taking potassium-depleting prescription drugs. Taking too many laxatives can also lead to deficiency. Alcoholism, severe burns, diabetes, and heart failure are other potential causes of deficiency.

Fatigue, abnormal heart rhythms, muscle weakness and spasm, depression, loss of appetite, listlessness, and potassium depletion can all result from a magnesium deficiency.

How Much Should I Take?

Most people do not consume enough magnesium. Many nutritionally oriented doctors recommend 250–350 mg per day for adults.

Are There Any Side Effects?

Taking too much magnesium often leads to diarrhea. For some people, this can happen at amounts as low as 350–500 mg per day. Severe excess is more serious but rarely results from taking magnesium supplements. People with kidney disease should not take magnesium supplements without consulting a doctor.

Are There Any Interactions with Other Nutrients?

Magnesium increases the amount of **vitamin B6** (page 214) that can enter cells. As a result, these two nutrients are often taken together. Magnesium may compete for absorption with other minerals, particularly **calcium** (page 144). Taking a **multiple mineral supplement** (page 187) avoids this potential problem.

MANGANESE

MANGANESE is needed for healthy skin, bone, and cartilage formation as well as glucose tolerance. It also helps activate superoxide dismutase (SOD), an important antioxidant enzyme.

Where Is It Found?

Nuts, wheat germ, wheat bran, leafy green vegetables, beet tops, pineapple, and seeds are all good sources of manganese.

In What Condition Might Manganese Be Supportive?

- Osteoporosis (page 100)

Who Is Likely to Be Deficient?

Many people consume less than the 2.5–5 mg of manganese currently considered safe and adequate. Nonetheless, clear deficiencies are rare. Individuals with osteoporosis sometimes have low blood levels of manganese, suggestive of deficiency.

How Much Should I Take?

Several minerals, such as **calcium** (page 144) and **iron** (page 173), reduce the absorption of manganese.[1] Including 5–15 mg per day found in a **multiple vitamin/mineral** (page 187) supplement should prevent a deficiency caused by mineral competition.

Are There Any Side Effects?

Amounts found in supplements (5–20 mg) have not been linked with any toxicity. Excessive intake of manganese can lead to the rare side effects of dementia and psychiatric symptoms. Preliminary research suggests that individuals with cirrhosis may not be able to properly excrete manganese; until more is known, these people should not supplement with manganese.[2]

Are There Any Interactions with Other Nutrients?

Calcium, iron, and possibly **zinc** (page 224) reduce the absorption of manganese. Zinc and **copper** (page 151) work together with manganese to activate superoxide dismutase.

MEDIUM CHAIN TRIGLYCERIDES

MEDIUM CHAIN TRIGLYCERIDES are a class of fatty acids. Their chemical composition is of a shorter length than the long-chain fatty acids present in most other fats and oils, which accounts for their name. While other dietary fats supply nine calories per gram, medium chain triglycerides provide slightly less at 8.3 calories per gram. Another difference between medium chain triglycerides and other fats is that the medium chain triglycerides are more rapidly absorbed and burned as energy.

Where Are They Found?

Medium chain triglycerides are found in coconut oil and butter.

In What Conditions Might Medium Chain Triglycerides Be Supportive?

- Athletic performance (page 14)

Who Is Likely to Be Deficient?

Most people consume adequate or excessive fat in their diets, so extra fat intake as medium chain triglycerides is unnecessary. However, the body metabolizes medium chain triglycerides slightly differently than ordinary fats, so it may be more likely that medium chain triglycerides will be burned as energy—not stored as fat.[1]

How Much Should I Take?

The best amount of medium chain triglycerides to take is currently unknown. Many experts believe that this nutrient should not be used except for certain situations in which they are recommended by a nutritionally oriented physician.

Are There Any Side Effects?

Consuming medium chain triglycerides on an empty stomach can lead to gastrointestinal upset. Anyone with cirrhosis or other liver problems should not use medium chain triglycerides.

MELATONIN

MELATONIN is a natural hormone that regulates the human biological clock. Double-blind research with young adults shows that melatonin facilitates sleep.[1] Another study of healthy, young adults reports that melatonin significantly shortens the time needed to go to sleep, reduces the number of night awakenings, and improves sleep quality.[2]

Melatonin is also helpful in relieving symptoms of jet lag. One double-blind trial, involving fifty-two international flight crew members taking either melatonin or a placebo for three days before and five days after an international flight, found that the melatonin significantly reduced symptoms of jet lag and resulted in a quicker recovery of pre-flight energy levels and alertness.[3]

Less than 1 mg of melatonin has lowered pressure within the eyes of healthy people,[4] but studies have not yet been published on the effects of using melatonin with people who have glaucoma.

Where Is It Found?

Melatonin is produced by the pineal gland, located within the brain. Levels of melatonin in the body correspond with the cycles of night and day, with the highest melatonin levels produced at night. Melatonin appears in foods only in trace amounts.

In What Conditions Might Melatonin Be Supportive?

- **Glaucoma** (page 58)
- **Insomnia** (page 79)
- Jet lag

Who Is Likely to Be Deficient?

The body produces less melatonin with advancing age, which may explain why elderly people often have difficulty sleeping[5] and why melatonin supplements improve sleep in the elderly.[6] Adults with insomnia have lower melatonin levels.[7] Frequent travelers and shift workers are also likely to benefit from melatonin for the resynchronization of their sleep schedules.[8]

How Much Should I Take?

Normally, the body makes melatonin for several hours per night—an effect best duplicated with time-release supplements. Studies using time-release melatonin have reported good results.[9] Many doctors of natural medicine suggest 1–3 mg of melatonin taken one to two hours before bedtime. Melatonin should not be taken during the day.

Are There Any Side Effects?

There are few side effects with melatonin; however, there are reports of morning grogginess, undesired drowsiness, and sleepwalking and disorientation. It has been hypothesized that certain individuals should not use melatonin supplements, including pregnant or breast-feeding women, individuals with depression or schizophrenia, and those with autoimmune disease, including lupus.

Special United Kingdom Considerations

Melatonin is either not available or may require a prescription. Please check with your nutritionally oriented physician.

METHIONINE

METHIONINE is one of the essential amino acids (building blocks of protein). It supplies sulfur and other compounds required by the body for normal metabolism and growth. Methionine also belongs to a group of compounds called lipotropics; the others in this group include **choline** (page 176), **inositol** (page 170), and betaine. Methionine helps prevent excessive fat accumulation in the liver.[1] It is also one of the three amino acids needed by the body to manufacture **creatine** (page 153), a compound essential for energy production and muscle building.

Where Is It Found?

Meat, fish, and dairy are all good sources of methionine.

In What Conditions Might Methionine Be Supportive?

- Liver support

Who Is Likely to Be Deficient?

Most people consume plenty of methionine through a typical diet.

How Much Should I Take?

Amino acid requirements vary according to body weight, but average-size adults require approximately 800–1,000 mg of methionine per day—an amount exceeded by most Western diets.

Are There Any Side Effects?

It has been hypothesized that diets high in methionine, in the presence of B vitamin deficiencies, may increase the risk for **atherosclerosis** (hardening of the arteries) (page 11) by increasing blood levels of **cholesterol** (page 62) and a compound called homocysteine.[2]

Are There Any Interactions with Other Nutrients?

Excessive methionine intake, in the presence of inadequate intake of **folic acid** (page 163), **vitamin B6** (page 214), and **vitamin B12** (page 216), can increase the conversion of methionine to homocysteine.

MULTIPLE VITAMIN/MINERAL

ONE-PER-DAY MULTIPLES focus primarily on **B-complex** (page 210) vitamins, with **vitamin A** (page 209) and **vitamin D** (page 219) sometimes being high and other times being low potency. The rest of the formula, including vitamins C and E and the minerals, tends to be low potency. It does not take much of some of the minerals—for example, **copper** (page 151), **zinc** (page 224), and **iron** (page 173)—to offer 100% or more of what people normally require.

When you read a label for a one-per-day multiple, evaluate it as primarily a B-complex with added A and D along with low potencies of most minerals except copper, zinc, and iron.

How Many Tablets or Capsules Are Required?

Since one-per-day formulas are hard to balance with adequate minerals and **vitamin C** (page 217) and **vitamin E** (page 220), it is usually better to take multiples that suggest 2–6 capsules or tablets a day. In general, it takes about six tablets or capsules to fit all that is in the one-per-day plus 800–1,000 mg of **calcium** (page 144), 350–500 mg of **magnesium** (page 182), and a reasonable amount of C (300–1,000 mg) and E (200–400 IU).

With two to six per-day multiples, the dose should be spread out over an entire day—instead of taking all of them at one sitting. It is easy to increase or decrease the amount of vitamins and minerals by taking more or fewer of the multiples.

Which Is Better— Capsule or Tablet?

Multiples are available as a powder inside a hard-shell pull-apart capsule, as a liquid inside a soft-gelatin capsule, or as a tablet.

Most multiples have all the ingredients mixed together. Sometimes the B vitamins react with the rest of the ingredients in the capsule or tablet. This reaction is sped up whenever there is moisture or heat. This reaction can cause the B vitamins to "bleed" through the tablet or capsule, discoloring it and also making the multiple smell. While the multiple is still safe and effective, the smell is off-putting and usually not very well tolerated. Liquid multiples in a soft-gel capsule—or tablets or capsules that are kept dry and cool—do not have this problem.

Many people find capsules easier to swallow. This is often a function of size. Capsules are usually not as large as a tablet.

Some people prefer vegetarian multiples. While some capsules are made from vegetarian sources, most come from animal gelatin. Vegetarians need to carefully read the label to insure they are getting a vegetarian product.

One concern people have with tablets is whether they will break down. Properly made tablets and capsules will both dissolve readily in the stomach.

Are Time-Released Forms Better?

Some multiple supplements are in time-released form. The theory is that if the vitamins and minerals can be slowly released into the body over a period of time, it is better than releasing all the nutrients at once. Except for work done on vitamin C—some of which showed time-released C was better absorbed than non-time-released—research has been lacking, so it is still not certain whether this is a good idea or not. Some doctors think time releasing may make some of the nutrients unavailable—by the time the nutrient is released, it may have moved too far down the digestive tract to be absorbed efficiently. Others think that for the water-soluble nutrients, such as vitamin C and the B vitamins, time-released products may be a good idea.

Do the Ingredients "Fight" with Each Other?

Another area of controversy is whether all the nutrients in a multiple would be better utilized if they were taken separately.

While it is true that certain nutrients compete with each other for absorption, this is also the case when the nutrients are supplied in food. It is known, for example, that magnesium, zinc, and calcium compete for absorption; copper and zinc also compete. However, the body is designed to cope with this problem, and taking many different pills at different times is awkward and unnecessary.

How About Chewables?

Unfortunately, multiples do not taste very good. In order to make chewable multiples palatable, whether for children or adults, some compromises must be made. First, bad-tasting ingredients (such as iron) must be reduced or eliminated. Second, the rest of the ingredients must be masked with a sweetener.

Unless an artificial sweetener like aspartame (NutraSweet) or saccharine is used, the only sweeteners available are sugars. No matter their source (sucrose in white table sugar or fructose from fruit), sugar is sugar, and it would be preferable to not have it in a dietary supplement.

Some chewables, such as vitamin C, contain more sugar than any other ingredient. In such products, the sweetener should be listed as the first ingredient but often is not. This means care needs to be exercised when reading labels about chewable vitamins. If it tastes sweet, it contains sugar or a synthetic sweetener.

When Should I Take My Multiple?

The best time to take vitamins or minerals—with the exception of amino acids—is with meals. Multiples taken between meals often cause stomach upset and are likely not as well absorbed.

N-ACETYL CYSTEINE

N-ACETYL CYSTEINE (NAC) is an altered form of the amino acid **cysteine** (page 154), which is commonly found in food and synthesized by the body. NAC helps break down mucus. For that reason, inhaled NAC is used in hospitals to treat bronchitis. NAC helps the body synthesize glutathione— an important **antioxidant** (page 8). In animals, the antioxidant activity of NAC protects the liver from exposure to several toxic chemicals. NAC also protects the body from acetaminophen (Tylenol) toxicity and is used at very high doses in hospitals for that purpose.

Where Is It Found?

Cysteine, the amino acid from which NAC is derived, is found in most high-protein foods. NAC is not found in the diet.

In What Conditions Might N-Acetyl Cysteine Be Supportive?

- Bronchitis
- **Chemotherapy support** (page 25)
- Emphysema

Who Is Likely to Be Deficient?

Deficiencies of NAC have not been defined and may not exist. Deficiencies of the related amino acid cysteine have been reported in HIV-infected patients.[1]

How Much Should I Take?

It is not known whether healthy people need to supplement with NAC. Optimal levels of supplementation remain unknown. Much of the research uses 250–1,500 mg per day.

Are There Any Side Effects?

No consistent adverse effects of NAC have been reported in humans. One small study found that daily amounts of 1.2 grams or more could lead to oxidative damage.[2] Extremely large amounts of cysteine, the amino acid from which NAC is derived, may be toxic to nerve cells in rats.

Are There Any Interactions with Other Nutrients?

NAC may increase urinary zinc excretion.[3] It would be prudent to add supplemental **zinc** (page 224) and **copper** (page 151) when supplementing with NAC for extended periods.

ORNITHINE

ORNITHINE, an amino acid, is manufactured by the body when another amino acid, **arginine** (page 137), is metabolized during the production of urea (a constituent of urine). Some experts have claimed that ornithine promotes muscle-building activity in the body, but other research does not support these claims.[1]

Where Is It Found?

As with amino acids in general, ornithine is predominantly found in meat, fish, dairy, and eggs. The body also produces ornithine.

In What Conditions Might Ornithine Be Supportive?

- **Athletic performance** (page 14)
- Wound healing

Who Is Likely to Be Deficient?

Since ornithine is produced by the body, a deficiency of this nonessential amino acid is unlikely. However, individuals undergoing surgery or confined to the hospital may find particular benefit from supplemental intake of this amino acid.[2]

How Much Should I Take?

In human research involving ornithine, several grams are typically used per day, sometimes combined with arginine.

Are There Any Side Effects?

There are no reported side effects from the use of ornithine.

Are There Any Interactions with Other Nutrients?

The presence of arginine is needed to produce ornithine in the body, so higher levels of this amino acid should increase ornithine production.

ORNITHINE ALPHA-KETOGLUTARATE

THE AMINO ACIDS ornithine (page 190) and **glutamine** (page 166) are combined to form ornithine alpha-ketoglutarate (OKG). OKG enhances the body's release of the muscle-building hormones such as growth hormone and insulin and increases arginine and glutamine levels in muscle. OKG also encourages synthesis of polyamine, helps prevent the breakdown of muscle, increases muscle growth, and improves immune function.[1 2]

Where Is It Found?

Although the amino acids that comprise OKG are present in protein foods such as meat, poultry, and fish, the OKG compound is found only in supplements.

In What Conditions Might Ornithine Alpha-Ketoglutarate Be Supportive?

- **Athletic performance** (page 14)
- Wound healing

Who Is Likely to Be Deficient?

A deficiency of OKG has not been reported.

How Much Should I Take?

Optimal levels remain unknown, though some people take 2–4 grams of OKG three times per day with meals.

Are There Any Side Effects?

There are no reported side effects from the use of OKG.

Are There Any Interactions with Other Nutrients?

No clear interaction between OKG and any nutrients has been established.

PABA (PARAAMINOBENZOIC ACID)

PABA is the abbreviation for paraaminobenzoic acid, a compound that is loosely considered to be a member of the vitamin B-complex. PABA appears to enhance the effects of cortisone,[1] estrogen, and possibly other hormones by delaying their breakdown in the liver. PABA also prevents or even reverses the accumulation of abnormal fibrous tissue.

Some infertile women may have increased their ability to become pregnant after taking PABA.[2] Certain autoimmune or connective tissue disorders, such as scleroderma,[3][4] dermatomyositis,[5] and Peyronie's disease (accumulation of abnormal fibrous tissue in the penis)[6] have been relieved by PABA.

This vitamin may be helpful for two skin diseases: pemphigus, a severe blistering disease,[7] and **vitiligo** (page 122), a disorder in which patches of skin lose their pigmentation. An isolated study found that PABA darkened gray hair in some elderly (but not younger) individuals; however, other studies failed to show an effect of PABA on gray hair.[8]

Where Is It Found?

PABA is found in grains and animal foods.

In What Conditions Might PABA Be Supportive?

- Dermatomyositis
- **Infertility (female)** (page 75)
- Pemphigus
- Peyronie's disease
- Scleroderma
- **Vitiligo** (page 122)

Who Is Likely to Be Deficient?

Deficiencies of PABA have not been described in humans, and most conventional nutritionists do not consider it an essential nutrient.

How Much Should I Take?

Small amounts of PABA are present in some B-complex vitamins and **multiple vitamin** (page 187) formulas. The amount of PABA used for the conditions described on the previous page ranges from 300 mg per day and up to 12 grams per day for auto-immune, connective tissue, or skin disorders. Anyone taking more than 400 mg of PABA per day should consult a nutritionally oriented physician.

Are There Any Side Effects?

No serious side effects have been reported with 300–400 mg per day. Larger amounts (such as 8 grams per day or more) may cause low blood sugar, rash, fever, and (on rare occasions) liver damage.

Are There Any Interactions with Other Nutrients?

There are no known interactions between PABA and other nutrients. However, PABA interferes with sulfa drugs (a class of antibiotics) and therefore should not be taken when these medications are being used.

PANTOTHENIC ACID (VITAMIN B5)

PANTOTHENIC ACID, sometimes called vitamin B5, is involved in the Kreb's cycle of energy production and is needed to make the neurotransmitter acetylcholine. It is also essential in producing, transporting, and releasing the energy from fats. Synthesis of cholesterol (needed for vitamin D and hormone synthesis) depends on pantothenic acid. Pantothenic acid also activates the adrenal glands.[1] Pantethine—a variation of pantothenic acid—has been reported to lower blood levels of cholesterol and triglycerides.

Where Is It Found?

Liver, yeast, and salmon have high levels of pantothenic acid, but most other foods, including vegetables, dairy, eggs, grains, and meat, also provide some pantothenic acid.

In What Conditions Might Pantothenic Acid or Pantethine Be Supportive?

- **Athletic performance** (page 14) (pantothenic acid)
- **High cholesterol** (page 62) (pantethine)
- **Hypertriglyceridemia (high triglycerides)** (page 69) (pantethine)
- **Rheumatoid arthritis** (page 115) (pantothenic acid)

Who Is Likely to Be Deficient?

Pantothenic acid deficiencies may occur in people with alcoholism but are generally believed to be rare.

How Much Should I Take?

Most people do not need to supplement with pantothenic acid. However, the 10–25 mg found in many **multiple vitamin** (page 187) supplements might be beneficial in improving pantothenic acid status (so-called primitive human diets provided greater amounts of this nutrient than found in modern diets).

Are There Any Side Effects?

Toxicity has not been reported at supplemental doses. Very large amounts of pantothenic acid (several grams per day) can cause diarrhea.

Are There Any Interactions with Other Nutrients?

Pantothenic acid works together with **vitamins B1** (page 211), **B2** (page 212), and **B3** (page 213) to help make ATP—the fuel the body runs on.

PHENYLALANINE (L-PHENYLALANINE AND DL-PHENYLALANINE, DLPA)

L-PHENYLALANINE serves as a building block for the various proteins that are produced in the body. L-phenylalanine can be converted to L-**tyrosine** (page 207), another amino acid, and subsequently to L-dopa, norepinephrine, and epinephrine (three compounds that are involved in the functioning of the nervous system).

L-phenylalanine can also be converted (through a separate pathway) to phenylethylamine, a substance that occurs naturally in the brain and appears to elevate mood.

D-phenylalanine is not normally found in the body and cannot be converted to L-tyrosine, L-dopa, or norepinephrine. As a result, D-phenylalanine is converted primarily to phenylethylamine (the potential mood elevator). D-phenylalanine also appears to influence certain chemicals in the brain that relate to pain sensation.

DLPA is a mixture of the essential amino acid L-phenylalanine and its mirror image D-phenylalanine. DLPA (or the D- or L-form alone) has been used to treat depression.[1][2] D-phenylalanine may be helpful for some individuals with Parkinson's disease.[3] D-phenylalanine has been used to treat chronic pain—including **osteoarthritis** (page 97) and **rheumatoid arthritis** (page 115)—with both positive[4] and negative[5] results. For conditions where

D-phenylalanine alone has been shown to be effective, DLPA should also work, as it contains 50% D-phenylalanine.

Where Is It Found?

L-phenylalanine is found in most foods that contain protein. D-phenylalanine does not normally occur in food. However, when phenylalanine is synthesized in the laboratory, half appears in the L-form and the other half in the D- form. It is possible (although expensive) to separate these two compounds. However, the combination supplement (DLPA) is often used because both components exert different health-enhancing effects.

In What Conditions Might Phenylalanine or DLPA Be Supportive?

- **Depression** (page 36) (phenylalanine and DLPA)
- **Osteoarthritis** (page 97) (DLPA)
- Pain (DLPA)
- Parkinson's disease (phenylalanine)
- **Rheumatoid arthritis** (page 115) (DLPA)
- **Vitiligo** (page 122) (phenylalanine)

Who Is Likely to Be Deficient?

Individuals whose diets are very low in protein may develop a deficiency of L-phenylalanine, though this is believed to be very uncommon. However, one does not necessarily have to be deficient in L-phenylalanine in order to benefit from a DLPA supplement.

How Much Should I Take?

DLPA has been used in amounts ranging from 75–1,500 mg per day. As this compound can have powerful effects on mood and on the nervous system, DLPA should be taken only under medical supervision.

Are There Any Side Effects?

Ingestion of very large quantities of individual amino acids can cause nerve damage. The maximum amount of DLPA that is safe is unknown, but nerve damage has not been reported with 1,500 mg per day or less of DLPA. When taken in the quantities mentioned above, DLPA has occasionally caused mild side effects, such as nausea, heartburn, or transient headaches. Less is known about possible untoward effects of L-phenylalanine.

Are There Any Interactions with Other Nutrients?

L-phenylalanine competes with several other amino acids for attachment on a common amino acid carrier in the body. Therefore, it should not be taken with protein-containing foods. DLPA may interact with some antidepressants or stimulant drugs. Individuals taking prescription or over-the-counter medications should consult a nutritionally oriented physician before taking DLPA.

Phenylalanine

PHOSPHATIDYLSERINE

PHOSPHATIDYLSERINE (PS) belongs to a special category of fat-soluble substances called phospholipids. Phospholipids in general are essential components of cell membranes, and phosphatidylserine in particular is found in high concentrations in the brain. Phosphatidylserine may support mental function.[1]

Where Is It Found?

Phosphatidylserine is found in only trace amounts in a typical diet. Very small amounts are present in **lecithin** (page 176). The body manufactures phosphatidylserine from phospholipid building blocks. The research into PS has been done using material derived from a bovine source. Currently, the source of PS being used is soy. Since the soy product has not been used in research, it has not been conclusively shown to work. However, clinicians in the field report that it appears to work as well.

In What Conditions Might Phosphatidylserine Be Supportive?

- **Alzheimer's disease** (page 6)
- **Depression** (page 36)
- Mental function

Who Is Likely to Be Deficient?

Adults age fifty and older, especially those with age-related declines in mental function such as memory loss, are most likely to benefit from phosphatidylserine.

How Much Should I Take?

Phosphatidylserine (100 mg three times per day) has been shown to improve mental function in individuals with Alzheimer's disease.[2]

Are There Any Side Effects?

No side effects associated with phosphatidylserine have been reported.

Are There Any Interactions with Other Nutrients?

Phosphatidylserine works together with other phospholipids to build cell membranes.

POTASSIUM

POTASSIUM is needed to regulate water balance, levels of acidity, blood pressure, and neuromuscular function. It is also required for carbohydrate and protein metabolism.

Where Is It Found?

Most fruits are excellent sources of potassium. Beans, milk, and vegetables contain significant amounts.

In What Conditions Might Potassium Be Supportive?

- Congestive heart failure (page 30)
- Hypertension (**high blood pressure**) (page 67)
- Kidney stones (page 83)

Who Is Likely to Be Deficient?

So-called primitive diets provided much greater levels of potassium; modern diets may provide too little. Gross deficiencies, however, are rare except in cases of prolonged vomiting, diarrhea, or use of potassium-depleting diuretic drugs. Anyone taking one of these drugs should be informed by their doctor to take potassium. Prescription levels of potassium are higher than the amount sold over the counter but not more than the amount found in several pieces of fruit.

How Much Should I Take?

The best way to get extra potassium is to eat several pieces of fruit per day. The amount allowed in supplements—99 mg per tablet or capsule—is very low, considering that one banana can contain 500 mg. It is not wise to take multiple potassium pills in an attempt to get a higher amount, as they can irritate the stomach—a problem not encountered with the potassium in fruit.

Are There Any Side Effects?

Taking more than 99 mg by taking multiple potassium pills can produce stomach irritation. Potassium in fruit is safe for almost everyone, except for individuals with kidney failure or those taking potassium-sparing drugs used to treat high blood pressure. Individuals on these drugs should consult a nutritionally oriented doctor before taking potassium supplements or increasing fruit intake.

Are There Any Interactions with Other Nutrients?

Potassium and sodium work together in the body to maintain muscle tone, blood pressure, water balance, and other functions. Many researchers believe that part of the blood pressure problem caused by too much salt (which contains sodium) is made worse by too little dietary potassium.

PREGNENOLONE

PREGNENOLONE is one of the hormones produced by the body. Once circulating in the bloodstream, it is converted into other hormones, including progesterone and **dehydroepiandrosterone** (page 155), or DHEA.

Where Is It Found?

The body produces pregnenolone primarily in the adrenal glands. Supplements containing pregnenolone are also available in some countries.

Who Is Likely to Be Deficient?

As with hormones in general, older individuals produce less pregnenolone than younger individuals.

How Much Should I Take?

Pregnenolone supplementation is a controversial issue. Some experts believe that approximately 30 mg of pregnenolone, depending on age, gender, and other individual factors, may be a beneficial amount to take. Other experts, however, do not feel that pregnenolone or other hormones should be taken as supplements. It would be prudent to consult a nutritionally oriented doctor to have pregnenolone levels monitored before and during supplementation.

Are There Any Side Effects?

Pregnenolone is a hormone, and as such there are serious concerns about its inappropriate use. A nutritionally oriented physician should be consulted before using this hormone as a supplement.

Are There Any Interactions with Other Nutrients?

Pregnenolone is converted into other hormones by the body, including progesterone and DHEA.

PROANTHOCYANIDINS

Proanthocyanidins

PROANTHOCYANIDINS, also called OPCs for oligomeric proanthocyanidins, are a class of nutrients belonging to the flavonoid family. Two of the main functions of proanthocyanidins are as **antioxidants** (page 8) and in the stabilization of collagen and maintenance of elastin—two critical proteins in connective tissue, blood vessels, and muscle.[12]

Where Are They Found?

Proanthocyanidins can be found in many plants, most notably pine bark and grape seeds and skin. However, **bilberry** (page 234), **cranberry** (page 249), black currant, **green tea** (page 272), black tea, and other plants also contain this flavonoid. Nutritional supplements containing extracts of proanthocyanidins from various plant sources are available, alone or in combination with other nutrients, in herbal extracts, capsules, and tablets.

In What Conditions Might Proanthocyanidins Be Supportive?

- Chronic venous insufficiency

Who Is Likely to Be Deficient?

Flavonoids and proanthocyanidins are not classified as essential nutrients, since their absence does not induce a deficiency state. However, proanthocyanidins may have many health benefits, and anyone not eating a wide variety of plants will not derive these benefits.

How Much Should I Take?

Flavonoids (including proanthocyanidins and others) are a significant source of antioxidants in the average diet. Proanthocyanidins at 50–100 mg per day may be a reasonable supplemental level.

Are There Any Side Effects?

Flavonoids in general and proanthocyanidins specifically are free of side effects. Since they are water-soluble nutrients, excess intake is simply excreted in the urine.

Are There Any Interactions with Other Nutrients?

Proanthocyanidins as antioxidants may have a sparing effect on the body's stores of **vitamin C** (page 217).

PYRUVATE

PYRUVATE (in the form pyruvic acid) is created in the body during the metabolism of carbohydrates and protein. Pyruvate may aid weight loss efforts.[1] A clinical trial found that pyruvate supplements, compared to placebo, enhance weight loss and also result in a greater reduction of body fat in overweight adults consuming a low-fat diet.[2] Animal studies suggest that pyruvate leads to weight loss by increasing the resting metabolic rate.[3] A small number of clinical trials also indicate that pyruvate supplements improve exercise endurance.[4,5]

Preliminary research indicates that pyruvate functions as an antioxidant, inhibiting the production of harmful free radicals.[6,7,8] Due to its potential antioxidant function, preliminary research with animals suggests that pyruvate may inhibit the growth of cancer tumors.[9]

Where Is It Found?

In addition to being formed in the body during digestive processes, pyruvate is present in several foods, including red apples, cheese, dark beer, and red wine. Dietary supplements of pyruvate are also available.

In What Conditions Might Pyruvate Be Supportive?

- **Weight loss and obesity** (page 124)
- **Athletic performance** (page 14)

Who Is Likely to Be Deficient?

Because it is not an essential nutrient, pyruvate is not associated with a deficiency state.

How Much Should I Take?

Most human research with pyruvate and weight loss has used at least 30 grams per day.

Are There Any Side Effects?

High intakes of pyruvate can trigger gastrointestinal upset, such as gas, bloating, and diarrhea.

QUERCETIN

QUERCETIN belongs to a class of water-soluble plant pigments called bioflavonoids. Quercetin acts as an antihistamine and has anti-inflammatory activity. As an **anti-oxidant** (page 8), it protects LDL cholesterol (the "bad" cholesterol) from becoming damaged. Cardiologists believe that damage to LDL cholesterol is an underlying cause of heart disease. Quercetin blocks an enzyme that leads to accumulation of sorbitol, which has been linked to nerve, eye, and kidney damage in those with diabetes.

Where Is It Found?

Quercetin can be found in onions, apples, and black tea. Smaller amounts are found in leafy green vegetables and beans.

In What Conditions Might Quercetin Be Supportive?

- **Atherosclerosis** (page 11)
- **Cataracts** (page 24)
- **Diabetes** (page 39)
- **Hay fever** (page 59)
- **High cholesterol** (page 62)
- **Peptic ulcer** (page 103)

Who Is Likely to Be Deficient?

No clear deficiency of quercetin has been established.

How Much Should I Take?

Common supplemental intake of quercetin is 400 mg two to three times per day.

Are There Any Side Effects?

No clear toxicity has been identified. Early quercetin research suggested that large amounts of quercetin could cause cancer in animals,[1] but current research finds no effect on cancer risk[2] or protection from cancer.[3][4]

Are There Any Interactions with Other Nutrients?

Since bioflavonoids help protect and potentiate **vitamin C** (page 217), quercetin is often taken with vitamin C.

RESVERATROL

RESVERATROL, found primarily in red wine, is a naturally occurring **antioxidant** (page 8) that decreases the "stickiness" of blood platelets and helps blood vessels remain open and flexible.[1][2][3] A series of laboratory experiments suggest that resveratrol inhibits the development of cancer in animals as well as prevents the progression of cancer.[4] However, human research is still needed in this area. In another set of animal studies, resveratrol was shown to inhibit both the acute and chronic phases of inflammation.[5]

Where Is It Found?

Resveratrol is present in a wide variety of plants; of the edible plants, resveratrol is found mainly in grapes and peanuts.[6] Wine is the primary dietary source of resveratrol. Red wine contains much greater amounts of resveratrol than does white wine, since resveratrol is concentrated in the grape skin and the manufacturing process of red wine includes prolonged contact with grape skins.

In What Conditions Might Resveratrol Be Supportive?

- **Atherosclerosis** (page 11)
- Cancer risk reduction

Who Is Likely to Be Deficient?

Since it is not an essential nutrient, resveratrol is not associated with a deficiency state.

How Much Should I Take?

A glass of red wine provides 640 mcg of resveratrol, while a handful of peanuts provides 73 mcg of resveratrol. Resveratrol supplements (often found in combination with grape extracts or other antioxidants) are generally taken in the amount of 200–600 mcg per day. The amount used in animals to prevent cancer, however, would exceed 500 mg per human adult. Therefore, it is not reasonable to assume that the traces found in supplements or food would be protective.

Are There Any Side Effects?

There are no reported side effects with the use of resveratrol.

SELENIUM

SELENIUM activates an antioxidant enzyme called glutathione peroxidase, which may protect the body from cancer. A recent double-blind study following over 1,300 people found that those given 200 mcg of yeast-based selenium per day for seven years had a 50% drop in the cancer death rate compared with the placebo group.[1] Selenium is also needed to activate thyroid hormones.

Where Is It Found?

Brazil nuts are the best source of selenium. Yeast, whole grains, and seafood are also good sources.

In What Conditions Might Selenium Be Supportive?

- **Abnormal Pap smear** (page 102)
- **Atherosclerosis** (page 11)
- Cancer risk reduction
- **Macular degeneration** (page 85)
- **Osgood-Schlatter disease** (page 96)

Who Is Likely to Be Deficient?

While most people do not take in enough selenium, gross deficiencies are rare. Soils in some areas are selenium deficient, and people who eat foods grown primarily on selenium-poor soils are at risk for deficiency.

How Much Should I Take?

An adult dose of 200 mcg of selenium per day is recommended by many nutritionally oriented doctors.

Are There Any Side Effects?

Supplementing or eating 1,000 mcg of selenium per day may cause loss of fingernails, skin rash, and changes in the nervous system.

Are There Any Interactions with Other Nutrients?

Selenium enhances the antioxidant effect of **vitamin E** (page 220).

SOY

SOY, a staple food in many Asian countries, contains valuable constituents, including protein, isoflavones, saponins, and phytosterols. Soy protein provides most of the essential amino acids and can be used as well as animal protein by adults. It is also low in fat and cholesterol-free. The isoflavones in soy, primarily genistein and daidzein, have been well researched by scientists for their **antioxidant** (page 8) and phytoestrogenic properties.[1] Saponins enhance **immune function** (page 72) and bind to cholesterol to limit its absorption in the intestine. Phytosterols and other components of soy have been reported to lower cholesterol levels.

Isoflavones may reduce the risk of hormone-dependent cancers, such as breast and prostate cancer, as well as other cancers. A review study of soy research conducted by leading soy expert Mark Messina, Ph.D., found that 65% of twenty-six animal-based cancer studies showed a protective effect of soy or soy isoflavones.[2] Human research is also highly suggestive of a protective role of soy against cancer.[3][4]

A meta-analysis study that pooled thirty-eight trials for reanalysis reported that a soy diet led to cholesterol reductions in 89% of the studies. Increasing soy intake was associated with a 23 mg per deciliter drop in total cholesterol levels.[5]

The mild estrogen activity of soy isoflavones may ease menopause symptoms for some women, without creating estrogen-related problems. A group of fifty-eight menopausal women, who experienced an average of fourteen hot flashes per week, supplemented their diets with either wheat flour or soy flour every day for three months; the women taking the soy reduced their hot flashes by 40%.[6] In addition, soy may help regulate hormone levels in premenopausal women.[7]

Where Is It Found?

In addition to whole soybeans, foods derived from soy include tofu, tempeh, soy milk, textured and hydrolyzed vegetable protein, meat substitutes, soy flour, miso, and soy sauce. Soy is also available as a supplement, as soy protein or isoflavone in powder, capsule, or tablet form. High levels of soy-based isoflavones are in roasted soy nuts, tofu, tempeh, soy milk, and some soy protein isolates.

In What Conditions Might Soy Be Supportive?

- Cancer risk reduction
- **High cholesterol** (page 62)
- **Menopause** (page 87)
- **Pregnancy support** (page 107)

Who Is Likely to Be Deficient?

There is no deficiency as such, but people who do not consume soy foods will not gain the benefits of soy.

How Much Should I Take?

The ideal intake of soy is not known. Researchers suggest that the equivalent of one serving of soy foods per day supports good health, and the benefits increase as soy intake increases.[8]

Are There Any Side Effects?

Soy products and cooked soybeans are very safe at a wide range of intakes; however, a small percentage of people have allergies to soybeans and should, therefore, avoid soy products. Certain constituents in soy interfere with thyroid function,[9] but the clinical importance of this problem remains unclear.

Are There Any Interactions with Other Nutrients?

Soy contains a compound called phytic acid, which can interfere with mineral absorption.

SPIRULINA

SPIRULINA, or blue-green algae as it is also known, belongs to a group of 1,500 species of microscopic aquatic plants. The two most common species used for human consumption are *Spirulina maxima* and *Spirulina platensis*. Spirulina is particularly rich in protein, containing all of the essential amino acids (protein building blocks).

Spirulina also contains carotenoids, vitamins, minerals, and essential fatty acids. Most health benefits popularly based on spirulina supplementation come from anecdotes and not scientific research.

Where Is It Found?

Spirulina grows in some lakes, particularly those rich in salts, in Central and South America and Africa. It is also grown in outdoor tanks specifically to be harvested for nutritional supplements.

In What Conditions Might Spirulina Be Supportive?

- Protein supplementation
- **Weight loss and obesity** (page 124)

Who Is Likely to Be Deficient?

As it is not an essential nutrient, spirulina is not associated with a deficiency state. However, individuals who do not consume several servings of vegetables per day could benefit from the carotenoids and other nutrients in spirulina. Since it is a complete protein, it can be used in place of some of the protein in a healthy diet.

How Much Should I Take?

Spirulina can be taken as a powder, flakes, capsules, or tablets. The typical intake is 2,000–3,000 mg per day divided throughout the day.

Are There Any Side Effects?

There are no side effects reported with spirulina. However, since spirulina can accumulate heavy metals from contaminated water, consuming spirulina from such areas can increase the body's load of lead, mercury, and cadmium.[1] There are a few reports of allergic reactions to spirulina.

TAURINE

TAURINE is an amino acid (protein building block) as well as a component of bile acids, which are used to absorb fats and fat-soluble vitamins. Taurine also regulates heartbeat, maintains cell membrane stability, and helps prevent brain cell overactivity.

Where Is It Found?

Taurine is found mostly in meat and fish. Except for infants, the human body is able to make taurine from **methionine** (page 186), another amino acid.

In What Conditions Might Taurine Be Supportive?

- **Congestive heart failure** (page 30)
- **Diabetes** (page 39)
- **Hypertension (high blood pressure)** (page 67)
- Epilepsy
- Liver disease

Who Is Likely to Be Deficient?

Vegans (vegetarians who eat no dairy or eggs) consume virtually no taurine but usually make enough to avoid deficiency. Infants do not make enough, but taurine is found both in human milk and most infant formulas. Diabetics have lower blood levels of taurine.[1]

How Much Should I Take?

Most people, even vegans, do not need taurine supplements. While infants do require taurine, the level in either human milk or formula is adequate. If needed, nutritionally oriented doctors will typically recommend 2 grams taken three times per day for a total of 6 grams per day.

Are There Any Side Effects?

Taurine has not been consistently linked with any toxicity.

TYROSINE

TYROSINE is a nonessential amino acid (protein building block), which the body synthesizes from **phenylalanine** (page 194), another amino acid. Tyrosine is important to the structure of almost all proteins in the body. It is also the precursor of several neurotransmitters, including L-dopa, dopamine, norepinephrine, and epinephrine. Tyrosine, through its effect on neurotransmitters, may affect several health conditions, including Parkinson's disease, depression, and other mood disorders. Studies have suggested that tyrosine may help people with depression.[1]

Preliminary findings indicate a beneficial effect of tyrosine, along with other amino acids, in people affected by dementia including Alzheimer's disease.[2] Tyrosine may also ease the adverse effects of environmental stress.[3]

Tyrosine is formed by skin cells into melanin, the dark pigment that protects against the harmful effects of ultraviolet light. Thyroid hormones, which have a role in almost every process in the body, also contain tyrosine as part of their structure.

People born with the genetic condition phenylketonuria (PKU) are unable to metabolize the amino acid phenylalanine. Mental retardation and other severe disabilities can result. While phenylalanine restriction prevents these problems, it also leads to low tyrosine levels in many (but not all) people with PKU. Tyrosine supplementation may be beneficial in some people with PKU, although the evidence remains preliminary.[4]

Where Is It Found?

Dairy products, meats, fish, wheat, oats, and many other foods contain tyrosine.

In What Conditions Might Tyrosine Be Supportive?

- **Alzheimer's disease** (page 6)
- **Depression** (page 36)
- Phenylketonuria (PKU)

Who Is Likely to Be Deficient?

Some people affected by PKU are deficient in tyrosine. Tyrosine levels are sometimes low in depressed people.[5] Any person losing large amounts of protein, such as those with some kidney diseases, may be deficient in several amino acids, including tyrosine.[6]

How Much Should I Take?

Some human research uses the equivalent of 7 grams per day. A useful amount in PKU remains uncertain. Monitoring of blood levels by a nutritionally oriented physician is recommended.

Are There Any Side Effects?

Very high levels of tyrosine may cause diarrhea, nausea, vomiting, or nervousness; lessening tyrosine intake usually alleviates these problems.

Are There Any Interactions with Other Nutrients?

Vitamin B6 (page 214), **folic acid** (page 163), and **copper** (page 151) are necessary for conversion of tyrosine into neurotransmitters.

VANADIUM

VANADIUM is an ultra-trace mineral found in the human diet and body. It is essential for some animals, and deficiency symptoms in these animals include growth retardation, bone deformities, and infertility. However, vanadium has not been proven to be an essential mineral for humans. Vanadium may play a role in building bones and teeth.

Vanadyl sulfate, a form of this mineral, may improve glucose control in individuals with non-insulin-dependent diabetes mellitus (NIDDM), according to a study of eight diabetics supplemented with 100 mg of the mineral daily for four weeks.[1]

However, the researchers of this study caution that the long-term safety of such large doses of vanadium remains unknown. Many doctors of natural medicine expect that amounts this high will turn out to be unsafe.

Where Is It Found?

Vanadium is found in very small amounts in a wide variety of foods, including seafood, cereals, mushrooms, parsley, corn, **soy** (page 204), and gelatin.

In What Conditions Might Vanadium Be Supportive?

- **Diabetes** (page 39)

Who Is Likely to Be Deficient?

Deficiencies of the mineral vanadium have not been reported and appear unlikely.

How Much Should I Take?

Optimal intake of vanadium is unknown. The estimated requirement is probably less than 10 mcg per day; an average diet provides 15–30 mcg per day.

Are There Any Side Effects?

There is limited information about vanadium toxicity. Workers exposed to vanadium dust can develop toxic effects. High blood levels have been linked to manic-depressive mental disorders, but the meaning of this remains uncertain.[2] Vanadium sometimes inhibits, but at other times stimulates, cancer growth in animals. The effect in humans remains unknown.[3]

Are There Any Interactions with Other Nutrients?

Vanadium is not known to interact with other nutrients.

VITAMIN A AND BETA-CAROTENE

VITAMIN A helps cells reproduce normally—a process called differentiation. Cells that have not properly differentiated are more likely to undergo precancerous changes. Vitamin A, by maintaining healthy cell membranes, helps prevent invasion by disease-causing microorganisms. Vitamin A also stimulates immunity and is needed for formation of bone, protein, and growth hormone. Beta-carotene, a substance from plants that the body can convert into vitamin A, also acts as an **antioxidant** (page 8) and immune system booster.

Other members of the antioxidant carotene family include cryptoxanthin, alpha-carotene, zeaxanthin, **lutein** (page 179), and **lycopene** (page 180), but most of them do not convert to significant amounts of vitamin A.

Where Are They Found?

Dark green and orange-yellow vegetables are good sources of beta-carotene. Liver, dairy products, and cod liver oil provide vitamin A. Vitamin A can also be found in vegetarian supplements.

In What Conditions Might Vitamin A or Beta-Carotene Be Supportive?

- **Abnormal Pap smear** (page 102)
- **Acne** (page 5)
- **Cataracts** (page 24)
- **Chemotherapy support** (page 25)
- **Crohn's disease** (page 34)
- **Immune function** (page 72)
- **Macular degeneration** (page 85)

- Measles
- **Menorrhagia (heavy menstruation)** (page 89)
- **Night blindness** (page 95)
- **Peptic ulcer** (page 103)
- **Photosensitivity** (page 105)
- **Premenstrual syndrome** (page 109)
- **Recurrent ear infection** (page 47)
- **Urinary tract infection** (page 120)

Who Is Likely to Be Deficient?

Individuals who limit their consumption of liver, dairy foods, and vegetables can develop a vitamin A deficiency. The earliest deficiency sign is poor night vision. Deficiency symptoms can also include dry skin, increased risk of infections, and metaplasia (a precancerous condition).

How Much Should I Take?

In males and postmenopausal women, up to 25,000 IU (7,500 mcg) of vitamin A per day is considered safe. In women who could become pregnant, the safest intake level is being reevaluated; less than 10,000 IU (3,000 mcg) per day is widely accepted as safe.

The most common beta-carotene supplement intake is probably 25,000 IU (15 mg) per day, though some people take as much as 100,000 IU (60 mg) per day.

Are There Any Side Effects?

Women who are or could become pregnant should take less than 10,000 IU (3,000 mcg) per day of vitamin A to avoid the risk of birth defects. For other adults, intake above 25,000 IU (7,500 mcg) per day can—in rare cases—cause headaches, dry skin, hair loss, fatigue, bone problems, and liver damage.[1] Beta-carotene, however, does not cause any side effects, aside from excessive intake (more than 100,000 IU, or 60 mg, per day) sometimes giving the skin a yellow-orange hue.

Are There Any Interactions with Other Nutrients?

Individuals taking beta-carotene for long periods of time should also supplement with **vitamin E** (page 220), as beta-carotene may reduce vitamin E levels.[2]

Taking vitamin A and **iron** (page 173) together helps overcome iron deficiency more effectively than iron supplements alone.[3]

VITAMIN B-COMPLEX

OFTEN PEOPLE want to take one or more of the individual B vitamins.

Unless there is a reason to take a high dose of a single B vitamin—for example, taking **vitamin B6** (page 214) for **carpal tunnel syndrome** (page 23)—many nutritionally oriented doctors will recommend people take either a "balanced" B-complex or a **multiple vitamin/mineral** (page 187).

So-called balanced B-complexes usually contain 50–100 mg or mcg of the various B vitamins. For example, a "Balanced 50" might contain 50 mg of **B1** (page 211), **B2** (page 212), niacin or **B3** (page 213), **pantothenic acid** (page 193), B6, **PABA** (page 192), **methionine** (page 186), **choline** (page 176), and **inositol** (page 170); it might also contain 50 mcg of **folic acid** (page 163), **biotin** (page 141), and **B12** (page 216). The term "balanced" refers only to the way companies have traditionally formulated B-complexes.

Most multiple vitamin/mineral products have a B-complex included as part of the formula, so people taking multiples usually do not need to also take a B-complex.

VITAMIN B1 (THIAMIN)

VITAMIN B1 (also called thiamin) is needed to process carbohydrates, fat, and protein. Every cell of the body requires vitamin B1 to form ATP, the fuel the body runs on. Nerve cells require vitamin B1 in order to function normally.

Where Is It Found?

Wheat germ, whole wheat, peas, beans, so-called enriched flour, fish, peanuts, and meat are all good sources of vitamin B1.

In What Conditions Might Vitamin B1 Be Supportive?

- Canker sores (**mouth ulcers**) (page 21)
- **Fibromyalgia** (page 51)
- **Pregnancy support** (page 107)

Who Is Likely to Be Deficient?

Deficiency is most commonly found in alcoholics, people with malabsorption conditions, and those eating a very poor diet.

How Much Should I Take?

While ideal levels are somewhat uncertain, one study reports that the healthiest people eat more than 9 mg per day.[1] The amount found in many **multiple vitamin** (page 187) supplements (20–25 mg) is more than adequate.

Are There Any Side Effects?

Vitamin B1 is nontoxic, even in very high amounts.

Are There Any Interactions with Other Nutrients?

Vitamin B1 works hand in hand with several other B vitamins. Therefore, nutritionists usually suggest that vitamin B1 be taken as part of a **B-complex** (page 210) vitamin or other multivitamin supplement.

VITAMIN B2 (RIBOFLAVIN)

VITAMIN B2 (also called riboflavin) is needed to process amino acids and fats, activate **vitamin B6** (page 214) and **folic acid** (page 163), and help convert carbohydrates into ATP, the fuel the body runs on. Under some circumstances, vitamin B2 can act as an **antioxidant** (page 8).

Where Is It Found?

Dairy foods, eggs, and meat contain significant amounts of vitamin B2. Leafy green vegetables and whole and so-called enriched grains contain some vitamin B2.

In What Conditions Might Vitamin B2 Be Supportive?

- Athletic performance (page 14)
- Canker sores (mouth ulcers) (page 21)
- Cataracts (page 24)
- Migraine headaches (page 91)

Who Is Likely to Be Deficient?

Vitamin B2 deficiency can occur in alcoholics. Also, a deficiency may be more likely in people with cataracts[1][2] or sickle cell anemia.[3]

How Much Should I Take?

Ideal levels remain unknown, but surprisingly the recommended daily allowance might be too high. Vegans (vegetarians who eat no dairy or eggs) generally consume less than 1 mg per day of vitamin B2, yet they do not usually show any signs of deficiency. The amounts found in many **multiple vitamin** (page 187) supplements (20–25 mg) is more than adequate.

Are There Any Side Effects?

Vitamin B2 is nontoxic, even in high amounts.

Are There Any Interactions with Other Nutrients?

Vitamin B2 works with several other B vitamins; consequently, it makes sense to take vitamin B2 as part of a **B-complex** (page 210) supplement.

VITAMIN B3 (NIACIN, NIACINAMIDE)

THE BODY uses vitamin B3 in the process of releasing energy from carbohydrates. It is needed to form fat from carbohydrates and to process alcohol. The niacin form of vitamin B3 also regulates cholesterol.

Vitamin B3 comes in two basic forms—niacin (also called nicotinic acid) and niacinamide (also called nicotinamide). A variation on niacin, called inositol hexaniacinate, is also available in supplements. Because it has not been linked with any of the usual niacin toxicity in scientific research, inositol hexaniacinate is sometimes prescribed by European doctors for those who need high doses of niacin.

Where Is It Found?

The best food sources of vitamin B3 are peanuts, **brewer's yeast** (page 143), fish, and meat. Some vitamin B3 is also found in whole grains.

In What Conditions Might Vitamin B3 Be Supportive?

Niacin or Inositol Hexaniacinate:

- Bursitis (page 20)
- Cataracts (page 24)
- Diabetes (page 39)
- High cholesterol (page 62)
- Hypertriglyceridemia (**high triglycerides**) (page 69)
- Pregnancy support (page 107)

Niacinamide:

- Depression (page 36)
- Diabetes (page 39)
- Osteoarthritis (page 97)
- Photosensitivity (page 105)

Who Is Likely to Be Deficient?

Pellagra, the disease caused by a vitamin B3 deficiency, is rare in Western societies. Symptoms include loss of appetite, skin rash, diarrhea, mental changes, beefy tongue, and digestive and emotional disturbance.

How Much Should I Take?

In part because it is added to white flour, most people probably get enough vitamin B3 from their diets; however, 10–25 mg of the vitamin can be taken as part of a **B-complex** (page 210) or **multiple vitamin** (page 187) supplement.

Are There Any Side Effects?

Niacinamide is almost always safe to take, although rare liver problems have occurred at doses in excess of 1,000 mg per day. Niacin, at amounts as low as 50–100 mg, may cause flushing, headache, and stomachache in some people.

Cardiologists, in treating specific health problems, sometimes prescribe very high amounts of niacin—often several 1,000 mg per day. These doses can cause liver damage, diabetes, gastritis, eye damage, and elevated blood levels of uric acid (which can cause gout) and should never be taken without the supervision of a cardiologist or nutritionally oriented doctor.

Although the inositol hexaniacinate form of niacin has not been linked with side effects, the amount of research remains quite limited. Therefore, it makes sense for people taking this supplement in large amounts (1,000 mg or more per day) to be followed by a nutritionally oriented doctor.

Are There Any Interactions with Other Nutrients?

Vitamin B3 works with **vitamin B1** (page 211) and **vitamin B2** (page 212) to release energy from carbohydrates. Therefore, these vitamins are often taken together in a B-complex or multiple vitamin supplement (although most B3 research uses niacin or niacinamide by itself).

VITAMIN B6 (PYRIDOXINE)

VITAMIN B6 is the master vitamin in the processing of amino acids (the building blocks of all proteins and some hormones). Vitamin B6 helps to make and take apart many amino acids and is also needed to make serotonin, **melatonin** (page 185), and dopamine.

Vitamin B6 aids in the formation of several neurotransmitters and is therefore an essential nutrient in the regulation of mental processes and possibly mood.

Where Is It Found?

Potatoes, bananas, raisin bran, lentils, liver, turkey, and tuna are all good sources of vitamin B6.

In What Conditions Might Vitamin B6 Be Supportive?

- **Asthma** (page 9)
- **Atherosclerosis** (page 11)

- Athletic performance (page 14)
- Autism (page 17)
- Canker sores (mouth ulcers) (page 21)
- Carpal tunnel syndrome (page 23)
- Chemotherapy support (page 25)
- Depression (page 36)
- Diabetes (page 39)
- Fibrocystic breast disease (page 51)
- High cholesterol (page 62)
- Kidney stones (page 83)
- Morning sickness (page 93)
- MSG sensitivity (page 94)
- Osteoporosis (page 100)
- Photosensitivity (page 105)
- Premenstrual acne (page 5)
- Premenstrual syndrome (page 109)

Who Is Likely to Be Deficient?

Vitamin B6 deficiencies, although very rare, cause impaired immunity, skin lesions, and mental confusion. A marginal deficiency sometimes occurs in alcoholics, patients with kidney failure, and women using oral contraceptives. Many nutritionally oriented doctors believe that most diets do not provide optimal amounts of this vitamin.

How Much Should I Take?

The most common supplemental intake is 10–25 mg per day; however, higher amounts (200–500 mg per day) may be recommended for certain conditions.

Are There Any Side Effects?

Although side effects from vitamin B6 supplements are rare, at very high levels (200 mg or more per day) this vitamin can eventually damage sensory nerves, leading to numbness in the hands and feet as well as difficulty walking. Vitamin B6 supplementation should be stopped if any of these symptoms begin to develop.

Pregnant and lactating women should not take more than 100 mg of vitamin B6. For other adults, vitamin B6 is usually safe in amounts of 200–300 mg per day,[1] although occasional problems have been reported in this range.[2] Any adult taking more than 100–200 mg of vitamin B6 for more than a few months should consult a nutritionally oriented doctor. Side effects from vitamin B6 appear to be more common when intake reaches 2,000 mg per day; consequently no one should ever take more than 500 mg per day.[3]

Are There Any Interactions with Other Nutrients?

Since vitamin B6 increases the bioavailability of magnesium (page 182), these nutrients are sometimes taken together.

VITAMIN B12 (COBALAMIN)

VITAMIN B12 is needed for normal nerve cell activity, DNA replication, and production of the mood-affecting substance called SAM (S-adenosyl methionine). Vitamin B12 works with **folic acid** (page 163) to control homocysteine levels. An excess of homocysteine, which is an amino acid (protein building block), dramatically increases the risk of heart disease and perhaps osteoporosis.

Where Is It Found?

Vitamin B12 is found in all foods of animal origin, including dairy, eggs, meat, fish, and poultry. Inconsistent but small amounts occur in seaweed, including **spirulina** (page 205), and tempeh.

In What Conditions Might Vitamin B12 Be Supportive?

- **Asthma** (page 9)
- **Atherosclerosis** (page 11)
- **Bursitis** (page 20)
- **Crohn's disease** (page 34)
- **Depression** (page 36)
- **Diabetes** (page 39)
- **High cholesterol** (page 62)
- **Infertility (male)** (page 77)
- **Osteoporosis** (page 100)
- Pernicious anemia
- **Vitiligo** (page 122)

Who Is Likely to Be Deficient?

After several years, vegans (vegetarians who avoid dairy and eggs) frequently become deficient. People with malabsorption conditions suffer from vitamin B12 deficiency. Individuals suffering from pernicious anemia require high-dose supplements of vitamin B12.

How Much Should I Take?

Most people do not require vitamin B12 supplements. However, vegans should take at least 2–3 mcg per day. Treatment for pernicious anemia includes supplements of 1,000 mcg of vitamin B12 per day or vitamin B12 injections. In addition, the elderly may benefit from 10–25 mcg per day of vitamin B12.

Are There Any Side Effects?

Vitamin B12 supplements are not associated with side effects.

Are There Any Interactions with Other Nutrients?

If a person is deficient in vitamin B12 and takes 1,000 mcg of folic acid per day or more, the folic acid can improve anemia caused by the B12 deficiency but not affect neurological symptoms. This is not a toxicity but rather a partial solution to one of the problems caused by B12 deficiency. The other problems caused by a lack of vitamin B12 (mostly neurological) do not improve with folic acid supplements.

Vitamin B12 deficiencies often occur without anemia (even in people who do not take folic acid supplements). Some doctors do not know that the absence of anemia does not rule out a B12 deficiency. If this confusion delays diagnosis of a vitamin B12 deficiency, the patient could be injured, sometimes permanently. This problem is rare and should not happen with doctors knowledgeable in this area using correct testing procedures.

Anyone supplementing with more than 1,000 mcg per day of folic acid needs to be initially evaluated by a doctor of natural medicine to avoid this potential problem.

VITAMIN C (ASCORBIC ACID)

VITAMIN C is a water-soluble vitamin that functions as a powerful **antioxidant** (page 8). Vitamin C is needed to make collagen, the "glue" that strengthens many parts of the body, such as the muscles and blood vessels. Vitamin C also plays important roles in wound healing and as a natural antihistamine. This vitamin also aids in the formation of liver bile and helps to fight viruses and to detoxify alcohol and other substances.

Although vitamin C appears to have only a small effect in preventing the common cold, it reduces the duration and severity of a cold. Large amounts of vitamin C (e.g., 1–8 grams daily) taken at the onset of a cold episode may shorten the duration of illness by up to 23%.[1]

Where Is It Found?

Broccoli, red peppers, currants, Brussels sprouts, parsley, rose hips, acerola berries, citrus fruit, and strawberries are great sources of vitamin C.

In What Conditions Might Vitamin C Be Supportive?

- **Abnormal Pap smear** (page 102)
- Allergy
- **Asthma** (page 9)
- **Atherosclerosis** (page 11)
- **Athletic performance** (page 14)
- Backache
- **Cataracts** (page 24)
- **Chemotherapy support** (page 25)

- **Common cold/sore throat** (page 28)
- **Diabetes** (page 39)
- **Eczema** (page 49)
- **Gingivitis (periodontal disease)** (page 56)
- **Glaucoma** (page 58)
- **Hay Fever** (page 59)
- Hepatitis support
- **High cholesterol** (page 62)
- **Hypertension (high blood pressure)** (page 67)
- **Immune function** (page 72)
- Infections
- **Infertility (male)** (page 77)
- Iron deficiency
- **Macular degeneration** (page 85)
- **Menopause** (page 87)
- **Menorrhagia (heavy menstruation)** (page 89)
- **Morning sickness** (page 93)
- **Recurrent ear infection** (page 47)
- **Urinary tract infection** (page 120)
- **Vitiligo** (page 122)

Who Is Likely to Be Deficient?

Although scurvy (severe vitamin C deficiency) is uncommon in Western societies, many nutritionally oriented doctors believe that most people consume less than optimal amounts. Easy bruising and bleeding gums are early signs of vitamin C deficiency that occur long before symptoms of scurvy develop. Smokers have low levels of vitamin C and require a higher daily intake to maintain normal vitamin C levels.

How Much Should I Take?

A daily amount of at least 500–1,000 mg per day is often recommended for this vitamin; however, much greater dosages are not uncommon. For example, Linus Pauling took 18,000 mg per day for many years. The ideal level remains in debate.

Are There Any Side Effects?

Some individuals develop diarrhea after as little as a few thousand milligrams of vitamin C per day, while others are not bothered by ten times this amount. However, high levels of vitamin C can deplete the body of **copper** (page 151),[2] [3] an essential nutrient. It is prudent to ensure adequate copper intake at higher intakes of vitamin C. Copper is found in many **multiple vitamin/mineral** (page 187) supplements.

People with the following conditions should consult their doctor before supplementing with vitamin C:

- Glucose-6-phosphate dehydrogenase deficiency
- History of kidney stones
- History of surgery to the small intestines
- Iron overload (hemosiderosis or hemochromatosis)
- Kidney failure

Are There Any Interactions with Other Nutrients?

When large amounts (greater than 1,000 mg) of vitamin C are taken for more than a few weeks, copper should also be supplemented to guard against copper deficiency. Vitamin C probably increases the absorption of **iron** (page 173), although this effect may be mild. Vitamin C helps recycle the antioxidant **vitamin E** (page 220).

VITAMIN D (CHOLECALCIFEROL)

VITAMIN D'S most important role is maintaining blood levels of **calcium** (page 144), which it accomplishes by increasing absorption of calcium from food and reducing urinary calcium loss. Both effects keep calcium in the body and therefore spare the calcium that is stored in the bones. When necessary, vitamin D transfers calcium from the bone into the bloodstream, which does not benefit bones. Although the overall effect of vitamin D on the bones is complicated, some vitamin D is necessary for healthy bones and teeth.

Vitamin D plays a role in immunity and blood cell formation. Vitamin D also helps cells differentiate—a process that may reduce the risk of cancer.

Where Is It Found?

Cod liver oil is an excellent dietary source of vitamin D, as are vitamin D–fortified foods. Traces of vitamin D are found in egg yolks and butter. However, the majority of vitamin D in the body is created during a chemical reaction that starts with sunlight exposure to the skin.

In What Conditions Might Vitamin D Be Supportive?

- Crohn's disease (page 34)
- Migraine headaches (page 91)
- Osteoporosis (page 100)
- Psoriasis (page 112)
- Rickets (page 118)

Who Is Likely to Be Deficient?

Vitamin D deficiency, which causes abnormal bone formation, is more common after the winter due to restricted sunlight exposure in that season. Deficiencies are also more common in strict vegetarians (who avoid vitamin D–fortified dairy), dark-skinned individuals, people with malabsorption conditions, liver disease, or kidney disease, and alcoholics. People with liver and kidney disease can make vitamin D but cannot activate it.

How Much Should I Take?

People who get plenty of sun exposure do not require supplemental vitamin D. Otherwise, 400 IU per day is a safe adult dose.

Are There Any Side Effects?

Patients with sarcoidosis or hyperparathyroidism should not take vitamin D without consulting a physician. For most people, there is little reason to take more than 400 IU per day—a very safe adult dose. Excessive vitamin D intake (significantly more than 1,000 IU per day for long periods of time) can ultimately lead to headaches, weight loss, and kidney stones and, rarely, deafness, blindness, and death.

Are There Any Interactions with Other Nutrients?

Vitamin D increases both calcium and phosphorus absorption.

VITAMIN E (TOCOPHEROL)

VITAMIN E is a powerful **antioxidant** (page 8) that protects cell membranes and other fat-soluble parts of the body, such as LDL cholesterol (the "bad" cholesterol). Most cardiologists believe that only damaged LDL cholesterol increases the risk of heart disease; therefore protection of LDL cholesterol by vitamin E may reduce the risk of heart disease. Two studies published in the *New England Journal of Medicine* show that both men[1] and women[2] who supplement with at least 100 IU of vitamin E per day for at least two years have a 37–41% drop in the risk of heart disease. Even more impressive is the 77% drop in nonfatal heart attacks reported in the double-blind CHAOS study, in which people were given 400–800 IU vitamin E per day.[3]

The names of all types of vitamin E begin with either "d" or "dl," which refers to differences in chemical structure. The d form is natural and dl is synthetic. The natural form is more active. More synthetic vitamin E is added to supplements to compensate for the low level of activity. For example, 100 IU of vitamin E requires about 67 mg of the natural form but at least 100 mg of the synthetic. Little is known about how the synthetic dl form affects the body, though no clear toxicity has been discovered.

Most doctors of natural medicine advise people to use only the natural (d) form of vitamin E. After the d or dl designation, often the Greek letter alpha appears, which also describes the structure. Synthetic (dl) vitamin E is found only in the alpha form, as in dl-alpha tocopherol. Natural vitamin E can be found either as alpha (as in d-alpha tocopherol) or in combination with beta, gamma, and delta—this combination is labeled "mixed" (as in mixed natural tocopherols).

Human trials with vitamin E have almost always been done with the alpha (not gamma) form. Historically, the synthetic (dl) form was used in most trials but some trials are now using the natural (d) form. The reports mentioned above (men and women who supplement vitamin E have fewer heart attacks) were measuring alpha intake. The double-blind CHAOS trial mentioned above, showing a 77% reduction in nonfatal attacks, used alpha and not gamma. This strongly suggests that the alpha form is protective.

A group of researchers recently claimed that gamma might better protect against oxidative damage;[4] the evidence comes from a test tube study. The researchers hypothesize that alpha might interfere with the activity of gamma-tocopherol, a claim that remains unproven. They caution against alpha supplementation, a position not shared by most vitamin E researchers nor supported by most other research.

The issue of alpha versus gamma requires much more research before it can be fully understood. Almost all vitamin E research shows that positive results require hundreds of units per day—an amount easily obtained with supplements but impossible with food. Therefore, switching to food sources as suggested by these researchers is impractical. Until more is known, people seeking to add gamma tocopherol can find mixed natural tocopherol supplements. They contain a small amount of gamma, but the percentage remains much lower than that found in food.

Vitamin E forms are listed as either tocopherol or tocopheryl, followed by the name of what is attached to it, as in tocopheryl acetate. There is no great difference between the two, but tocopherol may absorb a little better, while tocopheryl forms may have slightly longer shelf life. Both forms are active when taken by mouth. However, there is no evidence that the skin can utilize the tocopheryl forms, so for those planning to apply vitamin E to the skin, it makes sense to buy tocopherol. In health food stores, the most common forms of vitamin E are d-alpha tocopherol and d-alpha tocopheryl (acetate or succinate). Both of these d (natural) alpha forms are frequently recommended by doctors of natural medicine.

Where Is It Found?

Wheat germ oil, nuts, seeds, vegetable oils, whole grains, egg yolks, and leafy green vegetables all contain vitamin E.

In What Conditions Might Vitamin E Be Supportive?

- Abnormal Pap smear (page 102)
- Alzheimer's disease (page 6)
- Angina pectoris
- Atherosclerosis (page 11)
- Athletic performance (page 14)

- Cataracts (page 24)
- Chemotherapy support (page 25)
- Diabetes (page 39)
- Dupuytren's contracture (page 46)
- Eczema (page 49)
- Fibrocystic breast disease (page 51)
- Fibromyalgia (page 53)
- High cholesterol (page 62)
- Infertility (female) (page 75)
- Infertility (male) (page 77)
- Macular degeneration (page 85)
- Menopause (page 87)
- Menorrhagia (heavy menstruation) (page 89)
- Osgood-Schlatter disease (page 96)
- Osteoarthritis (page 97)
- Photosensitivity (page 105)
- Premenstrual syndrome (page 109)
- Rheumatoid arthritis (page 115)
- Yellow nail syndrome (page 129)

Who Is Likely to Be Deficient?

Severe vitamin E deficiencies are rare.

How Much Should I Take?

The most commonly recommended dose of vitamin E for adults is 400 IU per day.

Are There Any Side Effects?

Vitamin E toxicity is very rare; supplements are widely considered to be safe.

Are There Any Interactions with Other Nutrients?

A diet high in unsaturated fat increases vitamin E requirements. Vitamin E and selenium (page 203) work together to protect fat-soluble parts of the body.

VITAMIN K (PHYLLOQUINONE)

VITAMIN K is needed for proper bone formation and blood clotting, in both cases by helping the body transport **calcium** (page 144).

Where Is It Found?

Leafy green vegetables are the best sources of vitamin K.

In What Conditions Might Vitamin K Be Supportive?

- Morning sickness (page 93)
- Osteoporosis (page 100)

Who Is Likely to Be Deficient?

A vitamin K deficiency, which causes uncontrolled bleeding, is rare, except in individuals with certain malabsorption diseases. All newborn infants receive vitamin K to prevent deficiencies that sometimes develop in breast-fed infants.

How Much Should I Take?

Many physicians suggest 65–80 mg of vitamin K per day—a level that can be achieved by eating vegetables.

Are There Any Side Effects?

Vitamin K interferes with the action of prescription blood thinners. People taking these drugs should never supplement vitamin K without consulting a physician. Phylloquinone—the natural vegetable form of vitamin K—has not been linked with any other side effects.

Are There Any Interactions with Other Nutrients?

Vitamin K facilitates the effects of calcium in building bone and proper blood clotting.

WHEY PROTEIN

WHEY PROTEIN is a dairy-based source of amino acids (protein building blocks). Whey protein provides the body with several amino acids, including **leucine** (page 177), isoleucine, and valine—the **branched-chain amino acids** (page 138), or BCAAs, needed for the maintenance of muscle tissue.

Where Is It Found?

During the process of making milk into cheese, whey protein is separated from the milk. This whey protein is then incorporated into ice cream, bread, canned soup, infant formulas, and other food products. Supplements containing whey protein are also available.

In What Conditions Might Whey Protein Be Supportive?

- Athletic performance (page 14)

Who Is Likely to Be Deficient?

Individuals who do not include dairy foods in their diets would not consume whey protein; however, the amino acids in whey protein are available from other sources, and a deficiency of these amino acids is unlikely. In fact, most Americans consume too much rather than too little protein.

How Much Should I Take?

Most people do not require extra protein such as whey protein. However, athletes in training sometimes take approximately 25 grams of whey protein per day.

Are There Any Side Effects?

People who are allergic to dairy products could react to whey protein and should therefore avoid it. Lactose-intolerant people will also react to whey protein. As with protein in general, long-term, excessive intake is associated with deteriorating kidney function and possibly osteoporosis. However neither kidney nor bone problems have been directly associated with whey protein, and the other dietary sources of protein typically contribute more protein to the diet than does whey protein.

ZINC

ZINC is a component of more than 300 enzymes that are needed to repair wounds, maintain fertility, synthesize protein, help cells reproduce, preserve vision, boost immunity, and protect against **free radicals** (page 8), among other functions.

Zinc gluconate lozenges, according to a double-blind clinical trial involving 100 men and women suffering from the common cold, shorten the duration of cold symptoms. Taking zinc gluconate lozenges (every two waking hours) has been reported to halve the number of days cold symptoms are present.[1]

Where Is It Found?

Good sources of zinc include oysters, meat, eggs, seafood, black-eyed peas, tofu, and wheat germ.

In What Conditions Might Zinc Be Supportive?

- **Acne** (page 5)
- Anorexia nervosa
- **Athletic performance** (page 14)
- **Benign prostatic hyperplasia** (page 18)
- **Common cold/sore throat** (page 28)
- **Crohn's disease** (page 34)
- **Diabetes** (page 39)
- Down's syndrome
- **Immune function** (page 72)
- **Infertility (male)** (page 77)
- **Macular degeneration** (page 85)
- **Night blindness** (page 95)
- **Osteoporosis** (page 100)
- **Peptic ulcer** (page 103)
- **Recurrent ear infection** (page 47)
- **Rheumatoid arthritis** (page 115)
- Sickle cell anemia
- **Wilson's disease** (page 126)
- Wound healing

Who Is Likely to Be Deficient?

Low-income pregnant women and pregnant teenagers are at risk for marginal zinc deficiencies. Supplementing with 25–30 mg per day improves pregnancy outcome in these groups.[2][3]

The average diet frequently provides less than the recommended daily allowance for zinc. A low-dose supplement (15 mg per day) can fill in dietary gaps. Zinc deficiencies are more common in alcoholics and individuals with sickle cell anemia, malabsorption problems, and chronic kidney disease.[4]

How Much Should I Take?

Moderate intakes of zinc, 15–25 mg, are adequate to prevent deficiencies. Higher doses (up to 50 mg taken three times per day) are reserved for treating certain health conditions, under the supervision of a nutritionally oriented doctor. For the alleviation of cold symptoms, lozenges providing 10–15 mg of zinc in the zinc gluconate form are generally used frequently throughout the day.

Are There Any Side Effects?

Zinc intake in excess of 300 mg per day may impair immune function.[5] Some people report that zinc lozenges lead to mild problems, such as stomachache, nausea, mouth irritation, and a bad taste.

Preliminary research had suggested that patients with **Alzheimer's disease** (page 6) should avoid zinc supplements until further studies clarify the role of zinc in this disease.[6] The latest research, however, suggests that zinc may actually help people with this condition.[7] Until more is known, people with Alzheimer's disease should consult a nutritionally oriented doctor before supplementing zinc.

Are There Any Interactions with Other Nutrients?

Zinc inhibits **copper** (page 151) absorption, which can lead to anemia and lower levels of HDL cholesterol (the "good" cholesterol).[8] [9] [10] Copper intake should be increased if zinc supplementation continues for more than a few days (except for individuals with Wilson's disease).[11] Many zinc supplements, to prevent copper inhibition, include copper in the formulation.

Zinc competes for absorption with **iron** (page 173),[12] [13] **calcium** (page 144),[14] and **magnesium** (page 182).[15] A **multiple mineral** (page 187) supplement will prevent mineral imbalances that can result from taking high doses of zinc for extended periods of time.

N-acetyl cysteine (page 189), or NAC, may increase urinary excretion of zinc.[16] Long-term users of NAC may consider adding supplements of zinc and copper.

Zinc

HERBS

ALFALFA *(Medicago sativa)*

ALFALFA is a member of the pea family and is native to western Asia and the eastern Mediterranean region. Alfalfa sprouts have become a popular food. Alfalfa herbal supplements primarily use the dried leaves of the plant.

In What Conditions Might Alfalfa Be Supportive?

- **High cholesterol** (page 62)
- Poor appetite

Historical or Traditional Use

Early Chinese physicians used young alfalfa leaves to treat disorders of the digestive tract.[1] In India, Ayurvedic physicians prescribed the leaves and flowering tops for poor digestion. It was also considered therapeutic for water retention and arthritis. North American Indians recommended alfalfa to treat jaundice and to encourage blood clotting.

Although conspicuously absent from many classic textbooks on herbal medicine, alfalfa did find a home in the texts of the Eclectic physicians as a tonic for indigestion, dyspepsia, anemia, loss of appetite, and poor assimilation of nutrients.[2] The plant was also recommended to stimulate lactation in nursing mothers. The seeds have also been traditionally made into a poultice for the treatment of boils and insect bites.

Active Constituents

The constituents in alfalfa are well studied. The leaves contain about 2–3% saponins.[3] Animal studies indicate that these constituents block absorption of cholesterol and prevent the formation of atherosclerotic plaques.[4] It should be noted that excess consumption of saponins may potentially cause damage to red blood cells in the body. The leaves also contain flavones, isoflavones, sterols, and coumarin derivatives. The isoflavones are probably the part of the plant responsible for the estrogen-like effects in animals. Although this has not been confirmed with human trials, it is used popularly to treat menopause

230

symptoms. Alfalfa also contains protein and vitamins A, B1, B6, C, E, and K. Nutrient analysis also demonstrates the presence of calcium, potassium, iron, and zinc.

How Much Should I Take?

Dried alfalfa leaf is available as a bulk herb and in tablets or capsules. It is also available in liquid extracts. No therapeutic dose of alfalfa has been established for humans. Some experts recommend 500–1,000 mg of the dried leaf per day or 1–2 ml of tincture.[5]

Are There Any Side Effects or Interactions?

Moderate use of the dried leaves of alfalfa is usually safe. There have been isolated reports of persons allergic to alfalfa. Ingestion of large amounts of the seed and/or sprouts has been linked to the onset of systemic lupus erythematosus (SLE) in animal studies.[6] SLE is a dangerous autoimmune illness that is characterized by inflamed joints and potential kidney damage. The chemical responsible for this effect is believed to be canavanine. Persons with SLE or with a history of SLE should avoid the use of alfalfa products.

ALOE *(Aloe vera, Aloe barbadensis)*

THE ALOE PLANT originally came from Africa. The leaves are used; they are long, green, fleshy, and have spikes along the edges. The fresh leaf gel and latex (the sticky residue left after the liquid from cut aloe leaves has evaporated) are used for many purposes.

In What Conditions Might Aloe Be Supportive?

- **Constipation** (page 32)
- **Diabetes** (page 39)
- Maintaining a healthy pancreas
- Minor burns
- Wound healing

Historical or Traditional Use

Aloe has been historically used for many of the same conditions it is used for today, particularly constipation and for minor cuts and burns. In India, it was also used to treat intestinal infections and for suppressed menses. The root was used for colic.

Active Constituents

The constituents that cause the cathartic laxative effects of aloe latex are known as anthraquinone glycosides. These molecules are split by the normal bacteria in the large intestines to form other molecules (aglycones), which exert the laxative action.

Aloe

Various constituents have been shown to have anti-inflammatory effects as well as to stimulate wound healing.[1] Preliminary evidence also suggests an antibacterial effect.[2]

How Much Should I Take?

For constipation, a single 50–200 mg capsule of aloe latex can be taken each day for a maximum of ten days.

Topically for minor burns, the stabilized aloe gel is applied to the affected area of skin three to five times per day. Treatment of more serious burns should only be done after first consulting a health care professional. For internal use of aloe gel, 30 ml three times per day is used by some people.

Are There Any Side Effects or Interactions?

Except in the rare person who is allergic to aloe, topical application of the gel is harmless. For any burn that blisters significantly or is otherwise severe, medical attention is absolutely essential. In some severe burns and wounds, aloe gel may actually impede healing.[3]

Laxative preparations, if used for more than ten consecutive days, can aggravate constipation and cause dependency. Constipation that does not resolve within a few days of use of laxatives may require medical attention.

ASIAN GINSENG *(Panax ginseng C.A. Meyer)*

COMMON NAMES: Korean ginseng, Chinese ginseng

ASIAN GINSENG is a member of the Araliaceae family, which also includes the closely related American ginseng, *Panax quinquefolius*, and less-similar Siberian ginseng, *Eleutherococcus senticosus*, also known as **eleuthero** (page 257). Asian ginseng commonly grows on mountain slopes and is usually harvested in the fall. The root is used.

In What Conditions Might Asian Ginseng Be Supportive?

- Aerobic capacity
- **Alzheimer's disease** (page 6)
- **Atherosclerosis** (page 11)
- **Athletic performance** (page 14)
- **Chemotherapy support** (page 25)
- Chronic fatigue syndrome
- **Common cold/sore throat** (page 28)
- **Diabetes** (page 39)
- Endurance and stress
- **Fibromyalgia** (page 53)
- Influenza (flu)
- Male reproductive system support

Historical or Traditional Use

Asian ginseng has been a part of Chinese medicine for over 2,000 years. The first reference to the health-enhancing use of Asian ginseng dates to the first century A.D., in which the writer mentions ginseng's use as follows: "It is used for repairing the five viscera, quieting the spirit, curbing the emotion, stopping agitation, removing noxious influence, brightening the eyes, enlightening the mind, and increasing wisdom. Continuous use leads one to longevity with light weight." Ginseng was commonly used by elderly persons in the Orient to improve mental and physical vitality.

Active Constituents

Ginseng's actions in the body are due to a complex interplay of constituents. The primary group are the ginsenosides, which are believed to increase energy, counter the effects of stress, and enhance intellectual and physical performance. Thirteen ginsenosides have been identified in Asian ginseng. Ginsenosides Rg1 and Rb1 have received the most attention.[1]

Other constituents include the panaxans, which help lower blood sugar, and the polysaccharides (complex sugar molecules), which support immune function.[2]

How Much Should I Take?

The best researched forms of ginseng are standardized herbal extracts that supply approximately 4–7% ginsenosides; more concentrated extracts may be less effective due to reduction of panaxan levels. People often take 100–200 mg per day. Nonstandardized extracts require a higher intake, generally 1–2 grams per day for tablets or 2–3 ml for fresh herb tincture. Ginseng is usually used for two to three weeks continuously, followed by a one- to two-week "rest" period before resuming.

Are There Any Side Effects or Interactions?

Used at the recommended dosage, ginseng is generally safe. In rare instances, it may cause overstimulation and possibly insomnia. Consuming caffeine with ginseng increases the risk of overstimulation and gastrointestinal upset. Persons with uncontrolled high blood pressure should not use ginseng. Long-term use of ginseng may cause menstrual abnormalities and breast tenderness in some women. Ginseng is not recommended for pregnant or lactating women.

ASTRAGALUS *(Astragalus membranaceus)*

COMMON NAME: Huang qi

ASTRAGALUS is native to northern China and the elevated regions of the Chinese provinces Yunnan and Sichuan. The portion of the plant used medicinally is the four- to seven-year-old dried root collected in the spring.

While there are over 2,000 types of astragalus worldwide, the Chinese version has been extensively tested, both chemically and pharmacologically.[1]

In What Conditions Might Astragalus Be Supportive?

- **Alzheimer's disease** (page 6)
- **Chemotherapy support** (page 25)
- **Common cold/sore throat** (page 28)
- **Immune function** (page 72)

Historical or Traditional Use

Shen Nong, the founder of Chinese herbal medicine, classified astragalus as a superior herb in his classical treatise *Shen Nong Pen Tsao Ching* (circa A.D. 100). The Chinese name huang qi translates as "yellow leader," referring to the yellow color of the root and its status as one of the most important tonic herbs. Traditional Chinese medicine utilized this herb for night sweats, deficiency of chi (e.g., fatigue, weakness, and loss of appetite), and diarrhea.[2]

Active Constituents

Astragalus contains numerous components, including flavonoids, polysaccharides, triterpene glycosides (e.g., astragalosides I–VII), amino acids, and trace minerals.[3] Research conducted by the M.D. Anderson Hospital in Houston, Texas, confirms this herb's immune-potentiating actions. Astragalus appears to restore T-cell (a specific type of white blood cell that is part of the lymphocyte family) counts to relatively normal ranges in some cancer patients.

How Much Should I Take?

Textbooks on Chinese herbs recommend taking 9–15 grams of the crude herb per day in decoction form. A decoction is made by boiling the root in water for a few minutes and then brewing the tea. Supplements typically contain 500 mg of astragalus. Two to three tablets or capsules or 3–5 ml of tincture three times per day are often recommended.

Are There Any Side Effects or Interactions?

Astragalus has no known side effects when used as recommended.

BILBERRY *(Vaccinium myrtillus)*

A CLOSE relative of American blueberry, bilberry grows in northern Europe, Canada, and the United States. The ripe berries are used. The leaves may also contain beneficial compounds.

In What Conditions Might Bilberry Be Supportive?

- **Atherosclerosis** (page 11)
- Bruising
- **Cataracts** (page 24)
- Circulation
- **Diabetes** (page 39)
- **Macular degeneration** (page 85)
- **Night blindness** (page 95)
- Retinopathy
- Varicose veins

Historical or Traditional Use

The dried berries and leaves of bilberry have been recommended for a wide variety of conditions, including scurvy, urinary tract infections, and kidney stones. Perhaps the most sound historical application is the use of the dried berries for the treatment of diarrhea. Modern research of bilberry was partly based on its use by British World War II pilots, who noticed that their night vision improved when they ate bilberry jam prior to night bombing raids.

Active Constituents

Anthocyanosides, the bioflavonoid complex in bilberries, are potent antioxidants.[1] They support normal formation of connective tissue and strengthen capillaries in the body. Anthocyanosides may also improve capillary and venous blood flow.

How Much Should I Take?

People often take 240–480 mg per day of bilberry herbal extract in capsules or tablets standardized to provide 25% anthocyanosides.

Are There Any Side Effects or Interactions?

In recommended amounts, there are no known side effects with bilberry extract. Bilberry does not interact with commonly prescribed drugs, and there are no known contraindications to its use during pregnancy or lactation.

BITTER MELON (Momordica charantia)

BITTER MELON grows in tropical areas, including parts of East Africa, Asia, the Caribbean, and South America, where it is used as a food as well as a medicine. The fruit of this plant lives up to its name—it tastes very bitter. Although the seeds, leaves, and vines of bitter melon have all been used, the fruit is the safest and most prevalent part of the plant used medicinally.

In What Conditions Might Bitter Melon Be Supportive?

- **Diabetes** (page 39)
- HIV support
- **Psoriasis** (page 112)

Historical or Traditional Use

Being a relatively common food item, bitter melon was traditionally used for a dazzling array of conditions by people in tropical regions. Numerous infections, cancer, and diabetes are among the most common conditions it was purported to improve.[1] The leaves and fruit have both been used occasionally to make teas and beer or to season soups in the Western world. The berries also produce wax, which can be made into candles.

Active Constituents

At least three different groups of constituents in bitter melon have been reported to have hypoglycemic (blood sugar lowering) or other actions of potential benefit in diabetes mellitus. These include a mixture of steroidal saponins known as charantin, insulin-like peptides, and alkaloids.[2] It is still unclear which of these is most effective or if all three work together. Two proteins, known as alpha- and beta-momorcharin, inhibit the AIDS virus, but this research has only been demonstrated in test tubes and not in humans.[3] An as yet unidentified constituent in bitter melon inhibits the enzyme guanylate cyclase, an act that may benefit people with psoriasis.

How Much Should I Take?

For those with a taste or tolerance for bitter flavor, a small melon can be eaten as food or up to 50 ml of fresh juice can be drunk per day. An option for those who do not care for the bitter taste are bitter melon tinctures, of which 5 ml is generally taken two to three times per day.

Are There Any Side Effects or Interactions?

Excessively high doses of bitter melon juice can cause abdominal pain and diarrhea. Small children or anyone with hypoglycemia should not take bitter melon because this herb could theoretically trigger or worsen low blood sugar (hypoglycemia). Furthermore, diabetics taking hypoglycemic drugs (such as chlorpropamide, glyburide, or phenformin) or insulin should use bitter melon only under medical supervision, as it may potentiate the effectiveness of the drugs and lead to severe hypoglycemia.

Special United Kingdom Considerations

Bitter melon is either not available or may require a prescription. Please check with your nutritionally oriented physician.

BLACK COHOSH *(Cimicifuga racemosa)*

BLACK COHOSH is a shrub-like plant native to the eastern deciduous forests of North America, ranging from southern Ontario to Georgia, north to Wisconsin and west to Arkansas.

The dried root and rhizome are the constituents utilized medicinally.[1] When wild harvested, the root is black in color. *Cohosh*, an Algonquin Indian word meaning "rough," refers to its gnarly root structure.[2]

In What Conditions Might Black Cohosh Be Supportive?

- **Menopause** (page 87)
- Painful menstruation
- Uterine spasms

Historical or Traditional Use

Native American Indians valued the herb and used it for many conditions, ranging from gynecological problems to rattlesnake bites. Some nineteenth-century American physicians used black cohosh for problems such as fever, menstrual cramps, arthritis, and insomnia.[3]

Active Constituents

Black cohosh contains several important ingredients, including triterpene glycosides (e.g., acetin and cimicifugoside) and isoflavones (e.g., formononetin). Other constituents include aromatic acids, tannins, resins, fatty acids, starches, and sugars. Formononetin is the active element in the herb that binds to estrogen receptor sites, inducing an estrogen-like activity in the body. As a woman approaches menopause, the signals between the ovaries and pituitary gland diminish, slowing down estrogen production and increasing luteinizing hormone (LH) secretions. Hot flashes can result from these hormonal changes. Clinical studies from Germany have demonstrated that an alcohol extract of black cohosh decreases LH secretions in menopausal women.[4]

How Much Should I Take?

Black cohosh can be taken in several forms, including crude, dried root, or rhizome (300–2,000 mg per day) or as a solid, dry powdered extract (250 mg three times per day). Tinctures can be taken at 2–4 ml per day.[5] Standardized extracts of the herb are available and contain 1 mg of deoxyacteine per tablet. The usual amount is 40 mg twice per day.[6] Black cohosh can be taken for up to six months, and then it should be discontinued.

Are There Any Side Effects or Interactions?

Black cohosh has an estrogen-like effect, and women who are pregnant or lactating should not use the herb. Large doses of this herb may cause abdominal pain, nausea, headaches, and dizziness. Women taking estrogen therapy should consult a physician before using black cohosh.

BLESSED THISTLE *(Cnicus benedictus)*

ALTHOUGH NATIVE to Europe and Asia, blessed thistle is now cultivated in many areas of the world, including the United States. The leaves, stems, and flowers are all used in herbal preparations.

In What Conditions Might Blessed Thistle Be Supportive?

- Indigestion and heartburn
- Poor appetite

Historical or Traditional Use

Folk medicine utilized blessed thistle tea for digestive problems, including gas, constipation, and stomach upset. This herb was also used for liver and gallbladder diseases, in a similar way as its well-known relative, **milk thistle** (page 290).[1]

Active Constituents

The sesquiterpene lactones, such as cnicin, provide the main beneficial effects of blessed thistle. The bitterness of these compounds stimulates digestive activity, including the flow of saliva and secretion of gastric juice, which leads to improved appetite and digestion.[2] There is some evidence that blessed thistle also has anti-inflammatory properties.

How Much Should I Take?

Many people take 2 ml three times per day of blessed thistle tincture. Approximately 2 grams of the dried herb can also be added to 250 ml (1 cup) of boiling water and steeped ten to fifteen minutes to make a tea. Three cups can be drunk each day.

Are There Any Side Effects or Interactions?

Blessed thistle is relatively safe and free from side effects. Anyone with allergies to plants in the daisy family should use blessed thistle cautiously.

BOSWELLIA *(Boswellia serrata)*

COMMON NAME: Salai guggal

BOSWELLIA is a moderate to large branching tree found in the dry, hilly areas of India. When the tree trunk is tapped, a gummy oleoresin is exuded. A purified extract of this resin is used in modern herbal preparations.

In What Conditions Might Boswellia Be Supportive?

- **Bursitis** (page 20)
- **Osteoarthritis** (page 97)
- **Rheumatoid arthritis** (page 115)

Historical or Traditional Use

In the ancient Ayurvedic medical texts of India, the gummy exudate from boswellia is grouped with other gum resins, which are referred to collectively as guggals. Historically, the guggals were recommended for a variety of conditions, including arthritis, diarrhea, dysentery, pulmonary disease, and ringworm.

Active Constituents

The gum oleoresin consists of essential oils, gum, and terpenoids. The terpenoid portion contains the boswellic acids that have been shown to be the active constituents in boswellia.[1] Today, extracts are typically standardized to contain 37.5–65% boswellic acids.

Studies have shown that the boswellic acids have an anti-inflammatory action—much like the conventional nonsteroidal anti-inflammatory drugs (NSAIDs) used by many for inflammatory conditions. Boswellia inhibits pro-inflammatory mediators in the body, such as leukotrienes.[2] As opposed to NSAIDs, long-term use of boswellia does not lead to irritation or ulceration of the stomach.

How Much Should I Take?

The standardized extract of the gum oleoresin of boswellia is recommended. For rheumatoid arthritis or osteoarthritis, many people take 150 mg three times per day. As an example, if an extract contains 37.5% boswellic acids, 400 mg of the extract should be taken three times per day. Treatment with boswellia generally lasts eight to twelve weeks.

Are There Any Side Effects or Interactions?

Boswellia is generally safe when used as directed. Rare side effects can include diarrhea, skin rash, and nausea. Any inflammatory joint condition should be closely monitored by a nutritionally oriented physician.

Special United Kingdom Considerations

Boswellia is either not available or may require a prescription. Please check with your nutritionally oriented physician.

BURDOCK (Arctium lappa)

BURDOCK is native to Asia and Europe. The root is the primary source of most herbal preparations. The root becomes very soft with chewing and tastes sweet, with a mucilaginous texture.

In What Conditions Might Burdock Be Supportive?

- Acne (page 5)
- Psoriasis (page 112)
- Rheumatoid arthritis (page 115)

Historical or Traditional Use

In traditional herbal texts, burdock root is described as a blood purifier or alterative.[1] Burdock root was believed to clear the bloodstream of toxins. It was used both internally and externally for eczema and psoriasis as well as to treat painful joints and as a diuretic. In traditional Chinese medicine, burdock root in combination with other herbs is used to treat sore throats, tonsillitis, colds, and even measles.[2] It is eaten as a vegetable in Japan and elsewhere.

Burdock root has recently become popular as part of a tea to treat cancer. To date, only minimal research has substantiated this application.[3]

Active Constituents

Burdock root contains high amounts of inulin and mucilage. This may explain its soothing effects on the gastrointestinal tract. Bitter constituents in the root may also explain the traditional use of burdock to improve digestion. It also contains polyacetylenes that have been shown to have antimicrobial activity.[4] Burdock root and fruit also have the ability to slightly lower blood sugar (hypoglycemic effect). Even though test-tube and animal studies have indicated some antitumor activity for burdock root, these results have not been duplicated in human studies.[5]

How Much Should I Take?

Traditional herbalists recommend 2–4 ml of burdock root tincture per day. For the dried root preparation in capsule form, the common amount to take is 1–2 grams three times per day. Many herbal preparations will combine burdock root with other alterative herbs, such as yellow dock, red clover, or cleavers.

Are There Any Side Effects or Interactions?

Use of burdock root in the dosages listed here is generally safe. However, burdock root in large quantities may stimulate the uterus and therefore should be used with caution during pregnancy.

BUTCHER'S BROOM (Ruscus aculeatus)

BUTCHER'S BROOM is a spiny, small-leafed evergreen bush native to the Mediterranean region and northwest Europe. It is a member of the lily family and is similar to asparagus in many ways. The roots and young stems of butcher's broom are used medicinally.

In What Conditions Might Butcher's Broom Be Supportive?

- **Atherosclerosis** (page 11)
- Chronic venous insufficiency
- **Hemorrhoids** (page 60)
- Varicose veins

Historical or Traditional Use

Butcher's broom is so named because the mature branches were bundled and used as brooms by butchers. The young shoots were sometimes eaten as food. Ancient physicians used the roots as a diuretic in the treatment of urinary problems.[1]

Active Constituents

Steroidal molecules called ruscogenin and neoruscogenin are responsible for the medicinal actions of butcher's broom.[2] Similar to diosgenin, found in **wild yam** (page 320), ruscogenins decrease vascular permeability—which accounts for the anti-inflammatory activity of this herb. Butcher's broom also causes small veins to constrict.[3][4]

How Much Should I Take?

Ointments and suppositories including butcher's broom are typically used for hemorrhoids. These are often applied or inserted at night before going to bed. Encapsulated butcher's broom extracts, often combined with vitamin C or flavonoids, can be used for systemic venous insufficiency in the amount of 1,000 mg three times per day. Alternatively, standardized extracts providing 50–100 mg of ruscogenins per day can be taken.

Are There Any Side Effects or Interactions?

There are no significant side effects or problems if butcher's broom is used in the amounts listed here.

Special United Kingdom Considerations

Butcher's broom is either not available or may require a prescription. Please check with your nutritionally oriented physician.

CALENDULA *(Calendula officinalis)*

COMMON NAME: Marigold

CALENDULA grows as a common garden plant throughout North America and Europe. The golden-orange or yellow flowers of calendula have been used as medicine for centuries.

In What Conditions Might Calendula Be Supportive?

- **Eczema** (page 49)
- Gastritis
- Minor burns (including sunburn)
- Wound healing

Historical or Traditional Use

Calendula flowers were historically considered beneficial for reducing inflammation, wound healing, and as an antiseptic. Calendula was used to treat various skin diseases, ranging from skin ulcerations to eczema.[1] Internally, the soothing effects of calendula have been used for stomach ulcers and inflammation. A sterile tea has also been applied in cases of conjunctivitis.

Active Constituents

The flavonoids, found in high amounts in calendula, account for much of its anti-inflammatory activity;[2]

triterpene saponins may also be important.[3] Calendula also contains carotenoids.

Investigations into anticancer and antiviral actions of calendula are continuing. At this time, there is insufficient evidence to recommend clinical use of calendula for cancer. There is evidence suggesting use of calendula for some viral infections. The constituents responsible for these actions are not entirely clear.

How Much Should I Take?

A tea of calendula can be made by pouring 200 ml of boiling water over 1–2 teaspoons of the flowers, which is steeped, covered for ten to fifteen minutes, strained, and then drunk. At least 3 cups of tea are generally drunk per day. Tincture is similarly used three times a day, taking 1–2 ml each time. The tincture can be taken in water or tea. Prepared ointments are often useful for skin problems, although wet dressings made by dipping cloth into the tea (after it has cooled) are also effective. Home treatment for eye conditions is not recommended, as absolute sterility must be maintained.

Are There Any Side Effects or Interactions?

Except for the very rare person who is allergic to calendula and therefore should not use it, there are no known side effects or interactions.

CAROB (Ceratonia siliqua)

COMMON NAME: St. John's bread

CAROB is originally from the Mediterranean region and the western part of Asia. Today it is grown mostly in Mediterranean countries. The pods are used. Carob pods come from evergreen trees; the gum from carob seeds is called locust bean gum.

In What Conditions Might Carob Be Supportive?

- Diarrhea (page 44)
- Indigestion and heartburn

Historical or Traditional Use

Carob has long been eaten as food. John the Baptist is said to have eaten it, and thus it is sometimes called St. John's bread. Carob pods have been used to treat diarrhea for centuries.

Active Constituents

The main constituents of carob are large carbohydrates (sugars) and tannins. The sugars make carob gummy and able to act as a thickener to absorb water and help bind together watery stools. Tannins from carob, being water insoluble, do not bind proteins as some tannins do. Carob tannins do bind to (and thereby inactivate) toxins and inhibit growth of bacteria—both of which are beneficial in the treatment of diarrhea. Dietary fiber and sugars may make food more viscous in the stomach and thus interfere with reflux of acid into the esophagus.[1]

How Much Should I Take?

Commonly, 15 grams of carob powder is mixed with applesauce for children. Adults should take at least 20 grams a day. The powder can be mixed in applesauce or with sweet potatoes. Carob should be taken with plenty of water. Please note that infant diarrhea must be monitored by a health care professional and that proper hydration with a high electrolyte fluid is critical during acute diarrhea.

Are There Any Side Effects or Interactions?

Carob is generally very safe; only rarely have allergic reactions been reported.

CASCARA *(Rhamnus purshiani cortex)*

COMMON NAMES: Cascara sagrada, sacred bark

CASCARA is a small- to medium-size tree native to the provinces and states of the Pacific coast, including British Columbia, Washington, Oregon, and Northern California. The bark of the tree is removed, cut into small pieces, and dried for one year before being used medicinally. Fresh bark has an emetic, or vomit-inducing, property and therefore is not used.

In What Conditions Might Cascara Be Supportive?

- Constipation (page 32)

Historical or Traditional Use

Northern California Indians introduced this herb, which they called sacred bark, to sixteenth-century Spanish explorers. Being much milder in its laxative action than the herb buckthorn, cascara became popular in Europe as a treatment for constipation. Cascara has been part of the *U.S. Pharmacopoeia* since 1890.[1]

Active Constituents

Cascara bark is high in hydroxyanthraquinone glycosides called cascarosides. Resins, tannins, and lipids make up the bulk of the other bark ingredients. Cascarosides have a cathartic action, inducing the large intestine to increase its muscular contraction (peristalsis), resulting in bowel movement.[2]

How Much Should I Take?

Only the dried form of cascara should be used. Two capsules containing dried cascara can be taken up to two times per day. As a tincture, 1–5 ml per day is generally taken. It is important to drink eight 6-ounce glasses of water throughout the day. Cascara should be taken for a maximum of eight to ten days.[3]

Are There Any Side Effects or Interactions?

Women who are pregnant or lactating should not use cascara without the advice of a physician. Those with an intestinal obstruction should not employ this herb. Long-term use or abuse of cascara may cause a loss of electrolytes (especially the mineral potassium) or weaken the colon. Loss of potassium may potentiate the action of digitalis-like medications with fatal consequences.

CATNIP (Nepeta cataria)

THE CATNIP PLANT grows in North America and Europe. The leaves and flowers are utilized as medicine.

In What Conditions Might Catnip Be Supportive?

- Cough
- **Insomnia** (page 79)

Historical or Traditional Use

Catnip is famous for inducing a delirious, stimulated state in felines. Throughout history, this herb has been used in humans to produce a sedative effect.[1] Catnip tea was a regular beverage in England before the introduction of tea from China.[2] Several other conditions (including cancer, toothache, corns, and hives) have been treated with catnip by traditional herbalists.

Active Constituents

The essential oil in catnip contains a monoterpene similar to the valepotriates found in valerian, an even more widely renowned sedative.[3] Animal studies (except those involving cats) have found it to increase sleep.[4] The monoterpenes also help with coughs.

How Much Should I Take?

A catnip tea can be made by adding 250 ml (1 cup) of boiling water to 1–2 teaspoons of the herb; cover, then steep for ten to fifteen minutes. Drink 2–3 cups per day. For children with coughs, 5 ml of tincture three times per day can be used.

Are There Any Side Effects or Interactions?

Using reasonable doses, no side effects with catnip have been noted.

CAT'S CLAW *(Uncaria tomentosa)*

CAT'S CLAW grows in the rain forests of the Andes mountains in South America, particularly in Peru. The root bark is used as medicine.

In What Conditions Might Cat's Claw Be Supportive?

- **Immune function** (page 72)
- Inflammation

Historical or Traditional Use

Cat's claw has been reportedly used by indigenous peoples in the Andes to treat inflammation, rheumatism, gastric ulcers, tumors, dysentery, and as birth control.[1] Cat's claw is popular in South American folk medicine for intestinal complaints, gastric ulcers, arthritis, and to promote wound healing.

Active Constituents

Oxyindole alkaloids appear to give cat's claw much of its activity, particularly to stimulate the immune system.[2] The alkaloids and other constituents, such as glycosides, may account for the anti-inflammatory and antioxidant actions of this herb.[3] [4]

Although cat's claw has become very popular in North America and is used for cancer and HIV, there is little scientific evidence to support the use of cat's claw for these conditions.

How Much Should I Take?

A cat's claw tea is prepared from 1 gram of root bark by adding 250 ml (1 cup) of water and boiling for ten

Cat's Claw

to fifteen minutes. After cooling and straining, one cup is drunk three times per day. Alternatively, 1–2 ml of tincture can be taken up to two times per day, or 20–60 mg of a standardized dry extract can be taken per day.

multiple sclerosis, and tuberculosis. European practitioners avoid combining this herb with hormonal drugs, insulin, or vaccines. Cat's claw, until proven safe, should be taken only with great caution by pregnant or lactating women.

Are There Any Side Effects or Interactions?

No serious adverse effects have yet been reported. Cat's claw is contraindicated in autoimmune illness,

CAYENNE *(Capsicum annuum, Capsicum frutescens)*

ORIGINALLY FROM South America, the cayenne plant has spread across the globe both as a food and as a medicine. Cayenne is very closely related to bell peppers, jalapeños, paprika, and other similar peppers. The fruit is used.

In What Conditions Might Cayenne Be Supportive?

- **Bursitis** (page 20)
- Diabetic neuropathy
- **Osteoarthritis** (page 97)
- **Psoriasis** (page 112)
- **Rheumatoid arthritis** (page 115)
- Shingles (herpes zoster)/postherpetic neuralgia

Historical or Traditional Use

The potent, hot fruit of cayenne has been used as medicine for centuries. It was considered helpful for various conditions of the gastrointestinal tract, including stomachaches, cramping pains, and gas. Cayenne was frequently used to treat diseases of the circulatory system. It is still traditionally used in herbal medicine as a circulatory tonic (a substance believed to improve circulation). Rubbed on the skin, cayenne is a traditional, as well as modern, remedy for rheumatic pains and arthritis due to what is termed a counterirritant effect. A counterirritant is something that causes irritation to a tissue to which it is applied, thus distracting from the original irritation (such as joint pain in the case of arthritis).

Active Constituents

Cayenne contains a resinous and pungent substance known as capsaicin. This chemical relieves pain and itching by acting on sensory nerves. Capsaicin temporarily stimulates release of various neurotransmitters from these nerves, leading to their depletion. Without the neurotransmitters, pain signals can no longer be sent.[1] The effect is temporary. Capsaicin and other constituents in cayenne have been shown to have several other actions, including reducing platelet stickiness and acting as antioxidants.

How Much Should I Take?

Creams containing 0.025–0.075% capsaicin are generally used. There may be a burning sensation for the first several times the cream is applied, but this should gradually decrease with each use. The hands must be carefully and thoroughly washed after use, or gloves should be worn, to prevent the cream from accidentally reaching the eyes, nose, or mouth, which would cause a burning sensation. Do not apply the cream to areas of broken skin. A cayenne tincture can be used in the amount of 0.3–1 ml three times daily.

Are There Any Side Effects or Interactions?

Besides causing a mild burning for the first few applications (or severe burning if accidentally placed in sensitive areas, such as the eyes), there are no side effects from use of the capsaicin cream. Very high intake of cayenne internally may cause ulcers, but the necessary amount is rarely achieved with sensible intake.

As with anything applied to the skin, some people may have an allergic reaction to the cream, so the first application should be to a very small area of skin.

CHAMOMILE *(Matricaria recutita)*

CHAMOMILE, a member of the daisy family, is native to Europe and western Asia. German chamomile is the most commonly used. The dried flowers are utilized medicinally.

In What Conditions Might Chamomile Be Supportive?

- Blocked tear duct
- **Canker sores (mouth ulcers)** (page 21)
- Colic
- **Diarrhea** (page 44)
- **Eczema** (page 49)
- **Gingivitis (periodontal disease)** (page 56)
- Indigestion and heartburn
- **Insomnia** (page 79)
- **Irritable bowel syndrome** (page 81)
- **Peptic ulcer** (page 103)
- Skin irritations

Historical or Traditional Use

Chamomile has been used for centuries as a medicinal plant, mostly for gastrointestinal complaints. This practice continues today.

Active Constituents

The flowers of chamomile provide 1–2% volatile oils containing alpha-bisabolol, alpha-bisabolol oxides A & B, and matricin (usually converted to chamazulene). Other active constituents include the bioflavonoids apigenin, luteolin, and **quercetin** (page 201).[1] These active ingredients contribute to chamomile's anti-inflammatory, antispasmodic, and smooth muscle-relaxing effects, particularly in the gastrointestinal tract.[2 3 4 5]

How Much Should I Take?

Chamomile is often taken as a tea that can be drunk three to four times daily between meals. Common alternatives are to use tablets, capsules, or tinctures. Many people take 2–3 grams of the capsules or tablets or 4–6 ml of the tincture three times per day between meals.

Are There Any Side Effects or Interactions?

Though rare, allergic reactions to chamomile have been reported. These reactions have included bronchial constriction with internal use and allergic skin reactions with topical use. While such side effects are extremely uncommon, persons with allergies to plants of the Asteraceae family (ragweed, aster, and chrysanthemum) should avoid use of chamomile. There are no contraindications to the use of chamomile during pregnancy or lactation.

CHICKWEED *(Stellaria media)*

THE UBIQUITOUS, small, green chickweed plant grows across the United States and originated in Europe. The leaves, stems, and flowers are used in botanical medicine.

In What Conditions Might Chickweed Be Supportive?

- **Eczema** (page 49)
- Insect stings and bites

Historical or Traditional Use

Chickweed was reportedly used at times for food.[1] Chickweed enjoys a reputation as treating a wide spectrum of conditions in folk medicine, ranging from asthma and indigestion to skin diseases. Traditional Chinese herbalists used a tea made from chickweed to treat nosebleeds.

Active Constituents

The active constituents in chickweed are largely unknown. It contains relatively high amounts of vitamins and flavonoids, which may explain some of its effect. Although some older information suggests a possible benefit for chickweed in rheumatic conditions, this has not been validated in clinical practice.[2]

How Much Should I Take?

Although formerly used as a tea, chickweed's main use today is as a cream applied liberally several times each day to rashes and inflammatory skin conditions (e.g., eczema) to ease itching and inflammation. As a tincture, 1–5 ml per day can be taken.

Are There Any Side Effects or Interactions?

No side effects with chickweed have been reported.

CRANBERRY *(Vaccinium macrocarpon)*

CRANBERRY is a member of the same family as bilberry. It is from North American and grows in bogs. The ripe fruit is used.

In What Conditions Might Cranberry Be Supportive?

- Urinary tract infection (page 120)

Historical or Traditional Use

Cranberry has been used to prevent kidney stones and "bladder gravel" as well as to remove toxins from the blood. Cranberry has long been recommended for persons with recurrent urinary tract infections (UTIs).

Active Constituents

Cranberry prevents *E. coli*, the most common cause of UTIs and recurrent UTIs, from adhering to the cells lining the wall of the bladder. This antiadherence action renders the bacteria harmless in the urinary tract.[1][2] The constituents in cranberry responsible for this antiadherence activity have yet to be identified.

How Much Should I Take?

People often take one capsule or tablet of a concentrated cranberry juice extract two to four times per day. Several glasses (16 ounces total) of a high-quality cranberry juice (not the cocktail) each day can approximate the effect of the cranberry concentrate.

Are There Any Side Effects or Interactions?

There are no known side effects with cranberry concentrate, and it is safe for use during pregnancy and lactation. Cranberry should not be used as a substitute for antibiotics during an acute urinary tract infection.

DAMIANA *(Turnera diffusa)*

THE LEAVES of damiana were originally used as medicine by the indigenous cultures of Central America, particularly Mexico. Today the plant is found in hot, humid climates, including parts of Texas.

In What Conditions Might Damiana Be Supportive?

- **Depression** (page 36)
- Impotence/**infertility** **(male)** (page 77)

Historical or Traditional Use

Damiana has been hailed as an aphrodisiac since ancient times, particularly by the native peoples of Mexico.[1] Other folk uses have included asthma, bronchitis, neurosis, and various sexual disorders.[2] It has also been promoted as a euphoria-inducing substance at various times.

Active Constituents

Most research has been done on the essential oil of damiana, which includes numerous small, fragrant substances called terpenes. As yet, it is unclear if the essential oil is truly the main active fraction of damiana. The leaves also contain the antimicrobial substance arbutin, alkaloids, and other potentially important compounds.[3]

How Much Should I Take?

To make a tea, add 250 ml (1 cup) boiling water to 1 gram of dried leaves; allow to steep ten to fifteen minutes. Drink three cups per day. To use in tincture form, take 2–3 ml three times per day. Tablets or capsules may also be used in the amount of 400–800 mg three times per day. Damiana is not usually used alone; it is believed to be more effective when combined with other herbs of similar or complementary activity.

Are There Any Side Effects or Interactions?

Higher doses of damiana may induce a mild sense of euphoria. The leaves have a minor laxative effect, which is more pronounced at higher intakes, and may cause loosening of stools.[4]

DANDELION *(Taraxacum officinale)*

CLOSELY RELATED to chicory, dandelion is a common plant worldwide and the bane of those looking for the perfect lawn. The plant grows to a height of about 12 inches, producing spatula-like leaves and yellow flowers that bloom year-round. Upon maturation, the flower turns into the characteristic puffball containing seeds that are dispersed in the wind. Dandelion is grown commercially in the United States and Europe. The leaves and root are used in herbal supplements.

In What Conditions Might Dandelion Be Supportive?

Leaves:
- **Constipation** (page 32)
- Indigestion and heartburn
- **Pregnancy support** (page 107)
- Water retention

Root:
- Alcoholism
- **Constipation** (page 32)
- Indigestion and heartburn
- Liver support
- **Pregnancy support** (page 107)

Historical or Traditional Use

Dandelion is commonly used as a food. The leaves are used in salads and teas, while the roots are often used as a coffee substitute. Dandelion leaves and roots have been used for hundreds of years to treat liver, gallbladder, kidney, and joint problems. In some traditions, dandelion is considered a blood purifier and is used for ailments as varied as eczema and cancer. As is the case today, dandelion has also been used historically to treat poor digestion, water retention, and diseases of the liver, including hepatitis.

Dandelion

Active Constituents

The principal constituents responsible for dandelion's effect on the digestive system and liver are the bitter principles. Previously referred to as taraxacin, these constituents are sesquiterpene lactones of the eudesmanolide and germacranolide type and are unique to dandelion.[1] Dandelion is also a rich source of vitamins and minerals. The leaves have a very high content of vitamin A as well as moderate amounts of vitamin D, vitamin C, various B vitamins, iron, silicon, magnesium, zinc, and manganese.[2] The leaves are a rich source of potassium, which is interesting since the leaves are used for their diuretic action. This may make dandelion the only naturally occurring potassium-sparing diuretic, although its diuretic action is likely different from that of pharmaceuticals.

At high doses, the leaves have been shown to possess diuretic effects comparable to the prescription diuretic frusemide (Lasix).[3] Since clinical data in humans is sparse, it is advisable to seek the guidance of a physician trained in herbal medicine before using dandelion leaves for water retention.

The bitter compounds in the leaves and root help stimulate digestion and are mild laxatives.[4] These bitter principles also increase bile production in the gallbladder and bile flow from the liver.[5] This makes them a particularly useful tonic for persons with sluggish liver function due to alcohol abuse or poor diet. The increase in bile flow will help improve fat (including cholesterol) metabolism in the body.

How Much Should I Take?

As a general liver/gallbladder tonic and to stimulate digestion, 3–5 grams of the dried root or 5–10 ml of a tincture made from the root can be used three times per day. Some experts recommend the alcohol-based tincture because the bitter principles are more soluble in alcohol.[6]

As a mild diuretic or appetite stimulant, 4–10 grams of dried leaves can be added to 250 ml (1 cup) of boiling water and drunk as a decoction; or 5–10 ml of fresh juice from the leaves or 2–5 ml of tincture made from the leaves can be used three times per day.

Are There Any Side Effects or Interactions?

Dandelion leaf and root should be used with caution by persons with gallstones. If there is an obstruction of the bile ducts, then dandelion should be avoided altogether. In cases of stomach ulcer or gastritis, dandelion should be used cautiously, as it may cause overproduction of stomach acid. Those experiencing fluid or water retention should consult a nutritionally oriented doctor before taking dandelion leaves. People taking the leaves should be sure that their doctors monitor potassium levels. The milky latex in the stem and leaves of fresh dandelion may cause an allergic rash in some individuals.

DEVIL'S CLAW *(Harpogophytum procumbens)*

DEVIL'S CLAW is a native plant of southern Africa, especially the Kalahari desert, Namibia, and the island of Madagascar. The name devil's claw is derived from the herb's unusual fruits, which seem to be covered with numerous small hooks. The secondary storage roots, or tuber, of the plant are employed in herbal supplements.[1]

In What Conditions Might Devil's Claw Be Supportive?

- Indigestion and heartburn
- **Rheumatoid arthritis** (page 115)

Historical or Traditional Use

Numerous tribes native to southern Africa have utilized devil's claw for a wide variety of conditions, ranging from gastrointestinal difficulties to arthritic conditions.[2] Devil's claw has been widely used in Europe as a treatment for arthritis.

Active Constituents

Devil's claw tuber contains three important constituents belonging to the iridoid glycoside family: harpagoside, harpagide, and procumbide. The secondary tubers of the herb contain twice as much harpagoside as the primary tubers. As such, these secondary tubers contain the preferable concentration of active ingredients.[3] Harpagoside and other iridoid glycosides found in the plant may be responsible for the herb's anti-inflammatory and analgesic actions. However, research has not entirely supported the use of devil's claw in alleviating arthritic pain symptoms.[4,5]

Devil's claw is also considered by herbalists to be a potent bitter. Bitter principles, like the iridoid glycosides found in devil's claw, stimulate the stomach to increase the production of acid, thereby helping to improve digestion.

How Much Should I Take?

For use as a digestive stimulant, the dose for the powdered secondary tuber is 1.5–2 grams per day.

For tincture, the recommended amount is 1–2 ml per day. For arthritis, many people take 4.5–10 grams per day. Again, recent studies do not support devil's claw as a treatment for arthritis.

Are There Any Side Effects or Interactions?

Because devil's claw promotes stomach acid, anyone with gastric or duodenal ulcers should not use the herb.

DONG QUAI *(Angelica sinensis)*

DONG QUAI is a member of the celery family. Greenish-white flowers bloom from May to August, and the plant is typically found growing in damp mountain ravines, meadows, riverbanks, and coastal areas. The root is used.

In What Conditions Might Dong Quai Be Supportive?

- Fibrocystic breast disease (page 51)
- Menopause (page 87)
- Premenstrual syndrome (page 109)

Historical or Traditional Use

Also known as dang-gui in traditional Chinese medicine, dong quai is often referred to as the "female ginseng." In traditional Chinese medicine, dong quai is often included in prescriptions for abnormal menstruation, suppressed menstrual flow, painful or difficult menstruation, and uterine bleeding. A traditional use of dong quai was for hot flashes associated with perimenopause. Dong quai is also used for both men and women with cardiovascular disease, including high blood pressure and problems with peripheral circulation.[1]

Active Constituents

Traditionally, dong quai is believed to have a balancing or adaptogenic effect on the female hormonal system. Contrary to the opinion of several authors, dong quai does not qualify as a phytoestrogen or have any hormone-like actions in the body. A large part of its actions with regard to premenstrual syndrome may be related to its antispasmodic actions, particularly on smooth muscles.[2]

How Much Should I Take?

The powdered root can be used in capsules, tablets, tinctures, or as a tea. Many women take 3–4 grams per day.

Are There Any Side Effects or Interactions?

Dong quai is generally considered to be of extremely low toxicity. It may cause some fair-skinned persons to become more sensitive to sunlight. Persons using it on a regular basis should limit prolonged exposure to the sun or other sources of ultraviolet radiation. Dong quai is not recommended for pregnant or lactating women.

ECHINACEA *(Echinacea purpurea, Echinacea angustifolia)*

COMMON NAME: Purple coneflower

ECHINACEA is a wildflower native to North America. While echinacea continues to grow and is harvested from the wild, the majority of that used for herbal supplements is from cultivated plants. The root or aboveground part of the plant during the flowering growth phase is used medicinally.

In What Conditions Might Echinacea Be Supportive?

- Canker sores (**mouth ulcers**) (page 21)
- **Common cold/sore throat** (page 28)
- **Crohn's disease** (page 34)
- **Gingivitis (periodontal disease)** (page 56)
- **Immune function** (page 72)
- Influenza (flu)
- **Recurrent ear infection** (page 47)
- **Yeast infection** (page 127)

Historical or Traditional Use

Echinacea was used by American Indians for a variety of conditions, including venomous bites and other external wounds. It was introduced into U.S. medical practice in 1887 and was touted for use in conditions ranging from colds to syphilis. Modern research started in the 1930s in Germany.

Active Constituents

Echinacea supports the immune system. Several constituents in echinacea team together to increase the production and activity of white blood cells, lymphocytes, and macrophages. Echinacea also increases production of interferon, an important part of the body's response to viral infections such as colds and flu.[1]

How Much Should I Take?

As an immune system stimulant, echinacea is best taken for a specific period of time. At the onset of a cold, it can be taken three to four times per day for ten to fourteen days. To prevent a cold, many people take echinacea tablets or capsules three times per day for six to eight weeks. A "rest" period is recommended after this, as echinacea's effects may diminish if used longer. If preferred, powdered echinacea, in about 900 mg amounts, can be taken. Liquid extracts are typically taken as 3–4 ml, three times per day.

Are There Any Side Effects or Interactions?

Echinacea is essentially nontoxic when taken orally. People should not take echinacea without consulting a physician if they have an autoimmune illness, such as lupus, or other progressive diseases, such as tuberculosis or multiple sclerosis. Those who are allergic to flowers of the daisy family should take echinacea with caution. There are no known contraindications to the use of echinacea during pregnancy or lactation.

ELDERBERRY (Sambucus nigra)

ELDER OR elderberry grows in Europe and North America. The flowers and berries are used therapeutically.

In What Conditions Might Elderberry Be Supportive?

- **Common cold/sore throat** (page 28)
- Herpes simplex
- Inflammation
- Influenza (flu)

Historical or Traditional Use

Elderberries have long been used as food, particularly in the dried form. Elderberry wine, pie, and lemonade are some of the popular ways to prepare this plant as food. The leaves were touted to be pain relieving and to promote healing of injuries when applied as a poultice.[1] Native Americans used the plant for infections, coughs, and skin conditions.

Active Constituents

The flavonoids, including **quercetin** (page 201), are believed to account for the therapeutic effects of the elderberry flowers and berries. According to laboratory research, an extract from the leaves, combined with **St. John's wort** (page 312) and soapwort, inhibits the influenza virus and herpes simplex virus.[2] A study in humans determined that an extract of elderberries is an effective treatment for influenza.[3] Animal studies have shown the flowers to have anti-inflammatory properties.[4]

How Much Should I Take?

Liquid elderberry extract is taken in amounts of 5 ml (for children) to 10 ml (for adults) twice per day.

A tea made from 3–5 grams of the dried flowers steeped in 250 ml (1 cup) boiling water for ten to fifteen minutes may also be drunk three times per day.

Are There Any Side Effects or Interactions?

There are no known adverse reactions to elderberry.

ELEUTHERO
(Eleutherococcus senticosus, Acanthopanax senticosus)

COMMON NAMES: Siberian ginseng, ci wu ju

ELEUTHERO belongs to the Araliaceae family and is a distant relative of Asian ginseng (*Panax ginseng*). Also known commonly as touch-me-not and devil's shrub, eleuthero has been most frequently nicknamed Siberian ginseng in this country. Eleuthero is native to the Taiga region of the Far East (southeastern part of Russia, northern China, Korea, and Japan). The root and the rhizomes (underground stem) are used.

In What Conditions Might Eleuthero Be Supportive?

- **Alzheimer's disease** (page 6)
- **Athletic performance** (page 14)
- Attention deficit disorder
- **Chemotherapy support** (page 25)
- Chronic fatigue syndrome
- **Common cold/sore throat** (page 28)
- **Diabetes** (page 39)
- **Fibromyalgia** (page 53)
- Influenza (flu)
- Stress and fatigue

Historical or Traditional Use

Although not as popular as Asian ginseng, eleuthero use dates back 2,000 years, according to Chinese medicine records. Referred to as ci wu ju in Chinese medicine, it was used to prevent respiratory tract infections as well as colds and flu. It was also believed to provide energy and vitality. In Russia, eleuthero was originally used by people in the Siberian Taiga

Eleuthero

region to increase performance and quality of life and to decrease infections.

In more modern times, eleuthero's ability to increase stamina and endurance led Soviet Olympic athletes to use it to enhance their training. Explorers, divers, sailors, and miners used eleuthero to prevent stress-related illness. After the Chernobyl accident, many Russian citizens were given eleuthero to counteract the effects of radiation.

Active Constituents

The constituents in eleuthero that have received the most attention are the eleutherosides.[1] Seven primary eleutherosides have been identified, with most of the research attention focusing on eleutherosides B and E.[2] Eleuthero also contains complex polysaccharides (a kind of sugar molecule).[3] These constituents play a critical role in eleuthero's ability to support immune function.

As an adaptogen, eleuthero helps the body adapt to stress. It does this by encouraging normal functioning of the adrenal glands, allowing them to function optimally when challenged by stress.[4]

Eleuthero has been shown to enhance mental acuity and physical endurance without the letdown that comes with caffeinated products.[5] Research has shown that eleuthero improves the use of oxygen by the exercising muscle. This means that a person is able to maintain aerobic exercise longer and recovery from workouts is much quicker.[6]

Another way that eleuthero reduces stress on the body is to combat harmful toxins. Eleuthero has shown a protective effect in animal studies against chemicals such as ethanol, sodium barbital, tetanus toxoid, and chemotherapeutic agents.[7] Eleuthero also reduces the side effects of radiation exposure.[8]

Evidence is also mounting that eleuthero enhances and supports the immune response. Eleuthero may be useful as a preventive measure during cold and flu season. Recent evidence also suggests that eleuthero may prove valuable in the long-term management of various diseases of the immune system, including HIV infection, chronic fatigue syndrome, and autoimmune illnesses such as lupus.[9]

How Much Should I Use?

Dried, powdered root and rhizomes of 2–3 grams per day can be used. Concentrated solid extract standardized on eleutherosides B and E, 300–400 mg per day, can also be used, as can alcohol-based extracts, 8–10 ml in two to three divided dosages. Historically, eleuthero is taken continuously for six to eight weeks, followed by a one- to two-week break before resuming.

Are There Any Side Effects or Interactions?

Reported side effects have been minimal with use of eleuthero. Mild, transient diarrhea has been reported in a very small number of users. Eleuthero may cause insomnia in some people if taken too close to bedtime. Eleuthero is not recommended for individuals with uncontrolled high blood pressure. It can be used during pregnancy or lactation. However, pregnant or lactating women using eleuthero should avoid products that have been adulterated with *Panax ginseng* or other related species that are contraindicated.

EPHEDRA *(Ephedra sinica, Ephedra intermedia, Ephedra equisetina)*

COMMON NAME: Ma huang

EPHEDRA is a shrublike plant found in desert regions throughout the world. It is distributed from northern China to Inner Mongolia. The dried green stems of the three Asian species (*E. sinica, intermedia, equisetina*) are the plant parts employed medicinally. The North American species of ephedra does not appear to contain the active ingredients of its Asian counterparts.

In What Conditions Might Ephedra Be Supportive?

- **Asthma** (page 9)
- Congestion
- Cough
- **Weight loss and obesity** (page 124)

Historical or Traditional Use

The Chinese have used ephedra medicinally for over 5,000 years. Ephedra is listed as one of the original 365 herbs from the classical first century A.D. text on Chinese herbalism by Shen Nong.[1] Ephedra's traditional medicinal uses include the alleviation of sweating, lung and bronchial constriction, and water retention. Coughing, shortness of breath, the common cold, and fevers without sweat are all indications for its use. While the active constituent, ephedrine, was isolated in 1887, it was not until 1924 that the herb became popular with physicians in the U.S. for its bronchodilating and decongesting properties.[2]

Active Constituents

Ephedra's active medicinal ingredients are the alkaloids ephedrine and pseudoephedrine. The stem contains 1–3% total alkaloids, with ephedrine accounting for 30–90% of this total, depending on the plant species employed.[3] Both ephedrine and its synthetic counterparts stimulate the central nervous system, dilate the bronchial tubes, elevate blood pressure, and increase heart rate. Pseudoephedrine (the synthetic form) is a popular over-the-counter remedy for relief of nasal congestion.

How Much Should I Take?

The crude powdered stems of ephedra (with less than 1% ephedrine) are employed at a dose of 1–4

Ephedra

grams per day in tea form. Tinctures of 1–4 ml three times per day can be taken. Over-the-counter drugs containing ephedrine can be safely used by adults at a dose of 12.5–25 mg every four hours. Adults should take no more than 150 mg every twenty-four hours. Pseudoephedrine is typically recommended at a dose of 60 mg every six hours.

Are There Any Side Effects or Interactions?

Ephedra has a long history of safe use at the recommended amount. However, abuse of the drug—especially for weight loss—can lead to amphetamine-like side effects, including elevated blood pressure, muscle disturbances, insomnia, dry mouth, heart palpitations, nervousness, and even death due to heart failure.

Anyone with high blood pressure, heart conditions, diabetes, glaucoma, thyroid disease, and those taking MAO-inhibiting antidepressants should consult with a physician before using any type of product with ephedra. Pseudoephedrine can cause drowsiness and should be used with caution if driving or operating machinery. Ephedra-based products should be avoided during pregnancy and lactation and used with caution in children under the age of six years.

Special United Kingdom Considerations

Ephedra is either not available or may require a prescription. Please check with your nutritionally oriented physician.

EYEBRIGHT *(Euphrasia officinalis)*

EUPHRASIA OFFICINALIS has been used to refer to a vast genus containing over 450 species. European wild plants grow in meadows, pastures, and grassy places in Bulgaria, Hungary, and the former Yugoslavia. Eyebright is also grown commercially in Europe. The plant flowers in late summer and autumn. The whole herb is used in commercial preparations.

In What Conditions Might Eyebright Be Supportive?

- Blepharitis (inflammation of the eyelids)
- Conjunctivitis
- Irritated eyes

Historical or Traditional Use

Eyebright was and continues to be used primarily as a poultice for the topical treatment of eye inflammations, including blepharitis, conjunctivitis, and styes. A compress made from a decoction of eyebright can give rapid relief from redness, swelling, and visual disturbances in acute and subacute eye infections.[1] A tea is usually given internally along with the topical treatment. It has also been used for the treatment of eye fatigue and disturbances of vision. In addition, herbalists have recommended eyebright for problems of the respiratory tract, including sinus infections, coughs, and sore throat.[2]

Active Constituents

Eyebright is high in iridoid glycosides, flavonoids, and tannins.[3] The plant has astringent properties that probably account for its usefulness as a topical treatment for inflammatory states and its ability to reduce mucous drainage.

How Much Should I Take?

Traditional herbal texts recommend a compress made with 1 tablespoon of the dried herb combined with 0.5 liter of water and boiled for ten minutes. The undiluted liquid is used as a compress after cooling. This was commonly combined with antimicrobial herbs, such as goldenseal. The current German monograph on eyebright does not support this application, due to potential bacterial concerns.[4]

Internally, eyebright tea, made using the same formula above, can be drunk in the amount of two to three cups per day. Dried herb, as 2–4 grams three times per day, may be taken. The tincture is typically taken in 2–6 ml doses three times per day.

Are There Any Side Effects or Interactions?

Due to limited information on the active constituents in eyebright and the need for sterility in substances used topically in the eyes, the traditional use of eyebright as a topical compress currently cannot be recommended. Used internally at the amounts listed above, eyebright is generally safe. However, its safety during pregnancy and lactation has not been proven.

FENNEL *(Foeniculum vulgare)*

THE FENNEL PLANT came originally from Europe, where it is still grown. Fennel is also cultivated in many parts of Asia and Egypt. Fennel seeds are utilized for medicinal purposes.

In What Conditions Might Fennel Be Supportive?

- Colic
- Indigestion
- **Irritable bowel syndrome** (page 81)

Historical or Traditional Use

One author reports that fennel may have bestowed immortality in the Greek legend of Prometheus.[1] Fennel seeds are a common cooking spice, particularly for use with fish. After meals, they are used in several cultures to prevent gas and upset stomach.[2] The seeds are also used in Latin America to increase the flow of breast milk. Fennel has also been used as a remedy for cough and colic in infants.

Active Constituents

The main active constituents, which includes the terpenoid anethole, are found in the volatile oil. Anethole and other terpenoids may have estrogen-like activity and inhibit spasms in smooth muscles, such as those in the intestinal tract. Recent studies have found fennel to possess diuretic, choleretic (increase in production of bile), pain-reducing, fever-reducing, and antimicrobial actions.[3]

How Much Should I Take?

Whole seeds may be chewed or used in tea. To make a tea, boil $1/2$ teaspoon of crushed seeds in 250 ml (1 cup) of water for ten to fifteen minutes, keeping the pot covered during the process. Cool, strain, and then drink three cups per day. As a tincture, 2–4 ml can be taken three times per day.

Are There Any Side Effects or Interactions?

No significant adverse effects have been reported. Pregnant or lactating women, as well as anyone with an estrogen-dependent cancer, should avoid fennel in large quantities until the importance of its estrogen-like activity is clarified.

FENUGREEK *(Trigonella foenum-graecum)*

ALTHOUGH ORIGINALLY from southeastern Europe and western Asia, fenugreek grows today in many parts of the world, including India, northern Africa, and the United States. The seeds of fenugreek contain the most potent medicinal effects of the plant.

In What Conditions Might Fenugreek Be Supportive?

- **Atherosclerosis** (page 11)
- **Constipation** (page 32)
- **Diabetes** (page 39)
- **High cholesterol** (page 62)
- **Hypertriglyceridemia (high triglycerides)** (page 69)

Historical or Traditional Use

A wide range of uses were found for fenugreek in ancient times. Medicinally it was used for the treatment of wounds, abscesses, arthritis, bronchitis, and digestive problems. Traditional Chinese herbalists used it for kidney problems and conditions affecting the male reproductive tract.[1] Fenugreek was, and remains, a food and a spice commonly eaten in many parts of the world.

Active Constituents

The steroidal saponins account for many of the beneficial effects of fenugreek, particularly the inhibition of cholesterol absorption and synthesis.[2] The seeds are rich in dietary **fiber** (page 159), which may be the main reason it can lower blood sugar levels in diabetes.[3]

How Much Should I Take?

Due to the somewhat bitter taste of fenugreek seeds, debitterized seeds or encapsulated products are preferred. The typical range of intake is 5–30 grams with each meal or 15–90 grams all at once with one meal.

Are There Any Side Effects or Interactions?

Use of more than 100 grams of seeds daily can cause intestinal upset and nausea. Otherwise, fenugreek is extremely safe.

FEVERFEW *(Tanacetum parthenium)*

FEVERFEW grows widely across Europe. The leaves are used.

In What Conditions Might Feverfew Be Supportive?

- **Migraine headaches** (page 91)

Historical or Traditional Use

Feverfew was mentioned in Greek medical literature as a remedy for inflammation and for menstrual discomforts. Traditional herbalists in Great Britain used it to treat fevers, arthritis, and other aches and pains.

Active Constituents

Feverfew contains a range of compounds known as sesquiterpene lactones. Over 85% of these are a compound called parthenolide. Parthenolide helps prevent excessive clumping of platelets and inhibits the release of certain chemicals, including serotonin and some inflammatory mediators.[1,2] This may reduce the severity, duration, and frequency of migraine headaches and improve blood vessel tone.

Feverfew

How Much Should I Take?

Feverfew leaf extracts with at least 0.2% parthenolide content are generally used. Herbal extracts in capsules or tablets providing at least 250 mg of parthenolide per day are taken. It may take four to six weeks before benefits are noticed.

Are There Any Side Effects or Interactions?

Taken as recommended, standardized feverfew causes minimal side effects. Minor side effects include gastrointestinal upset and nervousness. Feverfew is not recommended during pregnancy or lactation and should not be used by children under the age of two years.

FO-TI *(Polygonum multiflorum)*

COMMON NAME:

He-shou-wu

FO-TI is a plant native to China, where it continues to be widely grown. It is also grown extensively in Japan and Taiwan. The unprocessed root is sometimes used. However, once it has been boiled in a special liquid made from black beans, it is considered a superior and rather different medicine according to traditional Chinese medicine. The unprocessed root is sometimes called white fo-ti and the processed root red fo-ti.

In What Conditions Might Fo-Ti Be Supportive?

- **Atherosclerosis** (page 11)
- **Constipation** (page 32)
- Fatigue
- **High cholesterol** (page 62)
- **Immune function** (page 72)

Historical or Traditional Use

The Chinese common name for fo-ti, he-shou-wu, was the name of a Tang dynasty man whose infertility was supposedly cured by fo-ti; in addition, his long life was attributed to the tonic properties of this herb.[1] Since then, traditional Chinese medicine has used fo-ti to treat premature aging, weakness, vaginal discharges, numerous infectious diseases, angina pectoris, and impotence.

Active Constituents

The active constituents of fo-ti have yet to be determined. The whole root has been shown to lower cholesterol levels, according to animal and human research, as well as to decrease hardening of the arteries, or atherosclerosis.[2,3] Other fo-ti research has investigated this herb's role in strong immune function, red blood cell formation, and antibacterial action.[4] The unprocessed roots possess a mild laxative effect.

How Much Should I Take?

A tea can be made from processed roots by boiling 3–5 grams in 250 ml (1 cup) of water for ten to fifteen minutes. Three or more cups are drunk each day. Fo-ti tablets, each in the amount of 500 mg, are also available. Many people take five tablets three times per day.

Are There Any Side Effects or Interactions?

The unprocessed roots may cause mild diarrhea. Some people who are sensitive to fo-ti may develop a skin rash. Very high doses may cause numbness in the arms or legs.

GARLIC *(Allium sativum)*

GARLIC is closely related to onion and chives. The largest commercial garlic production is in central California. The bulb is used.

In What Conditions Might Garlic Be Supportive?

- **Atherosclerosis** (page 11)
- **Congestive heart failure** (page 30)
- **High cholesterol** (page 62)
- **Hypertension (high blood pressure)** (page 67)
- **Hypertriglyceridemia (high triglycerides)** (page 69)
- **Immune function** (page 72)
- Intermittent claudication
- **Recurrent ear infection** (page 47)
- **Yeast infection** (page 127)

Historical or Traditional Use

Garlic is mentioned in the Bible and the Talmud. Hippocrates, Galen, Pliny the Elder, and Dioscorides all mention the use of garlic for a large number of conditions, including parasites, respiratory problems, poor digestion, and low energy. Its use in China was first mentioned in A.D. 510. Louis Pasteur confirmed the antibacterial action of garlic in 1858.

Active Constituents

The sulfur compound allicin, produced by crushing or chewing fresh garlic, in turn produces other sulfur compounds: ajoene, allyl sulfides, and vinyldithiins.

Circulatory Effects

More than 250 publications have shown that garlic supports the cardiovascular system. It may lower cholesterol and triglyceride levels in the blood, inhibit platelet stickiness (aggregation), and increase fibrinolysis—which results in a slowing of blood coagulation. It is mildly antihypertensive and has antioxidant activity.[1,2]

Note: Garlic only keeps clotting in check, a benefit for persons at risk for cardiovascular disease. It cannot effectively replace stronger anticlotting drugs; its primary value is as a preventive.

Antimicrobial Actions

Garlic has antibacterial, antiviral, and antifungal activity.[3] It may work against some intestinal parasites. Garlic appears to have roughly 1% the strength of penicillin against certain types of bacteria. This means it is not a substitute for antibiotics, but it can be considered as a support against some bacterial infections. *Candida albicans* growth is inhibited by garlic, and garlic has shown long-term benefit for recurrent yeast infections.

Anticancer Actions

Human population studies show that eating garlic regularly reduces the risk of esophageal, stomach, and colon cancer.[4] This is partly due to garlic's ability to reduce the formation of carcinogenic compounds. Animal and test tube studies also show that garlic, and its sulfur compounds, inhibit the growth of different types of cancer—especially breast and skin tumors.

How Much Should I Take?

Some people chew one whole clove of raw garlic per day. For those who prefer it, odor-controlled, enteric-coated tablets or capsules with standardized allicin potential can be taken at 400–500 mg once or twice per day (providing up to 5,000 mcg of allicin). Alternatively, a tincture of 2–4 ml can be taken three times daily.

Are There Any Side Effects or Interactions?

Most people enjoy garlic. However, some individuals who are sensitive to it may experience heartburn and flatulence. Because of garlic's anticlotting properties, persons taking anticoagulant drugs should check with their nutritionally oriented doctor before taking garlic. Those scheduled for surgery should inform their surgeon if they are taking garlic supplements. There are no known contraindications to the use of garlic during pregnancy and lactation.

GENTIAN *(Gentiana lutea)*

THIS PLANT comes from meadows in Europe and Turkey. It is also cultivated in North America. The root is used medicinally. Several other similar species can be used interchangeably.

In What Conditions Might Gentian Be Supportive?

- Indigestion
- Poor appetite

Historical or Traditional Use

Gentian root and other highly bitter plants have been used for centuries in Europe as digestive aids (the well-known Swedish bitters often contain gentian). Other folk uses included topical use on skin tumors, decreasing fevers, and treatment of diarrhea.[1] Its ability to increase digestive function, including production of stomach acid, has since been validated in modern times.

Active Constituents

Gentian contains some of the most bitter substances known, particularly the glycosides gentiopicrin and amarogentin. The taste of these can be detected even when diluted 50,000 times.[2] Besides stimulating secretion of saliva in the mouth and hydrochloric acid in the stomach, gentiopicrin may protect the liver.[3]

How Much Should I Take?

Up to 20 drops of gentian tincture dissolved in a small glass of water should be sipped, at least fifteen minutes before meals.

Are There Any Side Effects or Interactions?

Gentian should not be used by people suffering from excessive stomach acid, heartburn, stomach ulcers, or gastritis.

GINGER *(Zingiber officinale)*

GINGER is a perennial plant that grows in India, China, Mexico, and several other countries. The rhizome (the underground stem) is used.

In What Conditions Might Ginger Be Supportive?

- **Atherosclerosis** (page 11)
- **Chemotherapy support** (page 25)
- **Migraine headaches** (page 91)
- **Morning sickness** (page 93)
- Motion sickness
- Nausea and vomiting following surgery
- **Rheumatoid arthritis** (page 115)

Historical or Traditional Use

Traditional Chinese medicine has recommended ginger for over 2,500 years. It is used for abdominal bloating, coughing, vomiting, diarrhea, and rheumatism. Ginger is commonly used in the Ayurvedic and Tibb systems of medicine for the treatment of inflammatory joint diseases, such as arthritis.

Active Constituents

The dried rhizome of ginger contains approximately 1–4% volatile oils. These are the medically active constituents of ginger; they are also responsible for ginger's characteristic odor and taste. The aromatic principles include zingiberene and bisabolene, while the pungent principles are known as gingerols and shogaols.[1] The pungent constituents are credited with the antinausea and antivomiting effects of ginger.

Digestive System Actions

Ginger is a classic tonic for the digestive tract. Classified as an aromatic bitter, it stimulates digestion. It also keeps the intestinal muscles toned.[2] This action eases the transport of substances through the digestive tract, lessening irritation to the intestinal walls.[3] Ginger may protect the stomach from the damaging effect of alcohol and nonsteroidal anti-inflammatory drugs (such as ibuprofen) and may help prevent ulcers.[4]

Antinausea/Antivomiting Actions

Research is inconclusive as to how ginger acts to alleviate nausea. Ginger may act directly on the gastrointestinal system or it may affect the part of the central nervous system that causes nausea.[5][6] It may be that ginger exerts a dual effect in reducing nausea and vomiting.

Circulatory Effects

Ginger also supports a healthy cardiovascular system. Like garlic, ginger makes blood platelets less sticky and less likely to aggregate, although not all human research has confirmed this. This action reduces a major risk factor for atherosclerosis.[7]

How Much Should I Take?

Most people take 2–4 grams of the dried rhizome powder two to three times per day or a tincture of 1.5–3 ml three times daily. For treatment of nausea, people try single doses of approximately 250 mg every two to three hours, for a total of 1 gram per day. For prevention of motion sickness, many people start taking ginger tablets, capsules, or liquid herbal extract two days before the planned trip.

Are There Any Side Effects or Interactions?

Side effects of ginger are rare when used as recommended. However, some people may be sensitive to the taste or may experience heartburn. Persons with a history of gallstones should consult a nutritionally oriented doctor before using ginger. Short-term use of ginger for nausea and vomiting during pregnancy appears to pose no safety problems; however, long-term use during pregnancy is not recommended. A doctor should be informed if ginger is used before surgery to counteract possible postanesthesia nausea.

GINKGO BILOBA *(Ginkgo biloba)*

COMMON NAME:

Maidenhair tree

GINKGO BILOBA is the world's oldest living species of tree; individual trees live as long as 1,000 years.

The leaves of the tree are used. Ginkgo grows most prominently in the southern and eastern United States and in China.

In What Conditions Might Ginkgo Biloba Be Supportive?

- Alzheimer's disease (page 6)
- Atherosclerosis (page 11)

- Cerebrovascular insufficiency
- **Congestive heart failure** (page 30)
- **Depression** (page 36)
- **Diabetes** (page 39)
- Impotence/**infertility** (**male**) (page 77)
- Intermittent claudication
- **Macular degeneration** (page 85)
- **Migraine headaches** (page 91)
- Multiple sclerosis
- Raynaud's phenomenon
- Tinnitus

Historical or Traditional Use

Medicinal use of ginkgo can be traced back almost 5,000 years in Chinese herbal medicine. It was recommended for respiratory tract ailments as well as memory loss in the elderly.

Active Constituents

The medical benefits of ginkgo biloba extract (GBE) rely on the proper balance of two groups of active components: the ginkgo flavone glycosides and the terpene lactones. The 24% ginkgo flavone glycoside designation on GBE labels indicates the carefully measured balance of bioflavonoids. These bioflavonoids are primarily responsible for GBE's **antioxidant** (page 8) activity and ability to inhibit platelet aggregation (stickiness). These two actions may help GBE prevent circulatory diseases, such as atherosclerosis, and support the brain and central nervous system.[1]

The unique terpene lactone components found in GBE, known as ginkgolides and bilobalide, increase circulation to the brain and other parts of the body as well as exert a protective effect on nerve cells. Ginkgolides may improve circulation and inhibit platelet-activating factor (PAF). Bilobalide protects the cells of the nervous system.[2] Recent animal studies indicate that bilobalide may help regenerate damaged nerve cells.[3]

GBE and Circulation

GBE increases circulation to both the brain and extremities of the body. In addition to inhibiting platelet stickiness, GBE regulates the tone and elasticity of blood vessels.[4] In other words, it makes circulation more efficient. This improvement in circulation efficiency extends to both large vessels (arteries) and smaller vessels (capillaries) in the circulatory system.[5]

Antioxidant Properties

GBE may have antioxidant properties in the brain, retina of the eye, and the cardiovascular system.[6] Its antioxidant activity in the brain and central nervous system may help prevent age-related declines in brain function. GBE's antioxidant activity in the brain is of particular interest. The brain and central nervous system are particularly susceptible to free radical attack. Free radical damage in the brain is widely accepted as being a contributing factor in many disorders associated with aging, including Alzheimer's disease.[7]

Nerve Protection and PAF Inhibition

One of the primary protective effects of the ginkgolides are their ability to inhibit a substance known as platelet-activating factor (PAF).[8] PAF is a mediator released from cells that causes platelets to aggregate (clump together). High amounts of PAF are associated with damage to nerve cells, poor blood flow to the central nervous system, inflammatory conditions, and bronchial constriction.[9] Much like free radicals, higher PAF levels are also associated with aging.[10] Ginkgolides and bilobalide protect nerve cells in the central nervous system from damage during periods of ischemia (lack of oxygen to tissues in the body).[11] This effect may be supportive for persons who have suffered a stroke.

How Much Should I Take?

Many people take 120–160 mg of GBE, standardized to contain 6% terpene lactones and 24% flavone glycosides, two to three times per day. Amounts up to 240 mg per day are used by some people with cerebrovascular insufficiency, confusion and memory loss, and resistant depression. GBE may need to be taken for six to eight weeks before desired effects are noticed. Ginkgo may also be taken as a tincture of 0.5 ml three times daily.

Are There Any Side Effects or Interactions?

Ginkgo biloba extract is essentially devoid of any serious side effects. Mild headaches lasting for a day or two and mild upset stomach have been reported in a very small percentage of people using GBE.

There are no known contraindications to the use of GBE by pregnant and lactating women.

It is important to remember that circulatory conditions in the elderly can involve serious disease. Individuals should seek proper medical care and accurate medical diagnosis prior to self-prescribing GBE.

GOLDENSEAL *(Hydrastis canadensis)*

GOLDENSEAL is native to eastern North America and is cultivated in Oregon and Washington. The dried root and rhizome are used.

In What Conditions Might Goldenseal Be Supportive?

- Common cold/sore throat (page 28)
- Crohn's disease (page 34)
- Recurrent ear infection (page 47)
- Urinary tract infection (page 120)

Historical or Traditional Use

Goldenseal was used by the American Indians as a treatment for irritations and inflammation of the mucous membranes of the respiratory, digestive, and urinary tracts. It was commonly used topically for skin and eye infections. Because of its antimicrobial activity, goldenseal has a long history of use for infectious diarrhea, upper respiratory tract infections, and vaginal infections. Goldenseal is often recommended in combination with echinacea for the treatment of colds and flu.

Active Constituents

The two primary alkaloids are hydrastine and berberine, along with smaller amounts of canadine. Berberine, which ranges from 0.5–6.0% of the alkaloids present in goldenseal root and rhizome, has been the most extensively researched. It appears to have a wide spectrum of antibiotic activity against pathogens, such as *Chlamydia* species, *E. coli*, *Salmonella typhi*, and *Entomeba histolytica*.[1]

How Much Should I Take?

Most people take 4–6 grams of powdered goldenseal root and rhizome supplements per day as tablets or capsules. For liquid herbal extracts, 4–6 ml are used. Continuous use should not exceed three weeks, with a break of at least two weeks between use. Goldenseal powder as a tea or tincture may soothe a sore throat.

Are There Any Side Effects or Interactions?

Taken as recommended, goldenseal is generally safe. However, as with all alkaloid-containing plants, high amounts may lead to gastrointestinal distress and possible nervous system effects. Goldenseal is not recommended for pregnant or lactating women.

GOTU KOLA *(Centella asiatica)*

THIS GROUND-HUGGING plant grows in a widespread distribution in tropical, swampy areas, including parts of India, Pakistan, Sri Lanka, Madagascar, and South Africa. It also grows in eastern Europe. The roots and leaves are both used medicinally.

In What Conditions Might Gotu Kola Be Supportive?

- Chronic venous insufficiency
- Mental function
- Minor burns
- Scars
- Scleroderma
- Skin ulcers
- Varicose veins
- Wound healing

Historical or Traditional Use

Gotu kola has been important in the medicinal systems of central Asia for centuries. It was purported in Sri Lanka to prolong life, as the leaves are commonly eaten by elephants. Numerous skin diseases, ranging from poorly healing wounds to leprosy, have been treated with gotu kola. Gotu kola also has a reputation for boosting cognitive function and for helping a variety of systemic illnesses, such as high blood pressure, rheumatism, fever, and nervous disorders. Some of its common uses in Ayurvedic medicine include treating heart disease, water retention, hoarseness, bronchitis, and coughs in children, and as a poultice for many skin conditions.[1]

Active Constituents

Saponins (also called triterpenoids) known as asiaticoside, madecassoside, and madasiatic acid are the primary active constituents.[2] These saponins beneficially affect collagen (the material that makes up connective tissue), for example, inhibiting its production in hyperactive scar tissue.

How Much Should I Take?

Dried gotu kola leaf can be made into a tea by adding 1–2 teaspoons to 150 ml of boiling water and allowing it to steep for ten to fifteen minutes. Three cups are usually drunk per day. Tincture can also be used at a dose of 10–20 ml three times per day. Standardized extracts containing up to 100% total triterpenoids are generally taken as 60 mg once or twice per day.

Are There Any Side Effects or Interactions?

Except for the rare person who is allergic to gotu kola, the only problems encountered are occasional nausea if excessively high doses are used. Gotu kola should be avoided in pregnancy and while breast-feeding.

GREEN TEA (Camellia sinensis)

ALL TEAS (green, black, and oolong) are derived from the same plant, *Camellia sinensis*. The difference is in how the plucked leaves are prepared. The leaves of the tea plant are used both as a social and medicinal beverage. Green tea, unlike black and oolong tea, is not fermented, so the active constituents remain unaltered in the herb.

In What Conditions Might Green Tea Be Supportive?

- Cancer risk reduction
- **Gingivitis (periodontal disease)** (page 56)
- **High cholesterol** (page 62)
- **Hypertension (high blood pressure)** (page 67)
- **Hypertriglyceridemia (high triglycerides)** (page 69)
- **Immune function** (page 72)
- Infection

Historical or Traditional Use

According to Chinese legend, tea was discovered accidentally by an emperor 4,000 years ago. Since then, traditional Chinese medicine has recommended green tea for headaches, body aches and pains, digestion, depression, immune enhancement, detoxification, as an energizer, and to prolong life. Modern research has confirmed many of these health benefits.

Active Constituents

Green tea contains volatile oils, vitamins, minerals, and caffeine, but the active constituents are polyphenols, particularly the catechin called epigallocatechin gallate (EGCG). The polyphenols are believed to be responsible for most of green tea's roles in promoting good health.[1]

Research demonstrates that green tea guards against cardiovascular disease in many ways. Green tea lowers total cholesterol levels and improves the cholesterol profile (the ratio of LDL cholesterol to HDL cholesterol), reduces platelet aggregation, and lowers blood pressure.[2][3][4][5] The polyphenols in green tea have also been shown to lessen the risk of several types of cancers, stimulate the production of several immune system cells, and have antibacterial properties—even against the bacteria that cause dental plaque.[6][7][8]

How Much Should I Take?

Much of the research documenting the health benefits of green tea is based on the amount of green tea typically drunk in Asian countries—about three cups per day (providing 240–320 mg of polyphenols). To brew green tea, 1 teaspoon of green tea leaves are combined with 250 ml (1 cup) of boiling water and steeped for three minutes. Tablets and capsules containing standardized extracts of polyphenols, particularly EGCG, are available; some are decaffeinated and provide up to 97% polyphenol content—which is equivalent to drinking four cups of tea.

Are There Any Side Effects or Interactions?

Green tea is extremely safe. The most common adverse effect reported from consuming large amounts of green tea is insomnia, anxiety, and other symptoms caused by the caffeine content in the herb.

GUARANÁ *(Paullinia cupana)*

THE VAST majority of guaraná is grown in a small area in northern Brazil. Guaraná gum or paste is derived from the seeds and is used in herbal supplements.

In What Conditions Might Guaraná Be Supportive?

- **Athletic performance** (page 14)
- Fatigue
- **Weight loss and obesity** (page 124)

Historical or Traditional Use

The indigenous people of the Amazon rain forest used crushed guaraná seed as a beverage and a medicine. Guaraná was said to treat diarrhea, decrease fatigue, reduce hunger, and help arthritis.[1] It also has a history of use in treating hangovers from alcohol abuse and headaches related to menstruation.

Active Constituents

Guaranine (which is nearly identical to caffeine) and the closely related alkaloids theobromine and theophylline make up the primary active agents in guaraná. Caffeine's effects (and hence those of guaranine) are well known and include stimulating the central nervous system, increasing metabolic rate, and having a mild diuretic effect.[2] One long-term study found no significant effects on thinking or mental function in humans taking guaraná.[3] Caffeine may have adverse effects on the blood vessels and other body systems as well as on a developing fetus, and presumably guaranine would have similar effects. Guaraná also contains tannins, which act as astringents and may prevent diarrhea.

How Much Should I Take?

A cup of guaraná, prepared by adding 1–2 grams of crushed seed or resin to 250 ml (1 cup) of water and boiling for ten minutes, can be drunk three times per day. Each cup may provide up to 50 mg of guaranine.

Are There Any Side Effects or Interactions?

As with any caffeinated product, guaraná may cause insomnia, trembling, anxiety, palpitations, urinary frequency, and hyperactivity. Guaraná should be avoided during pregnancy and lactation. Long-term use may cause decreased fertility, cardiovascular disease, and several forms of cancer, according to epidemiological studies of caffeine use.

GUGGUL *(Commiphora mukul)*

COMMON NAMES:

Gugulipid, gum guggulu

THE MUKUL MYRRH

(*Commiphora mukul*) tree is a small, thorny plant distributed throughout India. Guggul and gum guggulu are the names given to a yellowish resin produced by the stem of the plant. This resin has been used historically and is also the source of modern extracts of guggul.

In What Conditions Might Guggul Be Supportive?

- Atherosclerosis (page 11)
- High cholesterol (page 62)
- Hypertriglyceridemia (high triglycerides) (page 69)

Historical or Traditional Use

The classical treatise on Ayurvedic medicine, *Sushrita Samhita,* describes the use of guggul for a wide variety of conditions, including arthritis and obesity. One of its primary indications was a condition known as medoroga. This ancient diagnosis is very similar to the modern description of atherosclerosis. Guggul was primarily used to prevent this condition by lowering serum cholesterol and triglyceride levels.

Active Constituents

Guggul contains resin, volatile oils, and gum. The extract isolates ketonic steroid compounds known as guggulsterones. These compounds have been shown to provide the lipid-lowering actions noted for guggul.[1] Guggul significantly lowers serum triglycerides and cholesterol as well as LDL and VLDL cholesterols (the "bad" cholesterols).[2] At the same time, it raises levels of HDL cholesterol (the "good" cholesterol). Guggul has also been shown to reduce the stickiness of platelets—another effect that lowers the risk of coronary artery disease.[3]

How Much Should I Take?

Daily recommendations for guggul are typically based on the amount of guggulsterones in the extract. A common intake of guggulsterones is 25 mg three times per day. Most extracts contain 5–10% guggulsterones. Many people take the extracts daily for twelve to twenty-four weeks.

Are There Any Side Effects or Interactions?

Early studies with the crude oleoresin reported numerous side effects, including diarrhea, anorexia, abdominal pain, and skin rash. Modern extracts are more purified, and far fewer side effects (e.g., mild abdominal discomfort) have been reported with long-term use. Guggul should be used with caution by persons with liver disease and in cases of inflammatory bowel disease and diarrhea. A physician should be consulted for any case of elevated cholesterol and/or triglycerides.

Special United Kingdom Considerations

Guggul is either not available or may require a prescription. Please check with your nutritionally oriented physician.

GYMNEMA *(Gymnema sylvestre)*

COMMON NAME:

Gurmarbooti

GYMNEMA SYLVESTRE is a woody climbing plant that grows in the tropical forests of central and southern India. The leaves are used in herbal medicine preparations.

G. sylvestre is known as "periploca of the woods" in English and *meshasringi* (meaning "ram's horn") in Sanskrit. The leaves, when chewed, interfere with the ability to taste sweetness, which explains the Hindi name *gurmar*—"destroyer of sugar."

In What Conditions Might Gymnema Be Supportive?

- Diabetes (page 39)

Historical or Traditional Use

Gymnema has been used in India for the treatment of diabetes for over 2,000 years. The primary application was for adult-onset diabetes (NIDDM), a condition for which it continues to be recommended today in India. The leaves were also used for stomach ailments, constipation, water retention, and liver disease.

Active Constituents

The hypoglycemic (blood sugar–lowering) effect of gymnema leaves was first documented in the late 1920s.[1] This action is gradual in nature, differing from the rapid effect of many prescription hypoglycemic drugs. Gymnema leaves raise insulin levels, according to research in healthy volunteers.[2] The leaves are also noted for lowering serum cholesterol and triglycerides.[3] While studies have shown that a water-soluble acidic fraction of the leaves provides hypoglycemic actions, it is not yet clear what specific constituent in the leaves is responsible for this action. Some researchers have suggested gymnemic acid as one possible candidate.[4] Further research is needed to clearly determine which constituent is responsible for this effect. Gurmarin, another constituent of the leaves, and gymnemic acid have been shown to block sweet taste in humans.[5]

How Much Should I Take?

Recent studies in India have used 400 mg per day of a water-soluble acidic fraction of the gymnema leaves. In adult-onset diabetics, ongoing use for periods as long as eighteen to twenty months has proven successful.[6] In IDDM (juvenile onset) diabetic patients, a similar amount has been used as an adjunct to ongoing use of insulin. Traditionally, 2–4 grams of the leaf powder per day is used.

Are There Any Side Effects or Interactions?

Used at the amounts suggested, gymnema is generally safe and devoid of side effects. The safety of gymnema during pregnancy and lactation has not yet been determined. Persons with NIDDM should only use gymnema to lower blood sugar under the clinical supervision of a health care professional. Gymnema cannot be used in place of insulin to control blood sugar by persons with IDDM or NIDDM.

Special United Kingdom Considerations

Gymnema is either not available or may require a prescription. Please check with your nutritionally oriented physician.

HAWTHORN *(Crataegus laevigata or Crataegus oxyacantha, Crataegus monogyna)*

HAWTHORN is commonly found in Europe, western Asia, and nothern Africa.

Modern medicinal extracts use the leaves and flowers. Traditional preparations use the ripe fruit.

In What Conditions Might Hawthorn Be Supportive?

- Angina pectoris
- **Atherosclerosis** (page 11)

- **Congestive heart failure** (page 30)
- **Hypertension (high blood pressure)** (page 67)

Historical or Traditional Use

Dioscorides, a Greek herbalist, used hawthorn in the first century A.D. Although numerous passing mentions are made for a variety of conditions, support for the heart is the main benefit of hawthorn.

Active Constituents

The leaves, flowers, and berries of hawthorn contain a variety of bioflavonoid-like complexes that appear to be primarily responsible for the cardiac actions of the plant. Bioflavonoids found in hawthorn include **oligomeric procyanidins** (OPCs) (page 199), vitexin, **quercetin** (page 201), and hyperoside. The action of these compounds on the cardiovascular system has led to the development of leaf and flower extracts, which are widely used in Europe.

Hawthorn has numerous beneficial effects on the heart and blood vessels. It may improve coronary artery blood flow[1] and the contractions of the heart muscle.[2] Also, it may inhibit angiotensin-converting enzyme (ACE) and reduce production of the potent blood vessel–constricting substance angiotensin II. This reduces resistance in arteries and improves extremity circulation. The bioflavonoids in hawthorn are potent antioxidants.[3] Hawthorn extracts may mildly lower blood pressure in some individuals with high blood pressure but should not be thought of as a substitute for cardiac medications for this condition.

How Much Should I Take?

Extracts of the leaves and flowers are most commonly used by nutritionally oriented doctors. Hawthorn extracts standardized for total bioflavonoid content (usually 2.2%) or oligomeric procyanidins (usually 18.75%) are often used. Many people take 80–300 mg of the herbal extract in capsules or tablets two to three times per day or a tincture of 4–5 ml three times daily. If traditional berry preparations are used, the recommendation is at least 4–5 grams per day. Hawthorn may take one to two months for maximum effect and should be considered a long-term therapy.

Are There Any Side Effects or Interactions?

Hawthorn is extremely safe for long-term use. There are no known interactions with prescription cardiac medications or other drugs. There are no known contraindications to its use during pregnancy or lactation.

HOPS (Humulus lupulus)

THE HOPS PLANT, *Humulus lupulus,* is a climbing plant native to Europe, Asia, and North America.

Hops are the cone-like, fruiting bodies (strobiles) of the plant and are typically harvested from cultivated female plants. Hops are most commonly used as a flavoring agent in beer.

In What Conditions Might Hops Be Supportive?

- Anxiety
- **Insomnia** (page 79)

Historical or Traditional Use

Soothing the stomach and promoting healthy digestion have been the strongest historical uses of this herb. Hops tea was also recommended as a mild sedative and remedy for insomnia, particularly for those with insomnia resulting from an upset stomach.[1] It was also common for a pillow to be filled with hops to encourage sleep. Traditionally, hops were also thought to have a diuretic effect and to treat sexual neuroses. A poultice of hops was used topically to treat sores and skin injuries and to relieve muscle spasms and nerve pain.[2]

Active Constituents

Hops are high in bitter substances. The two primary bitter principles are known as humulone and lupulone.[3] These bitter principles are thought to be responsible for the appetite-stimulating properties of hops. Hops also contain about 1–3% volatile oils. Hops have been shown to have mild sedative properties. Many herbal preparations for insomnia combine hops with more potent sedative herbs, such as **valerian** (page 316).

How Much Should I Take?

The dried fruits can be made into a tea by pouring 150 ml of boiling water over 1–2 teaspoons of the fruit. Steep for ten to fifteen minutes before drinking. Tinctures can be taken in amounts of 1–2 ml two or three times per day. Dried hops in tablet or capsule form can also be taken at a dose of 500–1,000 mg two or three times per day. As mentioned above, many herbal preparations use hops in combination with herbal sedatives, including valerian, **passion flower** (page 295), and **scullcap** (page 308).

Are There Any Side Effects or Interactions?

Use of hops is generally safe, and there are no known contraindications or potential interactions with other medications. There are some reports of persons experiencing an allergic skin rash after handling the dried flowers; this is most likely due to a pollen sensitivity.

HORSE CHESTNUT *(Aesculus hippocastanum)*

THE HORSE CHESTNUT tree is native to Asia and northern Greece, but it is now cultivated in many areas of Europe and North America. The tree produces fruits that are made up of a spiny capsule containing one to three large seeds, known as horse chestnuts.

Traditionally, many of the aerial parts of the horse chestnut tree, including the seeds, leaves, and bark, were used in medicinal preparations. Modern extracts of horse chestnut are usually extracts of the seeds, which are high in the active constituent aescin.

In What Conditions Might Horse Chestnut Be Supportive?

- Chronic venous insufficiency
- Edema
- **Hemorrhoids** (page 60)

- Sprains and other injuries
- Varicose veins

Historical or Traditional Use

Horse chestnut leaves have been used as a cough remedy and to reduce fevers.[1] They were also believed to reduce pain and inflammation of arthritis and rheumatism. Poultices of the seeds were used topically to treat skin ulcers and skin cancer. Other uses include the internal and external application for problems of venous circulation, including varicose veins and hemorrhoids. The topical preparation was also used to treat phlebitis.

Active Constituents

Extracts of the seeds are the source of a saponin known as aescin, which has been shown to promote circulation through the veins.[2] Aescin promotes normal tone in the walls of the veins, thereby promoting return of blood to the heart. This has made both topical and internal horse chestnut extracts popular in Europe for the treatment of chronic venous insufficiency and varicose veins. Aescin also possesses anti-inflammatory properties and has been shown to reduce edema (swelling with fluid) following trauma, particularly those following sports injuries, surgery, and head injury.[3] A topical aescin preparation is very popular in Europe for the treatment of acute sprains during sporting events. Horse chestnuts also contain flavonoids, sterols, and tannins.

How Much Should I Take?

Traditionally, 0.2–1.0 grams of the dried seeds were used per day. However, only standardized extracts should be used internally. Horse chestnut seed extracts standardized for aescin content (16–21%) or isolated aescin preparations are often recommended at an initial dose of 90–150 mg of aescin per day.[4] Once improvement is noted, this is usually reduced to a maintenance dose of 35–70 mg of aescin per day. Topical aescin preparations are used in Europe for hemorrhoids, skin ulcers, varicose veins, sports injuries, and trauma of other kinds. A gel of aescin is typically applied to the affected area three to four times per day.

For hemorrhoids and varicose veins, horse chestnut is often combined with **witch hazel** (page 321).

Are There Any Side Effects or Interactions?

Internal use of purified horse chestnut extracts standardized for aescin at the doses listed here is generally safe. There have been two reports of kidney damage in persons consuming very large quantities of aescin. Horse chestnut should be avoided by anyone with liver or kidney disease. Its internal use is also contraindicated during pregnancy and lactation.[5] Topically, horse chestnut has been associated with rare cases of allergic skin reactions. Since circulation disorders and trauma associated with swelling may be the sign of a serious condition, a health care professional should be consulted before self-treating with horse chestnut.

Horse Chestnut

HORSERADISH *(Cochlearia armoracia)*

HORSERADISH likely origi-nated in eastern Europe, but today it is cultivated worldwide. The root is used as food and medicine.

In What Conditions Might Horseradish Be Supportive?

- Bronchitis
- **Common cold/sore throat** (page 28)
- Indigestion
- Sinus congestion

Historical or Traditional Use

Horseradish, known for its pungent taste, has been used as a medicine and condiment for centuries in Europe. Its name is derived from the common prac-tice of naming a food according to its similarity with another food (horseradish was considered a rough substitute for radishes).

Horseradish was used both internally and exter-nally. Applied to the skin, it causes reddening and was used on arthritic joints or irritated nerves. Inter-nally, it was considered primarily to be a diuretic and was used for kidney stones or edema. It was also rec-ommended as a digestive stimulant. In addition, it found use in the treatment of worms, coughs, and sore throats.[1]

Active Constituents

Horseradish contains many compounds similar to mustard, which is in the same botanical family. Among these constituents are volatile oil, isothio-cyanates, and glycosides. Horseradish has antibiotic properties, which may account for its easing of throat and upper respiratory tract infections.[2] The glycosides are responsible for the reddening effect (by increasing blood flow to the area) when horse-radish is applied topically.

How Much Should I Take?

The freshly grated root can be eaten in the amount of $1/2$–1 teaspoon three times per day. Horseradish tincture is also available and can be used in the amount of 2–3 ml three times per day.

Are There Any Side Effects or Interactions?

Very high doses of horseradish can cause vomiting or excessive sweating. Direct application to the skin or eyes may cause irritation and burning. Horseradish should be avoided by patients with hypothyroidism.

HORSETAIL *(Equisetum arvense)*

COMMON NAMES: Shave grass, scouring rush

HORSETAIL is widely distributed throughout the temperate climate zones of the northern hemisphere, including Asia, North America, and Europe.[1] Horsetail is a unique plant with two distinctive types of stems. One variety of stem grows early in spring and looks like asparagus, except for its brown color and the spore-containing cones on top. The mature form of the herb, appearing in summer, has branched, thin, green, sterile stems and looks very much like a feathery tail.

In What Conditions Might Horsetail Be Supportive?

- Brittle nails
- **Osteoarthritis** (page 97)
- **Osteoporosis** (page 100)
- **Rheumatoid arthritis** (page 115)
- Water retention

Historical or Traditional Use

Since it was recommended by the Roman physician Galen, several cultures have employed horsetail as a folk remedy for kidney and bladder troubles, arthritis, bleeding ulcers, and tuberculosis. Additionally, the topical use of horsetail is said to stop the bleeding of wounds and promote rapid healing. The use of this herb as an abrasive cleanser to scour pots or shave wood illustrates the origin of horsetail's common names—scouring rush and shave grass.[2]

Active Constituents

Horsetail is very rich in silicic acid and silicates, which provide approximately 2–3% elemental silicon. Potassium, aluminum, and manganese along with fifteen different types of bioflavonoids are also found in the herb. The presence of these bioflavonoids are believed to cause the diuretic action, while the silicon content is said to exert a connective tissue–strengthening and antiarthritic action.[3] Some experts have suggested that the element silicon is a vital component for bone and cartilage formation.[4] This would indicate that horsetail may be beneficial in preventing osteoporosis. Anecdotal reports suggest that horsetail may be of some use in the treatment of brittle nails.

How Much Should I Take?

Horsetail can be taken daily as a tea at 1–4 grams per day. A tincture can also be used at 2–6 ml per day.

Are There Any Side Effects or Interactions?

Horsetail is generally considered safe for non-pregnant adults at the recommended dose. The only concern would be that the correct species of horsetail is used; *Equisetum palustre* is another species of horsetail, which contains toxic alkaloids and is a well-known livestock poison.

The Canadian Health Protection Branch requires supplement manufacturers to document that their products do not contain the enzyme thiaminase, found in crude horsetail, which destroys the B vitamin thiamin. Since alcohol, temperature, and alkalinity neutralize this potentially harmful enzyme, tinctures, fluid extracts, or preparations of the herb subjected to 100°C temperatures during manufacturing should be the preferable form of the plant utilized for medicinal use.[5]

JUNIPER *(Juniperus communis)*

JUNIPER, a type of evergreen tree, grows mainly in the plains regions of Europe as well as in other parts of the world. The medicinal portion of the plant is referred to as a berry, but it is actually a dark blue-black scale from the cone of the tree. Unlike other pine cones, the juniper cones are fleshy and soft.

In What Conditions Might Juniper Be Supportive?

- **Urinary tract infection** (page 120)
- Water retention

Historical or Traditional Use

Aside from being used as the flavoring agent in gin, juniper trees have contributed to the making of everything from soap to perfume.[1] Medicinally, many conditions have been treated with juniper berries, including gout, warts and skin growths, cancer, upset stomach, and various urinary tract and kidney diseases.

Active Constituents

The volatile oils, particularly 4-terpineol, cause an increase in urine volume.[2] Some evidence suggests it may lower uric acid levels, although further study is required to confirm this. Although juniper lignans inhibit the herpes simplex virus in laboratory studies, treatment for human herpes infections by juniper has yet to be proven.[3] Juniper contains bitter substances, at least partly accounting for its traditional use in digestive upset and related problems.

How Much Should I Take?

To make a tea, 250 ml (1 cup) of boiling water is added to 1 tablespoon of juniper berries and allowed to steep for twenty minutes in a tightly covered container. One cup can be drunk each morning and night. Juniper is often combined with other diuretic and antimicrobial herbs. As a capsule or tablet, 1–2 grams can be taken three times per day, or 1–2 ml of tincture can be taken three times per day.

Are There Any Side Effects or Interactions?

Due to potential damage to the kidneys, juniper should never be taken for more than six weeks continuously. Anyone with serious kidney diseases or taking diuretic drugs should not take juniper. Application of the essential oil directly to skin can cause a rash. Pregnant women should avoid juniper, as it may cause uterine contractions.

KAVA *(Piper methysticum)*

KAVA is a member of the pepper family and is native to many Pacific Ocean islands. The rhizome (root stock) is used.

In What Conditions Might Kava Be Supportive?

• Anxiety

Historical or Traditional Use

A nonalcoholic drink made from the root of kava played an important role in a variety of ceremonies in the Pacific islands, including welcoming visiting royalty, at meetings of village elders, or as part of social gatherings. Kava was valued both for its mellowing effects and to encourage socializing. It was also noted for initiating a state of contentment, a greater sense of well-being, and enhanced mental acuity, memory, and sensory perception. Kava has also been used traditionally to treat pain.

Active Constituents

The kava-lactones, sometimes referred to as kava-pyrones, are important active constituents in kava herbal extracts. High-quality kava rhizomes contain

5.5–8.3% kava-lactones.[1] Medicinal extracts used in Europe contain 30-70% kava-lactones.

Kava-lactones may have antianxiety, analgesic (pain-relieving), muscle-relaxing, and anticonvulsant effects.[2] Studies suggest that kava directly influences the limbic system, the ancient part of the brain associated with emotions and other brain activities. [3]

How Much Should I Take?

Many people take kava extracts supplying 140–210 mg of kava-lactones per day. Alternatively, 1–3 ml of fresh liquid kava tincture can be taken.

Are There Any Side Effects or Interactions?

In recommended amounts, the only reported side effects from kava use are mild gastrointestinal disturbances in some people. Long-term consumption of very high doses of kava may turn the skin yellow temporarily. If this occurs, people should simply discontinue kava use. In rare cases, an allergic skin reaction, such as a rash, may occur.

Kava is not recommended for use by pregnant or lactating women. It should not be taken together with other substances that also act on the central nervous system, such as alcohol, barbiturates, antidepressants, and antipsychotic drugs.

KUDZU *(Pueraria lobata)*

COMMON NAME: Ge-gen

KUDZU is a coarse, high-climbing, twining, trailing, perennial vine. The huge root, which can grow to the size of a human body, is the source of medicinal preparations used in traditional Chinese medicine and modern herbal products.

Kudzu grows in most shaded areas in mountains, fields, along roadsides, thickets, and thin forests throughout most of China. The root of another Asian species of kudzu, *Pueraria thomsonii*, is also used for herbal products.

In What Conditions Might Kudzu Be Supportive?

- Alcoholism
- Angina pectoris
- **Hypertension (high blood pressure)** (page 67)

Historical or Traditional Use

Kudzu root has been known for centuries in traditional Chinese medicine as ge-gen. The first written mention of the plant as a medicine is in the ancient herbal text of Shen Nong (circa A.D. 100). In traditional Chinese medicine, kudzu root is used in prescriptions for the treatment of wei, or "superficial," syndrome (a disease that manifests just under the surface—mild, but with fever), thirst, headache, and stiff neck with pain due to high blood pressure.[1] It is also recommended for allergies, migraine headaches, inadequate measles eruptions in children, and diarrhea. It is interesting to note that the historical application for drunkenness has become a major focal point of modern research on kudzu. It is also used in modern Chinese medicine as a treatment for angina pectoris.

Active Constituents

Kudzu root is high in isoflavones, such as daidzein, as well as isoflavone glycosides, such as daidzin and puerarin. Depending on its growing conditions, the total isoflavone content varies from 1.77–12.0%, with puerarin in the highest concentration, followed by daidzin and daidzein.[2]

As is the case with other flavonoid-like substances, the constituents in kudzu root are associated with improved microcirculation and blood flow through the coronary arteries. A widely publicized 1993 animal study showed that both daidzin and daidzein inhibit the desire for alcohol.[3] The authors concluded that the root extract may in fact be useful in reducing the urge for alcohol and as treatment for alcoholism. This has not yet been proven in controlled clinical studies with humans.

How Much Should I Take?

The 1985 *Chinese Pharmacopoeia* suggests 9–15 grams per day of kudzu root.[4] In China, tablets of the standardized root (10 mg of weight per tablet equivalent to 1.5 grams of the crude root) are used for angina pectoris. This would equate to 30–120 mg two to three times per day.

Are There Any Side Effects or Interactions?

At the dosages recommended here, there have been no reports of kudzu toxicity in humans.

LEMON BALM *(Melissa officinalis)*

THE LEMON BALM plant originated in southern Europe and is now found throughout the world. The lemony smell and pretty white flowers of the plant have led to its widespread cultivation in gardens. The leaves, stems, and flowers of lemon balm are used medicinally.

In What Conditions Might Lemon Balm Be Supportive?

- Grave's disease (hyperthyroidism)
- Herpes simplex
- Indigestion
- **Insomnia** (page 79)
- Nerve pain

Historical or Traditional Use

Charlemagne once ordered that lemon balm be planted in every monastery garden, testifying to its importance and beauty.[1] It was used traditionally to treat gas, sleeping difficulties, and heart problems. Additionally, topical applications to the temples was sometimes used for insomnia or nerve pain.

Active Constituents

The terpenes, part of the pleasant smelling essential oil from lemon balm, produce this herb's relaxing and gas-relieving effects. Flavonoids, polyphenolics, and other compounds appear to be responsible for lemon balm's antiherpes and thyroid-regulating actions. These constituents actually block attachment to the thyroid cells by the antibodies that cause Grave's disease.[2] The brain's signal to the thyroid (thyroid-stimulating hormone, or TSH) is also blocked from further stimulating the excessively active thyroid gland in this disease.

How Much Should I Take?

A simple tea, made from 2 tablespoons of the herb steeped for ten to fifteen minutes in 150 ml of boiling water, is often used. A tincture can also be used at 2–3 ml three times per day. Highly concentrated topical extracts for herpes can be applied three to four times per day to the herpes lesions.[3]

Lemon balm is frequently combined with other medicinal plants. For example, **peppermint** (page 297) and lemon balm together are very effective for soothing an upset stomach. **Valerian** (page 316) is often combined with lemon balm for insomnia and nerve pain. Bugleweed (*Lycopus virginicus*) and lemon balm are usually used together for Grave's disease.

Are There Any Side Effects or Interactions?

No significant adverse effects from lemon balm have been reported. Unlike sedative drugs, lemon balm is safe even while driving or operating machinery. Lemon balm's sedating effects are not intensified by alcohol. Persons with glaucoma should avoid lemon balm essential oil, as animal studies show that it may raise pressure in the eye.[4]

LICORICE *(Glycyrrhiza glabra, Glycyrrhiza uralensis)*

ORIGINALLY FROM central Europe, licorice now grows all across Europe and Asia. The root is used medicinally.

In What Conditions Might Licorice Be Supportive?

- **Asthma** (page 9)
- Bronchitis
- **Canker sores (mouth ulcers)** (page 21) (DGL)
- Chronic fatigue syndrome
- **Eczema** (page 49)
- **Fibromyalgia** (page 53)
- Indigestion and heartburn (DGL)
- Herpes simplex
- **Peptic ulcer** (page 103) (DGL)

Historical or Traditional Use

Licorice has a long and highly varied record of uses. It was and remains one of the most important herbs in traditional Chinese medicine. Among the most consistent and important uses were as a demulcent (soothing, coating agent) in the digestive and urinary tracts, to help with coughs, to soothe sore throats, and as a flavoring. It has also been used to treat conditions ranging from diabetes to tuberculosis.

Active Constituents

The two most important constituents of licorice are glycyrrhizin and the flavonoids. Glycyrrhizin is anti-inflammatory and inhibits the breakdown of the cortisol produced by the body.[1][2] It also has antiviral properties. Licorice flavonoids, as well as the closely related chalcones, help digestive tract cells heal. They are also potent antioxidants and work to protect the cells of the liver.

How Much Should I Take?

A licorice preparation without the glycyrrhizin circumvents certain potential safety problems as explained below. The result is known as deglycyrrhizinated licorice (DGL), which is used for conditions of the digestive tract, such as ulcers. For best effects, one 200–300 mg tablet is chewed three times per day before meals and before bed. For mouth ulcers 200 mg of DGL powder can be mixed with 200 ml warm water, swished in the mouth for three minutes, and then spit out. Licorice may also be taken as a tincture in the amount of 2–5 ml, three times daily.

For respiratory infections, chronic fatigue syndrome, or topically for herpes, extracts containing glycyrrhizin should be used. Encapsulated licorice root capsules can be used, 5–6 grams per day. Alternatively, a tea can be made by boiling $1/2$ ounce of root in 1 pint of water for fifteen minutes, drinking two to three cups of this per day. Long-term internal use of high doses of glycyrrhizin-containing products should be taken only with caution and under the supervision of a nutritionally oriented doctor.

Licorice creams or gels can be applied directly to herpes sores three to four times per day.

Are There Any Side Effects or Interactions?

Licorice products that still contain the glycyrrhizin may increase blood pressure and cause water retention. Some people are more sensitive to this effect than others. Long-term intake of products containing more than 1 gram of glycyrrhizin (which is the amount in approximately 10 grams of root) daily is the usual amount required to cause these effects. As a result of these possible side effects, long-term intake of high levels of glycyrrhizin are discouraged and should only be undertaken if prescribed by a qualified health care professional.

Deglycyrrhizinated licorice extracts do not cause these side effects because there is no glycyrrhizin in them.

Special United Kingdom Considerations

Licorice is either not available or may require a prescription. Please check with your nutritionally oriented physician.

MAITAKE (Grifola frondosa)

MAITAKE is a very large mushroom (the size of a basketball), which grows deep in the mountains of northeastern Japan. Famous for its taste and renowned health benefits, maitake is also known as the "dancing mushroom."[1] Legend holds that those who found the rare mushroom began dancing with joy. Others attribute the name to the way the fruit bodies of the mushroom overlap each other, giving the appearance of dancing butterflies.

Maitake is extremely sensitive to environmental changes, which has presented many challenges to those cultivating this mushroom. Only recently have Japanese farmers succeeded in producing high-quality, organic maitake mushrooms, allowing for wider availability both in Japan and the United States. The fruiting body and the mycelium of maitake are used medicinally.

In What Conditions Might Maitake Be Supportive?

- **Chemotherapy support** (page 25)
- **Diabetes** (page 39)
- **High cholesterol** (page 62)
- **HIV support**
- **Hypertension (high blood pressure)** (page 67)
- **Hypertriglyceridemia (high triglycerides)** (page 69)
- **Immune function** (page 72)

Historical or Traditional Use

Historically, maitake has been used as a tonic and adaptogen. Along with other "medicinal" mushrooms, such as shiitake and reishi, maitake was used as a food to help promote wellness and vitality. Traditionally, consumption of the mushroom was thought to prevent high blood pressure and cancer—two applications that have been the focal point of modern research.

Active Constituents

A common denominator among mushroom and herbal adaptogens is the presence of complex polysaccharides in their structure. These active components have the unique ability to act as immunomodulators and, as such, are researched for their potential role in cancer and AIDS treatment. The polysaccharides present in maitake have a unique structure and are among the most powerful to be studied to date.[2] The primary polysaccharide, beta-D-glucan, is well absorbed when taken orally and is currently under review for the prevention and treatment of cancer and as a supportive tool for HIV infection.[3] [4]

Clinical research with maitake mushroom has increased dramatically in the past several years. In addition to cancer and HIV-infection studies, maitake is also being studied as a potential tool in the management of diabetes, hypertension, high cholesterol, and **obesity** (page 124).

the fruit body is higher in polysaccharides than the mycelium, which is why it is recommended. Many people take 3–7 grams of maitake supplements per day.

How Much Should I Take?

Maitake can be used as a food or tea. Maitake is also available as a capsule or tablet containing the whole fruiting body of maitake. For maitake,

Are There Any Side Effects or Interactions?

Used as recommended here, there have been no reports of any side effects with maitake.

MARSHMALLOW (Althea officinalis)

THE MARSHMALLOW
plant loves water and grows primarily in marshes. Originally from Europe, it now grows in the United States as well. The root and leaves are used.

In What Conditions Might Marshmallow Be Supportive?

- **Asthma** (page 9)
- **Common cold/sore throat** (page 28)
- **Crohn's disease** (page 34)
- **Diarrhea** (page 44)
- **Peptic ulcer** (page 103)

Historical or Traditional Use

Marshmallow (not to be confused with confectionery marshmallows, which are a product of the modern food industry) has long been used to treat coughs and sore throats.[1] Because of its high mucilage content, this plant is soothing and healing to inflamed mucous membranes. Additionally, it was used to treat chapped skin, chilblains, and even minor wounds.

Active Constituents

The active constituents in marshmallow are large carbohydrate (sugar) molecules, which make up mucilage. This smooth, slippery substance can soothe and protect irritated mucous membranes. Although marshmallow has primarily been used for the respiratory and digestive tracts, its high mucilage content may also provide some relief for the urinary tract and skin.[2]

How Much Should I Take?

Marshmallow can be made into a hot or cold water tea. Make a tea by adding roots and/or leaves and letting it steep. Drink three to five cups a day. Herbal extracts in capsules and tablets providing 5–6 grams of marshmallow per day can also be used, or it may be taken as a tincture in the amount of 5–15 ml, three times daily.

Are There Any Side Effects or Interactions?

Marshmallow is very safe. Reports of allergic reactions are extremely rare.

MILK THISTLE *(Silybum marianum)*

MILK THISTLE is commonly found growing wild in a variety of settings, including roadsides, worldwide. The seeds of the dried flower are used.

In What Conditions Might Milk Thistle Be Supportive?

- **Gallstones** (page 55)
- **Liver support**
- **Psoriasis** (page 112)

Historical or Traditional Use

Medical use of milk thistle can be traced back more than 2,000 years. Culpepper, the well-known eighteenth-century herbalist, cited its use for opening "obstructions" of the liver and spleen and recommended it for the treatment of jaundice. Milk thistle has also been used to relieve congestion of the liver, spleen, and kidneys.

Active Constituents

Milk thistle seeds contain a bioflavonoid complex known as silymarin. This constituent is responsible for the medical benefits of the plant.[1] Silymarin is made up of three parts: silibinin, silidianin, and silicristin. Silibinin is the most active and is largely responsible for the benefits attributed to silymarin.[2]

Milk thistle extract may protect the cells of the liver by blocking the entrance of harmful toxins and helping remove these toxins from the liver cells.[3][4] As with other bioflavonoids, silymarin is a powerful **antioxidant** (page 8).[5] Milk thistle also regenerates injured liver cells.[6]

How Much Should I Take?

Many people with liver disease and impaired liver function take 420 mg of silymarin per day from an herbal extract of milk thistle standardized to 70–80% silymarin content. According to research and clinical experience, improvement should be noted in about eight to twelve weeks. Once that occurs, intake is often reduced to 280 mg of silymarin per day. This lower amount may also be used for preventive purposes.

For those who prefer, 12–15 grams of milk thistle seeds can be ground and eaten or made into a tea. This should not be considered therapeutic for conditions of the liver, however.

Are There Any Side Effects or Interactions?

Milk thistle extract is virtually devoid of any side effects and may be used by a wide range of people, including pregnant and lactating women. Since silymarin does stimulate liver and gallbladder activity, it may have a mild, transient laxative effect in some individuals. This will usually cease within two to three days.

MULLEIN *(Verbascum thapsus)*

IN EUROPE, the flowers from *Verbascum phlomoides* or *Verbascum thapsiforme*, both close relatives of North American mullein, are the source of most mullein herbal products. The leaves and flowers of mullein are typically used in herbal preparations. The leaves are collected in midsummer and the flowers between July and September.

In What Conditions Might Mullein Be Supportive?

- **Asthma** (page 9)
- Bronchitis
- **Common cold/sore throat** (page 28)
- Cough
- **Recurrent ear infection** (page 47)

Historical or Traditional Use

Mullein is classified in the herbal literature as a expectorant and demulcent herb. Historically, mullein has been used as a remedy for the respiratory tract, particularly in cases of irritating coughs with bronchial congestion.[1] As such, bronchitis sufferers often find relief with this herb, particularly when combined with white horehound and lobelia. Some herbal texts extended the therapeutic use to pneumonia and asthma.[2] Because of its mucilage content, mullein was also used topically as a soothing emollient for inflammatory skin conditions and burns.

Active Constituents

Mullein contains about 3% mucilage and small amounts of saponins and tannins.[3] The mucilaginous constituents are primarily responsible for the soothing effects on mucous membranes noted for mullein. Many herbal experts feel that the saponins are responsible for the expectorant actions of mullein.[4]

How Much Should I Take?

A tea of mullein is made by pouring 250 ml (1 cup) of boiling water over 1–2 teaspoons of dried leaves or flowers and steeping for ten to fifteen minutes.

The tea can be drunk three to four times per day. For the tincture, 1–4 ml is taken three to four times per day. As a dried product, 1–2 grams is used three times per day. As mentioned above, mullein is usually combined with other demulcent or expectorant herbs when used to treat coughs and bronchial irritation.

Are There Any Side Effects or Interactions?

Mullein is generally safe, and there are no known contraindications to its use during pregnancy or lactation, except for rare reports of skin irritation.

MYRRH *(Commiphora molmol)*

MYRRH grows as a shrub in desert regions, particularly in northeastern Africa and the Middle East. The resin obtained from the stems is used in medicinal preparations.

In What Conditions Might Myrrh Be Supportive?

- Athlete's foot
- **Canker sores (mouth ulcers)** (page 21)
- **Common cold/sore throat** (page 28)
- **Gingivitis (periodontal disease)** (page 56)

Historical or Traditional Use

In ancient times, the red-brown resin of myrrh was utilized in the preservation of mummies. It was also used as a remedy for numerous infections, including leprosy and syphilis. Myrrh was also recommended for relief from bad breath and for dental conditions.[1] In traditional Chinese medicine, it has been used for bleeding disorders and wounds.

Active Constituents

The three main constituents of myrrh are the resin, the gum, and the volatile oil. All are important in myrrh's activity as an herbal medicine. The resin has been shown to kill various microbes and to stimulate macrophages (a type of white blood cell).[2] Myrrh also has astringent properties and has a soothing effect on inflamed tissues in the mouth and throat. Studies continue on the potential anticancer and pain-relieving effects of myrrh resin.[3][4]

How Much Should I Take?

Tincture of myrrh is usually taken at a dose of 1–2 ml three times per day. The tincture can also be applied topically for canker sores and athlete's foot. Due to the gummy nature of the product, a tea cannot be made from myrrh. Capsules, containing up to 1 gram of resin taken three times per day, can also be used.

Are There Any Side Effects or Interactions?

No adverse effects from myrrh usage have been reported.

NETTLE *(Urtica dioica)*

THE LATIN root of *Urtica* is *uro,* meaning "I burn." This is very appropriate, given that the little hairs on the leaves of this plant cause small stings that burn when contact is made with the skin. The root and leaves are used medicinally.

In What Conditions Might Nettle Be Supportive?

- Benign prostatic hyperplasia (page 18)
- Hay fever (page 59)
- Pregnancy support (page 107)

Historical or Traditional Use

Nettle has a long history of use. The tough fibers from the stem have been used to make cloth. Cooked nettle leaves were eaten as vegetables. From ancient Greece to the present, nettle has been documented for its use as a medicine for coughs and tuberculosis, to increase hair growth, and to treat arthritis.

Active Constituents

There has been a great deal of controversy regarding the identity of nettle's active constituents. One authoritative study came to the conclusion that polysaccharides (complex sugars) and lectins (large protein-sugar combination molecules) are probably the active constituents. The leaf has been shown to be anti-inflammatory by preventing the body from making inflammatory chemicals known as

Nettle

prostaglandins.[1] The root has complicated effects on hormones and proteins that carry sex hormones (such as testosterone or estrogen) in the human body. This may explain why it helps benign prostatic hyperplasia (BPH).[2]

How Much Should I Take?

Many people use two to three 300 mg nettle leaf capsules or tablets, or a 2–4 ml tincture three times per day during allergy season to help prevent and treat hay fever. For BPH, many people use 240 mg per day of the root extract in capsules or tablets. Many products for BPH will combine nettle root with **saw palmetto** (page 306) or **pygeum** (page 300) extracts.

Are There Any Side Effects or Interactions?

Allergic reactions to nettle are rare. However, when contact is made with the skin, fresh nettles can cause a rash.

OATS *(Avena sativa)*

THE COMMON OAT used in herbal supplements and foods is derived from wild species that have since been cultivated. For herbal supplements, the green or rapidly dried aerial parts of the plant are harvested just before reaching full flower. Many herbal texts refer to using the fruits (seeds) or green tops. Although some herbal texts discuss oat straw, there is little medicinal action in this part of the plant. Oats are now grown worldwide.

In What Conditions Might Oats Be Supportive?

- Anxiety
- **Eczema** (page 49)
- **High cholesterol** (page 62)
- **Hypertriglyceridemia (high triglycerides)** (page 69)
- **Insomnia** (page 79)
- Nicotine withdrawal

Historical or Traditional Use

In folk medicine as well as in current herbal treatments, oats are used to treat nervous exhaustion, insomnia, and "weakness of the nerves." A tea made from oats was thought to be useful in rheumatic conditions and to treat water retention. A tincture of the green tops of oats was also used to help with withdrawal from tobacco addiction.[1] Oats were often used in baths to treat insomnia and anxiety as well as a variety of skin conditions, including burns and eczema.

Active Constituents

The fruits (seeds) contain alkaloids, such as gramine and avenine, as well as saponins, such as avenacosides A and B.[2] The seeds are also rich in iron, manganese, and zinc. The straw is high in silica. Oat alkaloids are believed to account for oats' relaxing effect. It should be noted that this action of oats continues to be debated in Europe; the Commission E Monographs do not endorse this herb as a sedative.[3] However, an alcohol-based tincture of the fresh plant has proved useful in cases of nicotine withdrawal.

How Much Should I Take?

Oats can be eaten as a morning breakfast cereal. A tea can be made from a heaping tablespoonful of oats brewed with 250 ml (1 cup) of boiling water; after cooling and straining, the tea can be drunk several times a day or shortly before going to bed. As a tincture, oats are often taken at 3–5 ml three times per day. Encapsulated or tableted products can be used in the amount of 1–4 grams per day. A soothing bath to ease irritated skin can be made by running the bath water through a sock containing several tablespoons of oats.

Are There Any Side Effects or Interactions?

Oats are not associated with any adverse effects, although individuals with gluten sensitivity (celiac disease) should use oats with caution.

PASSION FLOWER (Passiflora incarnata)

THE BEAUTY of the passion flower has made this plant very popular. The plant is native to North, Central, and South America. While primarily tropical, some of its 400 species can grow in colder climates. The name passion flower dates back to the seventeenth century. The mystery of the beautiful blossom out of the unassuming bud was compared to the Passion of Christ. The leaves, stems, and flowers are used for medicinal purposes.

In What Conditions Might Passion Flower Be Supportive?

- Anxiety
- **Insomnia** (page 79)

Historical or Traditional Use

The historical use of passion flower was not dissimilar to its current use as a mild sedative. Medical use of the herb did not begin until the late nineteenth century in the United States. Passion flower was used to treat nervous restlessness and gastrointestinal spasms. In short, the effects of passion flower were believed to be primarily on the nervous system. Its effects were particularly touted for those with anxiety due to mental worry and overwork.[1]

Active Constituents

For many years, plant researchers believed that a group of harmane alkaloids were the active constituents in passion flower. Recent studies, however, have pointed to the flavonoids in passion flower as the primary constituents responsible for its relaxing and antianxiety effects.[2] European pharmacopoeias typically recommend passion flower products containing no less than 0.8% total flavonoids. The European literature involving passion flower recommends it primarily for antianxiety treatment; in this context, it is often combined with **valerian** (page 316), **lemon balm** (page 285), and other herbs with sedative properties.

How Much Should I Take?

The recommended intake of the dried herb is 4–8 grams three times per day.[3] To make a tea, 0.5–2.5 grams of the herb can be steeped with boiling water for ten to fifteen minutes and drunk two to three times per day. Alternatively, 2–4 ml of passion flower tincture can be taken per day. As mentioned, many European products combine passion flower with other sedative herbs to treat mild to moderate anxiety.

Are There Any Side Effects or Interactions?

Used in the amounts listed above, passion flower is generally safe and has not been found to negatively interact with other sedative drugs. However, some experts suggest not using passion flower with MAO-inhibiting antidepressant drugs. Passion flower has not been proven to be safe during pregnancy and lactation.

PAU D'ARCO *(Tabebuia impestiginosa)*

COMMON NAMES:

Lapacho, taheebo

VARIOUS RELATED species of pau d'arco trees grow in rain forests throughout Latin America. The bark is used for medical purposes.

In What Conditions Might Pau d'Arco Be Supportive?

- Infection
- **Yeast infection** (page 127)

Historical or Traditional Use

Native peoples in Central and South America reportedly use pau d'arco bark to treat cancer, lupus, infectious diseases, wounds, and many other health conditions.[1] Caribbean folk healers use the leaf of this tree in addition to the bark for the treatment of backache, toothache, sexually transmitted diseases, and as an aphrodisiac.

Active Constituents

Lapachol and beta-lapachone (known collectively as naphthaquinones) are two primary active compounds in pau d'arco. According to laboratory tests, both have antifungal properties as potent or more so than ketaconazole, a common antifungal drug.[2] Although these compounds also have anticancer properties, the effective dosage to achieve this effect is toxic.[3][4] Therefore, pau d'arco cannot currently be recommended as a treatment for cancer.

How Much Should I Take?

Because the naphthaquinone active constituents are not water soluble, a tea from pau d'arco bark is ineffective. Capsules or tablets providing 300 mg of powdered bark can be taken; usually three capsules are ingested three times per day.

Are There Any Side Effects or Interactions?

High doses of lapachol can cause uncontrolled bleeding, nausea, and vomiting.[5] Use of the whole bark is much safer than isolated lapachol—the whole bark has no known serious side effects.[6] Pregnant or lactating women should avoid use of pau d'arco.

PEPPERMINT (Mentha piperita)

PEPPERMINT is a hybrid of water mint and spearmint and was first cultivated near London in 1750. Peppermint grows almost everywhere. The two main cultivated forms are the black mint, which has violet-colored leaves and stems and a relatively high oil content, and the white mint, which has pure green leaves and a milder taste. The leaves are used.

In What Conditions Might Peppermint Be Supportive?

- Gingivitis (periodontal disease) (page 56)
- Headache (tension)
- Irritable bowel syndrome (page 81)

Historical or Traditional Use

Although not recognized until the early eighteenth century, the historical use of peppermint is not dramatically different than its use in modern herbal medicine. Classified as a carminative herb, peppermint has been used as a general digestive aid and employed in the treatment of indigestion and intestinal colic.[12]

Active Constituents

Peppermint leaves contain about 0.5–4.0% volatile oil that is composed of 50–78% free menthol and

5–20% menthol combined with other constituents.[3] Peppermint oil is classified as a carminative,[4] meaning that it helps ease intestinal cramping and tone the digestive system. It may also increase the flow of bile from the gallbladder.

Peppermint oil's relaxing effect also extends to topical use. When applied topically, it acts as a counterirritant and analgesic with the ability to reduce pain and improve blood flow to the affected area.[5]

How Much Should I Take?

For internal use, a tea can be made by pouring 250 ml (1 cup) of boiling water over 1 teaspoon (heaped) of the dried leaves and steeping for five to ten minutes; three to four cups daily between meals can relieve stomach and gastrointestinal complaints. Peppermint leaf tablets, capsules, and liquid extracts are often taken at 3–6 grams per day. For treatment of irritable bowel syndrome (IBS), 1–2 capsules of the enteric-coated capsules containing 0.2 ml of peppermint oil taken two to three times per day may be preferable.

For headaches, many people apply a combination of peppermint oil and eucalyptus oil diluted with base oil to the temples at the onset of the headache and every hour after that or until symptom relief is noted.

Are There Any Side Effects or Interactions?

Peppermint tea is generally considered safe for regular consumption. Peppermint oil, in large amounts, can cause burning and gastrointestinal upset in some people. It should be avoided by people with chronic heartburn. Some individuals using the enteric-coated peppermint capsules may experience a burning sensation in the rectum. Rare allergic reactions have been reported with topical use of peppermint oil. Peppermint tea should be used with caution in infants and young children, as they may choke in reaction to the strong menthol; **chamomile** (page 247) is usually a better choice for this group.

PHYLLANTHUS *(Phyllanthus niruri)*

COMMON NAMES:

Bahupatra, bhuiamla

PHYLLANTHUS is an herb common to central and southern India. It can grow to 30–60 centimeters in height and blooms with many yellow flowers.

All parts of the plant are employed therapeutically. Phyllanthus species are also found in other countries, including China (e.g., *Phyllanthus urinaria*), the Philippines, Cuba, Nigeria, and Guam.[1]

In What Conditions Might Phyllanthus Be Supportive?

• Hepatitis support

Historical or Traditional Use

Phyllanthus has been used in Ayurvedic medicine for over 2,000 years and has a wide number of traditional uses. This includes employing the whole plant for jaundice, gonorrhea, frequent menstruation, and diabetes, and using it topically as a poultice for skin ulcers, sores, swelling, and itchiness. The young shoots of the plant are administered in the form of an infusion for the treatment of chronic dysentery.[2]

Active Constituents

Phyllanthus primarily contains lignans (e.g., phyllanthine and hypophyllanthine), alkaloids, and bioflavonoids (e.g., quercetin). While it remains unknown as to which of these ingredients has an antiviral effect, research shows that this herb acts primarily on the liver. This action in the liver confirms its historical use as a remedy for jaundice.

Phyllanthus blocks DNA polymerase, the enzyme needed for the hepatitis B virus to reproduce. Fifty-nine percent of those infected with chronic viral hepatitis B lost one of the major blood markers of HBV infection (e.g., hepatitis B surface antigen) after using phyllanthus for thirty days.[3] While clinical studies on the outcome of phyllanthus and HBV have been mixed, the species *P. urinaria* and *P. niruri* seem to work far better than *P. amarus*.[4]

How Much Should I Take?

Research has utilized the powdered form of phyllanthus in amounts ranging from 900–2,700 mg per day for three months.

Are There Any Side Effects or Interactions?

No side effects have been reported using phyllanthus as recommended.

Special United Kingdom Considerations

Phyllanthus is either not available or may require a prescription. Please check with your nutritionally oriented physician.

PSYLLIUM *(Plantago ovata, Plantago ispaghula)*

COMMON NAME:

Plantago seed

PSYLLIUM is native to Iran and India and is currently cultivated in these countries. The seeds are used.

In What Conditions Might Psyllium Be Supportive?

- **Atherosclerosis** (page 11)
- **Constipation** (page 32)
- **Diarrhea** (page 44)
- **Hemorrhoids** (page 60)
- **High cholesterol** (page 62)
- **Hypertriglyceridemia (high triglycerides)** (page 69)
- **Irritable bowel syndrome** (page 81)
- **Psoriasis** (page 112)
- **Weight loss and obesity** (page 124)

Historical or Traditional Use

In addition to its traditional and current use for constipation, psyllium was also used topically to treat skin irritations, including poison ivy reactions and insect bites and stings. It has also been used in traditional herbal systems of China and India to treat diarrhea, hemorrhoids, bladder problems, and high blood pressure.

Active Constituents

Psyllium is a bulk-forming laxative and is high in both fiber and mucilage. Psyllium seeds contain 10–30% mucilage. The laxative properties of psyllium are due to the swelling of the husk when it comes in contact with water. This forms a gelatinous mass and keeps the feces hydrated and soft.

The resulting bulk stimulates a reflex contraction of the walls of the bowel, followed by emptying.[1]

How Much Should I Take?

Many people take 7.5 grams of the seeds or 5 grams of the husks one to two times per day, with water or juice. It is important to maintain adequate fluid intake when using psyllium.

Are There Any Side Effects or Interactions?

Using psyllium in recommended amounts is generally safe. People with chronic constipation should seek the advice of a health care professional. Side effects, such as allergic skin and respiratory reactions to psyllium dust, have largely been limited to people working in plants that manufacture psyllium products.

PYGEUM *(Pygeum africanum)*

PYGEUM is an evergreen tree found in the higher elevations of central and southern Africa. The bark is used.

In What Conditions Might Pygeum Be Supportive?

- Benign prostatic hyperplasia (page 18)

Historical or Traditional Use

The powdered bark was used as a tea for relief of urinary disorders. European scientists were so impressed with reports of pygeum's actions that they began laboratory investigations into the active constituents in the bark. This led to the development of the modern lipophilic (fat soluble) extract used today.

Active Constituents

Chemical analysis and pharmacological studies indicate that the lipophilic extract of pygeum bark has three categories of active constituents. The phytosterols, including beta-sitosterol, have anti-inflammatory effects by interfering with the formation of proinflammatory prostaglandins that tend to accumulate in the prostate of men with benign prostatic hyperplasia (BPH). The pentacyclic terpenes have an anti-edema, or decongesting, effect. The last group are the ferulic esters. These constituents reduce levels of the hormone prolactin and also block cholesterol in the prostate. Prolactin increases uptake of testosterone in the prostate, and cholesterol increases binding sites for testosterone and its more active form dihydrotestosterone.[1]

How Much Should I Take?

The accepted form of pygeum used in Europe for treatment of BPH is a lipophilic extract standardized to 13% total sterols (typically calculated as beta-sitosterol). The recommended dose is 50–100 mg two times per day. Pygeum should be monitored over at least a six- to nine-month period to determine efficacy. As is the case with all BPH treatments, close medical supervision is of the utmost importance.

Are There Any Side Effects or Interactions?

Side effects to the lipophilic extract of pygeum are rare. In clinical studies, there were very rare reports of mild gastrointestinal irritation in some patients.

RED CLOVER (Trifolium pratense)

THIS PLANT grows in Europe and North America. The flowering tops are used in botanical medicine. Another plant, white clover, grows in similar areas. Both have interesting white arrow-shaped patterns on their leaves.

In What Conditions Might Red Clover Be Supportive?

- Cancer risk reduction
- Cough
- Eczema (page 49)

Historical or Traditional Use

Traditional Chinese medicine and Western folk medicine used this plant for similar purposes. It was well regarded as a diuretic, to stop coughing, and as an alterative.[1] Alterative plants were considered beneficial for all manner of chronic conditions, particularly those afflicting the skin.

Active Constituents

Red clover contains isoflavone compounds, such as genistein, which have weak estrogen properties.[2]

Various laboratory studies show that these isoflavones may help prevent cancer.[3] Although the isoflavones in red clover may help prevent certain forms of cancer (e.g., breast and prostate), more clinical studies must be completed before red clover is recommended for cancer patients. The mechanism of action and responsible constituents for its purported benefit in skin conditions is unknown.

How Much Should I Take?

Usually, red clover is taken as a tea by adding 250 ml (1 cup) of boiling water to 2–3 teaspoons of dried flowers and steeping, covered, for ten to fifteen minutes. Three cups can be drunk each day. Red clover can also be used in capsule or tablet form in the amount of 2–4 grams of the dried flowers or 2–4 ml of tincture three times per day. Dried red clover tops are also available in capsules, tablets, and tinctures.

Are There Any Side Effects or Interactions?

Nonfermented red clover is relatively safe. However, fermented red clover should be avoided altogether.

RED RASPBERRY (Rubus idaeus)

ALTHOUGH MOST well known for its delicious berries, raspberry's leaves are used in botanical medicine. Raspberry bushes are native to North America and are also cultivated in Canada.

In What Conditions Might Raspberry Be Supportive?

- Common cold/sore throat (page 28)
- Diarrhea (page 44)
- Pregnancy support (page 107)

Historical or Traditional Use

Raspberry leaves, beyond their traditional use for diarrhea, have been connected to female health, including pregnancy. It was considered a remedy for excessive menstrual flow (menorrhagia) and as a "partus prepartor," or an agent used in pregnancy to help prevent complications.[1]

Active Constituents

Raspberry leaf is high in tannins and like its relative, blackberry, may relieve acute diarrhea.[2] The constituents that affect the smooth muscles such as those in the uterus have not yet been clearly identified.

How Much Should I Take?

Raspberry leaf tea is prepared by pouring 250 ml (1 cup) boiling water over 1–2 teaspoons of the herb and steeping for ten to fifteen minutes. Up to six cups per day may be necessary for acute problems, while less (two to three cups) is used for preventive use during pregnancy. By itself, raspberry is usually not a sufficient treatment for diarrhea. Tincture can be used in the amount of 4–8 ml three times per day.

Are There Any Side Effects or Interactions?

Raspberry may cause mild loosening of stools and nausea.

REISHI *(Ganoderma lucidum)*

COMMON NAMES: Ling chih, ling zhi

REISHI mushrooms grow wild on decaying logs and tree stumps in the coastal provinces of China. The fruiting body of the mushroom is employed medicinally. Reishi occurs in six different colors, but the red variety is most commonly used and commercially cultivated in North America, China, Taiwan, Japan, and Korea.[1]

In What Conditions Might Reishi Be Supportive?

- Altitude sickness
- **Chemotherapy support** (page 25)
- Fatigue
- Hepatitis support
- **Hypertension** (**high blood pressure**) (page 67)
- **Hypertriglyceridemia** (**high triglycerides**) (page 69)

Historical or Traditional Use

Reishi has been used in traditional Chinese medicine for more than 4,000 years.[2] The Chinese name ling zhi translates as the "herb of spiritual potency" and was highly prized as an elixir of immortality.[3] Its traditional Chinese medicine indications include treatment of general fatigue and weakness, asthma, insomnia, and cough.[4]

Active Constituents

Reishi contains several constituents, including sterols, coumarin, mannitol, polysaccharides, and triterpenoids called ganoderic acids. Ganoderic acids seem to help lower blood pressure as well as decrease low density lipoprotein (LDL) and triglyceride levels. These specific triterpenoids also help to reduce blood platelets from sticking together—an important factor in lowering the risk for coronary artery disease. While human research demonstrates some efficacy for the herb in treating altitude sickness and chronic hepatitis B, these uses still need to be confirmed.[5]

How Much Should I Take?

Many people take reishi in doses of 1.5–9 grams of the crude dried mushroom per day, 1–1.5 grams per day in powder form, 1 ml per day of tincture, or as a tea.

Are There Any Side Effects or Interactions?

Side effects from reishi can include dizziness, dry mouth and throat, nose bleeds, and abdominal upset; these rare effects may develop with continuous use over three to six months. Since it may increase bleeding time, reishi is not recommended for those taking anticoagulant (blood-thinning) medications. Pregnant or lactating women should consult a physician before taking reishi.

SANDALWOOD *(Santalum album)*

SANDALWOOD trees grow in India and Asia. The wood is renowned for being excellent for carving and also yields the medicinal oil.

In What Conditions Might Sandalwood Be Supportive?

- Infection

Historical or Traditional Use

Sandalwood oil was used traditionally to treat skin diseases, acne, dysentery, gonorrhea, and a number of other conditions.[1] In traditional Chinese medicine, sandalwood oil is considered an excellent sedating agent.

Active Constituents

The essential oil contains high amounts of alpha- and beta-santalol. These small molecules possess antibacterial and sedative properties.[2][3] Synthetic sandalwood does not contain the active ingredients.

How Much Should I Take?

Typically, a few drops of sandalwood oil are dissolved in water, and the infected area of skin is then soaked in the solution, or the diluted oil is applied directly.

Are There Any Side Effects or Interactions?

Some people may experience mild skin irritation from topical application of sandalwood oil.

SARSAPARILLA *(Smilax spp.)*

MANY DIFFERENT species are called by the general name sarsaparilla. Various species are found in Mexico, South America, and the Caribbean. The root is used therapeutically.

In What Conditions Might Sarsaparilla Be Supportive?

- Eczema (page 49)
- Psoriasis (page 112)
- Rheumatoid arthritis (page 115)

Historical or Traditional Use

In Mexico, sarsaparilla was used for arthritis, cancer, skin diseases, and a host of other conditions.[1] At the turn of the century, there were reports of its use in the treatment of psoriasis and leprosy.[2] Sarsaparilla also has a tradition of use in various women's health concerns and was rumored to have a progesterone-like effect. Sarsaparilla was formerly a major flavoring agent in root beer.

Active Constituents

Sarsaparilla contains steroidal saponins, such as sarsasapogenin, which may mimic the action of some human hormones; this property remains undocumented. Sarsaparilla also contains phytosterols, such as beta-sitosterol, which may contribute to the therapeutic effects of this herb. Reports have shown anti-inflammatory[3] and liver-protecting[4] effects for this herb.

How Much Should I Take?

Capsules or tablets should provide at least 9 grams of the dried root per day, usually taken in divided doses. Tincture is used in the amount of 3 ml three times per day. Invariably, sarsaparilla is used in conjunction with other therapeutic herbs.

Are There Any Side Effects or Interactions?

Sarsaparilla can cause nausea and kidney damage. Large doses for long periods of time are to be avoided. Since sarsaparilla can increase absorption and/or elimination of digitalis and bismuth, such combinations are contraindicated.[5]

SAW PALMETTO *(Serenoa repens, Sabal serrulata)*

SAW PALMETTO (sometimes referred to as sabal in Europe) is a native of North America. The berries of the plant are used.

In What Conditions Might Saw Palmetto Be Supportive?

• Benign prostatic hyperplasia (BPH) (page 18)

Historical or Traditional Use

In the early part of this century, saw palmetto berry tea was commonly recommended for benign enlargement of the prostate.[1][2][3][4][5] It was also used to treat chronic urinary tract infections. Some believed that the berry increased sperm production and sex drive in men.

Active Constituents

The lipophilic (fat-soluable) extract of saw palmetto provides sterols and the fatty acids caproic, lauric, and palmitic, which reduce the amount of dihydrotestosterone in the prostate. The fatty acids in saw palmetto also discourage the actions of inflammatory substances that otherwise contribute to BPH.

How Much Should I Take?

For early-stage BPH, many people take 320 mg per day of saw palmetto herbal extract in capsules or tablets—which are rich in fatty acids, sterols, and esters. It may take four to six weeks to see results with BPH; if improvement is noted, the saw palmetto can be continued. The powdered dried fruit can also be taken as a tea; since this is weaker than the herbal extract, 5–6 grams may be taken per day. Liquid extracts of whole herb at 5–6 ml per day may also be effective.

Are There Any Side Effects or Interactions?

No significant side effects have been noted in clinical studies with saw palmetto extracts. Saw palmetto extract is not believed to interfere with accurate measuring of prostate-specific antigen—a marker for prostate cancer. Please note that BPH can only be diagnosed by a physician; use of saw palmetto extract for this condition should only occur after a thorough workup and diagnosis by a doctor.

SCHISANDRA (Schisandra chinensis)

COMMON NAME: Wu-wei-zi

SCHISANDRA is a woody vine with numerous clusters of tiny, bright red berries. It is distributed throughout northern and northeast China and the adjacent regions of Russia and Korea.[1] The fully ripe, sun-dried fruit is used medicinally. It is purported to have sour, sweet, salty, hot, and bitter tastes. This unusual combination of flavors is reflected in schisandra's Chinese name wu-wei-zi, meaning "five taste fruit."

In What Conditions Might Schisandra Be Supportive?

- **Chemotherapy support** (page 25)
- **Common cold/sore throat** (page 28)
- Fatigue
- Hepatitis support
- Liver support
- Stress

Historical or Traditional Use

The classical treatise on Chinese herbal medicine, the *Shen Nong Pen Tsao Ching*, describes schisandra as a high-grade herbal drug useful for a wide variety of medical conditions—especially as a kidney tonic and lung astringent. Additionally, other textbooks on traditional Chinese medicine note that schisandra is useful for coughs, night sweats, insomnia, thirst, and physical exhaustion.[2]

Active Constituents

Schisandra contains a number of compounds, including essential oils, numerous acids, and lignans.

Schisandra

Lignans (schizandrin, deoxyschizandrin, gomisins, and pregomisin) are found in the seeds of the fruit and have a number of medicinal actions. Modern Chinese research suggests that lignans regenerate liver tissue damaged by harmful influences such as viral hepatitis and alcohol. Lignans lower blood levels of serum glutamic pyruvic transaminase (SGPT), a marker for infective hepatitis and other liver disorders.

Schisandra fruit may also have an adaptogenic action, much like the herbs **Asian ginseng** (page 232) and **eleuthero** (Siberian ginseng) (page 257), but with weaker effects. Laboratory work suggests that schisandra may improve work performance, build strength, and help to reduce fatigue.[3]

How Much Should I Take?

A daily dose of schisandra fruit ranges from 1–6 grams. The tincture, in the amount of 2–4 ml three times per day, can also be used.

Are There Any Side Effects or Interactions?

Side effects involving schisandra are uncommon but may include abdominal upset, decreased appetite, and skin rash.

SCULLCAP *(Scutellaria lateriflora)*

SCULLCAP is a member of the mint family. *Scutellaria lateriflora* grows in eastern North America and is most commonly used in U.S. and European herbal products containing scullcap. The aerial part of the plant is used in herbal preparations. *Scutellaria baicalensis* is grown in China and Russia. The root of this plant is used in traditional Chinese herbal medicines and has been the focus of most scientific studies on scullcap.

In What Conditions Might Scullcap Be Supportive?

- Anxiety
- **Insomnia** (page 79)

Historical or Traditional Use

As is the case in modern herbal medicine, scullcap was used historically as a sedative for persons with nervous tension and insomnia. It was, and continues to be, commonly combined with **valerian** (page 000) for insomnia.[1] It was also used as a remedy for epilepsy and nerve pain. Chinese scullcap is typically used in herbal combinations to treat inflammatory skin conditions, allergic diseases, high cholesterol and triglycerides, and high blood pressure.

Active Constituents

Few studies have been completed on the constituents of American scullcap. One of its constituents, scutellarian, has been shown to have mild sedative and antispasmodic actions.[2] The root of Chinese scullcap also contains a flavonoid substance, baicalin, that has been shown to have protective effects on the liver. Antiallergy effects and the inhibition of bacteria and viruses in test tube studies have been documented with Chinese scullcap.[3]

How Much Should I Take?

A scullcap tea can be made by pouring 250 ml (1 cup) of boiling water over 1–2 teaspoons of the dried herb and steeping for ten to fifteen minutes; this tea may be drunk three times per day. As a tincture, American scullcap can be taken in the amount of 2–4 ml three times per day. For the dried herb, 1–2 grams three times per day is often used. In traditional Chinese herbal medicine, scullcap is typically recommended as a tea made from 3–9 grams of the dried root.

Are There Any Side Effects or Interactions?

Use of scullcap in the amounts listed here is generally safe. Due to limited information on the safety of scullcap during pregnancy and lactation, it should be avoided by pregnant or lactating women. Recently, cases of liver damage were reportedly associated with intake of scullcap. On closer examination, it appears that these scullcap products actually contained germander, an herb known to cause liver toxicity.

SENNA (Cassia senna, Cassia angustifolia)

THE SENNA SHRUB grows in India, Pakistan, and China. The leaves and pods are used medicinally.

In What Conditions Might Senna Be Supportive?

- Constipation (page 32)

Historical or Traditional Use

People in northern Africa and southwestern Asia have used senna as a laxative for centuries. Because of its cathartic effect, it was considered a "cleansing" herb. Additionally, the leaves were sometimes made into a paste and applied to various skin diseases. Ringworm and acne were both treated in this way.

Active Constituents

Senna contains anthraquinone glycosides known as sennosides. These molecules are converted by the normal bacteria in the colon into rhein-anthrone, which in turn has two effects. It first stimulates colon activity and thus speeds bowel movements. Second, it increases fluid secretion by the colon.[1] Together, these actions work to get a sluggish colon functional again.

How Much Should I Take?

Many people use an herbal extract in capsules or tablets providing 10–60 mg of sennosides per day. This can be continued for up to ten days maximum. Use beyond ten days is strongly discouraged. If constipation is not alleviated within ten days, individuals should seek the help of a health care professional. Combination with herbal mint teas can help decrease cramping. Half the adult dose of senna can be safely used in children over the age of six as well.

Are There Any Side Effects or Interactions?

Senna can cause the colon to become dependent on it to move properly. Therefore, senna must not be used for more than ten consecutive days. Chronic senna use can also cause loss of fluids, low potassium levels, and diarrhea, all of which can lead to dehydration and negative effects on the heart and muscles. Senna is safe for use in pregnancy and lactation, but only under the supervision of a physician.[2][3] It is also safe for children over the age of six.

SHIITAKE *(Lentinan edodes)*

COMMON NAME: Hua gu

WILD SHIITAKE mushrooms are native to Japan, China, and other Asian countries and typically grow on fallen broadleaf trees. Shiitake is widely cultivated throughout the world, including the United States. The fruiting body is used medicinally.

In What Conditions Might Shiitake Be Supportive?

- Chemotherapy support (page 25)
- Hepatitis support
- HIV support

Historical or Traditional Use

Shiitake has been revered in Japan and China as both a food and medicinal herb for thousands of years. Wu Ri, a famous physician from the Chinese Ming Dynasty (A.D. 1368–1644), wrote extensively about this mushroom, noting its ability to increase energy, cure colds, and eliminate worms.[1]

Active Constituents

Shiitake contains proteins, fats, carbohydrates, soluble fiber, vitamins, and minerals. In addition, shiitake's key ingredient—found in the fruiting body—is a polysaccharide called lentinan. Commercial preparations employ the powdered mycelium of the mushroom before the cap and stem grow; this is called LEM (lentinan edodes mycelium extract). LEM is also rich in polysaccharides and lignans.

Research indicates that LEM helps decrease chronic hepatitis B infectivity, as measured by specific liver and blood markers. A highly purified intravenous form of lentinan has been employed in Japan for the treatment of recurrent stomach cancer, which increases survival with this cancer (particularly when used in combination with chemotherapy). These effects may be due to shiitake's ability to stimulate specific types of white blood cells called T-lymphocytes. Case reports from Japan are also highly suggestive that lentinan is helpful in treating individuals with HIV infection. However, large-scale clinical trials have not yet been performed confirming this action.[2]

How Much Should I Take?

The traditional intake of the whole, dried shiitake mushroom, in soups or as a decoction, is 6–16 grams per day. For LEM, the intake is 1–3 grams two to three times per day until the condition being treated improves. As LEM is the more concentrated and hence more potent extract, it is preferred over the crude mushroom. Tincture, in the amount of 2–4 ml per day, can also be used.

Are There Any Side Effects or Interactions?

Shiitake has an excellent record of safety but has been known to induce temporary diarrhea and abdominal bloating when used in high dosages. Its safety during pregnancy has not yet been established.

SLIPPERY ELM (Ulmus rubra)

THE SLIPPERY ELM tree is native to North America, where it still primarily grows. The inner bark of the tree provides the greatest therapeutic benefit.

In What Conditions Might Slippery Elm Be Supportive?

- **Common cold/sore throat** (page 28)
- Cough
- **Crohn's disease** (page 34)
- Gastritis

Historical or Traditional Use

Native Americans found innumerable medicinal and other uses for this handy tree. Canoes, baskets, and other household goods were made from the tree and its bark. Slippery elm was also used internally for everything from sore throats to diarrhea.[1] As a poultice, it was considered a remedy for almost any skin condition.

Active Constituents

The mucilage of slippery elm gives it the soothing effect for which it is known.[2] The bark contains a host of other constituents, but the carbohydrates that comprise the mucilage are the most important.

How Much Should I Take?

Two or more tablets or capsules (typically 400–500 mg each) can be taken three to four times per day. A tea is made by boiling 1–2 grams of the bark in 200 ml of water for ten to fifteen minutes, which is then cooled before drinking; three to four cups a day can be used. Tincture, 5 ml three times per day, can be taken. Slippery elm is also an ingredient of some cough lozenges and cough syrups.

Are There Any Side Effects or Interactions?

Slippery elm is quite safe, with no known side effects or interactions with any other medicines.

ST. JOHN'S WORT *(Hypericum perforatum)*

ST. JOHN'S WORT is found in Europe and the United States; it is especially abundant in northern California and southern Oregon. The flowering tops are used.

In What Conditions Might St. John's Wort Be Supportive?

- **Depression** (page 36)
- **Recurrent ear infection** (page 47)
- **Vitiligo** (page 122)

Historical or Traditional Use

In ancient Greece, the herb was used to treat many ailments, including sciatica and poisonous reptile bites. In Europe, St. John's wort was, and continues to be, very popular for the topical treatment of wounds and burns. It is also a folk remedy for kidney and lung ailments as well as depression.

Active Constituents

St. John's wort has a complex and diverse chemical makeup. Hypericin and pseudohypericin are believed to have antidepressive and antiviral properties.[1] Other constituents, such as xanthones and flavonoids, may also contribute to the medicinal actions of St. John's wort.[2]

The mechanism by which St. John's wort acts as an antidepressant is not fully understood. Early research indicated that this herb mildly inhibits the enzyme monoamine oxidase (MAO). MAO is responsible for the breakdown of two brain chemicals—serotonin and norepinephrine. By inhibiting MAO and increasing norepinephrine, St. John's wort may exert a mild antidepressive action. The antidepressant (or mood elevating) effects of St. John's wort were originally thought to be due solely to hypericin,[3] but hypericin does not act alone. As with many herbal medicines, St. John's wort relies on the complex interplay of many constituents (e.g., xanthones and flavonoids) for its antidepressant actions.[4] St. John's wort may also block the receptors that bind serotonin.[5]

How Much Should I Take?

Many people take 500 mg per day of herbal extract, tablets, or capsules of St. John's wort standardized to contain 0.2% hypericin. Higher intakes of St. John's wort extract, such as 900 mg per day, may be used in some instances. St. John's wort should be taken close to meals. If used to support depression treatment, its effectiveness should be assessed by a nutritionally oriented doctor after four to six weeks. Herbal tinctures are also available; they are often taken in doses of 1–2 ml three times per day.

Are There Any Side Effects or Interactions?

St. John's wort makes the skin more light-sensitive. Persons with fair skin should avoid exposure to strong sunlight and other sources of ultraviolet light, such as tanning beds. It is also advisable to avoid foods like red wine, cheese, yeast, and pickled herring. St. John's wort should not be used at the same time as prescription antidepressants. St. John's wort should not be used during pregnancy or lactation.

TEA TREE *(Melaleuca alternifolia)*

THE TEA TREE grows in Australia and Asia. This tall evergreen tree has a white, spongy bark. The oil from the leaves is used.

In What Conditions Might Tea Tree Be Supportive?

- **Acne** (page 5)
- Athlete's foot
- Vaginitis
- **Yeast infection** (page 127)

Historical or Traditional Use

Australian Aboriginals used the leaves to treat cuts and skin infections. They would crush the leaves and apply them to the affected area. Captain James Cook and his crew named the tree "tea tree," using its leaves as a substitute for tea as well as to flavor beer. Australian soldiers participating in World War I were given tea tree oil as a disinfectant, leading to a high demand for its production.

Active Constituents

The oil contains numerous chemicals known as terpenoids. Australian standards were established for the amount of one particular compound, terpinen-4-ol, which must make up at least 30% and preferably 40–50% of the oil for it to be medically useful. Another compound, cineole, should make up less than 15% and preferably 2.5% of the oil. The oil kills fungus and bacteria, including those resistant to some powerful antibiotics.[12]

How Much Should I Take?

Oil at a strength of 70–100% should be applied moderately in small areas at least twice per day to the affected areas of skin or nail. For topical treatment of acne, the oil is used at a dilution of 5–15%. Concentrations as strong as 40% may be used—with extreme caution and qualified advice—as vaginal douches.

Are There Any Side Effects or Interactions?

The oil should not be applied to broken skin or to areas affected by rashes not due to fungus. The oil may burn if it gets into eyes, the nose, mouth, or other tender areas. Some people have allergic reactions, including rashes and itching, when applying tea tree oil. For this reason, only a small amount should be applied when first using it. The oil should never be taken internally.

TURMERIC *(Curcuma longa)*

THE VAST majority of turmeric comes from India. Turmeric is one of the key ingredients in many curries, giving them color and flavor. The root and rhizome (underground stem) are used medicinally.

In What Conditions Might Turmeric Be Supportive?

- **Atherosclerosis** (page 11)
- **Bursitis** (page 20)
- Inflammation
- **Rheumatoid arthritis** (page 115)

Historical or Traditional Use

In Ayurvedic medicine (the traditional medicine of India), many different species similar to turmeric are used. It has been prescribed for treatment of many conditions, including poor vision, rheumatic pains, coughs, and to increase milk production. Native peoples of the Pacific sprinkled the dust on their shoulders during ceremonial dances, as well as using it for numerous medical problems ranging from constipation to skin diseases. It was used for numerous intestinal infections and ailments in Southeast Asia.

Active Constituents

The active constituent is known as curcumin. It has been shown to have a wide range of therapeutic effects. First, it protects against free radical damage because it is a strong **antioxidant** (page 8).[1] Second, it reduces inflammation. It accomplishes this by reducing histamine levels and possibly by increasing production of natural cortisone by the adrenal glands.[2] Third, it protects the liver from a number of toxic compounds.[3] Fourth, it has been shown to reduce platelets from clumping together, which in turn improves circulation and helps protect against atherosclerosis.[4] There are also numerous studies showing a cancer-preventing effect of curcumin. This may be due to its powerful antioxidant activity in the body.

How Much Should I Take?

Many people take 400 mg of curcumin three times per day in capsules or tablets. Turmeric as a spice can also be incorporated into the diet as a way to promote health.

Are There Any Side Effects or Interactions?

Turmeric is extremely safe. It has been used in large quantities as a food with no adverse reactions. However, persons with symptoms from gallstones should avoid turmeric.

UVA URSI *(Arctostaphylos uva-ursi)*

COMMON NAME: Bearberry

THE UVA URSI plant is found in colder, northern climates. It has red berries, which bears are said to be fond of. The flowers are also red. The leaf is used medicinally.

In What Conditions Might Uva Ursi Be Supportive?

- Urinary tract infection (page 120)

Historical or Traditional Use

The leaves and berries were used by numerous indigenous people from northern latitudes. Native Americans sometimes combined uva ursi with tobacco and smoked it. It was also used as a beverage tea in some places in Russia. The berries were considered beneficial as a weight-loss aid. It was found in wide use for infections of all parts of the body because of its astringent, or "drying," action.

Active Constituents

The glycoside arbutin is the active ingredient in uva ursi. Arbutin is present in fairly high amounts (up to 10%) in uva ursi. It has been shown to kill bacteria in the urine.[1] Before it can act, however, the sugar portion of arbutin and its attached small molecule (known as hydroquinone) must be broken apart. The urine must be alkaline for this to happen. Hydroquinone is a very powerful antimicrobial agent and is responsible for uva ursi's ability to treat urinary tract infections. Arbutin has also been shown to increase the anti-inflammatory effect of synthetic cortisone.[2]

How Much Should I Take?

For alcohol-based tinctures, many people take 5 ml three times per day. Herbal extracts in capsules or tablets (containing 20% arbutin) in an amount of 250–500 mg three times per day can also be taken. Use of uva ursi should be limited to no more than fourteen days. To ensure alkaline urine, 6–8 grams of sodium bicarbonate (baking soda) mixed in a glass of water can be drunk. Baking soda should not be taken for more than fourteen days; as well, individuals with high blood pressure should not take baking soda. People should not use uva ursi to treat an infection without first consulting a nutritionally oriented doctor.

Are There Any Side Effects or Interactions?

Some people may experience mild nausea after taking uva ursi. Long-term use of uva ursi is not recommended, due to possible side effects from excessive levels of hydroquinone. People should avoid taking acidic agents, such as fruit juice or vitamin C, while using uva ursi. Uva ursi is contraindicated in pregnant or lactating women and should be used in young children only with the guidance of a health care professional.

VALERIAN *(Valeriana officinalis)*

ALTHOUGH VALERIAN grows wild all over Europe, most valerian used for medicinal extracts is cultivated. The root is used.

In What Conditions Might Valerian Be Supportive?

- Insomnia (page 79)

Historical or Traditional Use

The Greek physician Dioscorides recommended valerian for a host of medical problems, including digestive problems, nausea, liver problems, and even urinary tract disorders. Use of valerian for insomnia and nervous conditions has been common for many centuries. By the eighteenth century, it was an accepted sedative and was also used for nervous disorders associated with a restless digestive tract.

Active Constituents

Valerian root contains many different constituents, including essential oils that appear to contribute to the sedating properties of the herb. Central nervous system sedation is regulated by receptors in the brain known as GABA-A receptors. Valerian may weakly bind to these receptors to exert a sedating effect.[1]

How Much Should I Take?

Many people take 300–500 mg of valerian root herbal extract in capsules or tablets one hour before bedtime for insomnia. As an alcohol-based tincture, 5 ml can be taken before bedtime. Combination products with **lemon balm** (page 285), **hops** (page 277), **passion flower** (page 295), and **scullcap** (page 308) can also be used. Children aged six to twelve often respond to half the adult dose.

Are There Any Side Effects or Interactions?

Valerian should not be taken with alcohol. Recent research indicates that valerian does not impair ability to drive or operate machinery. Valerian does not lead to addiction or dependence. There are no known contraindications to using valerian during pregnancy or lactation.

VITEX (Vitex)

COMMON NAMES: Agnus-castus, chaste tree, monk's pepper

VITEX grows in the Mediterranean countries and central Asia. The dried fruit, which has a pepper-like aroma and flavor, is used.

In What Conditions Might Vitex Be Supportive?

- **Fibrocystic breast disease** (page 51)
- **Infertility (female)** (page 75)
- **Menopause** (page 87)
- **Menorrhagia (heavy menstruation)** (page 89)
- Menstrual difficulties (secondary amenorrhea)
- **Premenstrual syndrome** (page 109)

Historical or Traditional Use

Hippocrates, Dioscorides, and Theophrastus mention the use of vitex for a wide variety of conditions, including hemorrhage following childbirth, and also to assist with the "passing of afterbirth." Decoctions of the fruit and plant were also used in sitz baths for diseases of the uterus. In addition, vitex was believed to suppress libido and inspire chastity, which explains one of its common names, chaste tree.

Vitex

Active Constituents

The whole fruit extract, which contains several different components, is thought to be medicinally active.[1] Vitex does not contain hormones; its benefits stem from its actions upon the pituitary gland—specifically on the production of luteinizing hormone. This increases progesterone production and helps regulate a woman's cycle. Vitex also keeps prolactin secretion in check.[2] The ability to decrease excessive prolactin levels may benefit infertile women.

How Much Should I Take?

Many people take 40 drops (in a glass of water) of the concentrated liquid herbal extract in the morning. Vitex is also available in powdered form in tablets and capsules, again to be taken in the morning.

With its emphasis on long-term balancing of a woman's hormonal system, vitex is not a fast-acting herb. For premenstrual syndrome or frequent or heavy periods, vitex can be used continuously for four to six months. Women with amenorrhea and infertility can remain on vitex for twelve to eighteen months, unless pregnancy occurs during treatment.

Are There Any Side Effects or Interactions?

Side effects are rare using vitex. Minor gastrointestinal upset and a mild skin rash with itching have been reported in less than 2% of the women monitored while taking vitex. Vitex is not recommended for use during pregnancy or lactation.

WHITE WILLOW (Salix alba)

THE WHITE WILLOW tree grows primarily in central and southern Europe, although it is also found in North America. As with many medicinal trees, the bark of white willow contains the active constituents.

In What Conditions Might White Willow Be Supportive?

- **Bursitis** (page 20)
- Fever
- Headache (tension)
- **Osteoarthritis** (page 97)
- **Rheumatoid arthritis** (page 115)

Historical or Traditional Use

White willow's Latin name is the source of the name for acetylsalicylic acid (aspirin) as well as the parent compound from which aspirin was eventually created. Willow bark was used traditionally for fever, headache, pain, and rheumatic complaints.[1]

Active Constituents

The glycoside salicin, from which the body can split off salicylic acid, is the basis of the anti-inflammatory and pain-relieving effects of willow.[2] The analgesic actions of willow are typically slow-acting but last longer than standard aspirin products. The bark is also high in tannins, suggesting that it may be of some use in gastrointestinal conditions. However, excessive use may also cause nausea and diarrhea.

How Much Should I Take?

A white willow tea can be prepared from 1–2 grams of bark boiled in 200 ml of water for ten minutes. Five or more cups of this tea can be drunk per day.

Tincture is also used, commonly in the amount of 1–2 ml three times per day. Willow extracts standardized for salicin content are also available. The daily intake of salicin is typically 60–120 mg per day.

Are There Any Side Effects or Interactions?

Long-term use of willow may possibly cause gastrointestinal irritation. As is the case with aspirin, willow should not be used to lower fevers in children. People who are allergic to aspirin should avoid white willow. Long-term use of willow is not advisable, as it may cause some of the same problems that aspirin does—primarily stomach ulcers. However, willow is much safer than aspirin.

WILD CHERRY *(Prunus serotina)*

ALTHOUGH NATIVE to North America, wild cherry trees now grow in many other countries. The bark of the wild cherry tree is used for medicinal preparations.

In What Conditions Might Wild Cherry Be Supportive?

- Cough

Historical or Traditional Use

There is a long tradition of using wild cherry syrups to treat coughs and other lung problems. It has also been used to treat diarrhea and for relief of pain.[1]

Active Constituents

Wild cherry bark contains cyanogenic glycosides, particularly prunasin. These glycosides, once broken apart in the body, act by quelling spasms in the smooth muscles lining bronchioles, thereby relieving coughs.[2]

Wild Cherry

How Much Should I Take?

Many people use wild cherry tincture or syrup, taking 2–4 ml three to four times per day.

Are There Any Side Effects or Interactions?

Very large amounts of wild cherry pose the theoretical risk of causing cyanide poisoning. However, this has not been observed in clinical practice, making it a very safe herbal remedy.

WILD YAM *(Dioscorea villosa)*

WILD YAM plants are found across the midwestern and eastern United States, Latin America (especially Mexico), and Asia. Several different species exist, all possessing similar constituents and properties. The root is used medicinally.

In What Conditions Might Wild Yam Be Supportive?

- Abdominal cramps
- **High cholesterol** (page 62)
- **Hypertriglyceridemia (high triglycerides)** (page 69)
- **Menopause** (page 87)
- Muscle pain or spasms

Historical or Traditional Use

Wild yam root has been used as an expectorant for people with coughs. It was also used for gastrointestinal upset, nerve pain, and morning sickness.[1] Eventually, it was discovered that the saponins from wild yam could be converted industrially into cortisone, estrogens, and progesterone-like compounds. Wild yam and other plants with similar constituents continue to be the main source of these drugs.

Active Constituents

The steroidal saponins (such as diosgenin) account for some of wild yam's activity. Another compound, dioscoretine, has been shown to lower blood sugar levels in diabetic rabbits.[2] An extract of wild yam was found to have antioxidant properties. It has also been shown to lower blood triglycerides and to raise HDL cholesterol (the "good" cholesterol).[3] Wild yam is also considered to be a strong antispasmodic and is potentially anti-inflammatory.

Contrary to popular claims, wild yam roots do not contain and are not converted into progesterone or dehydroepiandrosterone (DHEA) in the body.[4][5] However, wild yam saponins or other constituents may have properties similar to these compounds. Pharmaceutical progesterone is made from wild yam using a chemical conversion process. This can lead to confusion—while wild yam can be a source of progesterone, it cannot be used without this pharmaceutical conversion, which cannot be duplicated by the body. Women who require progesterone should consult their nutritionally oriented physician and not rely solely on wild yam or other herbs.

How Much Should I Take?

Many people take up to 2–3 ml of wild yam tincture three to four times per day. Alternatively, one or two capsules or tablets of the dried root can be taken three times per day.

Are There Any Side Effects or Interactions?

Some people may experience nausea when taking large amounts of wild yam.

WITCH HAZEL *(Hamamelis virginiana)*

ALTHOUGH NATIVE to North America, witch hazel now also grows in Europe. The leaves and bark of the tree are used as medicine.

In What Conditions Might Witch Hazel Be Supportive?

- Eczema (page 49)
- Hemorrhoids (page 60)
- Skin ulcers
- Varicose veins
- Wound healing

Historical or Traditional Use

Native Americans utilized poultices of witch hazel leaves and bark to treat hemorrhoids, wounds, painful tumors, insect bites, and ulcers.[1] Witch hazel is one of the clearest examples of how modern research has confirmed the traditional uses of a botanical medicine.

Active Constituents

Tannins and volatile oils are the main active constituents in witch hazel, giving it a strong astringent effect. Witch hazel has also been shown to have a beneficial effect on veins and to be anti-inflammatory.[2][3] Topical creams are currently used in Europe to treat inflammatory skin conditions, such as eczema.

How Much Should I Take?

In combination with warm, moist compresses, witch hazel extracts can be applied liberally at least twice each day (in the morning and at bedtime) to hemorrhoids. For other skin problems, ointment or cream can be applied twice a day, or as needed. For hemorrhoids and varicose veins, witch hazel is often combined with **horse chestnut** (page 278).

Are There Any Side Effects or Interactions?

Witch hazel may cause minor skin irritation in some people when applied topically. This herb is not typically recommended for internal use.

WORMWOOD *(Artemisia absinthium)*

THE WORMWOOD shrub grows wild in Europe, North Africa, and western Asia. It is now cultivated in North America as well. The leaves and flowers, and the oil obtained from them, are used as medicine.

In What Conditions Might Wormwood Be Supportive?

- Indigestion
- Inflammation of the gallbladder (cholecystitis)
- **Irritable bowel syndrome** (page 81)
- Poor appetite

Historical or Traditional Use

Wormwood is perhaps best known because of the use of its oil to prepare certain alcoholic beverages, most notably vermouth and absinthe. Absinthe, popular in the nineteenth century in Europe, caused several cases of brain damage and even death and was banned in most places in the early twentieth century.[1]

Wormwood oil continues to be used as a flavoring agent for foods, although in much smaller amounts than were found in absinthe. As a medicine, wormwood was traditionally used as a bitter to improve digestion, to fight worm infestations, and to stimulate menstruation.[2] It was regarded as a useful remedy for problems involving the liver and gallbladder.

Active Constituents

The aromatic oil of wormwood contains the toxins thujone and isothujone. Very little of this oil is present in ordinary wormwood teas or tinctures.[3] Although the oil destroys various types of worms, it may cause damage to the human nervous system. Also present in the plant are strong bitter agents known as absinthin and anabsinthin. These stimulate digestive function.

How Much Should I Take?

A wormwood tea can be made by adding 1 teaspoon of the herb to 250 ml (1 cup) of boiling water, allowing it to steep for ten to fifteen minutes. Many people drink three cups each day. Tincture can be used, in the amount of 10–20 drops in water, taken ten to fifteen minutes before each meal. Either preparation should not be used for more than four weeks consecutively.

Are There Any Side Effects or Interactions?

Long-term intake of the thujone-containing oil or alcoholic beverages (absinthe) made with the oil is strictly contraindicated—it is addictive and causes brain damage, seizures, and even death. Short-term use of the wormwood tea or tincture has not resulted in any reports of significant side effects. Longer-term use can cause nausea, vomiting, insomnia, restlessness, vertigo, tremors, and seizures.[4] Wormwood is contraindicated during pregnancy and lactation.

YOHIMBE *(Pausinystalia yohimbe)*

THE YOHIMBE tree grows primarily in western Africa. The bark of this African tree is used medicinally.

In What Conditions Might Yohimbe Be Supportive?

- **Depression** (page 36)
- Impotence/**infertility** (**male**) (page 77)

Historical or Traditional Use

Historically, yohimbe bark was used in western Africa for fevers, leprosy, and coughs.[1] It has also been used to dilate pupils, for heart disease, and as a local anesthetic. It has a more recent history of use as an aphrodisiac and a hallucinogen.

Active Constituents

The alkaloid known as yohimbine is the primary active constituent in yohimbe, although similar alkaloids may also play a role. Yohimbine blocks alpha-2 adrenergic receptors, part of the sympathetic nervous system.[2] It also dilates blood vessels. This has made the compound a useful substance for treating male sexual dysfunction. Yohimbine inhibits monoamine oxidase (MAO) and therefore may be of benefit in depressive disorders. However, it is not backed by the clinical research of other herbs used for depression, such as **St. John's wort** (page 312).

How Much Should I Take?

A tincture of the bark is often used in the amount of 5–10 drops three times per day. There are also standardized yohimbe products available for the treatment of impotence. A typical safe daily amount of yohimbine from any product is 15–30 mg. It is best to use yohimbine under the supervision of a nutritionally oriented doctor.

Are There Any Side Effects or Interactions?

Patients with kidney disease or peptic ulcer and pregnant or lactating women should not use yohimbe. Standard doses may sometimes cause dizziness, nausea, insomnia, or anxiety. Using more than 40 mg of yohimbine per day can cause dangerous side effects, including loss of muscle function, chills, and vertigo. Some people will also experience hallucinations when taking higher amounts of yohimbine.

Foods with high amounts of tyramine (such as cheese, red wine, and liver) should not be eaten while a person is taking yohimbe, as it may cause severe hypertension and other problems. Similarly, yohimbe should only be combined with other antidepressant drugs under the close supervision of a physician, although at least one study suggests it may benefit those who are not responding to serotonin reuptake inhibitors such as Prozac.[3]

YUCCA *(Yucca schidigera and other species)*

YUCCA grows primarily in the southwestern United States and is related to the Joshua tree. The stalk and root of this desert tree are used medicinally.

In What Conditions Might Yucca Be Supportive?

- **Osteoarthritis** (page 97)
- **Rheumatoid arthritis** (page 115)

Historical or Traditional Use

Native Americans used the soapy leaves from yucca for numerous conditions. Poultices or baths were used for skin sores and other diseases as well as for sprains. Inflammation of all sorts, including joint inflammations, and bleeding were also treated with yucca. Some report that the Native Americans washed their hair with yucca to fight dandruff and hair loss.

Active Constituents

The saponins from yucca are the main medicinal agents in the plant. They have both a water-soluble and fat-soluble end and therefore act like soap. The authors of the study looking at patients with osteoarthritis and rheumatoid arthritis speculate that yucca saponins block release of toxins from the intestines that inhibit normal formation of cartilage.[1] An extract of one species of yucca has been found to fight melanoma cells in test tube studies.[2]

How Much Should I Take?

Many people take two capsules or tablets of yucca saponins per day. Up to twice this dose has been used in some cases and may be required for more severe arthritis. Alternatively, $1/4$ ounce of the root can be boiled in a pint of water for fifteen minutes. Three to five cups can be drunk per day. If this causes loose stools, the amount of root in the tea should be decreased.

Are There Any Side Effects or Interactions?

Yucca and other saponins can cause red blood cells to burst (known as hemolysis) in test tubes. The level to which this occurs when the saponins are taken by mouth is unknown. However, yucca is approved for use in foods as a foaming agent (particularly in root beer). Since there have been no reports of problems with hemolysis in root beer drinkers, it can be assumed that yucca herbal supplements are generally safe.

HOMEOPATHIC REMEDIES

Homeopathy is a system of medicine that treats illness by the stimulation of the body's own healing powers. Homeopathy gently encourages the body to do more of what it is already trying to do to heal itself. Think of homeopathy as somewhat similar to the principle behind vaccines: A little bit of the "disease" is given in order to prompt the body to better heal itself. Homeopathy has the added advantage of using microdoses, which means that there are no side effects and no risk of toxicity.

Homeopathic therapy has three underlying rules:

1. Any pharmacologically active substance can cause a set of symptoms in an otherwise healthy individual.
2. Anyone suffering from a particular disease presents a set of symptoms that is characteristic of that disease.
3. A remission of the symptoms can be obtained by administration of a small quantity of the substance whose experimental effects are similar to the symptoms of the patient.

Homeopathic medicine is based on a principle called the Law of Similars, which says that if a natural substance in large amounts causes a symptom in a healthy person, it will, in small amounts, stimulate the body's own curative powers in the unhealthy individual.

An example of the Law of Similars is red onions. Imagine what happens when someone chops a red onion—watery eyes, runny nose, sneezing, and an irritated throat develops. A medicine can be made from the red onion, following a very specific laboratory process; this medicine will safely and effectively treat the symptoms of watery eyes, runny nose, sneezing, and throat irritation. According to the Law of Similars, the symptoms experienced by an individual do not need to be caused by the red onion; they can result from a mild allergy or the common cold, just as long as the symptoms are similar.

Understanding Homeopathy Potency

Homeopathic therapy involves the use of infinitesimally small doses. The first step in producing a homeopathic medication is to prepare a mother tincture (MT), which is the base substance derived from a natural source. Mother tinctures are made according to very strict guidelines and are different from regular tinctures in subtle but important ways.

Mother tinctures are the source for homeopathic preparations, which are designated as either "x" potency or "c" potency. Keep in mind that according to Roman numerals, x equals 10 and c equals 100. Therefore, x potencies are made in a homeopathic laboratory by diluting one part of the mother tincture with nine parts of water or alcohol. This new mixture (1:9) is then shaken vigorously. This is called succussion, and it is absolutely essential in the homeopathic manufacturing process. Succussion is the potentizing process; without succussion after each dilution, a homeopathic medicine would not be complete.

In the above example, the mother tincture was diluted once, so the result is called a 1x potency. In the next step, one part of the 1x is mixed with nine parts of water or alcohol, and after succussion, this new mixture is called 2x. This process is continued to produce 3x, 4x, and so on.

A similar process produces the c potencies. One part of the mother tincture is diluted in ninety-nine parts of water or alcohol and succussed to produce a 1c potency. One part of the 1c potency is then mixed with ninety-nine parts of water or alcohol and again this new bottle is shaken vigorously, yielding a 2c potency. This process can be continued to produce 3c, 4c, and so on.

Homeopathic Dosage

In cases where there are several remedies listed under the condition, choose the remedy that most closely matches your symptoms. Use the number of tablets as directed on the label or by your physician. For all of the following remedies, dissolve the pellet or tablet under your tongue unless directed otherwise.

REMEDIES FOR ACNE

ACNE (page 5), or the presence of pimples or blackheads, can be a problem on the face, chest, and back. Although it is most common during adolescence, acne can occur at other times in life. In women, acne may be triggered by hormonal shifts in the monthly cycle. Good hygiene and diet play an important role in resolving this complaint.

Sulfur 6c

Persistent cases of acne may respond well to Sulfur. This remedy is indicated when pimples become red, infected, and sore; often the skin condition is worse after washing with water, which may cause the skin to feel itchy. Sulfur 6c can be taken three times per day for ten to fourteen days, reducing the frequency as the condition improves.

Hepar Sulfuris 6c

This remedy is called for when there are large, red, painful eruptions similar to boils, or when the pimples have become infected and have a thick discharge. Quite often, individuals who could benefit from the use of Hepar sulfuris tend to be somewhat chilly and have a preference for warm drinks. Hepar sulfuris 6c can be taken three to four times per day for up to ten days, reducing the frequency as the symptoms improve.

REMEDIES FOR ALCOHOL WITHDRAWAL SUPPORT

WITHDRAWAL from the use of alcohol can be a complex matter. A physician or other health care professional should be consulted if alcohol has been consumed for a long period of time. The following remedies may ease the difficulties of the withdrawal process.

Nux Vomica 6c

This remedy is well known for its effectiveness in helping with the common hangover. It can also help individuals who are very irritable and sensitive to noises. Bright lights and strong odors are disturbing to people needing this remedy; they are also likely to be quite chilly, exhausted, and suffering from an upset stomach. Nux vomica 6c can be taken three times per day for several days.

Carbo Vegetabilis 6c

When withdrawal symptoms include a lot of gas and belching, with great fatigue, this remedy may bring relief. People needing this remedy will not want to be covered up, despite feeling chilly and having cold sweats, preferring light clothing and cool breezes instead. Carbo vegetabilis 6c can be taken three to four times per day for several days or until symptoms change.

Coffea Cruda 6c

This remedy may bring relief to individuals whose minds are running wild and full of ideas. Sleeplessness is a common problem. People will be quite sensitive to any stimulation and may experience headaches that are relieved by cold applications. Coffea cruda 6c can be taken three to four times per day for up to ten days.

REMEDIES FOR ANXIETY

EVERYONE SUFFERS from anxiety at times. Anxiety is a sensation of discomfort or apprehension, the cause of which is not always known. Homeopathy can be used for cases of general anxiety.

Gelsemium 30c

This remedy is known for its use in anticipatory anxiety, for example, fears that precede a visit to the dentist, a big audition, or delivering a speech. Individuals with this anxiety may experience a sensation of being paralyzed by fear, with trembling and weakness. Gelsemium 30c can be taken as needed, but no more than three to four doses per day.

Argentum Nitricum 6c

Like Gelsemium, this remedy can help with a panicky sensation that develops before a big event. Individuals may have diarrhea, along with stage fright, craving for sweets, and a perception of slow passage of time. Argentum nitricum 6c can be taken as needed, but no more than three to four doses per day.

Ignatia Amara 6c

This remedy is best known for helping in times of grief. People needing Ignatia will sigh often and exhibit changeable temperaments. It can help with melancholy that follows disappointment. Ignatia amara 6c can be taken up to four times per day.

Anxiety

REMEDIES FOR BACKACHE

MANY DIFFERENT factors can contribute to back pain. Homeopathy provides safe and effective pain relief for many types of backaches. Whether back pain develops from overwork, injury, or during menstruation, the following homeopathic remedies can be considered.

Arnica 6c

When back pain results from an injury or a blow, Arnica is the first remedy of choice. The affected area often feels bruised and can appear swollen. Arnica should also be considered whenever overexertion is the underlying cause of the problem. This remedy has a strong reputation for its usefulness after difficult pregnancies, extreme sports activities, or unexpected physical workouts. Arnica 6c can be taken four times per day for a two-day period.

Arnica Ointments and Gels

Arnica is a remedy with a well-known reputation for its usefulness in injuries and pain to soft tissue and muscles. Applied topically in either the gel or ointment form (and in conjunction with internal use of Arnica 6c), topical Arnica can be useful for relieving pain.

Rhus Toxicodendron 6c

This remedy can be useful for lower back pain, particularly when the pain worsens upon first movement but improves after gentle and continued motion. The aching may be brought on by cold, damp weather and is relieved by warm applications or showers. Even in pain, people needing this remedy may be unable to sit still, pacing restlessly about. Rhus toxicodendron 6c can be taken four times per day for a two-day period.

Actaea Racacemosa 6c

If severe aching and stiffness develops in the back during menstruation, extending down through the hips, buttocks, and thighs, Actaea racacemosa may offer relief. Muscles throughout the back feel heavy, sore, and cramped. People needing this remedy often appear agitated and irritable. Actaea racacemosa 6c can be taken every hour for three hours.

REMEDIES FOR BELL'S PALSY

BELL'S PALSY is a condition in which one side of the face becomes paralyzed. The muscles and nerves are rigid and swollen. Although it is uncomfortable and disconcerting to the person with this condition, it often resolves itself without treatment. However, two homeopathic remedies are known to bring relief. Other remedies may be useful; a homeopathic physician should be consulted.

Aconite Napellus 30c

This remedy may offer relief when the person's face has "frozen" after being exposed to a cold wind (for example, riding a bicycle in winter or driving a car with the window rolled down in frigid weather). People with this condition will likely be anxious, restless, and quite fearful about the condition. Aconite napellus 30c can be taken three times per day for three days; its use should be discontinued when symptoms diminish.

Causticum 30c

This remedy may be more helpful for Bell's palsy that develops on the right side of the face. Opening and closing the mouth may be difficult for individuals with this condition. In addition, they may be weak, restless, and feel better when warm. The problem may have started slowly, possibly due to emotional stress. Causticum 30c can be taken three times per day for three days; its use should be discontinued when symptoms diminish.

REMEDIES FOR BENIGN PROSTATIC HYPERPLASIA

BENIGN PROSTATIC

HYPERPLASIA (BPH) (page 18) is caused when the prostate gland enlarges or swells, putting pressure on the urethra and causing problems with urination.

In men over fifty years old, complaints concerning the prostate gland are common. Men should have regular examinations to ensure that their prostate problems are not indicative of a more serious condition, such as prostate cancer.

Lycopodium 6c

In cases where an enlarged prostate is coupled with impotence, this remedy may be effective. Urine is often slow in coming, and pain in the back ceases with urination. Flatulence is common. Warm drinks are preferred, and individuals generally feel worse between 4 P.M. and 8 P.M. Lycopodium 6c can be taken two times per day for three weeks.

Apis Mellifica 6c

When an enlarged prostate causes frequent and sometimes involuntary urination, this medicine may be helpful. There is a stinging and burning sensation with urination, often with the last drops causing the greatest pain. Individuals needing this remedy often feel worse from heat and in hot rooms and generally feel better in cool air or with a cool bath. Apis mellifica 6c is often taken three times per day for two weeks.

Sabal Serrulata 6c

When nightly visits to the bathroom become numerous and there is difficulty in passing urine, this remedy can be helpful. The sexual organ often feels cold. Sabal serrulata 6c can be taken two times per day for three weeks.

REMEDIES FOR BOILS

BOILS are most often the result of a bacterial infection of a hair follicle. Boils range in severity from a minor inconvenience to extreme pain. Homeopathic medicines can be quite useful in reducing the painfulness of boils and, in some cases, halting their growth altogether. If infection should spread, seek professional care.

Tarentula Cubensis 30c

This ominous-sounding medicine can bring relief when a boil appears suddenly and is accompanied by a burning, stinging painfulness. The area surrounding the boil is often purple or blue. People needing this remedy are likely to be very restless and unable to sit down for even a few minutes. Do not confuse this remedy with Tarentula hispanica. Tarentula cubensis 30c can be taken four times per day over a two-day period.

Hepar Sulfuris 6c

In cases where the boil is extremely sensitive to even slight touch, this remedy may be helpful. The boil also has a sharp or prickly pain. Persons benefiting from this remedy will likely be irritable and dislike cold drafts. Hepar sulfuris 6c can be taken four times per day over a two-day period.

Echinacea Angustifolia 30c

This well-known herb can be used in its homeopathic form to help with boils. People needing this remedy will likely be lethargic, chilly, and achy. A general sickliness is present. Echinacea angustifolia 30c can be taken four times per day over a two-day period.

Belladonna 6c

Belladonna can be used in the very early stages of inflammation, before pus formation. The area will be hot, throbbing, and tender to the touch, with violent stabbing pains. The boil may be made worse by movement and cold applications. Belladonna 6c can be taken once an hour for six doses, then three times per day for up to two weeks.

Silicea 6c

Silicea can be used when boils are a recurring problem and when pus formation has begun. Silicea will hasten the ripening of a boil and aid in the discharge of its contents. Silicea 6c can be taken every hour, for six doses, then three times per day for up to two weeks.

Hypericum MT

The liquid form of this remedy will serve well when applied undiluted to the unbroken boil to help relieve pain. It is often used in conjunction with the remedies mentioned above. If the boil has broken open, then the mother tincture should be diluted 1:10 (one part tincture to ten parts water) and applied to the open wound. Calendula MT can also be used on broken boils at a 1:25 dilution. The tincture should be applied three times daily.

REMEDIES FOR BROKEN BONE SUPPORT

A BROKEN BONE should always be treated by a licensed physician. Proper setting of a bone is essential. However, homeopathic remedies have a sound reputation for bringing relief from pain associated with broken bones as well as for accelerating the healing process.

In addition to the remedies described below, homeopathic doctors routinely give the following concurrently to ensure solid and speedy knitting of a broken bone.

- Calcarea phosphorica 6c: Two times per day for three days, then once daily for two weeks
- Symphytum 6c: Two times per day for three days, then once daily for two weeks

Arnica 30c

This remedy is often used immediately after a bone is broken. It can help relieve the pain that develops when tissue surrounding the broken bone is damaged. It may also help reduce swelling and act as a calming agent. Arnica 30c can be initially taken every fifteen to thirty minutes for an hour or two (for example, while driving to the hospital). Arnica 30c can then be continued three times per day for two days.

Ruta Graveolens 6c

Ruta graveolens can be of good use when the pain around the area of the fracture or break is extreme. This remedy is often given if Arnica does not provide relief. Ruta graveolens 6c can be taken three times per day.

REMEDIES FOR BURNS

FOR THE pain and blistering of burns that do not call for professional medical care, homeopathic remedies can be useful. "The sooner the better" is the motto when treating burns. Having these remedies on hand can save a lot of discomfort and expense.

Cantharis 6c

Given shortly after a scalding or a superficial burn, Cantharis may bring prompt relief. Homeopathic physicians note this remedy's reputation for preventing the formation of blisters. This remedy is called for when cold applications provide relief from pain. Cantharis 6c can be taken three to four times per day; use should be discontinued when symptoms diminish.

Calendula MT

This homeopathic liquid mother tincture can be useful in promoting the healing of a burn. Ten drops of Calendula MT are diluted into 1 ounce of water, then applied to the burn three times per day.

Urtica Urens 6c

When the burn is mild and only redness and stinging are prominent, this remedy may offer quick relief. Urtica urens can be given to individuals who have spent too much time in the sun and whose skin has developed hot, prickly, or stinging sensations. Urtica urens 6c can be taken three to four times per day for one to two days; its use should be discontinued when symptoms improve.

Causticum 6c

This remedy is noted for its special usefulness in relieving the pain of a scalded tongue. It can also be used when an old burn has not healed completely. The burned area, including the tongue, throat, or skin, will have a very raw soreness. Causticum 6c can be taken three to four times per day for one day.

REMEDIES FOR BURSITIS

BURSITIS (page 20) is a painful condition in which the bursa (a small, fluid-filled sac cushioning pressure points of the body) becomes inflamed. Homeopathic medicines can work effectively with many kinds of inflammation, thereby reducing or eliminating pain.

Rhus Toxicodendron 6c

Rhus toxicodendron, known as the "rusty gate" remedy, may be helpful for those who experience stiffness and pain when first getting up and moving about, which gradually improves after continued motion. The pain worsens with cold, damp weather and is relieved by warmth. Rhus toxicodendron 6c can be taken three to four times per day for three to four days, as needed.

Ruta Graveolens 6c

This remedy is known for its use to relieve symptoms of **carpal tunnel syndrome** (page 23). Symptoms noted are stiffness and aching. In addition, people may feel pain when stretching as well as weakness and fatigue. Like Rhus toxicodendron, pain is worse with cold and damp and better with warmth. Ruta graveolens 6c can be taken three to four times per day for three to four days, as needed.

Belladonna 6c

If there is a sensation of strong heat and throbbing pain in the joint, and if even a slight jolt to the area causes real discomfort, then this remedy may bring prompt relief. The joint may be swollen, red, and painful to even light touch. Heat can be felt radiating from the affected area. Belladonna 6c can be taken three to four times per day for one to two days.

REMEDIES FOR CANKER SORES

CANKER SORES (page 21), or mouth ulcers, are painful, ulcerated sores inside the mouth. They are usually caused by bacteria but may result from a combination of factors, including vitamin deficiencies and stress. Some commonly used homeopathic solutions are offered here.

Natrum Muriaticum 6c

People who may benefit from this remedy may also suffer at times from herpes on the lips. The mouth will be dry, often with a crack in the center of the lower lip. Dryness and tingling of the tongue, craving for salt, and an aversion to sun and heat may also be present. Natrum muriaticum 6c can be taken three to four times per day, then less often as symptoms improve.

Mercurius Sol 6c

Mercurius sol may be helpful if the breath is noticeably foul and salivation is greater than usual. The canker sores have a burning pain that worsens at night. In addition, thirst increases and, upon inspection, the tongue is indented on the sides. Mercurius sol 6c can be taken three to four times per day, then less often as symptoms improve.

Arsenicum Album 6c

Arsenicum album may be useful following stress, exhaustion, or anxiety. Persons who may benefit from this remedy typically have unhealthy, easily bleeding gums and burning, stinging ulcers with dry mouth. They are relieved by very hot drinks. Arsenicum album 6c can be taken three to four times per day, then discontinued when symptoms improve.

Borax 6c

Borax may help in cases in which the mouth is sensitive to acids (such as the acid in citrus fruits), the canker sores are on the inside of the cheeks and tongue, and the mouth feels dry yet still has saliva. If these symptoms are present in a child, the youngster may be sensitive to all noises and react very strongly to downward motion. Borax 6c can be taken three to four times per day; its use should be discontinued when symptoms improve.

Rhus Toxicodendron 6c

This remedy may be helpful for people whose whole mouth area is sore, inside and out, including the lips and gums. Also, ulceration and blistering occur at the corner of the mouth (these are often associated with cold sores). Rhus toxicodendron 6c can be taken three to four times per day, then less often as symptoms improve.

REMEDIES FOR CARPAL TUNNEL SYNDROME

CARPAL TUNNEL SYNDROME (page 23) is a condition of the forearm and wrist that results from overuse or stress to the muscles, for example, from working at a computer keyboard. Wear and tear on the nerves that move through the wrist can limit function of the forearm and hand. Symptoms may include weakness of the hand, wrist, and arm and sensations of numbness, tingling, or burning in these areas. A well-chosen homeopathic remedy can be useful in relieving the discomforts and limitations of this condition.

Ruta Graveolens 6c

Ruta graveolens may benefit individuals experiencing weakness in the wrists, particularly if it is accompanied by stiffness. Overuse of the arm and hand is often the culprit that brings on these symptoms, such as repetitive hammering for carpentry work or extensive use of a keyboard. The arm or wrist may feel sore and bruised and the pain is likely to be worse after using the limb. Ruta graveolens 6c can be taken three to four times per day, repeating as needed.

Rhus Toxicodendron 6c

Rhus toxicodendron is known as the "rusty gate" remedy. It may improve cases in which pain occurs with initial motion of the hand or wrist, then subsides with continued motion. The discomfort is likely to be relieved by heat and made worse by cold, damp weather, or an impending storm. The wrist joint may crack when the hand is moved in a circle. Rhus toxicodendron 6c can be taken three to four times per day for five to seven days, with reduced frequency as the discomfort is relieved.

REMEDIES FOR CHEMOTHERAPY SUPPORT

THE REMEDIES listed here are intended only for the relief of some of the unpleasant side effects of chemotherapy treatment. These remedies are not to be considered as a substitute for or an adjunct to cancer treatments. They are, however, safe and do not interfere with the chemotherapy treatment itself. See also the section on **chemotherapy support** (page 25).

Gelsemium 6c

This remedy is known for its usefulness in calming anticipatory anxiety, such as stage fright. It may prove helpful to people experiencing fear and anxiety prior to cancer treatment. Nervousness and weak trembling may be present, indicating the need for this remedy. Gelsemium 6c can be taken two to three times prior to chemotherapy treatment.

Ipecac 30c

Persistent nausea and vomiting are symptoms indicating the possible usefulness of this remedy. Individuals will likely have a clean tongue with a lot of saliva. They do not feel better when lying down or after vomiting. Ipecac 30c can be taken three to four times every fifteen to thirty minutes and discontinued when the nausea subsides.

Nux Vomica 6c

This remedy may be helpful for individuals with a hangover feeling accompanied by nausea and vomiting. They will likely be very sensitive to all loud noises, odors, and lights. Symptoms of chilliness and irritability may be present. Nux vomica 6c can be taken three to four times per day for one to two days and discontinued when symptoms diminish.

Cadmium Sulfuricum 30c

Cadmium sulfuricum is a little-known remedy for the vomiting and debilitating exhaustion that sometimes follows chemotherapy treatment. Individuals needing this remedy will be very chilly with intense nausea. Cadmium sulfuricum 30c can be taken three times per day for one to two days and discontinued when nausea and vomiting subside.

REMEDIES FOR CHICKEN POX

CHICKEN POX is caused by a highly contagious airborne virus. The disease appears ten to twenty-one days after exposure, and symptoms include fever, lethargy, and itching lesions. Homeopathy offers several good options to reduce the misery of this childhood disease.

Rhus Toxicodendron 6c

This remedy may be especially useful when tremendous itching and restlessness are present. In addition, there may be stiffness and muscular aching. Symptoms that improve with warmth also warrant this remedy. Rhus toxicodendron 6c can be taken four times per day for three to four days or until another remedy is indicated.

Note: Many homeopaths recommend several doses of Rhus toxicodendron at 30c or higher potency for people recently exposed to chicken pox, in order to provide a measure of resistence. Rhus toxicodendron 30c can be taken three times per day once a week for three weeks by adults and children.

Belladonna 30c

Belladonna may be useful at the onset of fever-burning hot skin with a pulsating headache. The face is hot and red, the pupils dilated, but the lips and mouth may be pale. Individuals who may benefit will have blisters that feel hot and painful. Belladonna 30c can be taken four times per day for three to four days or until the symptoms subside.

Sulfur 6c

Sulfur may be of help with people experiencing great itching and intense burning, often in patches. Individuals feel hot and cold, and they are drowsy in the afternoon but hot and bothered at night. In addition, they are aggravated by heat and contact with water. Sulfur 6c can be taken four times daily until symptoms improve.

Bryonia 30c

When a dry and persistent cough has developed and the temperature remains high, this remedy may help. Other indicative symptoms are increased thirst and irritability and when the expected course of the chicken pox has slowed. Bryonia 30c can be taken three to four times per day and discontinued when symptoms improve or change.

Antimonium Tartaricum 6c

This remedy may help a rattling cough accompanied by fussing and whining. It should also be used when the scabs are large. The itching in this case is less bothersome than the itching that is treated with Rhus toxicodendron, but the tongue may be coated thick and white, and individuals may desire cold water and fruit. Antimonium tartaricum 6c can be taken three to four times per day and discontinued when improvement is noted.

REMEDIES FOR COLIC

COLIC causes very painful spasmodic cramps. Homeopathy can bring relief to childhood colic as well as menstrual cramping. However, a physician should be seen if pain and discomfort persist.

Cuprum Metallicum 6c

If the abdominal pains are extreme (some describe it as sharp and stabbing) or if the abdomen is tense, and pain can be made either better or much worse by drinking cold water, then this remedy may be useful. This remedy can also be used for cramps in the calves and the soles of the feet, particularly in athletes or the elderly. Cuprum metallicum 6c can be taken three to four times as needed and discontinued when improvement is noted.

Chamomilla 6c

This remedy is noted for its usefulness in treating extremely painful (sometimes described by people as unbearable) colicky conditions and those that occur in sensitive or irritable people. Children needing this remedy will want to be carried and will feel worse in heat. Colic pain may center around the navel and be accompanied by diarrhea. Chamomilla is often sold as "teething granules." Chamomilla 6c can be taken three times per day for three to four days.

Colocynthis 30c

This remedy, made from bitter cucumber, is indicated when severe pain leads to doubling over. Pressing hard into the abdomen brings some relief to those who will benefit from this remedy. Individuals may become very irritable and angry. The pain is cutting and harshly contracting (some people describe feeling "clamped with iron bands"). Diarrhea may be present as well. Colocynthis 30c can be taken three times per day and discontinued when the pain diminishes.

Nux Vomica 6c

This remedy is indicated for colicky pains following overeating and overindulgences of all kinds. Symptoms include pinching pain and a hard abdomen that is not distended. Take Nux vomica 6c every fifteen minutes for up to one hour and discontinue when symptoms diminish.

Belladonna 6c

People who may benefit from this remedy feel a sudden onset of gripping pain and have hot, dry skin.

The pain worsens with movement but improves when the sufferer bends over. Pain may extend to bowels, creating a bloated feeling. Belladonna 6c can be taken in the amount of one dose every hour, up to six doses; its use should be reduced when improvement is noted.

Bryonia 6c

This remedy may help people who feel an extreme stitching pain accompanied by a bloated feeling. The individuals are also very irritable. For these people, the slightest movement causes pain—even breathing is difficult. Relief comes from warmth and doubling over. Bryonia 6c can be taken in the amount of one dose every hour, up to six doses; its use should be reduced when improvement is noted.

REMEDIES FOR THE COMMON COLD

THE COMMON COLD (page 28), a highly contagious viral infection, often strikes when immune resistance is compromised by overwork, stress, and anxiety. The most common symptoms are sneezing, watering of the eyes and nose, fever, lethargy, aching, sore throat, and coughing. Homeopathy offers a number of useful options in alleviating these symptoms.

Aconite 30c

This remedy can be taken at the first sign of a cold. The symptoms will come on very suddenly and violently, often following exposure to cold, dry wind (for example, after sitting in front of an air conditioner or riding a bicycle on a cool evening). The nose is dry, but individuals sneeze and have a scratchy sensation at the back of the throat. Aconite 30c can be taken in the amount of one dose every two hours, three times only.

Kali Bichromicum 6c

For later stages of a cold, this remedy may be useful when mucus discharge becomes thick, stringy, and difficult to clear from the head, nose, and throat. Mucus may be yellowish-green, and there is pain at the base of the nose as well as a hoarse cough with tenacious expectoration. Kali bichromicum 6c can be taken three to four times per day for two to three days.

Rhus Toxicodendron 6c

If the cold comes on as the season changes to cold and damp, people can look to this remedy. Early symptoms will be deep stiffness and body aches. There may also be restlessness, while continued motion somewhat relieves pain and anxiety. Symptoms should improve in a warm environment, such as a hot shower. Other possible symptoms that indicate the usefulness of this remedy are fever and a dry cough. Rhus toxicodendron 6c can be taken three times per day for one to two days.

Natrum Muriaticum 6c

This remedy may be helpful if sneezing is worse in the morning. People who may benefit often have cold sores and a headache and generally feel unwell. They see a watery discharge from the nose and experience a loss of taste and smell. Natrum muriaticum 6c can be taken in the amount of one dose every two hours, up to six doses.

Euphrasia 6c

People who may benefit from this remedy have streaming eyes and nose with much sneezing. Their eyes are red from burning tears. The symptoms are usually worse at night. Euphrasia 6c can be taken four times daily, until symptoms improve.

REMEDIES FOR CONJUNCTIVITIS

CONJUNCTIVITIS can have a variety of causes: a bacteria, a virus, a foreign body in the eye, or an allergic reaction. Although homeopathy can address this condition effectively, a doctor should be consulted if a foreign body is lodged in the eye. A simple, acute episode of conjunctivitis can be treated with several homeopathic remedies; however, it is important to obtain medically qualified treatment if no improvement is seen in the first twelve hours.

Argentum Nitricum 6c

If discharge from the eye is profuse, nonirritating, and yellowish in color, with the inner corner of the eye appearing very red and swollen, then this remedy is indicated. In addition, eyes may be tired and achy, and pain is relieved by cool water or a cold compress. Individuals generally feel better in cool air, crave sweets, and may experience belching and gas. Argentum nitricum 6c can be taken three to four times per day for one to two days.

Mercurius Sol 6c

People needing this remedy will be tired, with an erratic body temperature that alternates between hot and chilly. The discharge from the eye will be greenish-yellow, causing abrasion to the lids and margins of the eye. In addition, individuals will be thirsty and have excessive saliva and foul breath. Mercurius sol 6c can be taken three to four times per day for one to two days.

Hepar Sulfuris 6c

This remedy is called for when the redness and swelling are pronounced in the eye. The eyes feel as if they have sand and grit in them, and they are very sensitive to cold air and breezes. Also, individuals are sensitive to any loud noises, strong smells, and bright lights. The discharge from the eyes is profuse and yellowish, being sticky and dried in the morning upon awakening. Improvement is noticed after application of a warm compress. Hepar sulfuris 6c can be taken three to four times per day for one to two days.

REMEDIES FOR CONSTIPATION

CONSTIPATION (page 32) is a problem for many people in today's busy world. There are nearly as many causes of constipation as there are people suffering from it. Although homeopathy offers several gentle alternatives to harsh laxatives, dietary and lifestyle changes may also be needed.

Nux Vomica 6c

This remedy is well known in homeopathic circles for helping in cases of constipation that develop in individuals who work too hard, exercise too little, and drink and eat too much. People benefiting from this remedy often have the urge to defecate but are unsuccessful, passing only a small quantity, although this does provide some relief. Nux vomica is also helpful for people who are dependent on laxatives and have headaches that accompany the constipation. Nux vomica 6c can be taken three times daily for up to ten days.

Sepia 30c

This remedy is useful for women who develop constipation just before or just after menstruation. It is also known for helping pregnant women with difficult bowel movements. This remedy is indicated if there is a heavy sensation in the rectum that remains even after a bowel movement, stools are hard and difficult to pass (although they may be small), exercise brings relief to the condition, and cold hands and feet are present. Sepia 30c can be taken in the amount of three doses in a twenty-four-hour period, once a month.

Sulfur 6c

Afflicted people may alternate between constipation and diarrhea. They have dry, hard stools at intervals of a few days or more and an inflamed rectum with burning pain; no relief is experienced from passing the stool. Sulfur may be useful in pregnancy. Sulfur 6c can be taken three times daily for up to ten days; its use should be reduced when improvement is noted.

REMEDIES FOR DENTAL SUPPORT

HOMEOPATHIC remedies for dental support can be useful in a number of ways before and after a visit to the dentist. Remedies may prove helpful in alleviating painful dental conditions while a person is waiting to see a dentist.

Arnica 30c

This remedy may help in situations where bruising and damage to soft tissue has occurred. Dentists who use homeopathic remedies often use Arnica, recommending it before and after surgeries and following curettage (a surgical cutting or scraping with a medical instrument known as a curette). When soreness and aching follow dental procedures, Arnica may be useful. Arnica 30c can be taken once before the procedure and three times per day for two days following the procedure, and discontinued when the pain diminishes.

Gelsemium 6c

Gelsemium, made from the yellow jasmine, may be useful in reducing the apprehension and anxiety that often precedes a visit to the dentist. Individuals may appear dull and lethargic but fearful. A headache at the back of the head may also be present. Gelsemium 6c can be taken one to two times in the hours prior to the visit.

Calendula MT

Made from the marigold flower, this homeopathic liquid mother tincture may help in accelerating the healing process following tooth extractions. It can also help reduce tooth pain. The mother tincture should be diluted by mixing 25 drops into 4 ounces of water, which can then be used as a mouthwash. Do not swallow the tincture—rinse then spit it out.

Mercurius Sol 6c

People who may benefit from this remedy have excessive salivation. There is shooting pain radiating out to the ears and spongy, receding, tender gums that bleed easily. Bad breath is common, and teeth are often loose. Symptoms are generally worse at night. Mercurius sol 6c can be taken every thirty minutes for severe pain, for up to ten doses, and less frequently for chronic pain.

REMEDIES FOR DIARRHEA

DIARRHEA (page 44) can have many causes, including contaminated food, teething in infants, anxiety, dramatic changes in climate, and traveling. Homeopathic remedies can treat a whole host of gastrointestinal upsets and can be counted on in cases of uncomplicated diarrhea.

Arsenicum Album 6c

This remedy might work for cases of simultaneous diarrhea and vomiting, which can develop after a contaminated meal. Great anxiety, restlessness, and exhaustion may be seen in those who benefit from this homeopathic preparation. Individuals have watery and offensive diarrhea, often with burning pain, as well as being continually thirsty for sips of water. Arsenicum album 6c can be taken every thirty minutes for up to six doses, then three times daily until improvements are noted.

Argentum Nitricum 6c

Diarrhea may be anxiety related. This remedy may be of help if the diarrhea immediately follows eating or drinking, as if passing straight through. It is often worse at night and with much flatulence. Argentum nitricum 6c can be taken every hour for up to six doses; its use should be reduced when improvement is noted.

Podophyllum 30c

This remedy addresses profuse, gushing, and watery diarrhea, which is not usually accompanied by pain. In this case, a complete evacuation is soon followed by an urgent sense of having to use the bathroom again. The abdomen rumbles and gurgles before defecation. Diarrhea is worse in the morning, with some improvement as the day goes on. Podophyllum 30c can be taken three to four times per day for one to two days.

Pulsatilla 6c

Pulsatilla may be of help if the diarrhea occurs after eating rich and fatty foods. In this case, the diarrhea is worse at night and after drinking cold liquids or eating onions. Individuals will tend to be weepy and crave sympathy. Pulsatilla 6c can be taken every two hours for up to six doses.

Sulfur 6c

Sulfur may help in cases of painless diarrhea. The diarrhea is urgent—usually in the early morning, driving the person out of bed. It may be accompanied by hemorrhoids. This type of diarrhea is typical of pregnancy. Sulfur 6c can be taken every hour for up to six doses, then three times daily until symptoms improve.

REMEDIES FOR EAR INFECTIONS

EAR INFECTIONS (page 47) are most common in young children, although the infections can be an occasional problem at any age. Ear pain occurs when there is inflammation in the inner ear, often the result of blocked sinus passages during or following a cold. There may be a buildup of fluid in the ear, which dampens hearing, creates a sense of pressure, or is seen in a discharge from the ear. Localized ear pain may be accompanied by a fever. Not all ear infections are painful, and a child who shows no sign of pain may indicate a problem by tipping the head consistently to one side or tugging on an earlobe.

Aconite 30c

Aconite may be helpful in cases where ear pain appears somewhat suddenly in a child who showed no previous symptoms of illness, especially after exposure to cold, windy weather. The child may be fearful, restless with the pain, hot with fever, and thirsty for cold drinks. Even with a fever, a sense of chilliness and a pale face could indicate the usefulness of this remedy. Symptoms calling for Aconite are often at their worst around midnight (for example, a child wakes in the night with ear pain after going to bed feeling fine). Aconite 30c can be taken every thirty minutes, three to four times as needed, discontinuing as symptoms improve.

Belladonna 30c

Ear infections that may respond to Belladonna are also likely to appear rather swiftly and are more common in the right ear. The ear pain is often quite intense and throbbing, and the cry of a baby or child with this type of pain is likely to sound angry rather than fearful or whiny. A hot fever with a hot, red face suggests the use of Belladonna. Belladonna 30c can be taken every thirty minutes, up to four times, discontinuing when symptoms improve.

Pulsatilla 6c

Pulsatilla is the most likely remedy for children who arc unusually clingy, weepy, or whiny during an ear infection. They are typically comforted by rocking or walking, and the ear pain is often relieved by placing a cold, damp washcloth over the affected ear. These kinds of ear infections often appear during the later stages of a cold or nasal infection with a greenish discharge from the nose. Pulsatilla 6c can be taken three to four times daily, discontinuing when improvement is noted.

REMEDIES FOR EYE INJURIES/ EYE STRAIN

EYE STRAIN and minor eye injuries can sometimes be helped by using homeopathic remedies. Eye strain resulting from too many hours of looking at a computer screen, reading, or detailed work can produce tired eyes that ache and burn, water, have an increased sensitivity to light, or experience blurry vision. Minor eye irritations, from smoke, smog, or pollens, and slight injuries, such as a scratched cornea from a contact lens, dirt, or dust, may also be relieved by homeopathy. As always, if there is any doubt about the severity of a condition involving the eyes, it is best to check with a doctor.

Aconite 6c

When there is irritation from foreign matter in the eye, Aconite may bring relief from pain, watering, and heightened sensitivity to light. Aconite 6c can be taken three to four times per day and discontinued when the discomfort stops.

Ruta Graveolens 6c

Ruta is most likely to be helpful in cases of eye strain where the eyes burn and water after long periods of visual effort, such as reading, computer work, or embroidery. The eyelids may become somewhat swollen and itchy, and the eyes may be more sensitive to light than usual. Ruta graveolens 6c can be taken two to three times, a few hours apart, continuing only as long as symptoms persist.

Arnica 6c

If the eyes feel sore and bruised, especially after time spent looking off into the distance, then both rest and Arnica may offer some relief. The muscles of the eyes may ache and feel tired. Arnica 6c can be taken two to three times, a few hours apart, discontinuing as symptoms improve.

Apis Mellifica 6c

This remedy may be helpful in cases of rapid onset of very watery, burning, and stinging eyes. Symptoms are puffy eyelids and sensitivity to light. Apis mellifica is useful for symptoms caused by bright light (for example, snow blindness). Apis mellifica 6c can be taken in the amount of one dose every hour, up to six doses, then three times daily; its use should be reduced when improvement is noted.

REMEDIES FOR GOUT

GOUT is a painful condition resulting from the buildup of uric acid crystals in a joint. This is often caused by genetics, certain drugs, or a diet of rich foods. The homeopathic remedies listed below may provide a measure of relief for even the most painful attacks. A doctor should be consulted to prevent further episodes.

Nux Vomica 6c

This remedy may be indicated in individuals who also suffer from an acid stomach and constipation. They might be prone to indulgence in rich foods and alcoholic beverages and may be irritable and over-sensitive to noise and odors. Nux vomica 6c can be taken three to four times per day for one to two days, discontinuing when the pain subsides.

Belladonna 6c

When symptoms of burning and painful throbbing in a joint are present, this homeopathic remedy may bring relief. The joint will often appear red, swollen, and shiny. The pain will be sharp, and any pressure against the inflamed joint aggravates it greatly. Individuals may be quite thirsty and hot. Belladonna 6c can be taken three to four times per day for one to two days, discontinuing when the pain diminishes.

Calcarea Fluorica 6c

This remedy may be beneficial in conditions characterized by a stabbing pain in the affected joint, which may "crack" on movement. There are swollen, perhaps deformed joints. Pain is relieved by gentle movement and warmth. Calcarea fluorica 6c can be taken every two hours, up to six doses, in acute cases. Thereafter and in chronic cases, three to four doses can be taken daily until improvement is noted.

Colchicum 6c

This remedy may serve those with an extremely painful case of gout, where even slight movement worsens the pain. The pain is often worse at night,

Gout

and afflicted individuals will likely be very tired and chilly. Colchicum 6c can be taken three to four times per day for one to two days.

Rhus Toxicodendron 6c

This remedy may be helpful for joints that are hot, painful, and swollen. In this case, the big toe is often affected. The condition is generally improved on moving about and worsens when individuals are lying down and at rest. The pain is relieved by warmth. Rhus toxicodendron 6c can be taken every hour, up to six doses, in acute cases. Thereafter and in chronic cases, three to four doses can be taken daily until improvement is noted.

REMEDIES FOR HAY FEVER

ACUTE HAY FEVER (page 59) responds well to the following homeopathic remedies. The homeopathic view is that allergies are deep-seated problems requiring two to three seasons of good constitutional treatment under the care of a trained doctor in order to overcome them. However, homeopathy can be used to treat allergy symptoms.

Euphrasia 6c

Euphrasia may be helpful in cases where the eyes are swollen and water all the time, burning tears are present, a bland discharge comes from the nose, and symptoms worsen indoors. Euphrasia 6c can be taken every fifteen minutes for up to one hour; discontinue with significant improvement.

Allium Cepa 6c

This remedy may be beneficial in cases where the eye/nose symptoms are opposite those that call for treatment with Euphrasia: Individuals have watery eyes with nonirritating discharge, burning, runny nose discharge, and frequent, sudden sneezing. Allium cepa 6c can be taken every fifteen minutes for up to one hour; discontinue with significant improvement.

Sabadilla 6c

This homeopathic remedy can be tried by individuals experiencing violent sneezing; watery, swollen, and red eyes; and a sore throat that is soothed by warm drinks. The person's thinking is dull and slow. Sabadilla 6c can be taken every fifteen minutes for up to one hour; discontinue with significant improvement.

REMEDIES FOR HEMORRHOIDS

HEMORRHOIDS (page 60), also called piles, is a condition that can affect all ages and both sexes. Although few people are comfortable discussing this problem, many suffer from it as a result of overeating and inadequate exercise. Homeopathy is a safe and gentle treatment of this troublesome condition. A few remedies are listed below, but if the problem persists, people should consult a homeopath.

Hamamelis 6c

This remedy is indicated when a sore and bruised feeling is present in the affected area. The hemorrhoids can ooze blood, and the lower back may ache. The condition worsens with warmth. Hamamelis 6c can be taken three times per day for three days, discontinuing when improvement is noted.

Calcarea Fluorica 6c

A case of hemorrhoids that may be helped by this remedy will be accompanied by itching in the anal region, bleeding, and soreness in the lower back. Flatulence and constipation may also be present. Calcarea fluorica 6c can be taken three to four times per day for three to four days.

Arnica 30c

Although not often thought of as a remedy for hemorrhoids, Arnica may alleviate the effects of straining and overexertion; consequently, it may help women who suffer from hemorrhoids after childbirth. Arnica 30c can be taken four times per day for two to three days.

Aesculus Hippocastanum 30c

With this remedy, the bleeding is not so much the problem as the sharp, shooting pains felt in the rectum and back. The hemorrhoids are purple and painful. The sensation is described by some people as small sticks poking the rectum. Aesculus hippocastanum 30c can be taken three times per day for three days.

Hemorrhoids

Pulsatilla 6c

Pulsatilla may be helpful in cases where the hemorrhoids are bleeding, painful, and itchy. They may be protruding, and individuals may feel worse when lying down. This is a useful remedy duringpregnancy and is often associated with heartburn. Pulsatilla 6c can be taken every hour for the first six doses, then three times daily until improvement is noted.

REMEDIES FOR HERPES SIMPLEX

HERPES is a common virus that causes cold sores around the mouth as well as genital eruptions. These outbreaks tend to be painful sores; a burning or itching sensation may precede the outbreak by a few days. They are most likely to appear in times of stress, and the eruptions tend to reappear in the same locations.

Natrum Muriaticum 6c

For those who experience cold sores around the lips, especially after exposure to sun, Natrum muriaticum may be helpful. The eruptions may be in the corners of the mouth, and there may be a crack in the lip as well. Natrum muriaticum 6c can be taken three to four times per day for three to five days, discontinuing when symptoms improve.

Rhus Toxicodendron 6c

For herpes simplex outbreaks in any location, especially accompanied by burning and itching, Rhus toxicodendron may bring relief. Rhus toxicodendron 6c can be taken two to three times per day for one to two days.

Apis Mellifica 6c

When the herpes outbreak is accompanied by stinging pain and the area looks red and swollen, Apis mellifica could be helpful. A cold compress may bring relief and is another indication for trying this remedy. Apis mellifica 6c can be taken three to four times per day for two days.

REMEDIES FOR HERPES ZOSTER (SHINGLES)

HERPES ZOSTER, more commonly known as shingles, is a very painful and extremely uncomfortable nerve infection. Homeopathy offers a number of remedies for this aggravating problem. Homeopathic remedies do not interfere with other drugs prescribed by doctors for this condition. People with questions should consult their doctor.

Arsenicum Album 6c

When the shingles have a burning quality but the pain is relieved by hot applications, this remedy may be indicated. Restlessness, anxiety, and a worsening of symptoms around midnight are common in persons benefitting from this remedy. In addition, individuals are very thirsty but only for small sips at a time. Arsenicum album 6c can be taken three to four times per day; its use should be discontinued when improvement is noted.

Apis Mellifica 30c

Apis mellifica may be helpful if there is burning, stinging pain with intense itching and people are very sensitive to touch. Any form of heat severely aggravates the symptoms. Individuals are much relieved by cool air and cold applications. Apis mellifica 30c can be taken three to four times daily until improvement is noted.

Rhus Toxicodendron 6c

Rhus toxicodendron may be indicated if there is a red, itchy rash with vesicle formation. The scalp may also be involved. Warmth helps in this situation. Individuals are unhappy resting in bed and feel better walking about. There is little relief from scratching. Rhus toxicodendron 6c can be taken three to four times daily until improvement is noted.

Mezereum 30c

This remedy may help when the outbreak is bright red and burning, with almost intolerable itching. It worsens with cold air; a general achiness can be felt down to the bone. Mezereum 30c can be taken three to four times per day; its use should be discontinued when improvement is noted.

Ranunculus Bulbosus 30c

This remedy specifically addresses intercostal shingles—herpes zoster found mainly around the front and back of the rib cage area. Individuals experience extreme burning and itching and terrible soreness. There may or may not be blisters, but any contact with the affected area aggravates it. Ranunculus bulbosus 30c can be taken three to four times per day; its use should be discontinued when improvement is noted.

Other Remedies

Though not a homeopathic remedy, strictly speaking, Bach's "Rescue Remedy" can also be soothing for a case of shingles. Taken internally or applied directly onto the skin, it can have a calming effect on the sores and the individual.

REMEDIES FOR IMPOTENCE

FAILURE TO achieve or maintain an erection and premature ejaculation are problems that warrant professional attention. Many factors can contribute to impotence, including diet, physical activity level, and psychological issues. The homeopathic medicines described below may provide some help.

Lycopodium 30c

This remedy is considered useful when a man is no longer able to achieve an erection. An enlarged prostate may also be present. Men who may benefit from this remedy may lack self-confidence and be concerned about failing memory. Lycopodium 30c can be taken once per day for a week, and then once a week for the following month.

Argentum Nitricum 30c

If a man's erection fails when coitus is attempted, this medicine might provide a measure of assistance. This remedy is most useful for men who are anxious, very hurried, very warm-blooded, and have a noticeable craving for sweets and salt. Argentum nitricum 30c can be taken once per day for a week, and then once a week for the following month.

Selenium Metallicum 30c

This remedy is for men who still have an abundance of sexual fantasies but have lost their sexual ability. Men needing this remedy are often greatly exhausted by even slight effort and may be losing more hair than normal. Selenium metallicum 30c can be taken once daily for a week, then once a week for the following month.

REMEDIES FOR INDIGESTION AND GAS

FOR SIMPLE INDIGES- TION, homeopathy offers a number of safe remedies. Although uncomfortable and embarrassing, most cases of gas are fairly harmless. If pains are severe and persist for any length of time, however, people should not hesitate to consult a doctor.

Nux Vomica 6c

This remedy may help the overindulgent, when too much rich food and spirits have been consumed. Indicative symptoms are irritability, sensitivity to sound, and symptoms of the classic hangover. Other symptoms may include extreme nausea that is improved by vomiting, pain in the stomach area several hours after eating, stomach fluids backing up and burning the esophagus, and constipation. Nux vomica 6c can be taken as one dose every thirty minutes for two hours, after meals.

Carbo Vegetabilis 6c

This homeopathic treatment may help individuals who overeat, feel better sitting by an open window, have foul flatulence, and experience sour belching that brings only temporary relief from discomfort. Carbo vegetabilis 6c can be taken as one dose every thirty minutes for two hours, after meals.

Lycopodium 6c

This remedy might aid those who experience a sense of fullness after even a small meal and have rumbling gas in the lower abdomen. Trapped gas presses upward and makes breathing more difficult. In addition, there is sleepiness after meals, a worsening when lying down, and improvement after belching. Lycopodium 6c can be taken two to three times after meals, as needed.

Natrum Phosphoricum 6c

When indigestion or heartburn develop after eating too much sugar or milk products, this remedy may bring a measure of relief. There may also be a sour taste in the mouth; an acid, burning sensation; sour vomiting; regurgitated bits of food; and the back of the tongue may be coated yellow. Natrum phosphoricum 6c can be taken as one dose every thirty minutes for two hours, after meals.

Arsenicum Album 6c

This remedy may be helpful for indigestion that accompanies a poor appetite, perhaps with diarrhea and/or vomiting. Individuals feel restless and chilly, and symptoms worsen at night. Relief may be gained from warmth or warm drinks and from sitting up. Arsenicum album 6c can be taken every hour, up to six doses, then three times a day, reducing with improvement.

REMEDIES FOR INFLUENZA

INFLUENZA (or flu) causes a wide variety of symptoms. A flu may be experienced mainly in the digestive tract, with lots of vomiting and diarrhea, or with respiratory involvement that produces a cough. A different flu may be felt almost completely in the muscular system, with aching, fatigue, and fever. A homeopathic remedy that improves the symptoms of a particular flu may help others exposed to the same virus avoid developing symptoms.

Gelsemium 6c

Gelsemium may help when achiness and fatigue come on over a day or two. Individuals are likely to be dizzy, droopy, and sweaty with a mild fever and may have chills up and down the spine. A dull headache at the nape of the neck is another indication. If there is digestive upset, it is mild. Gelsemium 6c can be taken once every three to four hours for up to five days while symptoms persist.

Arsenicum Album 6c

This remedy is useful when vomiting and diarrhea are the most prevalent features of the illness. There may be a fever, but individuals are likely to feel chilly, wanting warm blankets and hot drinks. The head may feel hot, while the rest of the body feels chilly. There may be restlessness, burning pain in the stomach or abdomen, and digestive upset resembling the symptoms of food poisoning. Arsenicum album 6c can be taken four to six times per day for a few days while symptoms are present.

Aconite 6c

This remedy may help for a flu that develops suddenly with intense symptoms. The flu symptoms may follow exposure to cold temperatures. There may be fearful anxiety and restlessness, and symptoms are typically the worst around midnight. Aconite 6c can be taken once every hour for three to four hours; discontinue with significant improvement.

Bryonia 6c

When the main flu symptoms are a strong headache or a dry, hard cough, Bryonia may be helpful. This remedy is best indicated when individuals feel better from lying still and symptoms worsen with even slight motion. Digestive upset is minor, but irritability and thirst may be present. Bryonia 6c can be taken four to six times per day for a few days while symptoms are present.

Oscillococcinum

Oscillococcinum can be used preventively (over a short or long period) and curatively because it has strong antiviral effects. To prevent viral colds and flus, people take one unit dose per week. At the first onset of symptoms, one unit dose can be taken, followed by two more doses at six-hour intervals. Oscillococcinum can be taken concurrently with additional remedies for specific symptom relief. This remedy can be used by both children and adults, and should be taken in premeasured doses as directed.

REMEDIES FOR INJURIES

THE FOLLOWING homeopathic remedies should be in every first aid kit. When treating an injury, whether it is a shin banged into a coffee table, a head bumped in a car, or an injury caused by overexertion, people can try the best indicated remedy described below.

Arnica 30c

Whenever there has been a hard blow that could result in bruising, this remedy may help. It excels in reducing the painful soreness following overexertion and is especially useful for blows to the head. Arnica 30c can be taken three to four times per day for two to three days.

Ruta Graveolens 30c

For the unmistakable pain and damage from running an unprotected shinbone into a hard, sharp edge, this remedy may serve well. Ruta graveolens may also be useful when the eyeball has been injured and in treating injuries that feel better with warmth. Ruta graveolens 30c can be taken three to four times per day for two to three days.

Ledum 30c

When a blow to the nose area has brought on a black eye and the bruise lingers, this remedy may be indicated. If taken right after the blow, Ledum can prevent much of the bruising and skin discoloration. Individuals generally feel quite cold, as does the affected area. Ledum 30c can be taken three times per day for two to three days.

REMEDIES FOR INSECT BITES AND STINGS

HOMEOPATHIC remedies can be quite useful in addressing the pain and swelling that accompanies the bites and stings of insects and bees. Keeping a few of these remedies in a first aid kit may prove worthwhile. Any bite from a larger animal or snake, however, should be tended to by a doctor.

Apis Mellifica 30c

When a bee sting leaves the affected area puffy and swollen, pinkish or red in color, and hot to the touch, this remedy may prove useful. The area will be sore and sensitive to the slightest touch. The pain of the sting may be relieved by cold applications. Apis mellifica 30c can be taken three to four times every fifteen minutes and discontinued when symptoms subside.

Hypericum 30c

When an injury or bite has damaged a nerve-rich area of the body, such as the fingers, toes, or coccyx, and the pain is extreme, this remedy may bring considerable relief. Like Ledum, Hypericum is useful for the pain of puncture wounds. Injuries calling for this remedy often have radiating and shooting pain. Hypericum 30c can be taken three to four times in the hours following the injury and discontinued when the pain and swelling subside.

Aconitum Napellus 30c

This remedy may be beneficial if the affected area is red hot with a cutting, stabbing pain. Tingling and numbness are additional symptoms. Individuals are shocked, restless, and anxious. Aconitum napellus should be used early for best effects and followed with another remedy if necessary. Aconitum napellus 30c can be taken every fifteen minutes for up to four doses, then changed to the more appropriate remedy, if necessary.

Cantharis 30c

Cantharis may be indicated if there is intense burning and stinging, sometimes with itching. Blister formation is another possible symptom, and the area around the bite or sting is very red. This remedy is useful for gnat bites. Cantharis 30c can be taken in the amount of one dose every hour, up to six doses, then three times daily; its use should be reduced when improvement is noted.

Ledum 30c

This remedy may be helpful in relieving the pain and swelling from puncture wounds, notably spider bites.

The area surrounding the bite is often bluish in color and cold to the touch, although cold applications relieve the pain. General achiness can also be present. Ledum 30c can be taken three to four times in the hours following the bite, sting, or puncture wound.

REMEDIES FOR INSOMNIA

SOONER OR later, everyone has a difficult time getting to sleep at night. For many, a simple homeopathic remedy, which is effective and safe, is all that is needed for sleeplessness, also known as **insomnia** (page 79). It should not be necessary to take any medicine for weeks and months at a time for sleeping problems. If the inability to get a good night's sleep persists, a homeopath should be consulted.

Kali Phosphoricum 6c

If the cause of sleeplessness is nervous exhaustion from too much mental strain and exertion, this remedy may be useful. Individuals who might benefit from this remedy feel very weak, irritable, and in low spirits. Tasks seem to require great effort for these people, and the condition is helped by warmth. Kali phosphoricum 6c can be taken every fifteen minutes for up to one hour, until falling asleep.

Arsenicum Album 30c

Persons who may benefit from this remedy are restless and apprehensive. They often wake up after midnight, get up, and pace around. In addition, they may be very fussy and may sleep with their hands above their heads. Arsen album 30c can be taken in the amount of one dose four hours before bedtime and a second dose immediately before retiring.

Ignatia 30c

Persons who may benefit from this remedy are tired and yawn but are unable to sleep. When they do fall asleep, it is a light sleep only, with jerking and nightmares. These episodes may follow an emotional upset. Ignatia is useful for children and may be helpful during pregnancy. Ignatia 30c can be taken in the amount of one dose four hours before bedtime and a second dose immediately before retiring.

Insomnia

Coffea Cruda 6c

When nervous excitement, from either good news or bad, keeps people's minds from resting, they should try Coffea cruda. Symptoms are aggravated by cold air, and the mind and all the senses are fully alert. Individuals who may benefit from this remedy often awaken at 3 A.M. and are unable to return to sleep. Coffea cruda 6c can be taken every thirty minutes for up to one and a half hours.

Nux Vomica 30c

People who may benefit from this remedy experience a light and disturbed sleep—and always feel as though they need more sleep. Bad dreams occur, which are often due to overexertion or overindulgence in food and drink. Individuals wake up in the middle of the night (about 3 A.M.). Nux vomica 30c can be taken in the amount of one dose four hours before bedtime and a second dose immediately before retiring.

REMEDIES FOR MEASLES

MEASLES is a highly contagious viral infection that occurs most often in children under ten years of age. Early measles symptoms mimic the common cold, with a cough and watery eyes. Typically, the rash first appears on the face and is blotchy, red, and dotted. In the early stages, homeopathic medicines can be of great service. If any serious bronchial problems develop, a doctor should be consulted.

Aconite 30c

This remedy may help at the first sign of a dry fever with chilliness. There may be restlessness, hot but dry skin, thirst, and anxiety. These symptoms are more common during the late evening. Aconite 30c can be taken as one dose every hour, three to four times; its use should be discontinued when improvement is noted.

Euphrasia 6c

This remedy has an affinity for the eyes. With measles, the eyes will water profusely and be very sensitive to light; people benefiting from this remedy will prefer being in a darkened room. If tears are present, they are irritating and may be accompanied by a runny nose that produces a clear discharge. Euphrasia 6c can be taken four times per day for several days or until symptoms change.

Pulsatilla 6c

This remedy serves many purposes, but in this case it may bring relief to individuals who particularly desire company and to be coddled. They also feel better with fresh, cool air, are not usually thirsty, and have a cough that is dry at night and loose in the morning. Pulsatilla 6c can be taken every two hours, up to six doses, then three times daily until improvement is noted. Note: Pulsatilla may restore hearing lost as a result of measles.

REMEDIES FOR MENOPAUSE SYMPTOMS

WOMEN going through the hormonal life change of **menopause** (page 87) may experience mood swings, hot flashes, cold sweats, and irregular menstrual cycles. While these symptoms will go away on their own in time, a homeopathic remedy may help to ease them.

Calcarea Carbonica 6c

When weight gain accompanies or follows menopause, Calcarea carbonica may be helpful. Other typical indications for Calcarea carbonica include sleeplessness and worry, joint stiffness, and foot and leg cramps, which have developed after menopause. There may be hot flashes and cold sweats in women who are generally chilly and do not like drafts. Calcarea carbonica 6c can be taken three times per day for up to two weeks.

Pulsatilla 6c

Some women experience mood swings and weepiness during or following menopause. These women may benefit by using Pulsatilla. Recent weight gain may be a problem, and women may feel hot one moment and chilly the next. They generally feel better in the fresh air and worse in a stuffy room. Pulsatilla 6c can be taken three times per day for up to two weeks.

Ignatia 30c

Ignatia is very useful for emotional symptoms during menopause. In this case, there is a tendency to bottle up feelings and be easily hurt. Women who may benefit from this remedy have a low pain threshold and suffer from hot flashes. Ignatia 30c can be taken three to four times daily for up to three weeks.

Lachesis 6c

Hot flashes that bring out a sweat, especially in women who have high blood pressure, can improve with the use of Lachesis. Women who find help with this remedy are likely to be talkative and in touch with their emotions; they may have a tendency to become jealous or suspicious of others. The throat is often a sensitive area for these women, who may have an aversion to snug collars or necklaces. Lachesis 6c can be taken two to three times per day for ten to fourteen days; its use should be discontinued when symptoms improve.

Sepia 30c

Sepia may be helpful in cases where a woman's periods vary—either late and scanty or flooding. Women who may benefit from this remedy experience hot flashes with sweating but are otherwise chilly and irritable. They feel better with exercise but are worse in the morning. Sepia 30c can be taken three to four times daily for up to three weeks. ~

REMEDIES FOR MENSTRUAL PROBLEMS (PMS AND MENORRHAGIA)

MENSTRUAL CYCLES
seem to come and go easily for some women; others face a monthly challenge. Women who experience difficulty with menstruation, such as **premenstrual syndrome** (page 109) and **menorrhagia** (page 89), may find some relief by using a homeopathic remedy.

Sepia 30c

Sepia may be helpful when the menstrual cycle is accompanied by a sense of weight or heaviness in the pelvis or lower back. Prior to menstruation, women may experience weepiness, irritability, or depression, along with a sense of dealing with too many demands of life and a desire to be left alone. Women who may benefit from Sepia are often chilly and dislike stuffy rooms, preferring fresh air. Sepia 30c can be taken two to three times per day for one day only.

Pulsatilla 30c

For women who experience substantial weight fluctuations around their menstrual cycle, Pulsatilla may be helpful. A feeling of bloating or water retention before the flow begins or a craving for sweet or creamy foods may be present. Mood swings, periods of crying easily with a desire to be cared for or consoled by others, or a strong sense of loneliness are experienced by those who may benefit from Pulsatilla. Often the menstrual cycle is irregular, for example, coming early one month and late the next; the flow may be changeable as well, sometimes light and other times very heavy. Pulsatilla 30c can be taken two to three times per day for one day only.

Cimicifuga 6c

Cimicifuga is used for both irregular and painful periods, always with cramplike pains in the pelvic region. This condition may be linked with backache and headache—often prior to flow, which may be profuse with signs of clotting. Cimicifuga 6c can be taken in the amount of three to four doses daily for up to six days.

REMEDIES FOR MIGRAINE HEADACHES

MIGRAINE HEADACHES (page 91) are usually quite painful, if not completely debilitating. Symptoms often include throbbing pain on one side of the head, nausea, vomiting, and visual disturbances. The remedies described below should provide a measure of relief. However, people should not hesitate to consult a homeopath if the problem persists.

Belladonna 6c

If the head pain is noted for its throbbing, pulsing sensation with accompanying heat, redness of the face, and burning, this remedy may be indicated. In addition, attacks come on quickly, pupils are dilated, jarring exacerbates the pain, and symptoms are usually worse on the right side of the head. At the first sign of the headache, Belladonna 6c can be taken every thirty minutes for up to one and a half hours; discontinue with significant improvement.

Bryonia 6c

Headaches that may be eased by this remedy are described as "splitting," as if the head might burst. Any motion worsens the pain, irritability develops, and individuals experience dry mouth, excessive thirst, and nausea when trying to sit up. Symptoms improve when individuals are lying down and remaining still; sometimes they feel better with an ice pack and pressure. At the onset of pain, Bryonia 6c can be taken every thirty minutes for up to one and a half hours; discontinue with significant improvement.

Gelsemium 30c

This remedy may help pain that is focused in the back of the head (the occipital region) or in cases that feel as though a tight band were wrapped around the head. The headache may be preceded by diminished vision or even blindness. There can be heaviness and achiness in the eyes, neck, and shoulders. At the first sign of the headache, Gelsemium 30c can be taken every thirty minutes for up to one and a half hours; discontinue with significant improvement.

Kali Bichromicum 6c

This remedy may be beneficial if the pain is preceded by impaired vision, which gradually improves as the headache worsens. The condition is often accompanied by nausea and vomiting. Pain is aggravated by noise, light, and movement and is worse generally at night. Kali bichromicum 6c can be taken in the amount of one dose hourly for six doses, then one dose three times a day, reducing with improvement.

REMEDIES FOR MORNING SICKNESS

FOR NEARLY 200 years, homeopathy has served the needs of pregnant women. The safety and efficacy of these remedies make them ideal choices during this often delicate time. A homeopath should be consulted if there are any questions or doubts about use of these homeopathic remedies. See also the **morning sickness** section on page 93.

Sepia 30c

The nausea indicating the use of this homeopathic remedy worsens in the morning and at the sight and smell of food, although eating can help ease the nausea. There is only occasional vomiting, improvement with vigorous exercise, and often constipation. The hands and feet can be quite cold. Sepia 30c can be taken in the amount of one dose every hour, up to six doses, or until symptoms are relieved, if sooner.

Ipecac 6c

Ipecac may be helpful when persistent nausea and vomiting are present and vomiting does not relieve the nausea. Women who may benefit from this remedy are often exhausted after vomiting. The tongue is usually clean, and women feel better in the open air but feel worse after movement. Ipecac 6c can be taken in the amount of one dose every hour, up to six doses, then three to four doses daily until improvement is noted.

Phosphorus 6c

This remedy may be beneficial for a woman who is unusually fearful, very sensitive to all stimuli, and who vomits shortly after drinking water. The need to vomit often comes on suddenly, and the individual feels better in a warm environment. Phosphorus 6c can be taken in the amount of one dose every hour, up to six doses, or until relieved, if sooner.

REMEDIES FOR MUMPS

MUMPS, a common childhood disease, affects the parotid glands in the neck, which become inflamed and swollen. Fever, headache, pain around the ears, and excessive salivation are common symptoms. The following homeopathic remedies may be of help.

Mercurius Sol 6c

Mercurius sol may be beneficial if there is excess salivation, especially if the saliva has a sour or foul odor, and the right side of the jaw appears to be more swollen. Children may be more sensitive to temperature changes than usual and may pull the blankets on, only to find that the bed is too warm, or throw the covers off, only to find that it is too cold. They are likely to be sweaty. Mercurius sol 6c can be taken four to six times per day for two to four days; its use should be discontinued as symptoms improve.

Belladonna 30c

When the illness appears very quickly and a high fever is present, Belladonna may be called for. The child may have a red face, which radiates the heat of the fever. Typically, there will be more pain on the right side of the jaw, or the pain will begin first on the right and then move on to the left. Belladonna 30c can be taken three to four times per day for two to three days; its use should be discontinued when the symptoms improve or change.

Pulsatilla 6c

When mumps is contracted by an adult, there may be uncomfortable swelling of the ovaries or testicles in addition to the other symptoms normally experienced by children. In these cases, Pulsatilla may offer relief. Pulsatilla 6c can be taken four to six times per day for two to three days, reducing the frequency as the condition is relieved.

Calcarea Carbonica 6c

This remedy may be indicated if individuals are feverish and sweating. The head and feet feel cold and damp (head sweats cause a wet pillow). The pupils are dilated, with a sensitivity to light. Individuals also have swollen glands. Calcarea carbonica 6c can be taken in the amount of one dose every hour, for six doses, then three to four times daily; its use should be reduced when improvement is noted.

REMEDIES FOR OSTEOARTHRITIS

OSTEOARTHRITIS (page 97) leads to the breakdown of cartilage at the ends of bones, where joints meet. The subsequent pain and inflammation result as the bones thicken and in some cases become knotted and misshapen. The spine, the hips, and the knees are often affected. Homeopathic remedies may offer a measure of relief for painful or acute flare-ups.

Rhus Toxicodendron 6c

This remedy may prove useful in cases where the pain is aggravated when first moving, but then improves with continued motion. Hot applications or a hot bath often bring relief, but the stiffness forces individuals to keep moving. An anxious restlessness is often seen in people needing this remedy. Rhus toxicodendron 6c can be taken in the amount of one dose three times per day for two weeks.

Ledum 6c

Should the smaller joints (toes, fingers, and wrists) prove to be the most troublesome, this remedy may help. The joints crack and pop, and cold applications ease the pain somewhat. The pains can be quite severe and shift from joint to joint. Ledum 6c can be taken in the amount of one dose four times per day for two weeks.

Belladonna 6c

This remedy may be helpful when the pain has a strong, throbbing character and heat and redness are obvious. The affected area seems to be pulsing with pain. Belladonna 6c is often taken in the amount of one dose per day for two weeks.

Apis Mellifica 6c

This remedy may be helpful in acute conditions with redness and swelling, in which the joints feel hot to the touch and have stinging pain. In these individuals, often the hands and knees are affected and the symptoms are aggravated by warm applications. Apis mellifica 6c can be taken in the amount of one dose three times per day for up to two weeks.

Bryonia 6c

Bryonia may be helpful for individuals with severe, throbbing pain that is aggravated by movement but feels better when pressure is applied to the affected area and when resting. Cold applications may ease the pain. Bryonia 6c can be taken in the amount of one dose three times per day for up to two weeks.

Pulsatilla 6c

When pain moves unpredictably from one joint to another, this remedy may be useful. In addition, individuals may feel the worst pain when starting to move, but the pain lessens with continued gentle activity. Pulsatilla 6c can be taken in the amount of one dose three times per day for up to two weeks.

Ruta Graveolens 6c

This remedy is called for when mainly the large joints are affected, as well as the surrounding tendons and ligaments. Individuals often feel stiff and bruised and feel worse at night and when cold. Ruta graveolens 6c can be taken in the amount of one dose three times per day for up to two weeks.

REMEDIES FOR OSTEOPOROSIS

OSTEOPOROSIS (page 100) has many contributing factors, including inadequate exercise, excessive animal protein in the diet, excessive intake of carbonated drinks, certain drugs, and the aging process. Although homeopathic medicines cannot reverse bone loss, the remedies listed below have some history of successful use in speeding the knitting of broken bones and easing the pain of some bone problems. It is very important to examine diet and exercise in cases of osteoporosis and make any recommended changes.

Calcarea Phosphorica 6c

Calcarea phosphorica speeds the knitting of broken bones. Combined with other therapies for osteoporosis, this medicine may provide additional help. Persons needing this remedy may suffer rheumatic pains during colder weather, with noted weakness in the hips. Calcarea phosphorica 6c can be taken once at bedtime, every night for one month, followed by one time per week.

Calcarea Carbonica 6c

Calcarea carbonica may prove useful to people who are overweight, prone to worrying, and who tend to feel chilly. Weak ankles and swollen joints are common. Calcarea carbonica 6c can be taken once per day for one month, followed by once weekly.

Strontium Carbonica 6c

This little-known remedy may help persons who easily sprain their ankles, suffer bone pain that comes and goes erratically, and experience hot flashes. Strontium carbonica 6c can be taken once per day for a week, followed by one time per week.

REMEDIES FOR POSTPARTUM DEPRESSION

FOR A SMALL percentage of women, the weeks following childbirth can be emotionally devastating. Some women are wrought with anxiety, depression, and irritability rather than the anticipated joy and elation of new motherhood. This condition is known as postpartum depression. Homeopathy can help during these times. However, if the remedies do not bring improvement or if the symptoms worsen, medical advice should be sought immediately.

Sepia 30c

This remedy may be of help for the new mother who prefers that her husband and close friends, and even her newborn, keep their distance from her. She is irritable and cross, finds even the least effort overwhelming, and cries easily. Constipation may also be a problem. Vigorous exercise may temporarily lighten her mood. Sepia 30c can be taken three times per day for two weeks.

Ignatia 30c

A woman needing this remedy will experience alternating moods, such as tears followed by laughter, and she may sigh more than usual. This new mother may describe herself as feeling grief stricken. She is tense and difficult to comfort. Ignatia 30c can be taken three times per day for two weeks.

Pulsatilla 30c

This remedy may help the highly emotional woman who needs and seeks affection and attention. She cries very easily. Warm rooms aggravate her, while the cool outdoors relieves her condition. Pulsatilla 30c can be taken three times per day for two weeks.

Natrum Muriaticum 30c

This remedy may be called for when a woman wants to be left alone, is sad and sensitive, and does not want consolation or sympathy. However, she resents lack of attention. In addition, she may be resentful, aggressive, and guarded. Natrum muriaticum 30c can be taken three times per day for up to two weeks, or until symptoms improve.

REMEDIES FOR PREGNANCY AND DELIVERY SUPPORT

IT IS BEST to consult with a physician before taking any medicine or remedies during pregnancy. However, the homeopathic remedies listed below are safe and may be useful in the following pregnancy support and delivery support situations described. See also the section on **pregnancy support** (page 107).

Other remedies for the relief of the nausea of pregnancy can be found in the section on homeopathic remedies for **morning sickness** (page 368). See also the **morning sickness** section on page 93.

Ferrum Phosphoricum 6c

When anemia is a problem, this remedy may help the pregnant mother. Although made from iron phosphate, it does not cause constipation or nausea, as some iron supplements do. (However, the woman's diet should be examined for possible nutritional insufficiencies.) The woman may appear lethargic and have poor skin color. Ferrum phosphoricum 6c can be taken once per day for two weeks; its use should be discontinued when symptoms diminish.

Nux Vomica 6c

This remedy may be useful for the indigestion and heartburn often associated with pregnancy. There may be a bitter or sour taste with the heartburn. The woman will often be chilly, irritable, and constipated. Nux vomica 6c can be taken one to two times per day, after meals, for one to two days only. Should the indigestion continue, a physician may be consulted.

Arnica 30c

This remedy is indicated for the relief of physical exertion and strained muscles. Bruising can also be minimized with this remedy. Arnica may also relieve hemorrhoidal problems that follow childbirth. Arnica 30c can be taken one to two times prior to delivery, then three to four times per day for two days after delivery; its use should be discontinued when soreness subsides.

REMEDIES FOR RASHES

SKIN ERUPTIONS or rashes can be very uncomfortable. Some, such as from poison ivy contact or allergic reactions, have known causes; others appear spontaneously without apparent cause. Itching or stinging may occur either with or without a visible rash or skin welts. Some rashes, despite angry appearances, do not have any sensation of discomfort to go with them. Many of these various types of skin symptoms can be relieved by using one of the homeopathic remedies described here.

Rhus Toxicodendron 6c

This remedy is the first one to think of for poison oak or ivy or for rashes from other causes that bring on similar symptoms. Individuals are likely to feel restless. There can be intense itching that feels worse after scratching. Surprisingly, laying a very hot, damp cloth over the rash often brings relief from the itching for those who improve with Rhus toxicodendron. The rash may be more uncomfortable when exposed to cold. Rhus toxicodendron 6c can be taken three to four times per day; its use should be discontinued when the condition improves.

Sulfur 6c

Sulfur is most useful with skin rashes that itch and burn and that are especially bad after bathing or exposure to water. The itching may be particularly annoying when warm or exposed to wool. Scratching is likely to bring temporary relief, followed by increased itching or a burning sensation. The skin rash may be moist or weepy. Sulfur 6c can be taken three to four times per day; its use should be discontinued when the symptoms are relieved.

Apis Mellifica 30c

Apis mellifica may be helpful in cases where the skin rash seems to be the result of an allergic reaction to food or chemicals (such as a new laundry detergent) and the result is hives. Rashes characterized by patches of red, swollen skin that sting or burn and are relieved by applying cold to the rash may be helped by Apis mellifica. Apis mellifica 30c can be taken every thirty minutes, up to six times per day.

REMEDIES FOR RAYNAUD'S PHENOMENON

RAYNAUD'S PHENOME-NON is a disorder in which the circulation to fingers and toes is diminished when exposed to cold. This effect, which is more common in women than in men, is caused by spasmodic contractions in the tiny blood vessels of the hands and feet. It can produce chilled hands and feet, which turn white, or even blue, with cold. These very chilly hands and feet can be painful and difficult to restore to warmth. Fortunately, homeopathic remedies can aid in relieving the discomfort of Raynaud's phenomenon.

Carbo Vegetabilis 6c

When the skin looks mottled with a blue cast and feels icy cold, this remedy may be helpful. The symptoms may improve when individuals are being fanned or are breathing deeply, and they may express a desire for fresh air. Sometimes there is a tendency toward indigestion and bloating in those who may need this remedy. They are likely to feel chilly all over, not just on the hands and feet, and may feel as if they are never able to get truly warm. Carbo vegetabilis 6c can be taken once each hour, four to six times; its use should be discontinued as symptoms diminish.

Arsenicum Album 6c

Sometimes the symptoms of coldness and blanching are accompanied by localized swelling, and the affected areas itch or burn. For people experiencing these symptoms, Arsenicum album could be helpful. Those who benefit from Arsenicum album are often restless, anxious, and prefer warm drinks. Arsenicum album 6c can be taken every thirty minutes for up to three hours; discontinue with significant improvement.

Pulsatilla 6c

If the fingers and toes are icy cold, yet applying heat to warm them up increases the discomfort, then Pulsatilla may be indicated. As odd as it seems, the symptoms may actually be improved by applying cold. When the condition causes chilblains or blisters to form on the skin, or when the hands and feet feel worse by letting the arms or legs hang down, this remedy can be considered. Pulsatilla 6c can be taken every thirty minutes for up to three hours; discontinue with significant improvement.

REMEDIES FOR RESTLESS LEG SYNDROME

RESTLESS LEG SYN-DROME causes an unpleasant creeping sensation and urge to move the legs; it usually begins shortly after going to bed. Restless leg syndrome is an irritating condition, particularly since it results in loss of sleep. Homeopathic medicines can bring a measure of relief. If symptoms persist, a professional homeopath should be consulted for further advice.

Zincum Metallicum 6c

When legs are very restless, people should try this remedy first. Nervous exhaustion often precedes the need for this medicine. Individuals may also suffer headaches in the back of the head and be sensitive to noises. Zincum metallicum 6c can be taken three times per day for one week.

Ignatia 6c

When an emotional, tense person has restless and jerking arms and legs at bedtime, this remedy may serve well. People needing this homeopathic medicine will sigh often and have difficulty expressing their emotions freely. Ignatia 6c can be taken two times per day for three weeks.

Aconite 6c

Fears and anxieties can lead to restlessness in the extremities as well as restlessness of the mind. Typically, there is a feeling of numbness and tingling in the legs and feet. For those (often elderly) people who suffer from restless legs and deeply troubling thoughts, Aconite may be beneficial. Aconite 6c can be taken two times per day for three weeks.

REMEDIES FOR RHEUMATOID ARTHRITIS

RHEUMATOID ARTHRITIS (page 115) sufferers are plagued with the greatest number of symptoms during cold and damp seasons. Muscular pains caused by rheumatoid arthritis are often lessened by homeopathic medicines. Homeopathy can be helpful for acute flare-ups, but a homeopathic physician should be consulted for long-term care.

Rhus Toxicodendron 30c

This remedy can be used when muscular aches are relieved by hot applications or hot showers or baths. People who may benefit from this remedy are stiffest when first trying to move after being still for a period of time, although slow, gradual movement tends to diminish the pain. They often feel quite restless and unable to find a comfortable position when sitting. Rhus toxicodendron 30c can be taken in the amount of one dose three times per day for two weeks.

Bryonia 6c

When aches and pains are made worse from even small movements but improve by applying pressure to the sore area, then this remedy may prove useful. Cold, dry weather often brings on the soreness. Individuals can be very irritable and cranky. Bryonia 6c can be taken in the amount of one dose four times per day for two weeks.

Ruta Graveolens 6c

If the pain is centered in the joints and tendons and feels like long strings of pain, this remedy can help. This homeopathic medicine can be used for nonspecific bursitis pain as well. Ruta graveolens 6c can be taken in the amount of one dose four times per day for two weeks.

Pulsatilla 30c

For persons whose pains seem to wander from place to place and who feel greater discomfort in warm rooms, Pulsatilla may bring a measure of relief. Individuals who may benefit from this remedy are often emotional, with a tendency to cry easily; also, their digestion is disturbed by fatty foods. Pulsatilla 30c can be taken in the amount of one dose three times per day for two weeks.

Arnica Ointments and Gels

Arnica gels or ointments may be applied externally for any muscular ache, especially those that follow an injury to the painful area.

REMEDIES FOR SURGERY AND RECOVERY SUPPORT

IN CASES of surgery, all medicines or remedies should be discussed with the doctor in charge. The homeopathic remedies described below are safe and will not interfere with conventional surgical procedures.

Aconite Napellus 30c

For individuals deeply fearful of an upcoming surgery, with great anxiety and restlessness, this remedy may bring relief. These people may be quite sensitive to sounds and odors and startle easily. Other symptoms that may occur are a dry throat and mouth and excessive thirst. Aconite napellus 30c can be taken one to two times in the hours prior to surgery.

Arnica 30c

When surgery is associated with swelling, bruising, and pain, this remedy may be counted on for a measure of relief, particularly if the skin is black and blue and individuals do not want to be touched or even approached. In addition, they may complain that the hospital bed is too hard and have an overall feeling of soreness. Arnica 30c can be taken once prior to surgery and three times per day for two days afterward; its use should be discontinued when pain and swelling subside.

Phosphorus 6c

For people reacting to anesthesia with nausea and vomiting, this remedy may bring relief. Symptoms indicated for the use of this remedy may include lightheadedness, disorientation, and excessive bleeding. Individuals may ask for ice water but vomit shortly after drinking it. Phosphorus 6c can be taken two to three times in the hours following surgery; its use should be discontinued when nausea and vomiting subside.

Gelsemium 6c

This remedy may be helpful before surgery, for apprehensive individuals who tremble at the thought of surgery and feel weak in the knees. These people feel lethargic, nervous, and restless, and they prefer to be alone. Gelsemium 6c can be taken in the amount of three to four doses daily for two to three days before surgery.

Staphysagria 30c

This remedy may prove helpful when a sharp, stinging pain persists at the site of the surgical incision (often in surgeries involving the abdomen and stomach). Gas and bloating may occur as well. Staphysagria 30c can be taken two to three times for one day.

REMEDIES FOR TEETHING

CUTTING TEETH can be an uncomfortable time for babies and toddlers. Localized mouth pain may be accompanied by irritability, fever, diarrhea, or symptoms of nasal congestion. An appropriate homeopathic remedy may assist in relieving the discomfort and preventing sleepless nights.

Chamomilla 6c

When teething is very painful and the child becomes quite cranky, satisfied with nothing and pacified only by being carried, then Chamomilla may help. Sometimes, the child seeking some relief from the discomfort will demand one thing after another, rejecting each one when it does not give relief. Children who could benefit from this remedy are very irritable, with a cry that sounds as if they are in pain. Chamomilla 6c can be taken every thirty minutes, up to six times per day, while symptoms persist.

Mercurius Sol 6c

This remedy may be of help in cases where teething is accompanied by excessive salivation and drooling. In addition, the gums are likely to be red and sore, and the child may have diarrhea with a foul smell to it. Mercurius sol 6c can be taken four to six times per day for two to three days; its use should be discontinued when the symptoms diminish.

Belladonna 30c

For children who tend to develop a fever with a flushed, red face when they are cutting teeth, Belladonna may be a good choice. Often, the eyes have a glassy look, due to the dilation of the pupils. The child may be irritable and crying as if angry. Belladonna 30c can be taken every thirty minutes, up to four times per day, while symptoms continue.

Calcarea Carbonica 6c

When children are finally cutting teeth that have been late in erupting, Calcarea carbonica could be helpful. This remedy is often helpful with "late bloomers," babies who develop a little more slowly, crawling, walking, and cutting teeth on their own schedule, weeks or months later than some other babies or toddlers. Children likely to benefit from Calcarea carbonica often have sweaty heads and feet and may have a tendency to develop cradle cap or yeast infections. With teething, they often do not show the extreme irritability that calls for Chamomilla or the fever that indicates Belladonna, but they may have teeth that seem permanently on the verge of breaking through the surface. Calcarea carbonica 6c can be taken three times per day, for up to ten days; its use should be discontinued when symptoms improve.

REMEDIES FOR TINNITUS (RINGING IN THE EARS)

THIS CONDITION is more commonly seen in the elderly, but it can be extremely irritating to anyone unfortunate enough to suffer from continuous ringing, buzzing, or humming in the ears. Homeopathy offers several sure and safe alternatives to solving this frustrating problem.

Cimicifuga 6c

People who are likely to benefit from this remedy are sensitive to noise. Often, they are depressed and despondent, but their outlook improves when they are eating or warm. The condition may be accompanied by rheumatic pains (in the back and neck) and headache. Cimicifuga 6c can be taken in the amount of three to four doses daily, then reduced with improvement.

Carbo Vegetabilis 6c

In this case, symptoms are accompanied by vertigo and nausea. Individuals likely to benefit from this remedy feel worse during damp weather but feel better in cold, fresh air. The condition is sometimes triggered by a previous illness; it is worse in the evenings and at night. Carbo vegetabilis 6c can be taken in the amount of three to four doses daily, then reduced with improvement.

Graphites 6c

This remedy may be beneficial for tinnitus with associated deafness. Individuals hear hissing and clicking sounds in their ears; they also have dry skin inside their ears and moist eruptions behind the earlobes. Graphites 6c can be taken in the amount of three to four doses daily, then reduced with improvement.

Chininum Sulfuricum 30c

If there is reason to believe that the condition has come on after taking quinine tablets (as elderly people often do for nightly leg cramps), then this remedy might help. There is characteristic buzzing and ringing, at times becoming so loud as to render the afflicted persons nearly deaf. Vertigo is also present. Chininum sulfuricum 30c can be taken three times per day for two to three days.

Salicylic Acid 30c

This remedy may be useful when the tinnitus has come on from taking too much aspirin (a situation associated primarily with the elderly). There is a loud roaring and ringing in the ears. Salicylic acid 30c can be taken three times per day for two to three days; discontinue with significant improvement.

Natrum Salicylicum 30c

This remedy may be beneficial if the ringing in the ears is like a low, dull hum. Loss of hearing and vertigo may also be present. Natrum salicylicum 30c can be taken three times per day for two to three days.

Lycopodium 6c

Lycopodium may be helpful if there is a humming and roaring in the ears, along with impaired hearing. In this case, sounds seem to echo in the ears, and this condition may be associated with discharge from the ear and/or digestive or urinary complaints. Lycopodium 6c can be taken in the amount of three to four doses daily, then reduced on improvement.

REMEDIES FOR URINARY TRACT INFECTION

HOMEOPATHIC remedies are very helpful for women suffering from a **urinary tract infection** (page 120). For the occasional acute episode of cystitis (bladder infection), individuals can try the medicine described below that is the closest match for the symptoms.

Frequent urinary tract infections or infections associated with kidney pain should be seen by a doctor. Often, however, the right homeopathic medicine and extra glasses of water or unsweetened cranberry juice clears up cases of urinary tract infection.

Cantharis 30c

Most homeopaths try this remedy first in cases of a sudden onset of symptoms. Symptoms can include frequent or continual urges to urinate, even though only a few drops of urine are passed at one time; feelings that the bladder does not empty fully; and burning pain upon urination. Cantharis 30c can be taken three times per day for two days; discontinue with significant improvement.

Sepia 30c

This remedy is helpful for cases in which the urine has a strong odor (sometimes almost like ammonia), there is a sensation that urine will leak if urination is delayed, and there is pain in the urethra after urinating. Sepia 30c can be taken three times per day for two days; discontinue with significant improvement.

Belladonna 6c

This remedy may be beneficial if there is constant urging with burning pains—even after passing urine. Often, the condition has a rapid onset, with burning, hot skin and possibly a throbbing headache. The urine is a dark color. Belladonna 6c can be taken in the amount of one dose every two hours, for up to six doses. Thereafter, three to four doses can be taken daily. Usage should be reduced with improvement.

Staphysagria 12c

This medicine is called the "honeymooner's remedy" for its use in treating bouts of cystitis that develop after intercourse. It is also useful for cystitis resulting from hospital procedures, such as catheterization. Often, there is a sensation that a drop of urine is running through the urethra with a constant burning feeling. Staphysagria 12c can be taken three times per day for two days; discontinue with significant improvement.

Nux Vomica 6c

In this case, there is a burning pain in the bladder area, especially at night. Also, individuals experience burning and itching in passing urine. They feel a constant urge to urinate, but only a small quantity is produced. This remedy may be useful during pregnancy. Nux vomica 6c can be taken in the amount of one dose every two hours for up to six doses. Thereafter, three to four doses can be taken daily. Usage should be reduced with improvement.

REMEDIES FOR VARICOSE VEINS

WHEN THE valves inside the veins become weak, they are no longer able to keep blood from drifting backward. This can cause a pooling of blood in the vein, which becomes enlarged, purple, and lumpy.

This condition is called varicose veins. Usually, this happens in the legs, but it may also occur in the rectum, in which case it is called hemorrhoids. The legs may ache or swell, and the varicose veins may become tender or itchy. Homeopathic remedies may help to ease the discomfort varicose veins can cause.

Pulsatilla 6c

When varicose veins appear during pregnancy, Pulsatilla may be useful. Symptoms are made worse by hanging the legs down without support and also by applying warmth, such as a hot bath. Often, women who may benefit from this remedy feel chilly and enjoy lots of fresh air. Pulsatilla 6c can be taken three times per day for up to three weeks.

Arnica 30c

When the legs feel and look bruised in areas surrounding the varicose veins as well as the veins themselves, people should consider Arnica. Arnica 30c can be taken three times per day for up to five days; its use should be discontinued when the condition improves.

Aconitum Napellus 6c

This remedy may be beneficial in cases that are usually brought on by long periods of standing. Afflicted persons have painful, uncomfortable, restless legs as well as a feeling of fatigue. Aconitum napellus 6c can be taken in the amount of one dose every two hours for up to six doses. Thereafter, three to four doses can be taken daily. Usage should be reduced on improvement.

Carbo Vegetabilis 6c

This remedy may be beneficial in conditions that are accompanied by poor circulation. Individuals have mottled skin and cold extremities, which are much worse at night. This condition is often seen in the elderly. Carbo vegetabilis 6c can be taken in the amount of one dose every two hours for up to six doses. Thereafter, three to four doses can be taken daily. Usage should be reduced on improvement.

Hamamelis 6c

This remedy may help when there is a sore, bruised feeling with the varicose veins, and the discomfort may be worse from stepping sharply in a way that jars the leg. Individuals may have a tendency to develop hemorrhoids as well. Hamamelis 6c can be taken three to four times per day for two to three weeks.

REMEDIES FOR YEAST INFECTIONS

YEAST IS an organism that seizes an opportunity and makes the best of it. When a pH imbalance, overload of sugar, or worn-down immune system provides a chance, then a **yeast infection** (page 127) in any warm, moist place may result.

Sometimes, it occurs in the digestive tract, resulting in bloating. Nursing women may get yeast infections on their nipples and in their babies' mouths. More commonly, women experience vaginal yeast infections. Regardless of location, there is usually itching, often soreness or swelling, and sometimes a discharge. Choosing a homeopathic remedy is easiest after defining the type of discomfort that arises and the type of discharge that is produced.

Note: If this is the first time you have had vaginal itch and discomfort, consult your doctor. If you have had a doctor diagnose a vaginal yeast infection before and have the same symptoms, try the remedies below as directed. If you have any of the following symptoms, contact your doctor right away (you may have a more serious illness): Fever (higher than 100°F orally); pain in the lower abdomen, back, or either shoulder; a vaginal discharge that smells bad.

Pulsatilla 6c

For women who experience symptoms that are worse just before and after their menstrual periods and have vaginitis with a changeable discharge, which ranges from clear and watery to thick, creamy, and yellow, this remedy may be helpful. The discharge may be very irritating, itchy, and burning. Pulsatilla 6c can be taken four to six times per day for up to four days.

Kali Bichromicum 6c

In cases where there is much itching, with a discharge that has a greenish tinge to it, Kali bichromicum may be helpful. Kali bichromicum 6c can be taken four to six times each day for up to four days; its use should be discontinued when symptoms improve.

Sulfur 6c

This remedy may be beneficial if there is burning, stinging, and itching. Symptoms are aggravated by heat and bathing. Scratching gives temporary relief but is rapidly followed by rawness and burning. Sulfur 6c can be taken in the amount of one dose every hour, for up to six doses. Thereafter, three to four doses can be taken daily. Usage should be reduced on improvement.

REFERENCES

Conditions

Acne

1. Hillstrom L et al. Comparison of oral treatment with zinc sulfate and placebo in acne vulgaris. *Br J Dermatol* 1977; 97:679–84.

2. Michaelsson G et al. A double blind study of the effect of zinc and oxytetracycline in acne vulgaris. *Br J Dermatol* 1977; 97:561–66.

3. Kligman AM et al. Oral vitamin A in acne vulgaris. *Int J Dermatol* 1981; 20:278–85.

4. Snider B, Dietman DF. Pyridoxine therapy for premenstrual acne flare. *Arch Dermatol* 1974;110:130–31.

5. Bassett IB, Pannowitz DL, Barnetson RS. A comparative study of tea-tree oil versus benzoyl peroxide in the treatment of acne. *Med J Austral* 1990;53: 455–58.

6. Hoffman D. *The Herbal Handbook: A User's Guide to Medical Herbalism.* Rochester, VT: Healing Arts Press, 1988, 23–24.

Alzheimer's Disease

1. Priest ND. Satellite symposium on Alzheimer's disease and dietary aluminium. *Proc Nutr Soc* 1993;52:231–40.

2. Crook T et al. Effects of phosphatidylserine in Alzheimer's disease. *Psychopharmacol Bull* 1992;28:61–66.

3. Gindin J et al. The effect of plant phosphatidylserine on age-associated memory impairment and mood in the functioning elderly. Rehovot, Israel: Geriatric Institute for Education and Research, and Department of Geriatrics, Kaplan Hospital, 1995.

4. Cucinotta D et al. Multicenter clinical placebo-controlled study with acetyl-L-carnitine (LAC) in the treatment of mildly demented elderly patients. *Drug Development Res* 1988;14:213–16.

5. Sano M, Ernesto C, Thomas RG, et al. A controlled trial of selegiline, alpha-tocopherol, or both as treatment for Alzheimer's disease. *N Engl J Med* 1997; 336:1216–22.

6. Meyer JS, Welch KMA, Deshmuckh VD, et al. Neurotransmitter precursor amino acids in the treatment of multi-infarct dementia and Alzheimer's disease. *J Am Ger Soc* 1977;7:289–98.

7. Bush AI, Pettingell WH, Multhaup G, et al. Rapid induction of alzheimer A8 amyloid formation by zinc. *Science* 1994; 265:1464–65.

8. Sardi B. Winning over the public—the battle between pharmaceuticals and nutritional supplements. *Townsend Letter for Doctors and Patients* 1996;156:74–79.

9. Hofferberth B. The efficacy of EGb 761 in patients with senile dementia of the Alzheimer type: A double-blind, placebo-controlled study on different levels of investigation. *Human Psychopharmacol* 1994;9:215–22.

10. Kanowski S, Herrmann WM, Stephan K, et al. Proof of efficacy of the *Ginkgo biloba* special extract EGb 761 in outpatients suffering from mild to moderate primary degenerative dementia of the Alzheimer type or multi-infarct dementia. *Pharmacopsychiatr* 1996;29:47–56.

11. D'Angelo L, Grimaldi R, et al. A double-blind, placebo-controlled clinical study of a standardized ginseng extract on psychomotor performance in healthy volunteers. *J Ethnopharmacol* 1986;16:15–22.

12. Owen RT. Ginseng—a pharmacological profile. *Drugs Today* 1981;17: 343–51.

Antioxidants and Free Radicals

1. Ames BN, Shigenaga MK, Hagen TM. Oxidants, antioxidants, and the degenerative diseases of aging. *Proc Natl Acad Sci USA* 1993;90:7915–22.

Asthma

1. Rowe AH, Young EJ. Bronchial asthma due to food allergy alone in ninety-five patients. *JAMA* 1959;169:1158.

2. Collipp PJ et al. Tryptophane metabolism in bronchial asthma. *Ann Allergy* 1975;35:153–58.

3. Weir MR et al. Depression of vitamin B6 levels due to theophylline. *Ann Allergy* 1990;65:59–62.

4. Collipp PJ et al. Pyridoxine treatment of childhood bronchial asthma. *Ann Allergy* 1975;35:93–97.

5. Reynolds RD, Natta CL. Depressed plasma pyridoxal phosphate concentrations in adult asthmatics. *Am J Clin Nutr* 1985;41:684–88.

6. Haury VG. Blood serum magnesium in bronchial asthma and its treatment by the administration of magnesium sulfate. *J Lab Clin Med* 1940;26:340–44.

7. Skobeloff EM et al. Intravenous magnesium sulfate for the treatment of acute asthma in the emergency department. *JAMA* 1989;262:1210–13.

8. Zuskin E et al. Byssinosis and airway responses due to exposure to textile dust. *Lung* 1976;154:17–24.

9. Ruskin SL. Sodium ascorbate in the treatment of allergic disturbances. The role of adrenal cortical hormone-sodium-vitamin C. *Am J Dig Dis* 1947; 14:302–6.

10. Anibarro B et al. Asthma with sulfite intolerance in children: A blocking study with cyanocobalamin. *J Allerg Clin Immunol* 1992;90:103–9.

11. Johnson JL et al. Molybdenum cofactor deficiency in a patient previously characterized as deficient in sulfite oxidase. *Biochem Med Metabol Biol* 1988; 40:86–93.

12. *Ann Int Med* 1973;78:271–76.

13. Soyka F, Edmonds A. *The Ion Effect.* New York: Bantam, 1977.

14. Leung AY, Foster S. *Encyclopedia of Common Natural Ingredients Used in Foods, Drugs, and Cosmetics,* 2d ed. New York: John Wiley and Sons, 1996, 227–29.

Atherosclerosis

1. Raloff J. Oxidized lipids: A key to heart disease? *Sci News* 1985;127:278.

385

2. Ornish D, Brown SE, Scherwitz LW, et al. Can lifestyle changes reverse coronary heart disease? *Lancet* 1990; 336:129–33.

3. Lawson LD, Ransom DK, Hughes BG. Inhibition of whole blood platelet-»aggregation by compounds in garlic clove extracts and commercial garlic products. *Thrombosis Res* 1992;65:141–56.

4. Mansell P, Reckless JPD. Garlic—effects on serum lipids, blood pressure, coagulation, platelet aggregation, and vasodilatation. *BMJ* 1991;303:379–80 (editorial).

5. Belcher JD, Balla J, Balla G, et al. Vitamin E, LDL, and endothelium: Brief oral vitamin supplementation prevents oxidized LDL-mediated vascular injury in vitro. *Arterioscler Thromb* 1993;13: 1779–89.

6. Stephens NG, Parsons A, Schofield PM, et al. Randomised controlled trial of vitamin E in patients with coronary disease: Cambridge Heart Antioxidant Study (CHAOS). *Lancet* 1996;347:781–86.

7. Frei B. Ascorbic acid protects lipids in human plasma and low-density lipoprotein against oxidative damage. *Am J Clin Nutr* 1991;54:1113S–18S.

8. Salonen JT et al. Association between cardiovascular death and myocardial infarction and serum selenium in a matched-pair longitudinal study. *Lancet* 1982;ii:175.

9. Shamberger RJ, Willis CE. Epidemiological studies on selenium and heart disease. *Fed Proc* 1976;35:578 (abstract #2061).

10. Korpela H, Kumpulainen J, Jussila E, et al. Effect of selenium supplementation after acute myocardial infarction. *Res Comm Chem Pathol Pharmacol* 1989; 65:249–52.

11. Ronzio RA. Antioxidants, nutraceuticals and functional foods. *Townsend Letter for Doctors and Patients* Oct 1996: 34–35 (review).

12. Hertog MGL, Feskens EJM, Hollman PCH, et al. Dietary antioxidant flavonoids and risk of coronary heart disease: The Zutphen Elderly Study. *Lancet* 1993;342:1007–11.

13. Hertog MGL, Kromhout D, Aravanis C, et al. Flavonoid intake and long-term risk of coronary heart disease and cancer in the Seven Countries Study. *Arch Intern Med* 1995;155:381–86.

14. Knekt P, Jarvinen R, Reunanen A, Maatela J. Flavonoid intake and coronary mortality in Finland: A cohort study. *BMJ* 1996;312:478–81.

15. Rimm EB, Katan MB, Ascherio A, et al. Relation between intake of flavonoids and risk for coronary heart disease in male health professionals. *Ann Intern Med* 1996;125:384–89.

16. Stampfer MJ, Malinow R, Willett WC, et al. A prospective study of plasma homocyst(e)ine and risk of myocardial infarction in US physicians. *JAMA* 1992; 268:877–81.

17. Selhub J, Jacques PF, Wilson PW, et al. Vitamin status and intake as primary determinants of homocysteinemia in an elderly population. *JAMA* 1993; 270:2693–98.

18. Ubbink JB, Hayward WJ, van der Merwe A, et al. Vitamin requirements for the treatment of hyperhomocysteinemia in humans. *J Nutr* 1994;124:1927–33.

19. Manson JB, Miller JW. The effects of vitamin B12, B6, and folate on blood homocysteine levels. *Ann NY Acad Sci* 1992;669:197–204 (review).

20. Franken DG, Boers GHJ, Blom HJ, et al. Treatment of mild hyperhomocysteinemia in vascular disease patients. *Arterioscler Thromb* 1994; 14: 465–70.

21. Ubbink JB, Vermaak WJH, van der Merwe A, et al. Vitamin requirements for the treatment of hyperhomocysteinemia in humans. *J Nutr* 1994;124: 1927–33.

22. Ubbink JB, van der Merwe A, Vermaak WJH, Delport R. Hyperhomocysteinemia and the response to vitamin supplementation. *Clin Investig* 1993;71: 993–98.

23. Morrison LM, Branwood AW, Ershoff BH, et al. The prevention of coronary arteriosclerotic heart disease with chondroitin sulfate A: Preliminary report. *Exp Med Surg* 1969;27:278–89.

24. Morrison LM, Enrick NL. Coronary heart disease: Reduction of death rate by chondroitin sulfate A. *Angiology* 1973;24:269–82.

25. Bertelli AA, Giovanninni L, Bernini W, et al. Antiplatelet activity of cis-resveratrol. *Drugs Exp Clin Res* 1996; 22(2):61–63.

26. Chen CK and Pace-Asciak CR. Vasorelaxing activity of resveratrol and quercetin in isolated rat aorta. *Gen Pharm* 1996;27(2):363–66.

27. Pace-Asciak CR, Rounova O, Hahn SE, et al. Wines and grape juices as modulators of platelet aggregation in healthy human subjects. *Clin Chim Acta* 1996; 246(1–2):163–82.

Athletic Performance

1. Dekkers JC, van Doornen LJ, Kemper HC. The role of antioxidant vitamins and enzymes in the prevention of exercise-induced muscle damage. *Sports Med* 1996; 21(3):213–38.

2. Keith R, Alt L. Riboflavin status of female athletes consuming normal diets. *Nutr Res* 1991;11(7):727–34.

3. Lukaski H, Hoverson B, Gallagher S, et al. Physical training and copper, iron, and zinc status of swimmers. *Am J Clin Nutr* 1990;51:1093–99.

4. Page TG, Ward TL, Southern LL. Effect of chromium picolinate on growth and carcass characteristics of growing-finishing pigs. *J Animal Sci* 1991;69:356.

5. Lefavi R, Anderson R, Keith R, et al. Efficacy of chromium supplementation in athletes: Emphasis on anabolism. *Int J Sport Nutr* 1992;2:111–22.

6. McCarty MF. The case for supplemental chromium and a survey of clinical studies with chromium picolinate. *J Appl Nutr* 1991;43:59–66.

7. Rogers MA. *Medicine and Science in Sports and Exercise* 1996;28(2).

8. Weaver C, Rajaram S. Exercise and iron status. *J Nutr* 1992;122:782–87.

9. Drilla L, Haley T. Effect of magnesium supplementation on strength training in humans. *J Am Col Nutr* 1992;11(3): 326–29.

10. Blomstrand E, Hassmen P, Ek S, et al. Influence of ingesting a solution of branched-chain amino acids on perceived exertion during exercise. *Acta Physiol Scand* 1997;159:41–49.

11. Giamberardino MA et al. Effects of prolonged L-carnitine administration on delayed muscle pain and CK release after eccentric effort. *Int J Sports Med* 1996; 17:320–24.

12. Stanko RT, Robertson RJ, Galbreath RW, et al. Enhanced leg exercise endurance with a high-carbohydrate diet and dihyroxyacetone and pyruvate. *J Appl Phys* 1990;69(5):1651–56.

13. Stanko RT, Robertson RJ, Spina RJ, et al. Enhancement of arm exercise endurance capacity with dihydroxyacetone and pyruvate. *J Appl Phys* 1990; 68(1):119–24.

14. Kelly GS. Sports nutrition: A review of selected nutritional supplements

for bodybuilders and strength athletes. *Alt Med Rev* 1997;2(3):184–201.

15. Starling RD, Trappe TA, Short KR, et al. Effect of inosine supplementation on aerobic and anaerobic cycling performance. *Med Sci Sports Ex* 1996;28(9): 1193–98.

16. Bucci LR, Hickson JF, Wolinsky I, et al. Ornithine supplementation and insulin release in bodybuilders. *Int J Sport Nutr* 1992;2:287–91.

17. Jeevanandam M, Holaday NJ, Petersen SR. Ornithine-alpha-ketoglutarate (OKG) supplementation is more effective than its component salts in traumatized rats. *J Nutr* 1996;126(9):2141–50.

18. Le Bricon T, Cynober L, Baracos VE. Ornithine alpha-ketoglutarate limits muscle protein breakdown without stimulating tumor growth in rats bearing Yoshida ascites hepatoma. *Met Clin Exp* 1994;43(7):899–905.

19. Greenhaff PL, Bodin K, Soderlund K, et al. Effect of oral creatine supplementation on skeletal muscle phosphocreatine resynthesis. *Am J Physiol* 1994; 266:E725–30.

20. Greenhaff PL. Creatine and its application as an ergogenic aid. *Int J Sport Nutr* 1995;5:94–101.

21. Earnest CP, Snell PG, Rodriguez R, et al. The effect of creatine monohydrate ingestion on anaerobic power indices, muscular strength, and body composition. *Acta Physiol Scand* 1995;153:207–9.

22. Rosenbloom C, Millard-Stafford M, Lathrop J. Contemporary ergogenic aids used by strength/power athletes. *J Am Diet Assoc* 1992;92(10):1264–65.

23. Jeukendrup AE, Saris WHM, van Diesen RAJ, et al. Exogenous MCT oxidation from carbohydrate–medium chain triglyceride supplements during moderate intensity exercise. *Clin Sci* 1994;87:33.

Autism

1. Martineau J, Garreau B, Barthelemy C, et al. Effects of vitamin B6 on averaged evoked potentials in infantile autism. *Biol Psychiatr* 1981;16:627–39.

2. Lelord G, Muh JP, Barthelemy C, et al. Effects of pyridoxine and magnesium on autistic symptoms: Initial observations. *J Autism Developmental Disorders* 1981; 11:219–29.

3. Rimland B, Callaway E, Dreyfus P. The effect of high doses of vitamin B6 on autistic children: A double-blind crossover study. *Am J Psychiatr* 1978;135:472–75.

4. Rimland B. Vitamin B6 versus Fenfluramine: A case-study in medical bias. *J Nutr Med* 1991;2:321–22.

5. Martineau J, Barthelemy C, Garreau B, Lelord G. Vitamin B6, magnesium, and combined B6-Mg: Therapeutic effects in childhood autism. *Biol Psychiatr* 1985; 20:467–78.

Benign Prostatic Hyperplasia

1. Hart JP, Cooper WL. Vitamin F in the treatment of prostatic hypertrophy. Report Number 1, Lee Foundation for Nutritional Research, Milwaukee, WI, 1941.

2. Bush IM et al. Zinc and the prostate. Presented at the annual meeting of the American Medical Association, Chicago, 1974.

3. Fahim MS et al. Zinc treatment for reduction of hyperplasia. *Fed Proc* 1976; 35(3):361.

4. Damrau F. Benign prostatic hypertrophy: Amino acid therapy for symptomatic relief. *J Am Geriatrics Soc* 1962; 10(5):426–30.

5. Berges RR, Windeler J, Trampisch HJ, et al. Randomized, placebo-controlled, double-blind clinical trial of beta-sitosterol in patients with benign prostatic hyperplasia. *Lancet* 1995;345: 1529–32.

6. Chandra RK. Excessive intake of zinc impairs immune responses. *JAMA* 1984;252(11):1443.

7. Bush AI, Pettingell WH, Multhaup G, et al. Rapid induction of alzheimer A8 amyloid formation by zinc. *Science* 1994; 265:1464–65.

8. Sardi B. Winning over the public: The battle between pharmaceuticals and nutritional supplements. *Townsend Letter for Doctors and Patients* 1996;156:74–79.

9. Broun ER, Greist A, Tricot G, Hoffman R. Excessive zinc ingestion: A reversible cause of sideroblastic anemia and bone marrow depression. *JAMA* 1990; 264:1441–43.

10. Reiser S et al. Effect of copper intake on blood cholesterol and its lipoprotein distribution in men. *Nutr Rep Internat* 1987;36(3):641–49.

11. Sandstead HH. Requirements and toxicity of essential trace elements, illustrated by zinc and copper. *Am J Clin Nutr* 1995;61(suppl):621S–24S (review).

12. Fischer PWF, Giroux A, Labbe MR. Effect of zinc supplementation on copper

status in adult man. *Am J Clin Nutr* 1984;40(4):743–46.

13. Dawson EB, Albers J, McGanity WJ. Serum zinc changes due to iron supplementation in teen-age pregnancy. *Am J Clin Nutr* 199;50:848–52.

14. Crovton RW, Gvozdanovic D, Gvozdanovic S, et al. Inorganic zinc and the intestinal absorption of ferrous iron. *Am J Clin Nutr* 1989;50:141–44.

15. Argiratos V, Samman S. The effect of calcium carbonate and calcium citrate on the absorption of zinc in healthy female subjects. *Er J Clin Nutr* 1994; 48:198–204.

16. Spencer H, Norris C, Williams D. Inhibitory effects of zinc on magnesium balance and magnesium absorption in man. *J Coll Nutr* 1994;13:479–84.

17. Schneider HJ, Honold E, Mashur T. Treatment of benign prostatic hyperplasia. Results of a surveillance study in the practices of urological specialists using a combined plant-base preparation. *Fortschr Med* 1995;113:37–40.

18. Koch E, Biber A. Pharmacological effects of sabal and urtica extracts as a basis for a rational medication of benign prostatic hyperplasia. *Urologe* 1994;334: 90–95.

19. Braeckman J. The extract of Serenoa repens in the treatment of benign prostatic hyperplasia: A multicenter open study. *Cur Ther Res* 1994;55(7):776–85.

20. Ross RK et al. 5-alpha-reductase activity and risk of prostate cancer among Japanese and US white and black males. *Lancet* 1992;339:887–89.

21. Andro MC, Riffaud JP. *Pygeum africanum* extract for the treatment of patients with benign prostatic hyperplasia: A review of 25 years of published experience. *Curr Ther Res* 1995;56:796–817.

22. Koch E, Biber A. Pharmacological effects of sabal and urtica extracts as a basis for a rational medication of benign prostatic hyperplasia. *Urologe* 1994;334: 90–95.

Bursitis

1. Klemes IS. Vitamin B12 in acute subdeltoid bursitis. *Indust Med Surg* 1957; 26:290–92.

2. Kellman M. Bursitis: A new chemotherapeutic approach. *J Am Osteopathic Assoc* 1962;61:896–903.

Canker Sores

1. Hay KD, Reade PC. The use of an elimination diet in the treatment of

recurrent aphthous ulceration of the oral cavity. *Oral Surg Oral Med Oral Pathol* 1984;57:504–7.

2. Wray D. Gluten-sensitive recurrent aphthous stomatitis. *Dig Dis Sci* 1981; 26:737–40.

3. Wright A et al. Food allergy or intolerance in severe recurrent aphthous ulceration of the mouth. *BMJ* 1986;292:1237.

4. Wray D et al. Food allergens and basophil histamine release in recurrent aphthous stomatitis. *Oral Surg Oral Med Oral Pathol* 1982;54:338–95.

5. Porter SR et al. Hematologic status in recurrent aphthous stomatitis compared to other oral disease. *Oral Surg Oral Med Oral Pathol* 1988;66:41–44.

6. Palopoli J, Waxman J. Recurrent aphthous stomatitis and vitamin B12 deficiency. *South Med J* 1990;83:475–77.

7. Wray D et al. Nutritional deficiencies in recurrent aphthae. *J Oral Pathol* 1978;7:418–23.

8. Nolan A et al. Recurrent aphthous ulceration. *J Oral Pathol Med* 1991;20: 389–91.

9. Haisraeli-Shalish M, Livneh A, Katz J, et al. Recurrent aphthous stomatitis and thiamine deficiency. *Oral Surg Oral Med Oral Pathol Oral Radiol Endod* 1996; 82:634–36.

10. James APR. Common dermatologic disorders. *CIBA Clin Symposia* 1967; 19:38–64.

11. Werbach MR. *Nutritional Influences on Illness*, 2d ed. Tarzana, CA: Third Line Press, 1993, 56 (review).

12. Gerenrich RL, Hart RW. Treatment of oral ulcerations with Bacid (Lactobacillus acidophilus). *Oral Surg* 1970;30: 196–200.

13. Das SK, Gulati AK, Singh VP. Deglycyrrhizinated licorice in apthous ulcers. *J Assoc Physicians India* 1989;37:647.

14. Kamillosan NT. Therapy in dermatology. *Z Allgemeinmed* 1975;25:1105–6.

Carpal Tunnel Syndrome

1. Fuhr JF, Farrow A, Nelson HS. Vitamin B6 levels in patients with carpal tunnel syndrome. *Arch Surg* 1989;124:1329–30.

2. Ellis JM, Azuma J, Watanbe T, Folkers K. Survey and new data on treatment with pyridoxine of patients having a clinical syndrome including the carpal tunnel and other defects. *Res Comm Chem Path Pharm* 1977;17(1):165–77.

3. Ellis JM. Vitamin B6 deficiency in patients with a clinical syndrome including the carpal tunnel defect. Biochemical and clinical response to therapy with pyridoxine. *Res Comm Chem Path Pharm* 1976;13(4):743–57.

4. D'Souza M. Carpal tunnel syndrome: Clinical or neurophysiological diagnosis. *Lancet* 1985;I:1104–5.

5. Driskell JA, Wesley RL, Hess IE. Effectiveness of pyridoxine hydrochloride treatment on carpal tunnel syndrome patients. *Nutr Rep Internat* 1986; 34(4): 1031–39.

6. Ellis JM. Treatment of carpal tunnel syndrome with vitamin B6. *Southern Med J* 1987;80(7):882–84.

7. Smith GP et al. Biochemical studies of pyridoxal and pyridoxal phosphate status and therapeutic trial of pyridoxine in patients with carpal tunnel syndrome. *Ann Neurol* 1984;15:104–7.

8. Amadio PC. Pyridoxine as an adjunct in the treatment of carpal tunnel syndrome. *J Hand Surg* 1985;10A(2):237–41.

9. Stransky M et al. Treatment of carpal tunnel syndrome with vitamin B6: A double-blind study. *Southern Med J* 1989;82(7):841–42.

10. Gaby AR. Literature review & commentary. *Townsend Letter for Doctors* June 1990;338–39.

11. Parry G, Bredesen DE. Sensory neuropath with low-dose pyridoxine. *Neurology* 1985;35:1466–68.

12. Schaumburg H, Kaplan J, Windebank A, et al. Sensory neuropathy from pyridoxine abuse. *N Engl J Med* 1983; 309(8):445–48.

Cataracts

1. Kahn HA, Leibowitz HM, Ganley JP, et al. The Framingham Eye Study: I. Outline and major prevalence findings. *Am J Epidemiol* 1977;106:17–32.

2. Schocket SS, Esterson J, Bradford B, et al. Induction of cataracts in mice by exposure to oxygen. *Isr J Med Sci* 1972; 8:1596–1601.

3. Palmquist B, Phillipson B, Barr P. Nuclear cataract and myopia during hyperbaric oxygen therapy. *Br J Ophthalmol* 1984;68:113–17.

4. Jacques PF, Chylack LT Jr. Epidemiologic evidence of a role for the antioxidant vitamins and carotenoids in cataract prevention. *Am J Clin Nutr* 1991; 53:352S–55S.

5. Knekt P, Heliovaara M, Rissanen A, et al. Serum antioxidant vitamins and risk of cataract. *BMJ* 1992;305:1392–94.

6. Taylor A, Jacques PF, Nadler D, et al. Relationship in humans between ascorbic acid consumption and levels of total and reduced ascorbic acid in lens, aqueous humor, and plasma. *Curr Eye Res* 1991; 10:751–59.

7. Reddy VN. Glutathione and its function in the lens—An overview. *Exp Eye Res* 1990;150:771–78.

8. Packer JE, Slater TF, Willson RL. Direct observation of a free radical interaction between vitamin E and vitamin C. *Nature* 1979;278:737–38.

9. Taylor A. Cataract: Relationship between nutrition and oxidation. *J Am Coll Nutr* 1993;12:138–46 (review).

10. Taylor A, Jacques PF, Nadler D, et al. Relationship in humans between ascorbic acid consumption and levels of total and reduced ascorbic acid in lens, aqueous humor, and plasma. *Curr Eye Res* 1991; 10:751–59.

11. Jacques PF, Chylack LT Jr. Epidemiologic evidence of a role for the antioxidant vitamins and carotenoids in cataract prevention. *Am J Clin Nutr* 1991; 53:352S–55S.

12. Jacques PF, Chylack LT, McGandy RB, Hartz SC. Antioxidant status in persons with and without senile cataract. *Arch Ophthalmol* 1988;106:337–40.

13. Robertson J McD, Donner AP, Trevithick JR. Vitamin E intake and risk of cataracts in humans. *Ann NY Acad Sci* 1989;570:372–82.

14. Robertson J McD, Donner AP, Trevithick JR. A possible role for vitamins C and E in cataract prevention. *Am J Clin Nutr* 1991;53:346S–51S.

15. Hankinson SE, Stampfer MJ, Seddon JM, et al. Nutrient intake and cataract extraction in women: A prospective study. *BMJ* 1992;305:335–39.

16. Trevithick JR, Creighton MO, et al. Modelling cortical cataractogenesis: 2. *In vitro* effects on the lens of agents preventing glucose- and sorbitol-induced cataracts. *Can J Ophthalmol* 1981;16: 32–38.

17. Robertson J McD, Donner AP, Trevithick JR. A possible role for vitamins C and E in cataract prevention. *Am J Clin Nutr* 1991;53:346S–51S.

18. Hankinson SE, Stampfer MJ, Seddon JM, et al. Nutrient intake and cataract extraction in women: A prospective study. *BMJ* 1992;305:335–39.

19. Hankinson Se, Stampfer MJ, Seddon JM, et al. Nutrient intake and

cataract extraction in women: A prospective study. *BMJ* 1992;305:335–39.

20. Bhat KS. Nutritional status of thiamine, riboflavin and pyridoxine in cataract patients. *Nutr Rep Internat* 1987; 36:685–92.

21. Prchal JT, Conrad ME, Skalka HW. Association of presenile cataracts with heterozygosity for galactosaemic states and with riboflavin deficiency. *Lancet* 1978;I:12–13.

22. Sperduto RD, Hu TS, Milton RC, et al. The Linxian cataract studies. *Arch Ophthalmol* 1993;111:1246–53.

23. Varma SD et al. Diabetic cataracts and flavonoids. *Science* 1977;195:205.

24. Sanstead HH. Copper bioavailability and requirements. *Am J Clin Nutr* 1982;35:809-14 (review).

25. van Acker SA, van den Berg DJ, Tromp MN, et al. Structural aspects of antioxidant activity of flavonoids. *Free Rad Biol Med* 1996;20:331–42.

26. Salvayre R, Braquet P, et al. Comparison of the scavenger effect of bilberry anthocyanosides with various flavonoids. *Proceed Intl Bioflavonoids Symposium*, Munich, 1981, 437–42.

27. Bravetti G. Preventive medical treatment of senile cataract with vitamin E and anthocyanosides: Clinical evaluation. *Ann Ottamol Clin Ocul* 1989; 115:109.

Chemotherapy Support

1. de Blasio F et al. N-acetyl cysteine (NAC) in preventing nausea and vomiting induced by chemotherapy in patients suffering from inoperable non-small-cell lung cancer (NSCLC). *Chest* 1996;110(4, Suppl):103S.

2. Meyer K, Schwartz J, Crater D, Keyes B. *Zingiber officinale* (ginger) used to prevent 8-Mop associated nausea. *Dermatol Nurs* 1995;7:242–44.

3. Pace JC. Oral ingestion of encapsulated ginger and reported self-care actions for the relief of chemotherapy-associated nausea and vomiting. *Dissertaion Abstr Internat* 1987;8:3297.

4. Wadleigh RG, Redman RS, Graham ML, et al. Vitamin E in the treatment of chemotherapy-induced mucositis. *Am J Med* 1992;92:481–84.

5. Nakagawa M, Hamaguchi T, Ueda H, et al. Potentiation by vitamin A of the action of anticancer agents against murine tumors. *Jpn J Cancer Res* 1985;76:887–94.

6. Prasad KN, Edwards-Prasad J, Ramanujam S, et al. Vitamin E increases the growth inhibitory and differentiating effects of tumor therapeutic agents in neuroblastoma and glioma cells in culture. *Proc Soc Ex Biol Med* 1980;164:158–63.

7. Taper HS, de Gerlache J, et al. Nontoxic potentiation of cancer chemotherapy by combined C and K3 vitamin pre-treatment. *Int J Cancer* 1987;40:575–79.

8. Jaakkola K, Lahteenmaki P, Laakso J, et al. Treatment with antioxidant and other nutrients in combination with chemotherapy and irradiation in patients with small-cell lung cancer. *Anticancer Res* 1992;12:599–606.

9. Folkers K, Wolaniuk A. Research on coenzyme Q10 in clinical medicine and in immunomodulation. *Drugs Exptl Clin Res* 1985;11:539–45.

10. Fujita K, Shinpo K, Yamada K, et al. Reduction of Adriamycin toxicity by ascorbate in mice and guinea pigs. *Cancer Res* 1982;42:309–16.

11. Perez Ripoll EA, Rama BN, Webber MM. Vitamin E enhances the chemotherapeutic effects of adriamycin on human prostatic carcinoma cells in vitro. *J Urol* 1986;136:529–31.

12. Wood LA. Possible prevention of adriamycin-induced alopecia by tocopherol. *N Engl J Med* 1985;312:1060 (letter).

13. Myers C, McGuire W, Young R. Adriamycin amelioration of toxicity by alpha-tocopherol. *Cancer Treat Rep* 1976; 60:961–62.

14. Ogura R, Humon Y, Yoon S. Antioxidative effect of vitamin B2 in cardiac mitochondria affected with Adriamycin. *J Mol Cell C* 1985;17:R48.

15. Buckley JE, Clark VL, Meyer TJ, Pearlman NW. Hypomagnesemia after cisplatin combination chemotherapy. *Arch Intern Med* 1984;144:2347–48.

16. Flombaum CD. Hypomagnesemia associated with cisplatin combination chemotherapy. *Arch Intern Med* 1984; 144:2336–37 (editorial).

17. Cascinus S, Cordella L, Del Ferro E, et al. Neuroprotective effect of reduced glutathione on cioplatin based chemotherapy in advanced gastric cancer: A randomized double-blind placebo-controlled trial. *J Clin Oncol* 1995;13:26–32.

18. Smythe JF, Bowman A, Perren T, et al. Glutathione reduces the toxicity and improves quality of life of women diagnosed with ovarian cancer treated with cisplatin: Results of a double-blind, randomized trial. *Ann Oncol* 1997;8:569–73.

19. Vukelja SJ, Lombardo F, James WD, Weiss RB. Pyroxidine [*sic*] for the palmar-plantar erythrodysesthesia syndrome. *Ann Intern Med* 1989;111:688–89 (letter).

20. Molina R, Fabian C, Slavik M, Dahlberg S. Reversal of palmar-plantar erythrodysesthesia (PPE) by B6 without loss of response in colon cancer patients receiving 200/mg/m2/day continuous 5-FU. *Proc Am Soc Clin Oncol* 1987;6:90 (abstract).

21. Foster S, Chongxi Y. *Herbal Emissaries: Bringing Chinese Herbs to the West*. Rochester, VT: Healing Arts Press, 1992, 27–33.

22. Yarameko KV. The main aspects of the use of eleutherococcus extract in oncology. In *New Data on Eleutherococcus and Other Adaptogens*. Vladivostok: The Far Eastern Scientific Center, USSR Academy of Sciences, 1981, 75–78.

23. Brown DJ. *Herbal Prescriptions for Better Health*. Rocklin, CA: Prima Publishing, 1996, 129–38.

Common Cold/Sore Throat

1. Sanchez A, Reeser JL, Lau HS, et al. Role of sugars in human neutrophilic phagocytosis. *Am J Clin Nutr* 1973;26: 1180–84.

2. Hemil H. Does vitamin C alleviate the symptoms of the common cold? A review of current evidence. *Scand J Infect Dis* 1994;26:1–6.

3. Anderson TW, Reid DB, Beaton GH. Vitamin C and the common cold: A double-blind trial. *CMAJ* 1972;107:503–8.

4. Anderson TW, Suranyyi G, Beaton GH. The effect on winter illness of large doses of vitamin C. *CMAJ* 1974;111: 31–36.

5. Eby G, Davis DR, Halcomb WW. Reduction in duration of common colds by zinc gluconate lozenges in a double-blind study. *Antimicrobial Agents Chemotherapy* 1984;25:20–24.

6. Al-Nakib W, Higgins PG, Barrow I, et al. Prophylaxis and treatment of rhinovirus colds with zinc gluconate lozenges. *J Antimicrobial Chemotherapy* 1987;20:893–901.

7. Godfrey JC, Sloane BC, Smith DS, et al. Zinc gluconate and the common cold: A controlled clinical study. *J Intern Med Res* 1992;20:234–36.

8. Sandstead HH. Copper bioavailability and requirements. *Am J Clin Nutr* 1982;35:809–14 (review).

9. Finley EB, Cerklewski FL. Influence of ascorbic acid supplementation on copper status in young adult men. *Am J Clin Nutr* 1983;37:553–56.

10. Chandra RK. Excessive intake of zinc impairs immune responses. *JAMA* 1984;252(11):1443.

11. Leuttig B, Steinmüller C, et al. Macrophage activation by the polysaccharide arabinogalactan isolated from plant cell cultures of Echinacea purpurea. *J Natl Cancer Inst* 1989;81:669–75.

12. Schoenberger D. The influence of immune-stimulating effects of pressed juice from Echinacea purpurea on the course and severity of colds. *Forum Immunol* 1992;8:2–12.

13. Murray MT. *The Healing Power of Herbs*. Rocklin, CA: Prima Publishing, 1995, 162–72.

14. Bradley PR, ed. *British Herbal Compendium*, vol. 1. Bournemouth, Dorset, UK: British Herbal Medicine Association, 1992, 119–20.

Congestive Heart Failure

1. Coats AJS. Effects of physical training in chronic heart failure. *Lancet* 1990;335:63–66.

2. Mortensen SA, Vadhanavikit S, Baandrup U, Folkers K. Long-term coenzyme Q10 therapy: A major advance in the management of resistant myocardial failure. *Drug Exptl Clin Res* 1985;11:581–93.

3. Morisco C, Trimarco B, Condorelli M. Effect of coenzyme Q10 in patients with congestive heart failure: A long-term multicenter randomized study. *Clin Invest* 1993;71:S134–36.

4. Bartels GL, Remme WJ, Pillay M, et al. Effects of L-propionylcarnitine on ischemia-induced myocardial dysfunction in men with angina pectoris. *Am J Cardiol* 1994;74:125–30.

5. Suzuki Y, Masumura Y, Kobayashi A, et al. Myocardial carnitine deficiency in chronic heart failure. *Lancet* 1982;i:116 (letter).

6. Bashir Y, Sneddon JF, Staunton A, et al. Effects of long-term oral magnesium chloride replacement in congestive heart failure secondary to coronary artery disease. *Am J Cardiol* 1993;72:1156–62.

7. Packer M, Gottlieb SS, Kessler PD. Hormone-electrolyte interactions in the pathogenesis of lethal cardiac arrhythmias in patients with congestive heart failure. *Am J Med* 1986;80(suppl 4A):23–29.

8. Azuma J, Sawamura A, Awata N, et al. Double-blind randomized crossover trial of taurine in congestive heart failure. *Curr Ther Res* 1983;34(4):543–57.

9. Azuma J, Hasegawa H, Sawamura N, et al. Taurine for treatment of congestive heart failure. *Int J Cardiol* 1982;2:303–4.

10. Azuma J, Hasegawa H, Sawamura A, et al. Therapy of congestive heart failure with orally administered taurine. *Clin Ther* 1983;5(4):398–408.

11. Azuma J, Takihara K, Awata N, et al. Taurine and failing heart: Experimental and clinical aspects. *Prog Clin Biol Res* 1985;179:195–213.

12. Rector TS, Bank A, Mullen KA, et al. Randomized, double-blind, placebo controlled study of supplemental oral L-arginine in patients with heart failure. *Circulation* 1996;93:2135–41.

13. Leuchtgens H. *Crataegus* special extract (WS 1442) in cardiac insufficiency. *Fortschr Med* 1993;111:352–54.

14. Schmidt U, Kuhn U, et al. Efficacy of the hawthorn (*Crataegus*) preparation LI 132 in 78 patients with chronic congestive heart failure defined as NYHA functional class II. *Phytomed* 1994;1:17–24.

15. Maevers VW, Hensel H. Changes in local myocardial blood flow following oral administration of a *Crataegus* extract to non-anethesized dogs. *Arzneim-Forsch Drug Res* 1974;24:783–85.

16. Weikl A, Noh HS. The influence of *Crataegus* on global cardiac insufficiency. *Herz Gerfässe* 1992;11:516–24.

17. Bahorun T, Trotin F, et al. Antioxidant activities of *Crataegus monogyna* extracts. *Planta Med* 1994;60:323–28.

Constipation

1. Müller-Lissner SA. Effect of wheat bran on weight of stool and gastrointestinal transit time: A meta analysis. *BMJ* 1988;296:615–17.

2. Marcus SN, Heaton KW. Effects of a new, concentrated wheat fibre preparation on intestinal transit, deoxycholic acid metabolism and the composition of bile. *Gut* 1986;27:893–900.

3. Cheskin LK, Kamal N, Crowell MD, et al. Mechanisms of constipation in older persons and effects of fiber compared with placebo. *J Am Geriatr Assoc* 1995;43:666–69.

4. Oettl GJ. Effect of moderate exercise on bowel habit. *Gut* 1991;32:941–44.

5. Bingham SA, Cummings JH. Effect of exercise and physical fitness on large intestinal function. *Gastroenterol* 1989;97:1389–99.

6. Passmore AP, Wilson-Davies K, et al. Chronic constipation in long stay elderly patients: A comparison of lactulose and senna-fiber combination. *Br Med J* 1993;307:769–71.

Crohn's Disease

1. Mayberry JF, Rhodes J. Epidemiological aspects of Crohn's disease: A review of the literature. *Gut* 1984;886–99.

2. Shoda R, Masueda K, Yamato S, Umeda N. Epidemiologic analysis of Crohn's disease in Japan: Increased dietary intake of n-6 polyunsaturated fatty acids and animal protein relates to the increased incidence of Crohn's disease in Japan. *Am J Clin Nutr* 1996;63:741–45.

3. Riordan AM, Hunter JO, Cowan RE, et al. Treatment of active Crohn's disease by exclusion diet: East Anglian Multicentre Controlled Trial. *Lancet* 1993;342:1131–34.

4. Wantke F, Gotz M, Jarisch R. *Lancet* 1994;343:113 (letter).

5. Cottone M, Rosselli M, Orlando A, et al. Smoking habits and recurrence in Crohn's disease. *Gastroenterol* 1994;106:643–48.

6. Imes S, Plinchbeck BR, Dinwoodie A, et al. Iron, folate, vitamin B-12, zinc, and copper status in out-patients with Crohn's disease: Effect of diet counseling. *J Am Dietet Assoc* 1987;87:928–30.

7. Dvorak AM. Vitamin A in Crohn's disease. *Lancet* 1980;I:1303–4.

8. Rachet AJ, Busson A. Treatment of ulcerative rectocolitis by vitamin A. *Paris Medical* 1935;1:308–11.

9. Skogh M, Sundquist T, Tagesson C. Vitamin A in Crohn's disease. *Lancet* 1980;i:766 (letter).

10. Leichtmann GA, Bengoa JM, Bolt MJG, Sitrin MD. Intestinal absorption of cholecalciferol and 25-hydrocycholecalciferol in patients with both Crohn's disease and intestinal resection. *Am J Clin Nutr* 1991;54:548–52.

11. Harris AD, Brown R, Heatley RV, et al. Vitamin D status in Crohn's disease: Association with nutrition and disease activity. *Gut* 1985;26:1197–1203.

12. Driscoll RH, Meredith SC, Sitrin M, Rosenberg IH. Vitamin D deficiency

and bone disease in patients with Crohn's disease. *Gastroenterol* 1982;83:1252–58.

13. Belluzzi A, Brignola C, Campieri M, et al. Effect of an enteric-coated fish-oil preparation on relapses in Crohn's disease. *N Engl J Med* 1996;334:1557–60.

Depression

1. Gettis A. Food sensitivities and psychological disturbance: A review. *Nutr Health* 1989;6:135–46.

2. King DS. Can allergic exposure provoke psychological symptoms? A double-blind test. *Biol Psychiatr* 1981;16:3–19.

3. Brown M, Gibney M, Husband PR, Radcliffe M. Food allergy in poly-symptomatic patients. *Practitioner* 1981; 225:1651–54.

4. Christensen L. Psychological distress and diet-effects of sucrose and caffeine. *J Applied Nutr* 1988;40:44–50.

5. Martinsen EW. Benefits of exercise for the treatment of depression. *Sports Med* 1990;9:380–89.

6. Martinsen EW, Medhus A, Sandivik L. Effects of aerobic exercise on depression: A controlled study. *BMJ* 1985;291: 109.

7. Adams PW, Wynn V, Rose DP, et al. Effect of pyridoxine hydrochloride (Vitamin B6) upon depression associated with oral contraception. *Lancet* 1973; I:897–904.

8. Russ CS, Hendricks TA, Chrisley BM, et al. Vitamin B-6 status of depressed and obsessive-compulsive patients. *Nutr Rep Internat* 1983;27:867–73.

9. Gunn ADG. Vitamin B6 and the premenstrual syndrome (PMS). *Internat J Vit Nutr Res* 1985;(suppl 27):213–24 (review).

10. Kleijnen J, Riet GT, Knipschild P. Vitamin B6 in the treatment of the premenstrual syndrome—a review. *Brit J Obstet Gynaecol* 1990;97:847–52.

11. Lindenbaum J, Healton EB, Savage DG, et al. Neuropsychiatric disorders caused by cobalamin deficiency in the absence of anemia or macrocytosis. *N Engl J Med* 1988;318:1720–28.

12. Holmes JM. Cerebral manifestations of vitamin B12 deficiency. *J Nutr Med* 1991;2:89–90.

13. Ellis FR, Nasser S. A pilot study of vitamin B12 in the treatment of tiredness. *BR J Nutr* 1973;30:277–83.

14. Reynolds E et al. Folate deficiency in depressive illness. *Brit J Psychiatr* 1970; 117:287–92.

15. Coppen A, Chaudhry S, Swade C. Folic acid enhances lithium prophylaxis. *J Affective Disorders* 1986;10:9–13.

16. Di Palma C, Urani R, Agricola R, et al. Is methylfolate effective in relieving major depression in chronic alcoholics? A hypothesis of treatment. *Curr Ther Res* 1994;55:559–67.

17. Rose DP, Cramp DG. Reduction of plasma tyrosine by oral contraceptives and oestrogens: A possible consequence of tyrosine aminotransferase induction. *Clin Chem Acta* 1970;29:49–53.

18. Moller SE. Tryptophan and tyrosine availability and oral contraceptives. *Lancet* 1979;ii:472 (letter).

19. Kishimoto H, Hama Y. The level and diurnal rhythm of plasma tryptophan and tyrosine in manic-depressive patients. *Yokohama Med Bull* 1976;27:89–97.

20. Gelenberg AJ, Wojcik JD, Growdon JH, et al. Tyrosine for the treatment of depression. *Am J Psychiatr* 1980; 137:622–23.

21. Sabelli HC, Fawcett J, Gustovsky F, et al. Clinical studies on the phenylethyl-amine hypothesis of affective disorder: Urine and blood phenylacetic acid and phenylalanine dietary supplements. *J Clin Psychiatr* 1986;47:66–70.

22. Sabelli HC, Fawcett J, Gustovsky F, et al. Clinical studies on the phenylethyl-amine hypothesis of affective disorder: Urine and blood phenylacetic acid and phenylalanine dietary supplements. *J Clin Psychiatry* 1986;47:66–70.

23. Beckman H, Strauss MA, Ludolph E. DL-Phenylalanine in depressed patients: An open study. *J Neural Transmission* 1977;41:123–34.

24. Maggioni M, Picotti GB, Bondiolotti GP, et al. Effects of phosphatidylserine therapy in geriatric patients with depressive disorders. *Acta Psychiatr Scand* 1990;81:265–70.

25. Wright J. Treatment of chronic anxiety and associated physical complaints with niacinamide and essential fatty acids: Two cases. *J Ortho Mol Med* 1992;7(3):182–85.

26. Wolkowitz OM, et al. Dehydroepiandrosterone (DHEA) treatment of depression. *Biol Psychiatr* 1997;41:311–8.

27. Harrer G, Sommer H. Treatment of mild/moderate depressions with Hypericum. *Phytomed* 1994;1:3–8.

28. Ernst E. St. John's wort, an antidepressant? A systemic, criteria-based review. *Phytomed* 1995;2:67–71.

29. Vorbach EU, Hübner WD, Arnoldt KH. Effectiveness and tolerance of the *Hypericum* extract LI 160 in comparison with imipramine: Randomized double-blind study with 135 outpatients. *J Ger Psyciatr Neruol* 1994;7(suppl 1):S19–23.

Diabetes

1. Colagiuri S, Miller JJ, Edwards RA. Metabolic effects of adding sucrose and aspartame to the diet of subjects with noninsulin-dependent diabetes mellitus. *Am J Clin Nutr* 1989;50:474–78.

2. Abraira C, Derler J. Large variations of sucrose in constant carbohydrate diets in type II diabetes. *Am J Med* 1988; 84:193–200.

3. Loghmani E, Rickard K, Washburne L, et al. Glycemic response to sucrose-containing mixed meals in diets of children with insulin-dependent diabetes mellitus. *J Pediatr* 1991;119:531–37.

4. Wright DW, Hansen RI, Mondon CE, Reaven GM. Sucrose-induced insulin resistance in the rat: modulation by exercise and diet. *AM J Clin Nutr* 1983; 38:879–83.

5. Lettle GJ, Emmett PM, Heaton KW. Glucose and insulin responses to manufactured and whole-food snacks. *Am J Clin Nutr* 1987;45:86–91.

6. Florholmen J, Arvidsson-Lenner R, Jorde R, Burhol PG. The effect of Metamucil on postprandial blood glucose and plasma gastric inhibitory peptide in insulin-dependent diabetics. *Acta Med Scand* 1982;212:237–39.

7. Landin K, Holm G, Tengborn L, Smith U. Guar gum improves insulin sensitivity, blood lipids, blood pressure, and fibrinolysis in healthy men. *Am J Clin Nutr* 1992;56:1061–65.

8. Schwartz SE, Levine RA, Weinstock RS, et al. Sustained pectin ingestion: Effect on gastric emptying and glucose tolerance in non-insulin-dependent diabetic patients. *Am J Clin Nutr* 1988;48:1413–17.

9. Hallfrisch J, Scholfield DJ, Behall KM. Diets containing soluble oat extracts improve glucose and insulin responses of moderately hypercholesterolemic men and women. *Am J Clin Nutr* 1995;61:379–84.

10. Doi K, Matsuura M, Kawara A, Baba S. Treatment of diabetes with glucomannan (konjac mannan). *Lancet* 1979; i:987–88 (letter).

11. Sharma RD, Raghuram TC. Hypoglycaemic effect of fenugreek seeds in

non-insulin-dependent diabetic subjects. *Nutr Res* 1990;10:731–39.

12. Raghuram TC, Sharma RD, et al. Effect of fenugreek seeds on intravenous glucose disposition in non-insulin dependent diabetic patients. *Phytother Res* 1994; 8:83–86.

13. Story L, Anderson JW, Chen W-JL, et al. Adherence to high-carbohydrate, high-fiber diets: Long-term studies on non-obese diabetic men. *J Am Dietet Assoc*; 1985;85:1105–10.

14. Del Toma E, Clementi A, Marcelli M, et al. Food fiber choices for diabetic diets. *Am J Clin Nutr* 1988;47:243–46.

15. Hagander B, Asp N-G, Efendic S, et al. Dietary fiber decreases fasting blood glucose levels and plasma LDL concentration in noninsulin-dependent diabetes mellitus patients. *Am J Clin Nutr* 1988; 47:852–58.

16. Beattie VA, Edwards CA, Hosker JP, et al. Does adding fibre to a low energy, high carbohydrate, low fat diet confer any benefit to the management of newly diagnosed overweight type II diabetics? *BMJ* 1988;296:1147–49.

17. Feskens EJM, Bowles CH, Kromhout D. Inverse association between fish intake and risk of glucose intolerance in normoglycemic elderly men and women. *Diabetes Care* 1991;14:935–41.

18. Zak A, Zeman M, Hrabak P, et al. Changes in the glucose tolerance and insulin secretion in hypertriglyceridemia: Effects of dietary n-3 fatty acids. *Nutr Rep Internat* 1989;39:235–42.

19. Popp-Snijders C, Schouten J, et al. Dietary supplementation of omega-3 fatty acids improves insulin sensitivity in non-insulin dependent diabetes. *Neth J Med* 1985;28:531–32.

20. Popp-Snijders C, Schouten JA, Heine RJ, et al. Dietary supplementation of omega-3 polyunsaturated fatty acids improves insulin sensitivity in non-insulin-dependent diabetes. *Diabetes Res* 1987; 4:141–47.

21. Albrink MJ, Ullrich IH, Blehschmidt NG, et al. The beneficial effect of fish oil supplements on serum lipids and clotting function of patients with type II diabetes mellitus. *Diabetes* 1986;35 (suppl 1):43A (abstract #172).

22. Wei I, Ulchaker M, Sheehan J. Effect of omega-3 fatty acids (FA) in non-obese non-insulin dependent diabetes (NIDDM). *Am J Clin Nutr* 1988;47:775 (abstract #70).

23. Vandongen R, Mori TA, Codde JP, et al. Hypercholesterolaemic effect of fish oil in insulin-dependent diabetic patients. *Med J Austral* 1988;148:141–43.

24. Schectman G, Kaul S, Kissebah AH. Effect of fish oil concentrate on lipoprotein composition in NIDDM. *Diabetes* 1988;37:1567–73.

25. Stackpoole PW, Alig J, Kilgore LL, et al. Lipodystrophic diabetes mellitus. Investigations of lipoprotein metabolism and the effects of omega-3 fatty acid administration in two patients. *Metabol* 1988;37:944–51.

26. Glauber H, Wallace P, Griver K, Brechtel G. Adverse metabolic effect of omega-3 fatty acids in non-insulin-dependent diabetes mellitus. *Ann Intern Med* 1988;108:663–68.

27. Snowdon DA, Phillips RL. Does a vegetarian diet reduce the occurrence of diabetes? *Am J Publ Health* 1985;75:507–12.

28. Crane MG, Sample CJ. Regression of diabetic neuropathy with vegan diet. *Am J Clin Nutr* 1988;48:926 (abstract #P28).

29. Crane MG, Sample C. Regression of diabetic neuropathy with total vegetarian (vegan) diet. *J Nutr Med* 1994; 4:431–39.

30. Cohen D, Dodds R, Viberti G. Effect of protein restriction in insulin dependent diabetics at risk of nephropathy. *BMJ* 1987;294:795–98.

31. Evanoff G, Thompson C, Bretown J, Weinman E. Prolonged dietary protein restriction in diabetic nephropathy. *Arch Intern Med* 1989;149:1129–33.

32. Gin H, Aparicio M, Potauz L, et al. Low-protein, low-phosphorus diet and tissue insulin sensitivity in sinulin-dependent diabetic patients with chronic renal failure. *Nephron* 1991;57:411–15.

33. Garg A, Bananome A, Grundy SM, et al. Comparison of a high-carbohydrate diet with a high-monounsaturated-fat diet in patients with non-insulin dependent diabetes mellitus. *N Engl J Med* 1988; 319:829–34.

34. Dahl-Jorgensen K, Joner G, Hanssen KF. Relationship between cows' milk consumption and incidence of IDDM in childhood. *Diabetes Care* 1991;14:1081–83.

35. Coleman DL, Kuzava JE, Leiter EH. Effect of diet on incidence of diabetes in nonobese diabetic mice. *Diabetes* 1990; 39:432–36.

36. Gerstein H. Cow milk exposure and type I diabetes mellitus. *Diabetes Care* 1994;17:13–19.

37. Karajalainen J, Martin JM, Knip M, et al. A bovine albumin peptide as a possible trigger of insulin-dependent diabetes mellitus. *N Engl J Med* 1992;327: 302–7.

38. Scott FWE, Norris JM, Kolb H. Milk and type I diabetes. *Diabetes Care* 1996;19:379–83 (review).

39. Atkinson, MA, Bowman MA, Kao K-J, et al. Lack of immune responsiveness to bovine serum albumin in insulin-dependent diabetes. *N Engl J Med* 1993; 329:1853–58.

40. Pettit DJ, Forman MR, Hanson RL, et al. Breast feeding and incidence of non-insulin-dependent diabetes mellites in Pima Indians. *Lancet* 1997;350:166–68.

41. Isida K, Mizuno A, Murakami T, Shima K. Obesity is necessary but not sufficient for the development of diabetes mellitus. *Metabol* 1996;45:1288–95.

42. Casassus P, Fontbonne A, Thibult N, et al. Upper-body fat distribution: A hyperinsulinemia-independent predictor of coronary heart disease mortality. *Arterioscler Throm* 1992;1387–92.

43. Karter AJ, Mayer-Davis EJ, Selby JV, et al. Insulin sensitivity and abdominal obesity in African-American, Hispanic, and non-Hispanic white men and women. *Diabetes* 1996;45:1547–55.

44. Park KS, Hree BD, Lee K-U, et al. Intra-abdominal fat is associated with decreased insulin sensitivity in healthy young men. *Metabol* 1991;40:600–3.

45. Long SD, Swanson MS, O'Brien K, et al. Weight loss in severely obese subjects prevents the progression of impaired glucose tolerance to type II diabetes. *Diabetes Care* 1994;17:372.

46. Pi-Sunyer FX. Weight and non-insulin-dependent diabetes mellitus. *Am J Clin Nutr* 1996;63(suppl):426S–29S.

47. Wing RR, Marcuse MD, Blair EH, et al. Caloric restriction per se is a significant factor in improvements in glycemic control and insulin sensitivity during weight loss in obese NIDDM patients. *Diabetes Care* 1994;17:30.

48. Henry RR, Gumbiner B. Benefits and limitations of very-low-calorie diet therapy in obese NIDDM. *Diabetes Care* 1991;14:802–23.

49. Hersey III WC, Graves JE, Pollack ML, et al. Endurance exercise training improves body composition and plasma

insulin responses in 70- to 79-year-old men and women. *Metabol* 1994;43:847–54.

50. Rasmussen OW, Lauszus FF, Hermansen K. Effects of postprandial exercise on glycemic response in IDDM subjects. *Diabetes Care* 1994;17:1203.

51. Helmrich SP, Ragland DR, Leung RW, Paffenbarger RS. Physical activity and reduced occurrence of non-insulin-dependent diabetes mellitus. *N Engl J Med* 1991; 325:147–52.

52. Grimm J-J, Muchnick S. Type I diabetes and marathon running. *Diabetes Care* 1993;16:1624 (letter).

53. Bell DSH. Exercise for patients with diabetes—benefits, risks, precautions. *Postgrad Med* 1992;92:183-96 (review).

54. Kiechl S, Willeit J, Poewe W, et al. Insulin sensitivity and regular alcohol consumption: Large, prospective, cross sectional population study Bruneck study. *BMJ* 1996;313:1040–44.

55. Facchini F, Chen Y-DI, Reaven GM. Light-to-moderate alcohol intake is associated with enhanced insulin sensitivity. *Diabetes Care* 1994;17:115.

56. Rimm EB, Chan J, Stampfer MJ, et al. Prospective study of cigarette smoking, alcohol use, and the risk of diabetes in men. *BMJ* 1995;310:555–59.

57. Stampfer MJ, Colditz GA, Willett WC, et al. A prospective study of moderate alcohol drinking and risk of diabetes in women. *Am J Epidemiol* 1988;128:549–58.

58. Goden G, Chen X, Desantis R, et al. Effects of ethanol on carbohydrate metabolism in the elderly. *Diabetes* 1993; 42:28–34.

59. Ben G, Gnudi L, Maran A, et al. Effects of chronic alcohol intake on carbohydrate and lipid metabolism in subjects with type II (non-insulin-dependent) diabetes. *Am J Med* 1991;90:70.

60. Young RJ, McCulloch DK, Prescott RJ, Clarke PF. Alcohol: Another risk factor for diabetic retinopathy? *BMJ* 1984; 288:1035.

61. Connor H, Marks V. Alcohol and diabetes. A position paper prepared by the Nutrition Subcommittee of the British Diabetic Association's Medical Advisory Committee and approved by the Executive Council of the British Diabetic Association. *Human Nutr Appl Nutr* 1985; 39A:393–99.

62. Stegmayr B, Lithner F. Tobacco and end stage diabetic nephropathy. *BMJ* 1987; 295:581–82.

63. Scala C, LaPorte RE, Dorman JS, et al. Insulin-dependent diabetes mellitus mortality—the risk of cigarette smoking. *Circulation* 1990;82:37–43.

64. Rimm EB, Manson JE, Stampfer MJ, et al. Cigarette smoking and the risk of diabetes in women. *Am J Public Health* 1993;83:211–14.

65. Salonen JT, Nyssonen K, Tuomainen T-P, et al. Increased risk of non-insulin dependent diabetes mellitus at low plasma vitamin E concentrations: A four year follow up study in men. *BMJ* 1995; 311:1124–27.

66. Bierenbaum ML, Noonan FJ, Machlin LJ, et al. The effect of supplemental vitamin E on serum parameters in diabetics, post coronary and normal subjects. *Nutr Rep Internat* 1985;31:1171–80.

67. Paolisso G, D'Amore A, Giugliano D, et al. Pharmacologic doses of vitamin E improve insulin action in healthy subjects and non-insulin dependent diabetic patients. *Am J Clin Nutr* 1993;57:650–56.

68. Paolisso G, D'Amore A, Galzerano D, et al. Daily vitamin E supplements improve metabolic control but not insulin secretion in elderly type II diabetic patients. *Diabetes Care* 1993;16:1433–37.

69. Paolisso G, Di Maro G, Galzerano D, et al. Pharmacological doses of vitamin E and insulin action in elderly subjects. *Am J Clin Nutr* 1994;59:1291–96.

70. Paolisso G, Gambardella A, Galzerano D, et al. *Lancet* 1994;343:596 (letter).

71. Colette C, Pares-Herbute N, Monnier LH, Cartry E. Platelet function in type I diabetes: Effects of supplementation with large doses of vitamin E. *Am J Clin Nutr* 1988;47:256–61.

72. Gisnger C, Jeremy J, Speiser P, et al. Effect of vitamin E supplementation on platelet thromboxane A2 production in type I diabetic patients: Double-blind crossover trial. *Diabetes* 1988;37: 1260–64.

73. Ross WM, Creighton MO, Stewart-DeHaan PJ, et al. Modelling cortical cataractogenesis: 3. In vivo effects of vitamin E on cataractogenesis in diabetic rats. *Can J Ophthalmol* 1982;17:61.

74. Ceriello A, Giugliano D, Quatraro A, et al. Vitamin E reduction of protein glycosylation in diabetes. *Diabetes Care* 1991;14:68–72.

75. Duntas L, Kemmer TP, Vorberg B, Scherbaum W. Administration of d-alpha-tocopherol in patients with insulin-

dependent diabetes mellitus. *Curr Ther Res* 1996;57:682–90.

76. Reaven PD, Barnett J, Herold DA, Edelman S. Effect of vitamin E on susceptibility of low-density lipoprotein and low-density lipoprotein subfractions to oxidation and on protein glycation in NIDDM. *Diabetes Care* 1995;18:807.

77. Cunningham JJ, Ellis SL, McVeigh KL, et al. Reduced mononuclear leukocyte ascorbic acid content in adults with insulin-dependent diabetes mellitus consuming adequate dietary vitamin C. *Metabol* 1991;40:146–49.

78. Davie SJ, Gould BJ, Yudkin JS. Effect of vitamin C on glycosylation of proteins. *Diabetes* 1992;41:167–73.

79. Will JC, Tyers T. Does diabetes mellitus increase the requirement for vitamin C? *Nutr Rev* 1996;54:193–202 (review).

80. Eriksson J, Kohvakka A. Magnesium and ascorbic acid supplementation in diabetes mellitus. *Ann Nutr Metabol* 1995;39:217–23.

81. Paolisso G, Balbi V, Volpe C, et al. Metabolic benefits deriving from chronic vitamin C supplementation in aged non-insulin dependent diabetics. *J Am Coll Nutr* 1995;14:387–92.

82. Will JC, Tyers T. Does diabetes mellitus increase the requirement for vitamin C? *Nutr Rev* 1996;54:193–202 (review).

83. Wilson RG, Davis RE. Serum pyridoxal concentrations in children with diabetes mellitus. *Pathol* 1977;9:95–99.

84. Davis RE, Calder JS, Curnow DH. Serum pyridoxal and folate concentrations in diabetics. *Pathol* 1976;8:151–56.

85. McCann VJ, Davis RE. Serum pyridoxal concentrations in patients with diabetic neuropathy. *Austral NZ Med* 1978; 8:259–61.

86. Spellacy WN, Buhi WC, Birk SA. Vitamin B6 treatment of gestational diabetes mellitus. *Am J Obstet Gynecol* 1977; 127:599–602.

87. Coelingh HJT, Schreurs WHP. Improvement of oral glucose tolerance in gestational diabetes by pyridoxine. *BMJ* 1975;3:13–15.

88. Spellacy WN, Buhi WC, Birk SA. The effects of vitamin B6 on carbohydrate metabolism in women taking steroid contraceptives: Preliminary report. *Contraception* 1972;6:265–73.

89. Passariello N, Fici F, Giugliano D, et al. Effects of pyridoxine alpha-ketoglutarate on blood glucose and lactate in type

I and II diabetics. *Internat J Clin Pharmacol Ther Toxicol* 1983;21:252–56.

90. Solomon LR, Cohen K. Erythrocyte O2 transport and metabolism and effects of vitamin B6 therapy in type II diabetes mellitus. *Diabetes* 1989; 38:881–86.

91. Rao RH, Vigg BL, Rao KSJ. Failure of pyridoxine to improve glucose tolerance in diabetics. *J Clin Endocrinol Metabol* 1980;50:198–200.

92. Yamane K, Usui T, Yamamoto T, et al. Clinical efficacy of intravenous plus oral mecobalamin in patients with peripheral neuropathy using vibration perception thresholds as an indicator of improvement. *Curr Ther Res* 1995;56:656–70 (review).

93. Coggeshall JC, Heggers JP, Robson MC, Baker H. Biotin status and plasma glucose in diabetics. *Ann NY Acad Sci* 1985;447:389–92.

94. Maebashi M, Makino Y, Furukawa Y, et al. Therapeutic evaluation of the effect of biotin on hyperglycemia in patients with non-insulin dependent diabetes mellitus. *J Clin Biochem Nutr* 1993;14:211–18.

95. Koutsikos D, Agroyannis B, Tzanatos-Exarchou H. Biotin for diabetic peripheral neuropathy. *Biomed Pharmacother* 1990;44:511–14.

96. Molnar GD, Berge KG, Rosevear JW, et al. The effect of nicotinic acid in diabetes mellitus. *Metabol* 1964;13:181–89.

97. Gaut ZN, Pocelinko R, Solomon HM, Thomas GB. Oral glucose tolerance, plasma insulin, and uric acid excretion in man during chronic administration in nicotinic acid. *Metabol* 1971:1031–35.

98. Clearly JP. The importance of oxidant injury as a cause of impaired mitochondrial oxidation in diabetes. *J Orthomol Med* 1988;3:164–74.

99. Clearly JP. Vitamin B3 in the treatment of diabetes mellitus: Case reports and review of the literature. *J Nutr Med* 1990;1:217–25.

100. Lewis CM, Canafax DM, Sprafka JM, Bazrbosa JJ. Double-blind randomized trail of nicotinamide on early-onset diabetes. *Diabetes Care* 1992;15:121–23.

101. Chase HP, Butler-Simon N, Garg S, et al. A trial of nicotinamide in newly diagnosed patients with type 1 (insulin-dependent) diabetes mellitus. *Diabetologia* 1990;33:444–46.

102. Mendola G, Casamitjana R, Gomis R. Effect of nicotinamide therapy upon B-cell function in newly diagnosed type 1 (insulin-dependent) diabetic patients. *Diabetologia* 1989;32:160–62.

103. Schroeder HA. Serum cholesterol and glucose levels in rats fed refined and less refined sugars and chromium. *J Nutr* 1969;97:237–42.

104. Herepath WB, *Journal Provincial Med Surg Soc* Apr 28, 1854:374.

105. Offenbacher EG, PLi-Sunyer FX. Improvement of glucose tolerance and blood lipids in elderly subjects. *Am J Clin Nutr* 1980;33:916 (abstract).

106. Evans GW. The effect of chromium picolinate on insulin controlled parameters in humans. *Int J Biosocial Med Res* 1989;11:163–80.

107. Gaby AR, Wright JV. Diabetes. In *Nutritional Therapy in Medical Practice: Reference Manual and Study Guide*. Kent, WA: Wright/Gaby Seminars, 1996, 54–64 (review).

108. Anderson RA, Polansky MM, Bryden NA, Canary JJ. Supplemental-chromium effects on glucose, insulin, glucagon, and urinary chromium losses in subjects consuming controlled low-chromium diets. *Am J Clin Nutr* 1991;54:909–16.

109. Jovanovic-Peterson L, Gutierrez M, Peterson CM. Chromium supplementation for gestational diabetic women improves glucose tolerance and decreases hyperinsulinemia. *J Am Coll Nutr* 1995;14:530 (abstract #26).

110. Anderson RA, Polansky MM, Bryden NA, et al. Chromium supplementation of human subjects: Effects on glucose, insulin, and lipid variables. *Metabol* 1983;32:894–99.

111. Urberg M, Zemel MB. Evidence for synergism between chromium and nicotinic acid in the control of glucose tolerance in elderly humans. *Metabol* 1987;36:896–99.

112. Lee NA, Reasner CA. Beneficial effect of chromium supplementation on serum triglyceride levels in NIDDM. *Diabetes Care* 1994;17:1449–52.

113. Gaby AR, Wright JV. Nutritional protocols: Diabetes mellitus. In *Nutritional Therapy in Medical Practice: Protocols and Supporting Information*. Kent, WA: Wright/Gaby Seminars, 1996, 10.

114. Paolisso G, Scheen A, D'Onofrio FD, Lefebvre P. Magnesium and glucose homeostasis. *Diabetologia* 1990;33:511–14 (review).

115. Eibl NL, Schnack CJ, Kopp H-P, et al. Hypomagnesemia in type II diabetes: Effect of a 3-month replacement therapy. *Diabetes Care* 1995;18:188.

116. Paolisso G, Sgambato S, Pizza G, et al. Improved insulin response and action by chronic magnesium administration in aged NIDDM subjects. *Diabetes Care* 1989;12:265–69.

117. Paolisso G, Sgambato S, Gambardella A, et al. Daily magnesium supplements improve glucose handling in elderly subjects. *Am J Clin Nutr* 1992;55:1161–67.

118. Smellie WS, O'Reilly D St J, Martin BJ, Santamaria J. Magnesium replacement and glucose tolerance in elderly subjects. *Am J Clin Nutr* 1993;57:594–95 (letter).

119. Sjorgren A, Floren CH, Nilsson A. Oral administration of magnesium hydroxide to subjects with insulin dependent diabetes mellitus. *Magnesium* 1988;121:16–20.

120. McNair P, Christiansen C, Madsbad S, et al. Hypomagnesemia, a risk factor in diabetic retinopathy. *Diabetes* 1978;27:1075–77.

121. Mimouni F, Miodovnik M, Tsang RC, et al. Decreased maternal serum magnesium concentration and adverse fetal outcome in insulin-dependent diabetic women. *Obstet Gynecol* 1987;70:85–89.

122. American Diabetes Association. Magnesium supplementation in the treatment of diabetes. *Diabetes Care* 1992;15:1065–67.

123. Nakamura T, Higashi A, Nishiyama S, et al. Kinetics of zinc status in children with IDDM. *Diabetes Care* 1991;14:553–57.

124. Mcchegiani E, Boemi M, Fumelli P, Fabris N. Zinc-dependent low thymic hormone level in type I diabetes. *Diabetes* 1989;12:932–37.

125. Rao KVR, Seshiah V, Kumar TV. Effect of zinc sulfate therapy on control and lipids in type I diabetes. *JAPI* 1987;35:52 (abstract).

126. Pidduck HG, Wren PJJ, Price Evans DA. Hyperzincuria of diabetes mellitus and possible genetic implications of this observation. *Diabetes* 1970;19:240–47.

127. Shigeta Y, Izumi K, Abe H. Effect of coenzyme Q7 treatment on blood sugar and ketone bodies of diabetics. *J Vitaminology* 1966;12:293–98.

128. Salway JG, Whitehead L, Finnegan JA, et al. Effect of *myo*-inositol on peripheral-nerve function in diabetes. *Lancet* 1978;II:1282–84.

129. Packer L, Witt EH, Tartschler HJ. Alpha-lipoic acid as a biological anti-

oxidant. *Free Radical Biol Med* 1995; 19:227–50.

130. Abdel-Aziz MT, Abdou MS, Soliman K, et al. Effect of carnitine on blood lipid pattern in diabetic patients. *Nutr Rep Internat* 1984;29:1071–79.

131. Onofrj M, Fulgente T, Mechionda D, et al. L-acetylcarnitine as a new therapeutic approach for peripheral neuropathies with pain. *Int J Clin Pharmacol Res* 1995;15:9–15.

132. Franconi F, Bennardini F, Mattana A, et al. Plasma and platelet taurine are reduced in subjects with insulin-dependent diabetes mellitus: Effects of taurine supplementation. *Am J Clin Nutr* 1995; 61:1115–19.

133. Reichert R. Evening primrose oil and diabetic neuropathy. *Quarterly Rev Natural Med* Summer 1995:129–33 (review).

134. Halberstam M, Cohen N, Shlimovich P, et al. Oral vanadyl sulfate improves insulin sensitivity in NIDDM but not in obese nondiabetic subjects. *Diabetes* 1996; 45:659–66.

135. Ringsdorf WM, Cheraskin E. Medical complications from ascorbic acid: A review and interpretation (part two). *J Holistic Med* 1984;6:173–83 (review).

136. Cunningham JJ, Fu A, Mearkle P, Brown G. Hyperzincuria in individuals with insulin-dependent diabetes mellitus: Concurrent zinc status and the effect of high-dose zinc supplementation. *Metabol* 1994;43:1558–62.

137. Niewoener CB, Allen JI, Boosalis M, et al. Role of zinc supplementation in type II diabetes mellitus. *Am J Med* 1988; 63–68.

138. Gaby AR. Literature review and commentary. *Townsend Letter for Doctors and Patients* Jan 1997:25 (review).

139. Baskaran K, Ahmath BK, Shanmugasundaram KR, Shanmugasundaram ERB. Antidiabetic effect of a leaf extract from *Gymnema sylvestre* in non-insulin-dependent diabetes mellitus patients. *J Ethnopharmacol* 1990;30:295–305.

140. Shanmugasundaram ERB, Rajeswari G, Baskaran K, et al. Use of *Gymnema sylvestre* leaf extract in the control of blood glucose insulin-dependent diabetes mellitus. *J Ethnopharmacol* 1990; 30:281–94.

141. Zhang T, Hoshino M, et al. Ginseng root: Evidence for numerous regulatory peptides and insulinotropic activity. *Biomed Res* 1990;11:49–54.

142. Suzuki Y, Hikino H. Mechanisms of hypoglycemic activity of panaxans A and B, glycans of *Panax ginseng* roots: Effects on plasma levels, secretion, sensitivity and binding of insulin in mice. *Phytother Res* 1989;3:20–24.

143. Waki I, Kyo H, et al. Effects of a hypoglycemic component of ginseng radix on insulin biosynthesis in normal and diabetic animals. *J Pharm Dyn* 1982;5:547–54.

144. Sotaniemi EA, Haapakoski E, Rautio A. Ginseng therapy in non-insulin-dependent diabetic patients. *Diabetes Care* 1995;18:1373–75.

Diarrhea

1. Hyams JS, Etienne NL, Leichtner AM, Theuer RC. *Pediatr* 1988;82:64–68.

2. Barness LA. Safety considerations with high ascorbic acid dosage. *Ann NY Acad Sci* 1975;258:523–28 (review).

3. Eherer AH, Santa Ana CA, Porter J, Fordtran JS. Effect of psyllium, calcium polycarbophil, and wheat bran on secretory diarrhea induced by phenolphthalein. *Gastroenterol* 1993;104:1007–12.

4. Babb RR. Coffee, sugars and chronic diarrhea. *Postgrad Med* 1984; 75:82, 86–87.

5. Bowie MD, Hill ID, Mann MD. Response of severe infantile diarrhea to soya-based feeds. *S Afr Med J* 1988; 73:343–45.

6. Haffejee IE. Effect of oral folate on duration of acute infantile diarrhoea. *Lancet* 1988;ii:334–35 (letter).

7. Pothoulakis C, Kelly CP, Joshi MA, et al. Saccharomyces boulardii inhibits Clostridium difficile Toxin A binding and enterotoxicity in rat ileum. *Gastroenterol* 1993;104:1108–15.

8. Surawicz CM, Elmer GW, Speelman P, et al. Prevention of antibiotic-associated diarrhoea by Saccharomyces boulardii: A prospective study. *Gastroenterol* 1989;96:981–88.

9. Schellenberg D, Bonington A, Champion C, et al. Treatment of Clostridium difficile diarrhea with brewer's yeast. *Lancet* 1994;343:171–72 (letter).

10. Poupard JA, Hussain J, Norris RF. Biology of the bifidobacteria. *Bact Rev* 1973;37:136–65.

11. Rasic JL. Bifidobacteria and diarrhoea control in infants and young children. *Internat Clin Nutr Rev* 1992; 12: 27–30 (review).

12. Saavedra JM, Bauman NA, Oung I, et al. Feeding of Bifidobacterium bifidum and Streptococcus thermophilus to infants in hospital for prevention of diarrhoea and shedding of rotavirus. *Lancet* 1994; 344:1046–49.

13. Colombel JF, Cortot A, Neut C, Romond C. Horhurt with Bifidobacterium longum reduces erythromycin-induced gastrointestinal effects. *Lancet* 1987;ii:43 (letter).

14. Bhatia SJ, Kochar N, Abraham P, et al. Lactobacillus acidophilus inhibits growth of Campylobacter pylori in vitro. *J Clin Microbiol* 1989;27:2328–30.

15. Montes RG, Perman JA. Lactose intolerance. *Postgrad Med* 1991;89:175–84 (review).

16. Werbach MR. *Nutritional Influences on Illness*, 2d ed. Tarzana, CA: Third Line Press, 1993, 256–61 (review).

17. Loeb H, Vandenplas Y, et al. Tannin-rich pod for treatment of acute-onset diarrhea. *J Pediatr Gastroenterol Nutr* 1989;8:480–85.

18. Achterrath-Tuckerman U, Kunde R, et al. Pharmacological investigations with compounds of chamomile. V. Investigations on the spasmolytic effect of compounds of chamomile and Kamillosan® on isolated guinea pig ileum. *Planta Med* 1980;39:38–50.

19. Tyler VE. *Herbs of Choice: The Therapeutic Use of Phytomedicinals*. New York: Pharmaceutical Products Press, 1994, 51–54.

Dupuytren's Contracture

1. Thomson GR. Treatment of Dupuytren's contracture with vitamin E. *BMJ* Dec 17, 1949:1382–83.

2. Richards HJ. Dupuytren's contracture treated with vitamin E. *BMJ* Jun 21,1952:1328.

3. Kirk JE, Chieffi M. Tocopherol administration to patients with Dupuytren's contracture: Effect on plasma tocopherol levels and degree of contracture. *Pro Soc Exp Biol Med* 1952;80:565 (review).

Ear Infections

1. Cantekin EI, McGuire TW, Griffith TL. Antimicrobial therapy for otitis media with effusion (secretory otitis media). *JAMA* 1991;266:3309–17.

2. Le CT, Freeman DW, Fireman BH. Evaluation of ventilating tubes and myringotomy in the treatment of recurrent or persistent otitis media. *Pediatr Infect Dis J* 1991;10:2–11.

3. McMahan JT, Calenoff E, Croft J, et al. Chronic otitis media with effusion and allergy: Modified RAST analysis of 119 cases. *Otolaryngol Head Neck Surg* 1981; 89:427–31.

4. Nsouli TM, Nsouli SM, Linde RE, et al. Role of food allergy in serous otitis media. *Ann Allerg* 1994;73:215–19.

5. McGovern JP, Haywood TH, Fernandez AA. Allergy and secretory otitis media. *JAMA* 1967;200:134–38.

6. Roukonen J, Pagnaus A, Lehti H. Elimination diets in the treatment of secretory otitis media. *Internat J Pediatr Otorhinolaryngol* 1982;4:39–46.

7. Sanchez A, Reeser JL, Lau HS, et al. Role of sugars in human neutrophilic phagocytosis. *Am J Clin Nutr* 1973;26: 1180–84.

8. Bernstein J, Alpert S, Nauss KM, Suskind R. Depression of lymphocyte transformation following oral glucose ingestion. *Am J Clin Nutr* 1977;30:613 (abstract).

9. Uhari M, et al. Xylitol chewing gum in prevention of acute otitis media: Double blind randomised trial. *BMJ* 1996; 313:1180–84.

10. Etzel RA, Pattishall EN, Haley NJ, et al. Passive smoking and middle ear effusion among children in day care. *Pediatr* 1992;90:228–32.

11. Leibovitz B, Siegel BV. Ascorbic acid, neutrophil function, and the immune response. *Internat J Vit Nutr Res* 1978; 48:159–64.

12. Vojdani A, Ghoneum M. In vivo effect of ascorbic acid on enhancement of human natural killer cell activity. *Nutr Res* 1993;13:753–64.

13. Duchateau J, Delespesse G, Vereecke P. Influence of oral zinc supplementation on the lymphocyte response to mitogens of normal subjects. *Am J Clin Nutr* 1981;34:88–93.

14. Fraker PJ, Gershwin ME, Good RA, Prasad A. Interrelationships between zinc and immune function. *Fed Proc* 1986; 45:1474–79.

15. Glasziou PP, Mackerras DEM. Vitamin A supplementation in infectious diseases: A meta-analysis. *BMJ* 1993; 306:366–70.

16. Chandra RK. Excessive intake of zinc impairs immune responses. *JAMA* 1984;252:1443–46.

17. Brown DJ. *Herbal Prescriptions for Better Health*. Rocklin, CA: Prima Publishing, 1996, 213–14.

Eczema

1. Sampson HA, Scanlon SM. Natural history of food hypersensitivity in children with atopic dermatitis. *J Pediatr* 1989; 115:23–7.

2. Burks AW, Mallory SB, Williams LW, Shirrell MA. Atopic dermatitis: Clinical relevance of food hypersensitivity. *J Pediatr* 1988;113:447–51.

3. Atherton DJ. Diet and atopic eczema. *Clin Allerg* 1988;18:215–28 (review).

4. Veien NK, Hattel T, Justesen O, et al. Dermatoses in coffee drinkers. *Cutis* 1987; 40:421–22.

5. Manku MS, Horrobin DF, Morse NL, et al. Essential fatty acids in the plasma phospholipids of patients with atopic eczema. *Brit J Dermatol* 1984; 110:643–48.

6. Schalin-Karrila M, Mattila L, Jansen CT, et al. Evening primrose oil in the treatment of atopic eczema: Effect on clinical status, plasma phospholipid fatty acids and circulating blood prostaglandis. *Brit J Dermatol* 1987;117:11–19.

7. Lovell CR, Burton JL, Horrobin DF. Treatment of atopic eczema with evening primrose oil. *Lancet* 1981;i:278 (letter).

8. Wright S, Burton JL. Oral evening-primrose oil improves atopic eczema. *Lancet* 1982;ii:1120–22.

9. Morse PF, Horrobin DF, Manku MS, et al. Meta-analysis of placebo-controlled studies of the efficacy of Epogam in the treatment of atopic eczema. Relationship between plasma essential fatty acid changes and clinical response. *Brit J Dermatol* 1989;121:75–90.

10. Bamford JTM, Gibson RW, Renier CM. Atopic eczema unresponsive to evening primrose oil (linoleic and gamma-linolenic acids). *J Am Acad Dermatol* 1985;13:959–65.

11. Horrobin DF, Stewart C. Evening primrose oil in atopic eczema. *Lancet* 1990;I:864–65.

12. Cornbleet T. Use of maize oil (unsaturated fatty acids) in the treatment of eczema. *Arch Dermatol Syph* 1935; 31:224–34.

13. Hansen AE, Knott EM, Wiese HF, et al. Eczema and essential fatty acids. *Am J Dis Child* 1947;73:1–18.

14. Bjorneboe A, Soyland E, Bjorneboe G-E A, et al. Effect of dietary supplementation with eicosapentaenoic acid in the treatment of atopic dermatitis. *Brit J Dermatol* 1987;117:463–69.

15. Soyland E, Rajka G, Bjorneboe A, et al. The effect of eicosapentaenoic acid in the treatment of atopic dermatitis. A clinical study. *Arch Derm Venereol* (Stockh) 1989;144(suppl):139.

16. Olsen PE, Torp EC, Mahon RT, et al. Oral vitamin E for refractory hand dermatitis. *Lancet* 1994;343:672–73 (letter).

17. Anonymous. Severe atopic dermatitis responds to ascorbic acid. *Med World News* Apr 24,1989:41.

18. Sheehan MP, Atherton DJ. One-year follow up of children treated with Chinese medical herbs for atopic eczema. *Br J Dermatol* 1994;130:488–93.

19. Sheehan MP, Rustin MHA, et al. Efficacy of traditional Chinese herbal therapy in adult atopic dermatitis. *Lancet* 1992;340:13–17.

20. Evans FQ. The rational use of glycyrrhetinic acid in dermatology. *Br J Clin Pract* 1958;12: 269–79.

21. Laux P, Oschmann R. Witch hazel: *Hamamelis virgincia* L. *Zeitschrift Phytother* 1993;14:155–66.

22. Bradley PR, ed. *British Herbal Compendium*, vol. 1. Bounemouth, Dorset, UK: British Herbal Medicine Association, 1992, 194–96.

Fibrocystic Breast Disease

1. Minton JP, Foecking MK, Webster DJT, Matthew RH. Caffeine, cyclic nucleotides, and breast disease. *Surgery* 1979; 86:105–8.

2. Minton JP, Abou-Issa H, Reiches N, et al. Clinical and biochemical studies on methylxanthine-related fibrocystic breast disease. *Surgery* 1981;90:299–304.

3. Ernster VL, Mason L, Goodson WH, et al. Effects of a caffeine-free diet on benign breast disease: A randomized trial. *Surgery* 1982;91:263.

4. Allen S, Froberg DG. The effect of decreased caffeine consumption on benign proliferative breast disease: A randomized clinical trial. *Surgery* 1987; 101:720–30.

5. Marshall JM, Graham S, Swanson M. Caffeine consumption and benign breast disease: A case-control comparison. *Am J Publ Health* 1982;72(6):610–12.

6. Lubin F, Ron E, Wax Y, et al. A case-control study of caffeine and methylxanthines in benign breast disease. *JAMA* 1985;253(16):2388–92.

7. Boyle CA, Berkowitz GS, LiVoisi VA, et al. Caffeine consumption and fibrocystic breast disease: A case-control epidemi-

ologic study. *J Natl Cancer Inst* 1984; 72:1015–19.

8. Vecchia C, Franceschi S, Parazzini F, et al. Benign breast disease and consumption of beverages containing methylxanthines. *J Natl Cancer Inst* 1985;74: 995–1000.

9. Odenheimer DJ, Zunzunegui MV, King MC, et al. Risk factors for benign breast disease: A case-control study of discordant twins. *Am J Epidemiol* 1984;120: 565–71.

10. Rose DP, Boyar AP, Cohen C, Strong LE. Effect of a low-fat diet on hormone levels in women with cystic breast disease. I. Serum steroids and gonadotropins. *J Natl Cancer Inst* 1987;78: 623–26.

11. Woods MN, Gorbach S, Longcope C, et al. Low-fat, high-fiber diet and serum estrone sulfate in premenopausal women. *Am J Clin Nutr* 1989;49:1179–83.

12. Rose DP, Boyar A, Haley N, et al. Low fat diet in fibrocystic disease of the breast with cyclic mastalgia: A feasibility study. *Am J Clin Nutr* 1985;41(4):856 (abstract).

13. Boyd NF, McGuire V, Shannon P, et al. Effect of a low-fat high-carbohydrate diet on symptoms of cyclical mastopathy. *Lancet* 1988;ii:128–32.

14. Lubin F, Wax Y, Ron E, et al. Nutritional factors associated with benign breast disease etiology: A case-control study. *Am J Clin Nutr* 1989;50:551–56.

15. Prior JC, Vigna Y, Sciarretta D, et al. Conditioning exercise decreases premenstrual symptoms: A prospective, controlled 6-month trial. *Fertil Steril* 1987; 47(3):402–8.

16. Abrams AA. Use of vitamin E in chronic cystic mastitis. *N Engl J Med* 1965;272(20):1080–81.

17. London RS, Sundaram GS, Schultz M, et al. Endocrine parameters and alphatocopherol therapy of patients with mammary dysplasia. *Cancer Res* 1981;41: 3811–13.

18. Ernster VL, Goodson WH, Hunt TK, et al. Vitamin E and benign breast "disease": A double-blind, randomized clinical trial. *Surgery* 1985;97:490–94.

19. London RS, Sundaram GS, Murphy L, et al. The effect of vitamin E on mammary dysplasia: A double-blind study. *Obstet Gynecol* 1985;65:104–6.

20. Brush MG, Perry M. Pyridoxine and the premenstrual syndrome. *Lancet* 1985;I:1399.

21. Smallwood J, Ah-Kye D, Taylor I. Vitamin B6 in the treatment of pre-menstrual mastalgia. *Brit J Clin Pract* 1986; 40:532–33.

22. Krouse TB, Eskin BA, Mobini J. Age-related changes resembling fibrocystic disease in iodine-blocked rat breasts. *Arch Pathol Lab Med* 1979;103:631–34.

23. Ghent WR, Eskin BA, Low DA, Hill L. Iodine replacement in fibrocystic disease of the breast. *Canadian J Surg* 1993;36:453–60.

24. Gateley CA, Miers M, Mansel RE, Hughes LE. Drug treatments for mastalgia: 17 years experience in the Cardiff mastalgia clinic. *J Royal Soc Med* 1992; 85:12–15.

25. Mansel RE, Pye JK, Hughes LE. Effects of essential fatty acids on cyclical mastalgia and noncyclical breast disorders. In *Omega-6 Essential Fatty Acids: Pathophysiology and Roles in Clinical Medicine.* Alan R Liss: New York, 1990, 557–66.

26. Preece PE, Hanslip JI, Gilbert L, et al. Evening primrose oil (EFAMOL) for mastalgia. In *Clinical Uses of Essential Fatty Acids*, ed. DF Horrobin. Montreal: Eden Press, 1982, 147–54.

27. Gaby AR. Literature review and commentary. *Townsend Letter for Doctors and Patients* Jun 1990;338–39.

28. Parry G, Bredesen DE. Sensory neuropath with low-dose pyridoxine. *Neurol* 1985;35:1466–68.

29. Schaumburg H, Kaplan J, Windebank A, et al. Sensory neuropathy from pyridoxine abuse. *N Engl J Med* 1983; 309(8):445–48.

30. Böhnert KJ, Hahn G. Phytotherapy in gynecology and obstetrics—Vitex agnus castus. *Erfahrungsheilkunde* 1990; 39:494–502.

31. Dittmar FW, Böhnert KJ, et al. Premenstrual syndrome: Treatment with a phytopharmaceutical. *Therapiwoche Gynäkol* 1992;5:60–68.

32. Qi-bing M, Jing-yi T, Bo C. Advance in the pharmacological studies of radix Angelica sisnensis (oliv) diels (Chinese danggui). *Chin Med J* 1991;104: 776–81.

Fibromyalgia

1. Wolfe F, Ross K, Anderson J, Russell J. Aspects of fibromyalgia in the general population: Sex, pain threshold, and FM symptoms. *J Rheum* 1995;22(1): 151–55.

2. Anonymous. Is fibromyalgia caused by a glycolysis impairment? *Nutr Reviews* 1994;52(7):248–50.

3. Wilke W. Fibromyalgia: Recognizing and addressing the multiple interrelated factors. *Postgraduate Med* 1996; 100(1):153–70.

4. Carette S. Fibromyalgia 20 years later: What have we really accomplished? *J Rheum* 1995;22(4):590–94.

5. Mengshail AM, Komnaes HB, Forre O. The effects of 20 weeks of physical fitness training in female patients with fibromyalgia. *Clin Exp Rheum* 1992; 10:345–49.

6. Kaplan KH, Goldberg DL, Galvin-Naduea M. The impact of a meditation-based stress reduction program on fibromyalgia. *Gen Hosp Psychiatry* 1993; 15:284–89.

7. Deluze C, Bosia L, Zirbs A, et al. Electroacupuncture in fibromyalgia: Results of a controlled trial. *BMJ* 1992; 305:1249–52.

8. Abraham G, Flechas J. Management of fibromyalgia: Rationale for the use of magnesium and malic acid. *J Nutr Med* 1992;3:49–59.

9. Russell J, Michalek J, Flechas J, et al. Treatment of fibromyalgia syndrome with SuperMalic: A randomized, double-blind, placebo-controlled, crossover pilot study. *J Rheum* 1995;22(5):953–57.

10. Eisinger J, Zakarian H, Plantamura A, et al. Studies of transketolase in chronic pain. *J Adv Med* 1992;5:105–13.

11. Eisinger J, Bagneres D, Arroyo P, et al. Effects of magnesium, high energy phosphates, piracetam, and thiamin on erythrocyte transketolase. *Magnesium Res* 1994;7(1):59–61.

12. Steinberg CL. The tocopherols (vitamin E) in the treatment of primary fibrositis. *J Bone Joint Surg* 1942;24:411–23.

Gallstones

1. Lee DWT, Gilmore CJ, Bonorris G, et al. Effect of dietary cholesterol on biliary lipids in patients with gallstones and normal subjects. *Am J Clin Nutr* 1985; 42:414.

2. Andersen E, Hellstrom K. The effect of cholesterol feeding on bile acid kinetics and biliary lipids in normolipidemic and hypertriglyceridemic subjects. *J Lipid Res* 1979;20:1020–27.

3. Pixley F, Mann J. Dietary factors in the aetiology of gall stones: A case control study. *Gut* 1988;29:1511–15.

4. Pixley F, Wilson D, McPherson K, Mann J. Effect of vegetarianism on development of gall stones in women. *BMJ* 1985;291:11–12.

5. Heaton KW, Emmett PM, Symes CL, Braddon FEM. An explanation for gallstones in normal-weight women: Slow intestinal transit. *Lancet* 1993;341:8–10.

6. Marcus SN, Heaton KW. Intestinal transit, deoxycholic acid and the cholesterol saturation of bile—three interrelated factors. *Gut* 1986;27:550.

7. Breneman JC. Allergy elimination diet as the most effective gallbladder diet. *Ann Allerg* 1968;26:83.

8. Sarles H, Gerolami A, Cros RC. Diet and cholesterol gallstones. *Digestion* 1978; 17:121–27.

9. Kern F Jr. Epidemiology and natural history of gallstones. *Semin Liver Dis* 1983;3:87–96.

10. Stampfer MJ, Maclure KM, Colditz GA, et al. Risk of symptomatic gallstones in women with severe obesity. *Am J Clin Nutr* 1992;55:652–58.

11. Maclure KM, Hayes KC, Colditz GA, et al. Weight, diet, and the risk of symptomatic gallstones in middle-aged women. *N Engl J Med* 1989;321:563–69.

12. Thornton JR. Gallstone disappearance associated with weight loss. *Lancet* 1979;ii:478 (letter).

13. Everhart JE. Contributions of obesity and weight loss to gallstone disease. *Ann Intern Med* 1993;119:1029–35.

14. Scragg RKR. Diet, alcohol, and relative weight in gall stone disease: A case-control study. *BMJ* 1984;288:1113–19.

15. Morrison LM. The effects of a low fat diet on the incidence of gallbladder disease. *Am J Gastroenterol* 1956;25:158–63.

16. Capper WM, et al. Gallstones, gastric secretion and flatulent dyspepsia. *Lancet* 1967;I:413.

17. Toouli J, Jablonski P, Watts J McK. Gallstone dissolution in man using cholic acid and lecithin. *Lancet* 1975;ii:1124–26.

18. Tuzhilin SA, Dreiling D, Narodetskaja RV, Lukahs LK. The treatment of patients with gallstones by lecithin. *Am J Gastroenterol* 1976;165:231–35.

19. Holan KR, Holzbach T, Hsieh JYK, et al. Effect of oral administration of 'essential' phospholipid, 8-glycerophosphate, and linoleic acid on biliary lipids in patients with cholelithiasis. *Digestion* 1979;19:251–58.

20. Nassuato G, Iemmolo RM, et al. Effect of silibinin on biliary lipid composition. Experimental and clinical study. *J Hepatol* 1991;12:290–95.

Gingivitis (Periodontal Disease)

1. Krook L et al. Human periodontal disease. Morphology and response calcium therapy. *Cornell Vet* 1972;62:32–53.

2. Pack ARC. Folate mouthwash: Effects on established gingivitis in periodontal patients. *J Clin Periodontol* 1984; 11:619–28.

3. Vogel RI et al. The effect of topical application of folic acid on gingival health. *J Oral Med* 1978;33(1):20–22.

4. Vogel RI et al. The effect of folic acid on gingival health. *J Periodontol* 1976; 47:667–68.

5. Wilkinson EG et al. Bioenergetics in clinical medicine. VI. Adjunctive treatment of periodontal disease with coenzyme Q10. *Res Commun Chem Pathol Pharmacol* 1976;14:715–19.

6. El-Ashiry GM et al. Local and systemic influences in periodontal disease. II. Effect of prophylaxis and natural versus synthetic vitamin C upon gingivitis. *J Periodontol* 1964;35:250–59.

7. Serfaty R, Itic J. Comparative trial with natural herbal mouthwash versus chlorhexidine in gingivitis. *J Clin Dentistry* 1988;1:A34.

8. Yamnkell S, Emling RC. Two-month evaluation of Parodontax dentifrice. *J Clin Dentistry* 1988;1:A41.

Glaucoma

1. Berens C et al. Allergy in glaucoma. Manifestations of allergy in three glaucoma patients as determined by the pulse-diet method of Coca. *Ann Allerg* 1947; 5:526.

2. Raymond LF. Allergy and chronic simple glaucoma. *Ann Allerg* 1996;22:146.

3. Ringsdorf WM Jr, Cheraskin E. Ascorbic acid and glaucoma: A review. *J Holistic Med* 1981;3:167–72.

4. Boyd HH. Eye pressure lowering effect of vitamin C. *J Orthomol Med* 1995; 10:165–68.

5. Stocker FW. New ways of influencing the intraocular pressure. *NY State J Med* 1949;49:58–63.

6. Samples RJ et al. Effect of melatonin on intraocular pressure. *Curr Eye Res* 1988;7:649–53.

7. Gaspar AZ et al. The influence of magnesium on visual field and peripheral vasospasm in glaucoma. *Ophthalmologica* 1995;209:11–13.

Hay Fever

1. Holmes HM, Alexander W. Hay fever and vitamin C. *Science* 1942:96:497.

2. Ruskin SL. High dose vitamin C in allergy. *Am J Dig Dis* 1945;12:281.

3. Fortner BR Jr, Danziger RE, Rabinowitz PS, Nelson HS. The effect of ascorbic acid on cutaneous and nasal response to histamine and allergen. *J Aller Clin Immunol* 1982;69:484–88.

4. Middleton E, Drzewicki G. Effect of ascorbic acid and flavonoids on human basophil release. *J Allerg Clin Immunol* Jan 1992:278.

5. Soyka F, Edmonds A. *The Ion Effect.* New York: Bantam, 1977.

6. Mittman P. Randomized double-blind study of freeze-dried Urtica diocia in the treatment of allergic rhinitis. *Planta Med* 1990;56:44–47.

Hemorrhoids

1. Johanson JF, Sonnenberg A. Constipation is not a risk factor for hemorrhoids: A case-control study of potential etiological agents. *Am J Gastroenterol* 1994;89: 1981–86.

2. Johanson JF, Sonnenberg A. The prevalence of hemorrhoids and chronic constipation. *Gastroenterol* 1990;98: 380–86.

3. Deutsch AA, Kaufman Z, Reiss R. Hemorrhoids: A plea for nonsurgical treatment. *Isr J Med Sci* 1980;16:649–54.

4. Moesgaard F, Nielsen ML, Hansen JB, Knudsen JT. High-fiber diet reduces bleeding and pain in patients with hemorrhoids. *Dis Colon Rectum* 1982;25:454–56.

5. Eherer AJ, Santa Ana CA, Porter J, Fordtran JS. Effect of psyllium, calcium polycarbophil, and wheat bran on secretory diarrhea induced by phenolphthalein. *Gastroenterol* 1993;104:1007–12.

6. Wichtl M. *Herbal Drugs and Phytopharmaceuticals.* Boca Raton, FL: CRC Press, 1994, 268–70.

7. Leung AY, Foster S. *Encyclopedia of Common Natural Ingredients Used in Food, Drugs and Cosmetics.* New York: John Wiley & Sons, 1996, 427–29.

High Cholesterol

1. Kromhout D, Menotti A, Bloemberg B, et al. Dietary saturated and trans fatty acids and cholesterol and 25-year mortal-

ity from coronary heart disease: The Seven Countries Study. *Prev Med* 1995; 24:308–15.

2. Tell GS, Evans GW, Folsom AR, et al. Dietary fat intake and carotid artery wall thickness: The atherosclerosis risk in communities (ARIC) study. *Am J Epidemiol* 1994;139:979–89.

3. Ornish D, Brown SE, Scherwitz LW, et al. Can lifestyle changes reverse coronary heart disease? The Lifestyle Heart Trial. *Lancet* 1990;336:129–33.

4. Denke MA, Grundy SM. Comparison of effects of lauric acid and palmitic acid on plasma lipids and lipoproteins. *Am J Clin Nutr* 1992;56:895–98.

5. Zock PL, de Vries JHM, Katan MB. Impact of myristic acid versus palmitic acid on serum lipid and lipoprotein levels in healthy women and men. *Arterioscler Thromb* 1994;14:567–75.

6. Hepner G, Fried R, St Jeor S, et al. Hypocholesterolemic effect of yogurt and milk. *Am J Clin Nutr* 1979;19–24.

7. Santos MJ, Lopez-Jurado M, Llopis J, et al. Influence of dietary supplementation with fish on plasma total cholesterol and lipoprotein cholesterol fractions in patients with coronary heart disease. *J Nutr Med* 1992;3:107–15.

8. Kromhout D, Bosschieter EB, Coulander CDL, The inverse relation between fish consumption and 20-year mortality from coronary heart disease. *N Engl J Med* 1985;312:1205–9.

9. Ascherio A, Rimm EG, Stampfer MJ, et al. Dietary intake of marine n-3 fatty acids, fish intake, and the risk of coronary disease among men. *N Engl J Med* 1995;332:977–82.

10. Albert CM, Manson JE, O'Donnoell C, et al. Fish consumption and the risk of sudden death in the Physicians' Health Study. *Circulation* 1996;94(suppl 1):I-578 (abstract #3382).

11. Thorogood M, Carter R, Benfield L, et al. Plasma lipids and lipoprotein cholesterol concentrations in people with different diets in Britain. *BMJ* 1987; 295:351–53.

12. Burr ML, Sweetnam PM. Vegetarianism, dietary fiber and mortality. *Am J Clin Nutr* 1982;36:873–77.

13. Resnicow K, Barone J, Engle A, et al. Diet and serum lipids in vegan vegetarians: A model for risk reduction. *J Am Dietet Assoc* 1991;91:447–53.

14. Ornish D, Brown SE, Scherwitz LW, et al. Can lifestyle changes reverse coronary heart disease? The Lifestyle Heart Trial. *Lancet* 1990;336:129–33.

15. Connor SL, Connor WE. The importance of dietary cholesterol in coronary heart disease. *Prev Med* 1983; 12:115–23 (review).

16. Edington JD, Geekie M, Carter R, et al. Serum lipid response to dietary cholesterol in subjects fed a low-fat, high-fiber diet. *Am J Clin Nutr* 1989;50: 58–62.

17. Raloff J. Oxidized lipids: A key to heart disease? *Sci News* 1985;127:278.

18. Levy Y, Maor I, Presser D, Aviram M. Consumption of eggs with meals increases the susceptibility of human plasma and low-density lipoprotein to lipid peroxidation. *Ann Nutr Metabol* 1996;40: 243–51.

19. Shekelle RB, Stamler J. Dietary cholesterol and ischaemic heart disease. *Lancet* 1989;I:1177–79.

20. Anderson JW, Chen WJL. Legumes and their soluble fiber: Effect on cholesterol-rich lipoproteins. In *Unconventional Sources of Dietary Fiber*, ed. I Furda. Washington, DC: American Chemical Society, 1983.

21. Ripsin CM, Keenan JM, Jacobs DR, et al. Oat products and lipid lowering—A meta-analysis. *JAMA* 1992; 267:3317–25.

22. Williams CL, Bollella M, Spark A, Puder D. Soluble fiber enhances the hypocholesterolemic effect of the Step I diet in childhood. *J Am Coll Nutr* 1995;14: 251–57.

23. Glore SR, Van Treeck D, Knehans AW, Guild M. Soluble fiber and serum lipids: A literature review. *J Am Dietet Assoc* 1994;94:425–36.

24. Rimm EB, Ascherio A, Giovannucci E, et al. Vegetable, fruit, and cereal fiber intake and risk of coronary heart disease among men. *JAMA* 1996;275:447–51.

25. Anderson JW, Johnstone BM, Cook-Newell ME. Meta-analysis of the effects of soy protein intake on serum lipids. *N Engl J Med* 1995;3333:276–82.

26. Potter SM. Overview of proposed mechanisms for the hypocholesterolemic effect of soy. *J Nutr* 1995;606S–11S (review).

27. Yudkin J, Kang SS, Bruckdorfer KR. Effects of high dietary sugar. *BMJ* 1980;281:1396.

28. Reiser S. Effect of dietary sugars on metabolic risk factors associated with heart disease. *Nutr Health* 1985;3:203–16.

29. Urgert R, Schulz AGM, Katan MB. Effects of cafestol and kahweol from coffee grounds on serum lipids and serum liver enzymes in humans. *Am J Clin Nutr* 1995;61:149–54.

30. Superko HR, Bortz WM, Albers JJ, Wood PJ. Lipoprotein and apolipoprotein changes during a controlled trial of caffeinated and decaffeinated coffee drinking in men. *Circulation* 1989; 80:II–86.

31. Nygird O, Refsum H, Velanb PM, et al. Coffee consumption and plasma total homocysteine: The hordaland homocysteine study. *Am J Clin Nutr* 1997; 65:136–43.

32. Rosmarin PC, Applegate WB, Somes GW. Coffee consumption and serum lipids: A randomized, crossover clinical trial. *Am J Med* 1990;88:349–56.

33. Regular or decaf? Coffee consumption and serum lipoproteins. *Nutr Rev* 1992;50:175–78 (review).

34. Dai WS, Laporte RE, Hom DL, et al. Alcohol consumption and high density lipoprotein cholesterol concentration among alcoholics. *Am J Epidemiol* 1985; 122:620–27.

35. Marques-Vidal P, Ducimetiere P, Evans A, et al. Alcohol consumption and myocardial infarction: A case-control study in France and northern Ireland. *Am J Epidemiol* 1996;143:1089–93.

36. Rimm EB, Klatsky A, Grobbee D, Stampfer MJ. Review of moderate alcohol consumption and reduced risk of coronary heart disease: Is the effect due to beer, wine, or spirits? *BMJ* 1996; 312:731–36 (review).

37. Hendriks HF, Veenstra J, Wierik EJMV, Schaafsma G, Kluft C. Effect of moderate dose of alcohol with evening meal on fibrinolytic factors. *BMJ* 1994; 304:1003–6.

38. Doll R, Peto AR, Hall E, et al. Mortality in relation to consumption of alcohol: 13 years' observations on male British doctors. *BMJ* 1994;309:911–18.

39. Hein HO, Suadicani P, Gyntelberg F. Alcohol consumption, serum low density lipoprotein cholesterol concentration, and risk of ischaemic heart disease: Six year follow up in the Copenhagen male study. *BMJ* 1996;736–41.

40. Baggio G, Pagnan A, Muraca M, et al. Olive-oil-enriched diet: Effect on serum lipoprotein levels and biliary cholesterol saturation. *Am J Clin Nutr* 1988; 47: 960–64.

References

41. Grundy SM. Monounsaturated fatty acids and cholesterol metabolism: Implications for dietary recommendations. *J Nutr* 1989;119:529–33 (review).

42. Keys A, ed. Coronary heart disease in seven countries. *Circulation* 1970; 41(suppl q):I1–211.

43. Willett WC, Stampfer MJ, Manson JE, et al. Intake of *trans* fatty acids and risk of coronary heart disease among women. *Lancet* 1993;341:581–85.

44. Khosla P, Hayes KC. Dietary trans-monounsaturated fatty acids negatively impact plasma lipids in humans: Critical review of the evidence. *J Am Coll Nutr* 1996;15:235–39.

45. Warshafsky S, Kamer RS, Sivak SL. Effect of garlic on total serum cholesterol—A meta-analysis. *Ann Intern Med* 1993;119:599–605.

46. Lawson LD, Ransom DK, Hughes BG. Inhibition of whole blood platelet-aggregation by compounds in garlic clove extracts and commercial garlic products. *Thrombosis Res* 1992;65:141–56.

47. Mansell P, Reckless JPD. Garlic—effects on serum lipids, blood pressure, coagulation, platelet aggregation, and vasodilatation. *BMJ* 1991;303:379–80 (editorial).

48. Jenkins DJA, Khan A, Kenkins AL, et al. Effect of nibbling versus gorging on cardiovascular risk factors: Serum uric acid and blood lipids. *Metaboli* 1995; 44:549–55.

49. Edelstein SL, Barrett-Connor EL, Wingard DL, Cohn BA. Increased meal frequency associated with decreased cholesterol concentrations; Rancho Bernardo, CA, 1984–1987. *Am J Clin Nutr* 1992; 55:664–69.

50. Reaven PD, McPhillips JB, Barrett-Connor EL, Criqui MH. Leisure time exercise and lipid and lipoprotein levels in an older population. *J Am Geriatr Soc* 1990; 38:847–54.

51. Duncan JJ, Gordon NF, Scott CB. Women walking for health and fitness—How much is enough? *JAMA* 1991; 266:3295–99.

52. Pekkanen J, Marti B, Nissinen A, Tuomilehto J. Reduction of premature mortality by high physical activity: A 20-year follow-up of middle-aged Finnish men. *Lancet* 1987;1:1473–77.

53. Willich SN, Lewis M, Lowel H, et al. Physical exertion as a trigger of acute myocardial infarction. *N Engl J Med* 1993; 329:1684–90.

54. Hubert HB, Feinleib M, McNamara PM, Castelli WP. Obesity as an independent risk factor for cardiovascular disease: A 26-year follow-up of participants in the Framingham Heart Study. *Circulation* 1983;67:968–77.

55. Glueck CJ, Taylor HL, Jacobs D, et al. Plasma high-density lipoprotein cholesterol: association with measurements of body mass: the Lipid Research Clinics Program Prevalence Study. *Circulation* 1980; 62(suppl IV):IV62–69.

56. Wood PD, Stefanick ML, Dreon DM, et al. Changes in plasma lipids and lipoproteins in overweight men during weight loss through dieting as compared with exercise. *N Engl J Med* 1988; 319:1173–79.

57. Dwyer JH, Rieger-Ndakorerwa GE, Semmer NK, et al. Low-level cigarette smoking and longitudinal change in serum cholesterol among adolescents. *JAMA* 1988;2857–62.

58. Khosla S, Laddu A, Ehrenpreis S, Somberg JC. Cardiovascular effects of nicotine: Relation to deleterious effects of cigarette smoking. *Am Heart J* 1994; 127:1669–71 (editorial/review).

59. Nyboe J, Jensen G, Appleyard M, Schnohr P. Smoking and the risk of first acute myocardial infarction. *Am Heart J* 1991;122:438.

60. Kawachi I, Sparrow D, Spiro II A, et al. A prospective study of anger and coronary heart disease. *Circulation* 1996; 94:2090–95.

61. Jiang W, Babyak M, Krantz DS, et al. Mental stress-induced myocardial ischemia and cardiac events. *JAMA* 1996; 275:1651–56.

62. Bower B. Women take un-type A behavior to heart. *Sci News* 1993;144:244.

63. A perspective on type A behavior and coronary disease. *N Engl J Med* 1988;318:110–12 (editorial/review).

64. McCann BS, Warnick R, Knopp RH. Changes in plasma lipids and dietary intake accompanying shifts in perceived workload and stress. *Psychosomatic Med* 1990;52:97–108.

65. Lundberg U, Hedman M, Melin B, Frankenhaeuser M. Type A behavior in healthy males and females as related to physiological reactivity and blood lipids. *Psychosomatic Med* 1989;51: 113–22.

66. Friedman M, Theresen CE, Gill JJ, et al. Alteration of type A behavior and reduction in cardiac recurrences in postmyocardial infarction patients. *Am Heart J* 1984;108:237–48.

67. Brown WV. Niacin for lipid disorders. *Postgrad Med* 1995;98:185–93.

68. Head KA. Inositol hexaniacinate: A safer alternative to niacin. *Alt Med Rev* 1996;1:176–84 (review).

69. Murray M. Lipid-lowering drugs vs. inositol hexaniacinate. *Am J Natural Med* 1995;2:9–12 (review).

70. Dorner VG, Fisher FW. Zur Beinflussung der Serumlipide und Lipoproteine durch den Hexanicotinsäureester des m-Inositol. *Arzneimittel Forschung* 1961; 11:110–113.

71. Cloarec MJ, Perdriset GM, Lamberdiere FA, et al. a-tocopherol: Effect on plasma lipoproteins in hypercholesterolemic patients. *Isr J Med Sci* 1987; 23:869–72.

72. Kesaniemi YA, Grundy SM. Lack of effect of tocopherol on plasma lipids and lipoproteins in man. *Am J Clin Nutr* 1982;36:224–28.

73. Belcher JD, Balla J, Balla G, et al. Vitamin E, LDL, and endothelium: Brief oral vitamin supplementation prevents oxidized LDL-mediated vascular injury in vitro. *Arterioscler Thromb* 1993;13: 1779–89.

74. Stampfer MJ, Hennekens CH, Manson JE, et al. Vitamin E consumption and the risk of coronary disease in women. *N Engl J Med* 1993;328:1444–49.

75. Rimm EB, Stampfer MJ, Ascherio A, et al. Vitamin E consumption and the risk of coronary heart disease in men. *N Engl J Med* 1993;328:1450–56.

76. Stephens NG, Parsons A, Scho-field PM, et al. Randomised controlled trial of vitamin E in patients with coronary disease: Cambridge Heart Antioxidant Study (CHAOS). *Lancet* 1996; 347:781–86.

77. Frei B. Ascorbic acid protects lipids in human plasma and low-density lipoprotein against oxidative damage. *Am J Clin Nutr* 1991;54:1113S–18S.

78. Simon JA. Vitamin C and cardiovascular disease: A review. *J Am Coll Nutr* 1992;11:107–27.

79. Gatto LM, Hallen GK, Brown AJ, Samman S. Ascorbic acid induces a favorable lipoprotein profile in women. *J Am Coll Nutr* 1996;15;154–58.

80. Galeone F, Scalabrino A, Giuntoli F, et al. The lipid-lowering effect of pantethine in hyperlipidemic patients: A clinical investigation. *Curr Ther Res* 1983; 34:383–90.

81. Miccoli R, Marchetti P, Sampietro T, et al. Effects of pantethine on lipids and apolipoproteins in hypercholesterolemic diabetic and non diabetic patients. *Curr Ther Res* 1984;36:545–49.

82. Avogaro P, Bon B, Fusello M. Effect of pantethine on lipids, lipoproteins and apolipoproteins in man. *Curr Ther Res* 1983;33;488–93.

83. Ubbink JB, Hayward WJ, van der Merwe A, et al. Vitamin requirements for the treatment of hyperhomocysteinemia in humans. *J Nutr* 1994;124: 1927–33.

84. Heinecke JW, Rosen H, Suzuki LA, Chait A. The role of sulfur-containing amino acids in superoxide production and modification of low density lipoprotein by arterial smooth muscle cells. *Biol Chem* 1987;262:10098–103.

85. Ronzio RA. Antioxidants, nutraceuticals and functional foods. *Townsend Letter for Doctors and Patients* Oct 1996: 34–35 (review).

86. Hertog MGL, Feskens EJM, Hollman PCH, et al. Dietary antioxidant flavonoids and risk of coronary heart disease: The Zutphen Elderly Study. *Lancet* 1993; 342:1007–11.

87. Hertog MGL, Kromhout D, Aravanis C, et al. Flavonoid intake and long-term risk of coronary heart disease and cancer in the Seven Countries Study. *Arch Intern Med* 1995;155:381–86.

88. Knekt P, Jarvinen R, Reunanen A, Maatela J. Flavonoid intake and coronary mortality in Finland: A cohort study. *BMJ* 1996;312:478–81.

89. Rimm EB, Katan MB, Aschario A, et al. Relation between intake of flavonoids and risk for coronary heart disease in male health professionals. *Ann Intern Med* 1996;125:384–89.

90. Riales R, Albrink MJ. Effect of chromium chloride supplementation on glucose tolerance and serum lipids including high-density lipoprotein of adult men. *Am J Clin Nutr* 1981;34:2670–78.

91. Press RI, Geller J, Evans GW. The effect of chromium picolinate on serum cholesterol and apolipoprotein fractions in human subjects. *West J Med* 1990; 152:41–45.

92. Roeback JR, Hla KM, Chambless LE, Fletcher RH. Effects of chromium supplementation on serum high-density lipoprotein cholesterol levels in men taking beta-blockers. *Ann Intern Med* 1991; 115:917–24.

93. Wang MM, Fox EA, Stoecker BJ, et al. Serum cholesterol of adults supplemented with brewer's yeast or chromium chloride. *Nutr Res* 1989;9:989–98.

94. Newman HAI, Leighton RF, Lanese RR, Freedland NA. Serum chromium and angiographically determined coronary artery disease. *Clin Chem* 1978; 541–44.

95. Yacowitz H, Fleischman AI, Bierenbaum ML. Effects of oral calcium upon serum lipids in man. *BMJ* 1965;1: 1352–54.

96. Bell L, Halstenson CE, Halstenson CJ, et al. Cholesterol-lowering effects of calcium carbonate in patients with mild to moderate hypercholesterolemia. *Arch Intern Med* 1992;152:2441–44.

97. Denke MA, Fox MM, Schulte MC. Short-term dietary calcium fortification increases fecal saturated fat content and reduces serum lipids in men. *J Nutr* 1993;123:1047–53.

98. Davis WH, Leary WP, Reyes AJ, Olhaberry JV. Monotherapy with magnesium increases abnormally low high density lipoprotein cholesterol: A clinical assay. *Curr Ther Res* 1984;36:341–46.

99. Baxter GF, Sumeray MS, Walker JM. Infarct size and magnesium: Insights into LIMIT-2 and ISIS-4 from experimental studies. *Lancet* 1996;348:1424–26.

100. Galloe A, Rasmussen HS, Jorgensen LN, et al. Influence of oral magnesium supplementation on cardiac events among survivors of an acute myocardial infarction. *BMJ* 1993;307:585–87.

101. Pola P, Savi L, Grilli M, et al. Carnitine in the therapy of dyslipidemic patients. *Curr Ther Res* 1980;27:208–16.

102. Maebashi M, Kawamura N, Sato M, et al. Lipid-lowering effect of carnitine in patients with type-IV hyperlipoproteinaemia. *Lancet* 1978;ii:805–7.

103. Rossi CS, Siliprandi N. Effect of carnitine on serum HDL-cholesterol: Report of two cases. *Johns Hopkins Med J* 1982;150:51–54.

104. Pola P, Savi L, Grilli M, et al. Carnitine in the therapy of dyslipidemic patients. *Curr Ther Res* 1980;27:208–16.

105. Davini P et al. Controlled study on L-carnitine therapeutic efficacy in postinfarction. *Drugs Exptl Clin Res* 1992; 18:355–65.

106. Carrol KK, Kurowska EM. Soy consumption and cholesterol reduction: Review of animal and human studies. *J Nutr* 1995;125:594–75.

107. Izuka K, Murata K, Nakazawa K, et al. Effects of chondroitin sulfates on serum lipids and hexosamines in atherosclerotic patients: With special reference to thrombus formation time. *Japan Heart J* 1968;9:453–60.

108. Berge KG. Side effects of nicotinic acid in treatment of hypercholesteremia. *Geriatrics* August 1961:416–22 (review).

109. Silagy C, Neil A. Garlic as a lipid-lowering agent—A meta-analysis. *J R Coll Physicians London* 1994;28:39–45.

110. Holzgartner J, Schmidt U, Kuhn U. Comparison of the efficacy of a garlic preparation vs. bezafibrate. *Arzneim-Forsch Drug Res* 1992;42:1473–77.

111. Agarwal RC, Singh SP, Saran RK, et al. Clinical trial of gugulipid new hypolipidemic agent of plant origin in primary hyperlipidemia. *Indian J Med Res* 1986;84:626–34.

112. Nityanand S, Srivastava JS, Asthana OP. Clinical trials with Gugulipid—A new hypolipidemic agent. *J Assoc Phys India* 1989; 37:323–28.

113. Foster S, Chongxi Y. *Herbal Emissaries*. Rochester, VT: Healing Arts Press, 1992, 79–85.

114. Foster S. *Herbal Renaissance*. Layton, Utah: Gibbs Smith, 1993, 40–41.

115. Araghiniknam M, Chung S, Nelson-White T, et al. Antioxidant activity of dioscorea and dehydroepiandrosterone (DHEA) in older humans. *Life Sci* 1996; 11:147–57.

Hypertension (High Blood Pressure)

1. Stamler J et al. Findings of the international cooperative INTERSALT study. *Hypertension* 1991;17(suppl I):I9–I15.

2. MacGregor GA et al. Double-blind study of three sodium intakes and long-term effects of sodium restriction in essential hypertension. *Lancet* 1989;ii: 1244–47.

3. Margetts BM et al. Vegetarian diet in mild hypertension: A randomised controlled trial. *BMJ* 1986;293:1468–71.

4. Cappuccio FP, MacGregor GA. Does potassium supplementation lower blood pressure? A meta-analysis of published trials. *J Hypertens* 1991;9:465–73.

5. Rossner S, Andersson I-L, Ryttig K. Effects of a dietary fibre-supplement to a weight reduction programme on blood pressure. *Acta Med Scand* 1988; 223:353–57.

6. Rebello T, Hodges RE, Smith JL. Short-term effects of various sugars on antinatriuresis and blood pressure changes in normotensive young men. *Am J Clin Nutr* 1983;38(1):84–94.

7. Jeoung D-U, Dimsdale JE. The effects of caffeine on blood pressure in the work environment. *Am J Hypertens* 1990; 3:749–53.

8. Potter JF, Beevers DG. Pressor effect of alcohol in hypertension. *Lancet* 1984; I:119–22.

9. Silagy CA, Neil HA. A meta-analysis of the effect of garlic on blood pressure. *J Hypertension* 1994;12:463–68.

10. Grant ECG. Food allergies and migraine. *Lancet* 1979;I:966–69.

11. Pirkle JL, Schwartz H, Landis JR, et al. The relationship between blood lead levels and blood pressure and its cardiovascular risk implications. *Am J Epidemiol* 1985;121(2):246–58.

12. Narkiewicz K, Maraglino G, Biasion T, et al. Interactive effect of cigarettes and coffee on daytime systolic blood pressure in patients with mild essential hypertension. *J Hypertens* 1995;13: 965–70.

13. Kukkonen K, Rauramaa R, Voutilainene E, Lansimies E. Physical training of middle-aged men with borderline hypertension. *Ann Clin Res* 1982;14(suppl 34):139–45.

14. Alderman MH. Nonpharmacologic approaches treatment of hypertension. *Lancet* 1994;334:307–11 (review).

15. Bucher HC, Cook RJ, Guyatt GH, et al. Effects of dietary calcium supplementation on blood pressure—a meta-analysis of randomized controlled trials. *JAMA* 1996;275:1016–22.

16. Motoyama T, Sano H, Fukuzaki H, et al. Oral magnesium supplementation in patients with essential hypertension. *Hypertension* 1989;13:227–32.

17. Patki PS, Singh J, Gokhale SV, et al. Efficacy of potassium and magnesium in essential hypertension: A double-blind, placebo controlled, crossover study. *BMJ* 1990;301:521–23.

18. Dyckner T, Wester PO. Effect of magnesium on blood pressure. *BMJ* 1983; 286:1847–49.

19. Trout DL. Vitamin C and cardiovascular risk factors. *Am J Clin Nutr* 1991; 53(suppl):322S–25S.

20. Digiesi V, Cantini F, Bisi G, et al. Mechanism of action of coenzyme q10 in essential hypertension. *Curr Ther Res* 1992;51:668–72.

21. Morris MC, Sacks F, Rosner B. Does fish oil lower blood pressure? A meta-analysis of controlled trials. *Circulation* 1993;88:523–33.

22. Abe M, Shibata K, Matsuda T, Furukawa T. Inhibition of hypertension and salt intake by oral taurine treatment in hypertensive rats. *Hyperten* 1987;10:383–89.

23. Fujita T, Ando K, Noda H, et al. Effects of increased adrenomedullary activity and taurine in young patients with borderline hypertension. *Circulation* 1987; 75:525–32.

24. Clarke JTR, Cullen-Dean G, Reglink E, et al. Increased incidence of epistaxis in adolescents with familial hypercholesterolemia treated with fish oil. *J Pediatr* 1990;116:139–41.

25. Silagy C, Neil AW. A meta-analysis of the effect of garlic on blood pressure. *J Hypertens* 1994;12:463–68.

26. Blesken VR. Use of *Crataegus* in cardiology. *Fortschr Med* 1992;15:290–92.

Hypertriglyceridemia (High Triglycerides)

1. Steinberg D, Pearson TA, Kuller LH. Alcohol and atherosclerosis. *Ann Intern Med* 1991;114:967–76.

2. Reiser S. Effect of dietary sugars on metabolic risk factors associated with heart disease. *Nutr Health* 1985;3:203–16.

3. Szanto S, Yudkin J. The effect of dietary sucrose on blood lipids serum insulin, platelet adhesiveness and body weight in human volunteers. *J Postgrad Med* 1969;45:602–7.

4. Anderson JW, Gustafson NJ. High-carbohydrate, high-fiber diet. *Postgrad Med* 1987;82:40–55 (review).

5. Glore SR, van Treeck D, Knehans AW, Guild M. Soluble fiber and serum lipids: A literature review. *J Am Dietet Assoc* 1994;94:425–36.

6. Cominacini L, Zocca I, Garbin U, et al. Long-term effect of a low-fat, high carbohydrate diet on plasma lipids of patients affected by familial endogenous hypertriglyceridemia. *Am J Clin Nutr* 1988; 48:57–65.

7. West C, Sullivan DR, Katan MB, et al. Boys from populations with high-carbohydrate intake have higher fasting triglyceride levels than boys from populations with high-fat intake. *Am J Epidemiol* 1990;131:271–82.

8. Ullmann D, Connor WE, Hatcher LF, et al. Will a high-carbohydrate, low-fat diet lower plasma lipids and lipoproteins without producing hypertriglyceridemia? *Arterioscler Thromb* 1991;11:1059–67.

9. Consensus Development Panel. Treatment of hypertriglyceridemia. *JAMA* 1984;251:1196–200.

10. Burr ML et al. Effects of changes in fat, fish, and fibre intakes on death and myocardial reinfarction: Diet and reinfarction trial (DART). *Lancet* 1989; ii:757–61.

11. Kromhout D et al. The inverse relation between fish consumption and 20-year mortality from coronary heart disease. *New Engl J Med* 1985; 312(19):1205.

12. Ascherio A, Rimm EB, Stampfer MJ, et al. Dietary intake of marine n-3 fatty acids, fish intake, and the risk of coronary disease among men. *N Engl J Med* 1995;332:977–82.

13. Merril JR et al. Hyperlipemic response of young trained and untrained men after a high fat meal. *Arteriosclerosis* 1989;9:217–23.

14. Cowan LD, Wilcosky T, Criqui MH, et al. Demographic, behavioral, biochemical, and dietary correlates of plasma triglycerides. *Arteriosclerosis* 1985; 5:466–80.

15. Despres J-P, Tremblay A, Leblanc C, Bouchard C. Effect of the amount of body fat on the age-associated increase in serum cholesterol. *Prev Med* 1988; 17:423–31.

16. Prichard BN, Smith CCT, Ling KLE, Betteridge DJ. Fish oils and cardiovascular disease. *BMJ* 1995;310:819–20 (editorial/review).

17. Von Schacky C, Fischer S, Weber PC. Long-term effects of dietary marine omega-3 fatty acids upon plasma and cellular lipids, platelet function, and eicosanoid formation in humans. *J Clin Invest* 1985;76(4):626.

18. Leaf A, Weber PC. Cardiovascular effects of n-3 fatty acids. *N Engl J Med* 1988;318(9);549–57.

19. Adler AJ, Holub BJ. Effect of garlic and fish-oil supplementation on serum lipid and lipoprotein concentrations in hypercholesterolemic men. *Am J Clin Nutr* 1997;65:445–50.

20. Haglund O et al. The effects of fish oil on triglycerides, cholesterol, fibrinogen and malondialdehyde in humans supplemented with vitamin E. *J Nutr* 1991; 121:165–69.

21. Pola P et al. Carnitine in the therapy of dyslipidemic patients. *Curr Ther Res* 1980;27(2):208.

22. Abdi-Aziz MT et al. Effect of carnitine on blood lipid pattern in diabetic patients. *Nutr Rep Int* 1984;29(5):1071.

23. Arsenio L et al. Effectiveness of long-term treatment with pantethine in patients with dyslipidemia. *Clin Ther* 1986;8(5):537–45.

24. Avogaro P et al. Effect of pantethine on lipids, lipoproteins and apolipoproteins in man. *Curr Ther Res* 1983; 33(3):488–93.

25. Maggi GC et al. Pantethine: A physiological lipomodulating agent in the treatment of hyperlipidemias. *Curr Ther Res* 1982;32(3):380–86.

26. Brown WV. Niacin for lipid disorders. *Postgrad Med* 1995;98:183–93 (review).

27. Head KA. Inositol hexaniacinate: A safer alternative to niacin. *Alt Med Rev* 1996;1:176–84 (review).

28. Murray M. Lipid-lowering drugs vs. inositol hexaniacinate. *Am J Natural Med* 1995;2:9–12 (review).

29. Silagy C, Neil A. Garlic as a lipid-lowering agent: A meta-analysis. *J R Coll Physicians London* 1994;28:39–45.

30. Holzgartner J, Schmidt U, Kuhn U. Comparison of the efficacy of a garlic preparation vs. bezafibrate. *Arzneim-Forsch Drug Res* 1992;42:1473–77.

31. Agarwal RC, Singh SP, Saran RK, et al. Clinical trial of gugulipid new hypolipidemic agent of plant origin in primary hyperlipidemia. *Indian J Med Res* 1986;84:626–34.

32. Araghiniknam M, Chung S, Nelson-White T, et al. Antioxidant activity of dioscorea and dehydroepiandrosterone (DHEA) in older humans. *Life Sci* 1996; 11:147–57.

Immune Function

1. Sanchez A et al. Role of sugars in human neutrophilic phagocytosis. *Am J Clin Nutr* 1973;26:1180.

2. Ringsdorf WM et al. Sucrose, neutrophilic phagocytosis and resistance to disease. *Dental Survey* 1976;52(12):46.

3. Ahmed FE. Toxicological effects of ethanol on human health. *Crit Rev Tox* 1995;25(4):347–67.

4. Kubena KS, McMurray DN. Nutrition and the immune system: A review of nutrient-nutrient interactions. *J Am Diet Assoc* 1996;96(11):1156–64.

5. Cantekin EI, McGuire TW, Griffith TL. Antimicrobial therapy for otitis media with effusion (secretory otitis media). *JAMA* 1991;266:3309–17.

6. Le CT, Freeman DW, Fireman BH. Evaluation of ventilating tubes and myringotomy in the treatment of recurrent or persistent otitis media. *Pediatr Infect Dis J* 1991;10:2–11.

7. Pang LQ. The importance of allergy in otolaryngology. *Clin Ecology* 1982; 1(1):53.

8. Nieman DC. Exercise, upper respiratory tract infection, and the immune system. *Med Sci Sports Med* 1994; 26(2): 128–39.

9. Nieman DC, Henson DA, Gusewitch G, et al. Physical activity and immune function in elderly women. *Med Sci Sports Med* 1993;25(7):823–31.

10. Duchateau J, Delespesse G, Vereecke P. Influence of oral zinc supplementation on the lymphocyte response to mitogens of normal subjects. *Am J Clin Nutr* 1981;34:88–93.

11. Fraker PJ, Gershwin ME, Good RA, Prasad A. Interrelationships between zinc and immune function. *Fed Proc* 1986; 45:1474–79.

12. Mossad S et al. Zinc gluconate lozenges for treating the common cold. A randomized, double-blind, placebo-controlled study. *Ann Int Med* 1996; 125(2):81–88.

13. Glasziou PP, Mackerras DEM. Vitamin A supplementation in infectious diseases: A meta-analysis. *BMJ* 1993; 306:366–70.

14. Gerber WF et al. Effect of ascorbic acid, sodium salicylate, and caffeine on the serum interferon level in response to viral infection. *Pharmacology* 1975; 13:228.

15. Murata A. Virucidal activity of vitamin C for prevention and treatment of viral diseases. In *Proceedings of the First Intersectional Congress of IAMS,* vol. 3. Science Council Japan, 1975, 432.

16. Knodell RG, Tate MA, Akl BF, et al. Vitamin C prophylaxis for posttransfusion hepatitis: Lack of effect in a controlled trial. Am J Clin Nutr 1981; 34(1):20–23.

17. Hemila H. Vitamin C and the common cold. *Br J Nutr* 1992;67:3–16.

18. Fernandes CF, Shahani KM, Amer MA. Therapeutic role of dietary lactobacilli and lactobacillic fermented dairy products. *FEMS Micro Rev* 1987;46: 343–56.

19. Chandra RK. Excessive intake of zinc impairs immune responses. *JAMA* 1984;252:1443–46.

20. Brown DJ. *Herbal Prescriptions for Better Health.* Rocklin, CA: Prima Publishing, 1996, 213–14.

21. *Family Practice News* 1987;17(11): 21.

22. *Deutsche Zeitschrift Onkology* 1989;21:52–53.

23. Keplinger H. Oxindole alkaloids having properties stimulating the immunologic system and preparation containing same. US Patent no. 5,302,611, April 12, 1994.

24. Stoner GD, Mukhtar H. Polyphenols as cancer chemopreventive agents. *J Cell Bioch* 1995;22:169–80.

25. You SQ. Study on feasibility of Chinese green tea polyphenols (CTP) for preventing dental caries. *Chin J Stom* 1993; 28(4):197–99.

26. Hamilton-Miller JM. Antimicrobial properties of tea (*Camellia sinensis* L.). *Antimicro Ag Chemo* 1995; 39(11):2375–77.

27. Foster S, Chongxi Y. *Herbal Emissaries: Bringing Chinese Herbs to the West.* Rochester, VT: Healing Arts Press, 1992, 79–85.

Infertility (Female)

1. Grodstein F, Goldman MB, Ryan L, Cramer DW. Relation of female infertility to consumption of caffeinated beverages. *Am J Epidemiol* 1993;137:1353–60.

2. Hatch EE, Bracken MB. Association of delayed conception with caffeine consumption. *Am J Epidemiol* 1993;138: 1082–92.

3. Wilcox A, Weinberg C, Baird D. Caffeinated beverages and decreased fertility. *Lancet* 1988;ii:1453–56.

4. Williams MA, Monson RR, Goldman MG, et al. Coffee and delayed conception. *Lancet* 1990;335:1603 (letter).

5. Stanton CK, Gray RH. Effects of caffeine consumption on delayed conception. *Am J Epidemiol* 1995;142:1322–29.

6. Joesoef MR, Beral V, Rolfs RT, et al. Are caffeinated beverages risk factors for delayed conception? *Lancet* 1990; 335:136–37.

7. Fenster L, Bubbard A, Windham G, Hiatt R, et al. A prospective study of caffeine consumption and spontaneous abortion. *Am J Epidemiol* 1996;143 (11 suppl); 525 (abstract #99).

8. Cramer DW. Letter. *Lancet* 1990; 335:792.

9. Howe G, Westhoff C, Vessey M, Yeates D. Effects of age, cigarette smoking, and other factors on fertility: Findings in a large prospective study. *BMJ* 1985; 290:1697–99.

10. Weinberg CR, Wilcox AJ, Baird DD. Reduced fecundability in women with prenatal exposure to cigarette smoking. *Am J Epidemiol* 1989;129:1072–78.

11. Grodstein F, Goldman MB, Cramer DW. Infertility in women and moderate alcohol use. *Am J Public Health* 1994; 84:1429–32.

12. Florack EIM, Zielhuis GA, Rolland R. Cigarette smoking, alcohol consumption, and caffeine intake and fecundability. *Prev Med* 1994;23:175–80.

13. Green BB et al. Risk of ovulatory infertility in relation to body weight. *Fertil Steril* 1988;50:621–26.

14. Werbach MR. Female infertility. *Townsend Letter for Doctors and Patients* Aug 1995:34 (review).

15. Czeizel AE, Metneki J, Dudas I. The effect of preconceptional multivitamin supplementation on fertility. *Internat J Vit Nutr Res* 1996;66:55–58.

16. Thiessen DD et al. Vitamin E and sex behavior in mice. *Nutr Metabol* 1975;18:116–19.

17. Bayer R. Treatment of infertility with vitamin E. *Int J Fertil* 1960;5:70–78.

18. Rushton DH, Ramsay ID, Gilkes JJH, Norris MJ. Ferritin and fertility. *Lancet* 1991;337:1554 (letter).

19. Wiesel LL et al. The synergistic action of para-aminobenzoic acid and cortisone in the treatment of rheumatoid arthritis. *Am J Med Sci* 1951;222:243–48.

20. Sieve BF. The clinical effects of a new B-complex factor, para-aminobenzoic acid, on pigmentation and fertility. *South Med Surg* 1942(March);104:135–39.

21. Propping D, Katzorke T. Treatment of corpus luteum insufficiency. *Zeitschr Allgemeinmedizin* 1987;63:932–33.

Infertility (Male)

1. Fraga CG, Motchnik PA, Shigenaga MK, et all. Ascorbic acid protects against endogenous oxidative DNA damage in human sperm. *Proc Natl Acad Sci* 1991; 88:11003–6.

2. Dawson EB, Harris WA, Teter MC, Powell LC. Effect of ascorbic acid supplementation on the sperm quality of smokers. *Fertil Steril* 1992;58:1034–39.

3. Dawson EB, Harris WA, McGanity WJ. Effect of ascorbic acid on sperm fertility. *Fed Proc* 1983;42:531 (abstract #31403).

4. Dawson EB, Harris WA, Powell LC. Relationship between ascorbic acid and male fertility. In *Aspects of Some Vitamins, Minerals and Enzymes in Health and Disease,* ed. GH Bourne. *World Rev Nutr Diet* 1990;62:1–26 (review).

5. Hunt CD, Johnson PE, Herbel JOL, Mullen LK. Effects of dietary zinc depletion on seminal volume and zinc loss, serum testosterone concentrations, and sperm morphology in young men. *Am J Clin Nutr* 1992;56:148–57.

6. Netter A, Hartoma R, Nahoul K. Effect of zinc administration on plasma testosterone, dihydrotestosterone and sperm count. *Arch Androl* 1981;7:69–73.

7. Marmar JL et al. Semen zinc levels in infertile and postvasectomy patients and patients with prostatitis. *Fertil Steril* 1975:26:1057–63.

8. de Aloysio D, Mantuano R, Mauloni M, Nicoletti G. The clinical use of arginine aspartate in male infertility. *Acta Eur Fertil* 1982;13:133–67.

9. Tanimura J. Studies on arginine in human semen. Part II. The effects of medication with L-arginine-HCl on male infertility. *Bull Osaka Med School* 1967; 13:84–89.

10. Schacter A, Goldman JA, Zukerman Z. Treatment of oligospermia with the amino acid arginine. *J Urol* 1973; 110:311–13.

11. Schacter A et al. Treatment of oligospermia with the amino acid arginine. *Int J Gynaecol Obstet* 1973; 11:206–9.

12. Mroueh A. Effect of arginine on oligospermia. *Fertil Steril* 1970;21:217–19.

13. Pryor JP, Blandy JP, Evans P, Chaput De Saintonge DM, Usherwood M. Controlled clinical trial of arginine for infertile men with oligozoospermia. *Brit J Urol* 1978;50:47–50.

14. Tanimura J. Studies on arginine in human semen. Part III. The influences of several drugs on male infertility. *Bull Osaka Med School* 1967;13:90–100.

15. Thiessen DD et al. Vitamin E and sex behavior in mice. *Nutr Metabol* 1975;18:116–19.

16. Bayer R. Treatment of infertility with vitamin E. *Int J Fertil* 1960;5:70–78.

17. Sandler B, Faragher B. Treatment of oligospermia with vitamin B12. *Infertil* 1984;7:133–38.

18. Kumamoto Y, Maruta H, Ishigami J, et al. Clinical efficacy of mecobalamin in treatment of oligozoospermia. *Acta Urol Jpn* 1988;34:1109–32.

19. Costa M, Canale D, Filicori M, et al. L-carnitine in idiopathic asthenozoospermia: A multicenter study. *Andrologia* 1994;26:155–59.

20. Vitali G, Parente R, Melotti C. Carnitine supplementation in human idiopathic asthenospermia: Clinical results. *Drugs Exptl Clin Res* 1995;21:157–59.

21. Chandra RK. Excessive intake of zinc impairs immune responses. *JAMA* 1984;252:1443–46.

Insomnia

1. Weiss B, Laties VG. Enhancement of human performance by caffeine and the amphetamines. *Pharmacol Rev* 1962: 14:1–36.

2. Hollingworth HL. The influence of caffeine on mental and motor efficiency. *Arch Psychol* 1912;20:1–66.

3. Blum I, Vered Y, Graff E, et al. The influence of meal composition on plasma serotonin and norepinephrine concentrations. *Metabol* 1992;41:137–40.

4. Morin CM, Culbert JP, Schwartz SM. Nonpharmacological interventions for insomnia: A meta-analysis of treatment efficacy. *Am J Psychiatr* 1994;151: 1172–80.

5. Fuerst ML. Insomniacs give up stress and medications. *JAMA* 1983; 249:459–60.

6. Phillips BA, Danner FJ. Cigarette smoking and sleep disturbance. *Arch Intern Med* 1995;155:734–37.

7. Haimov I, Laudon M, Zisapel N, et al. Sleep disorders and melatonin rhythms in elderly people. *BMJ* 1994;309:167.

8. Singer C, McArthur A, Hughes R, et al. Melatonin and sleep in the elderly. *J Am Geriatr Soc* 1996;44:51 (abstract #A1).

9. Attenburrow MEJ, Dowling BA, Sharpley AL, Cowen PJ. Case-control study of evening melatonin concentration in primary insomnia. *BMJ* 1996;312: 1263–64.

10. Zhadanova IV, Wurtman RJ, Lynch HJ, et al. Sleep-inducing effects of low doses of melatonin ingested in the evening. *Clin Pharmacol Ther* 1995; 57:552–58.

11. Garfinkel D, Laudon M, Nof D, Zisapel N. Improvement of sleep quality in elderly people by controlled-release melatonin. *Lancet* 1995;346:541–44.

12. Leathwood PD, Chauffard F. Aqueous extract of valerian reduces latency to fall asleep in man. *Planta Medica* 1985; 51:144–48.

13. Leathwood PD, Chauffard F, et al. Aqueous extract of valerian root (*Valeriana officinalis* L.) improves sleep quality in man. *Pharmacol Biochem Behav* 1982; 17:65–71.

14. Dressing H, Riemann D, et al. Insomnia: Are valerian/balm combination of equal value to benzodiazepine? *Therapiewoche* 1992; 42:726–36.

15. Brown DJ. *Herbal Prescriptions for Better Health*. Rocklin, CA: Prima Publishing, 1996, 279.

Irritable Bowel Syndrome

1. Cann PA, Read NW, Holdsworth CD. What is the benefit of coarse wheat bran in patients with irritable bowel syndrome? *Gut* 1984;25:168–73.

2. Arfmann S, Andersen JR, Hegnhoj J, et al. Irritable bowel syndrome treated with wheat bran—a controlled double blind trial. *Scand J Gastroenterol* 1983;18 (S86):3.

3. Gaby AR. Commentary. *Nutrition and Healing,* Feb 1996:1,10–11 (review).

4. Bentley SJ, Pearson DJ, Rix KJ. Food hypersensitivity in irritable bowel syndrome. *Lancet* 1983;ii:295–97.

5. Alun Jones V, McLaughlan P, Shorthouse M, et al. Food intolerance: A major factor in the pathogenesis of irritable bowel syndrome. *Lancet* 1982;ii:1115–17.

6. Harvey RF. Individual and group hypnotherapy in treatment of refractory irritable bowel syndrome. *Lancet* 1989; i:424–26.

7. Houghton LA, Heyman D, Whorwell PJ. Hypnotherapy: effect on quality of life and economic consequences of irritable bowel syndrome. *Gut* 1994;35(suppl 5): (abstract #F231).

8. Cotterell CJ, Lee AJ, Hunter JO. Double-blind cross-over trial of evening primrose oil in women with menstrually-related irritable bowel syndrome. In

Omega-6 Essential Fatty Acids: Pathophysiology and Roles in Clinical Medicine. New York: Alan R Liss, 1990, 421–26.

9. Dew MJ, Evans BK, Rhodes J. Peppermint oil for the irritable bowel syndrome: A multi-center trial. *Br J Clin Pract* 1984;38:394–98.

10. Achterrath-Tuckerman U, Kunde R, et al. Pharmacological investigations with compounds of chamomile. V. Investigations on the spasmolytic effect of compounds of chamomile and Kamillosan® on isolated guinea pig ileum. *Planta Med* 1980;39:38–50.

11. Westphal J, Hörning M, Leonhardt K. Phytotherapy in functional abdominal complaints: Results of a clinical study with a preparation of several plants. *Phytomed* 1996;2:285–91.

Kidney Stones

1. Blacklock N. Renal stone. In *Western Diseases: Their Emergence and Prevention,* ed. DP Burkitt and HC Trowell. Cambridge, MA: Harvard Press, 1981, 60–70.

2. Massey LK, Roman-Smith H, Sutton RAL. Effect of dietary oxalate and calcium on urinary oxalate and risk of formation of calcium oxalate kidney stones. *J Am Dietet Assoc* 1993;93:901–6.

3. Massey LK, Roman-Smith H, Sutton RAL. Effect of dietary oxalate and calcium on urinary oxalate and risk of formation of calcium oxalate kidney stones. *J Am Dietet Assoc* 1993;93:901–6.

4. Brinkley L, McGuire J, Gregory J, Pak CYC, et al. Bioavailability of oxalate in foods. *Urol* 1981;17:534.

5. Hollingbery PW, Massey LK. Effect of dietary caffeine and sucrose on urinary calcium excretion in adolescents. *Fed Proc* 1986;45:375 (abstract #1280).

6. Kiel DP, Felson DT, Hannan MT, et al. Caffeine and the risk of hip fracture: The Framingham study. *Am J Epidemiol* 1990;132:675–84.

7. Curhan GC, Willett WC, Rimm EB, Stampfer MJ. A prospective study of dietary calcium and other nutrients and the risk of symptomatic kidney stones. *N Engl J Med* 1993;328:833–38.

8. Robertson WG, Peacock M, Marshall DH. Prevalence of urinary stone disease in vegetarians. *Eur Urol* 1982; 8:334–39.

9. Muldowney FP, Freaney R, Moloney MF. Importance of dietary sodium in the

hypercalciuria syndrome. *Kidney Int* 1982; 22:292–96.

10. Sabto J, Powell MJ, Gurr B, Gurr FW. Influence of urinary sodium on calcium excretion in normal individuals. *Med J Austral* 1984;140:354–56.

11. Silver J, Rubinger D, Friedlaender MM, Popovitzer MM. Sodium-dependent idiopathic hypercalciuria in renal-stone formers. *Lancet* 1983;ii:484–86.

12. Lehman J Jr, Pleuss JA, Gray RW, Hoffman RG. Potassium administration increases and potassium deprivation reduces urinary calcium excretion in healthy adults. *Kidney Int* 1991;39: 973–83.

13. Curhan GC, Willett WC, Rimm EB, Stampfer MJ. A prospective study of dietary calcium and other nutrients and the risk of symptomatic kidney stones. *N Engl J Med* 1993;328:833–8.

14. Shah PJR. Unprocessed bran and its effect on urinary calcium excretion in idiopathic hypercalciuria. *BMJ* 1980; 281:426.

15. Ebisuno S, Morimoto S, Yoshida T, et al. Rice-bran treatment for calcium stone formers with idiopathic hypercalciuria. *Brit J Urol* 1986;58:592–95.

16. Robertson WG, Peacock M, Heyburn PJ, Hanes FA. Epidemiological risk factors in calcium stone disease. *Scand J Urol Nephrol Supplement* 1980;53:15–30.

17. Shuster J, Jenkins A, Logan C, et al. Soft drink consumption and urinary stone recurrence: A randomized prevention trial. *J Clin Epidemiol* 1992; 45: 911–16.

18. Marshall RW, Cochran M, Hodginson A. Relationship between calcium and oxalic acid intake in the diet and their excretion in the urine of normal and renal-stone forming subjects. *Clin Sci* 1972; 43:91–99.

19. Curhan GC, Willett WC, Rimm EB, Stampfer MJ. A prospective study of dietary calcium and other nutrients and the risk of symptomatic kidney stones. *N Engl J Med* 1993;328:833–38.

20. Rao PN, Blacklock NJ. Hypercalciuria. *Lancet* 1983;ii:747 (letter).

21. Pak CYO. Nephrolithiasis from calcium supplementation. *J Urol* 1987;137: 1212–13 (editorial).

22. Levine BS, Rodman JS, Wienerman S, et al. Effect of calcium citrate supplementation on urinary calcium oxalate saturation in female stone formers:

Implications for prevention of osteoporosis. *Am J Clin Nutr* 1994;60:592–96.

23. Lindberg J, Harvey J, Pak CYC. Effect of magnesium citrate and magnesium oxide on the crystallization of calcium salts in urine: Changes produced by food-magnesium interaction. *J Urol* 1990;143:248–51.

24. Prien EL, Gershoff SF. Magnesium oxide-pyridoxine therapy for recurrent calcium oxalate calculi. *J Urol* 1974;112:509–12.

25. Johansson G, Backman U, Danielson BG, et al. Effects of magnesium hydroxide in renal stone disease. *J Am Col Nutr* 1982;1:179–85.

26. Ettiniger B, Citron JT, Livermore B, Dolman LI. Chlorthalidone reduces calcium oxalate calculus recurrence but magnesium hydroxide does not. *J Urol* 1988;139:679–84.

27. Wilson DR, Strauss AL, Manuel MA. Comparison of medical treatments for the prevention of recurrent calcium nephrolithiasis. *Urol Res* 1984;12:39–40.

28. Baggio B, Gambaro G, Marchini F, et al. Correction of erythrocyte abnormalities in idiopathic calcium-oxalate nephrolithiasis and reduction of urinary oxalate by oral glycosaminoglycans. *Lancet* 1991;338:403–5.

29. Bataille P, Charransol G, Gregoire I, et al. Effect of calcium restriction on renal excretion of oxalate and the probability of stones in the various pathophysiological groups with calcium stones. *J Urol* 1983;130:218–23.

30. Piesse JW. Nutritional factors in calcium containing kidney stones with particular emphasis on vitamin C. *Int Clin Nutr Rev* 1985;5(3):110–29 (review).

31. Ringsdorf WM, Cheraskin WM. Medical complications from ascorbic acid: A review and interpretation (part one). *J Holistic Med* 1984;6(1):49–63.

32. Hoffer A. Ascorbic acid and kidney stones. *Can Med Assoc J* 1985;32:320 (letter).

33. Wandzilak TR, D'Andre SD, Davis PA, Williams HE. Effect of high dose vitamin C on urinary oxalate levels. *J Urol* 1994;151:834–37.

Macular Degeneration

1. National Advisory Eye Council. Report of the Retinal and Choroidal Diseases Panel: Vision Research CA National Plan, 1983–1987. Bethesda, MD: US Dept of Health and Human Services, 1984. National Institutes of Health publication 83-2471.

2. Young RW. Solar radiation and age-related macular degeneration. *Surv Ophthalmol* 1988;32:252–69.

3. Katz ML, Parker KR, Handelman GJ, et al. Effects of antioxidant nutrient deficiency on the retina and retinal pigment epithelium of albino rats: A light and electron microscopic study. *Exp Eye Res* 1982;34:339–69.

4. West S, Vitale S, Hallfrisch J, et al. Are anti-oxidants or supplements protective of age-related macular degeneration? *Arch Ophthalmol* 1994;112:222–27.

5. Eye Disease Case-Control Study Group. Antioxidant status and neovascular age-related macular degeneration. *Arch Ophthalmol* 1993;111:104–9.

6. Goldberg J, Flowerdew G, Smith E, et al.: Factors associated with age-related macular degeneration. *Am J Epidemiol* 1988;128:700–10.

7. Bone RA, Landrum JT. Distribution of macular pigment components, zeaxanthin and lutein, in human retina. *Methods Enzymol* 1992;213:360–66.

8. Blumenkranz MS, Russell SR, Robey MG, et al. Risk factors in age-related maculopathy complicated by choroidal neovascularization. *Ophthalmol* 1986;96:552–58.

9. Mares-Perlman JA, Brady WE, Kleain R, et al. Serum antioxidants and age-related macular degeneration in a population-based case-control study. *Arch Ophthalmol* 1995;113:1518–23.

10. Seddon JM, Ajani UA, Sperduto RD, et al. Dietary carotenoids, vitamins A, C, and E, and advanced age-related macular degeneration. *JAMA* 1994;272:1413–20.

11. Newsome DA, Swartz M, Leone NC, et al. Oral zinc in macular degeneration. *Arch Ophthalmol* 1988;106:192–98.

12. Stur M, Tihl M, Reitner A, Meisinger V. Oral zinc and the second eye in age-related macular degeneration. *Invest Ophtholmol* 1966;37:1225–35.

13. Lebuisson DA, Leroy L, Reigal G. Treatment of senile macular degeneration with *Ginkgo biloba* extract: A preliminary double-blind study versus placebo. In *Rokan (Ginkgo biloba): Recent Results in Pharmacology and Clinic*, Fünfgeld FW, ed. Berlin: Springer-Verlag, 1988, 231–36.

14. Scharrer A, Ober M. Anthocyanosides in the treatment of retinopathies. *Klin Monatsbl Augenheikld Beih* 1981;178:386–89.

15. Mian E, Curri SB, et al. Anthocyanosides and the walls of microvessels: Further aspects of the mechanism of action of their protective in syndromes due to abnormal capillary fragility. *Minerva Med* 1977;68:3565–81.

Menopause

1. Knight DC, Eden JA. A review of the clinical effects of phytoestrogens. *Obstet Gynecol* 1996;87:897–904 (review).

2. Perloff WH. Treatment of the menopause. *Am J Obstet Gynecol* 1949;58:684–94.

3. Gozan HA. The use of vitamin E in treatment of the menopause. *NY State J Med* 1952;52:1289.

4. Blatt MHG et al. Vitamin E and climacteric syndrome: Failure of effective control as measured by menopausal index. *Arch Intern Med* 1953;91:792.

5. CJ Smith. Non-hormonal control of vaso-motor flushing in menopausal patients. *Chicago Med* Mar 7, 1964.

6. Duker EM. Effects of extracts from *Cimicifuga racemosa* on gonadotropin release in menopausal women and ovariectomized rats. *Planta Med* 1991;57:420–24.

Menorrhagia
(Heavy Menstruation)

1. Samuels, AJ. Studies in patients with functional menorrhagia: The antimenorrhagic effect of the adequate replication of iron stores. *Israel J Med Sci* 1965;1:851.

2. Taymor ML, Sturgis SH, Yahia C. The etiological role of chronic iron deficiency in production of menorrhagia. *JAMA* 1964;187:323–27.

3. Lithgow DM, Politzer WM. Vitamin A in the treatment of menorrhagia. *S Afr Med J* 1977;51:191–93.

4. Dasgupta PR, Dutta S, Banerjee P, Majumdar S. Vitamin E (alpha tocopherol) in the management of menorrhagia associated with the use of intrauterine contraceptive devices (ICUD). *Internat J Fertil* 1983;28(1):55–56.

5. Cohen JD, Rubin HW. Functional menorrhagia: treatment with bioflavonoids and vitamin C. *Curr Ther Res* 1960;2:539.

Migraine Headaches

1. Grant EC. Food allergies and migraine. *Lancet* 1979;I:966–69.

2. Monro J, Brostoff J, Carini C, Zilkha K. Food allergy in migraine. *Lancet* 1980;ii:1–4.

3. Egger J, Carter CM, Wilson J, et al. Is migraine food allergy? A double-blind controlled trial of oligoantigenic diet treatment. *Lancet* 1983;ii:865–69.

4. Hughs EC, Gott PS, Weinstein RC, Binggeli R. Migraine: A diagnostic test for etiology of food sensitivity by a nutritionally supported fast and confirmed by long-term report. *Ann Allergy* 1985; 55:28–32.

5. Egger J, Carter CM, Soothill JF, Wilson J. Oligoantigenic diet treatment of children with epilepsy and migraine. *J Pediatr* 1989;114:51–58.

6. Brainard JB. Angiotensin and aldosterone elevation in salt-induced migraine. *Headache* 1981;21:222–26.

7. Ratner D, Shoshani E, Dubnov B. Milk protein-free diet for nonseasonal asthma and migraine in lactase-deficient patients. *Israel J Med Sci* 1983;19(9):806–9.

8. Hanington E. Preliminary report on tyramine headache. *BMJ* 1967;2:550–51.

9. Perkine JE, Hartje J. Diet and migraine: A review of the literature. *J Am Dietet Assoc* 1983;83:459–63.

10. Smith I et al. A clinical and biochemical correlation between tyramine and migraine headache. *Headache* 1970; 10:43–51.

11. Hasselmark L, Malmgren R, Hannerz J. Effect of a carbohydrate-rich diet, low in protein-tryptophan, in classic and common migraine. *Cephalalgia* 1987; 7:87–92.

12. Unge G, Malmgren R, Olsson P, et al. Effects of dietary protein-tryptophan restriction upon 5-HT uptake by platelets and clinical symptoms in migraine-like headache. *Cephalalgia* 1983;3:213–18.

13. McCarren T, Hitzemann R, Allen C, et al. Amelioration of severe migraine by fish oil (omega-3) fatty acids. *Am J Clin Nutr* 1985;41(4):874 (abstract).

14. Glueck CJ, McCarren T, Hitzemann R, et al. Amelioration of severe migraine with omega-3 fatty acids: A double-blind placebo controlled clinical trial. *Am J Clin Nutr* 1986;43(4):710 (abstract).

15. Gallai V, Sarchielli P, Coata G, et al. Serum and salivary magnesium levels in migraine. Results in a group of juvenile patients. *Headache* 1992;32:132–35.

16. Weaver K. Magnesium and migraine. *Headache* 1990;30:168 (letter).

17. Mauskop A, Altura BT, Cracco RQ, Altura BM. Intravenous magnesium sulphate relieves migraine attacks in patients with low serum ionized magnesium levels: A pilot study. *Clin Sci* 1995; 89:633–36.

18. Facchinetti F, Sances G, Borella P, et al. Magnesium prophylaxis of menstrual migraine: Effects on intracellular magnesium. *Headache* 1991;31:298–301.

19. Thys-Jacobs S. Vitamin D and calcium in menstrual migraine. *Headache* 1994;34:544–46.

20. Thys-Jacobs S. Alleviation of migraines with therapeutic vitamin D and calcium. *Headache* 1994;34:590–92.

21. Schoenen J, Lenaerts M, Bastings E. High-dose riboflavin as a prophylactic treatment of migraine: Results of an open pilot study. *Cephalalgia* 1994;14:328–29.

22. Hepinstall S, White A, et al. Extracts of feverfew inhibit granule secretion in blood platelets and polymorphonuclear leukocytes. *Lancet* 1985;I:1071–74.

23. Murphy JJ, Hepinstall S, Mitchell JRA. Randomized double-blind placebo controlled trial of feverfew in migraine prevention. *Lancet* 1988;ii:189–92.

24. Johnson ES, Kadam NP, et al. Efficacy of feverfew as prophylactic treatment of migraine. *British Med J* 1985; 291:569–73.

25. Srivasta KC, Mustafa T. Ginger (*Zingiber officinale*) in migraine headache. *J Ethnopharmacol* 1992;39:267–73.

26. Lamant V, Mauco G, et al. Inhibition of the metabolism of platelet activating factor (PAF-acether) by three specific antagonist from *Ginkgo biloba*. *Biochem Pharmacol* 1987;36:2749–52.

Morning Sickness

1. Signorello LB, Harlow BL, Wang SP, Erick MA. Saturated fat intake and the risk of severe hyperemesis gravidarum. *Am J Epidemiol* 1996;143(11 suppl):S25 (abstract #97).

2. Merkel RL. The use of menadione bisulfite and ascorbic acid in the treatment of nausea and vomiting of pregnancy. *Am J Obstet Gynecol* 1952; 64:416–18.

3. Sahakian V, Rouse D, Sipes S, et al. Vitamin B6 is effective therapy for nausea and vomiting of pregnancy: A randomized, double-blind placebo-controlled study. *Obstet Gynecol* 1991;78:33–36.

4. Vutyavanich T, Wongtra-ngan S, Ruangsri R-A. Pyridoxine for nausea and vomiting of pregnancy: A randomized, double blind, placebo-controlled trial. *Am J Obstet Gynecol* 1995;173:881–84.

5. Fischer-Rasmussen W, Kjaer SK, et al. Ginger treatment of hyperemesis gravidarum. *Eur J Obstet Gynecol Reprod Biol* 1990;38:19–24.

6. Fischer-Rasmussen W, Kjaer SK, Dahl C, Asping U. Ginger treatment of hyperemesis gravidarum. *Eur J Obstet Gynecol Reproductive Biol* 1990;38:19–24.

MSG Sensitivity

1. Wen C-P, Gershoff SN. Effects of dietary vitamin B6 on the utilization of monosodium glutamate by rats. *J Nutr* 1972;102:835–40.

2. Folkers K, Shizukuishi S, Scudder SL, et al. Biochemical evidence for a deficiency of vitamin B6 in subjects reacting to monosodium-L-glutamate by the Chinese restaurant syndrome. *Biochem Biophys Res Comm* 1981;100:972–77.

Night Blindness

1. Anonymous. Zinc-responsive night blindness in sickle cell anemia. *Nutr Rev* 1982;40:175–77.

2. Alfieri R, Sole P. Influencedes anthocyanosides admintres parvoie parenterale su l'adaptoelectroretinogramme du lapin. *CR Soc Biol* 1964;15:2338.

3. Sala D, Rolando M, et al. Effect of anthocyanosides on visual performance at low illumination. *Minerva Oftalmol* 1979; 21:283–85.

Osgood-Schlatter Disease

1. Riech, CJ. Vitamin E, selenium, and knee problems. *Lancet* 1976;i:257 (letter).

2. Jonathan V Wright, MD, personal correspondence with author. April 1997.

Osteoarthritis

1. Warmbrand M. *How Thousands of My Arthritis Patients Regained Their Health.* New York: Arco Publishing, 1974.

2. Childers NF. A relationship of arthritis to the solanaceae (nightshades). *J Internat Acad Pre Med* Nov 1982:31–37.

3. Taylor MR. Food allergy as an etiological factor in arthropathies: A survey. *J Internat Acad Prev Med* 1983;8:28–38 (review).

4. Drovanti A, Bignamini AA, Rovati AL. Therapeutic activity of oral glucosamine sulfate in osteoarthritis: A placebo-controlled double-blind investigation. *Clin Ther* 1980;3(4):260–72.

5. Vaz AL. Double-blind clinical evaluation of the relative efficacy of ibuprofen and glucosamine sulphate in the

management of osteoarthritis of the knee in out–patients. *Curr Med Res Opin* 1982;8(3):145–49.

6. D'Ambrosio E, Casa B, Bompani G, et al. Glucosamine sulphate: A controlled clinical investigation in arthrosis. *Pharmatherapeutica* 1981;2(8):504–8.

7. Pujalte JM, Llavore EP, Ylescupidez FR. Double-blind clinical evaluation of oral glucosamine sulphate in the basic treatment of osteoarthrosis. *Curr Med Res Opin* 1980;7(2):110–14.

8. McAlindon TE, Jacques P, Azang Y. Do antioxidant micronutrients protect against the development and progression of knee osteoarthritis? *Arthrit Rheum* 1996;39:648–56.

9. Machtey I, Ouaknine L. Tocopherol in osteoarthritis: A controlled pilot study. *J Am Geriatr Soc* 1978;25(7):328–30.

10. Blankenhorn G. Klinische Wirtsamkeit von Spondyvit (vitamin E) bei aktiverten arthronsen. *Z Orthop* 1986; 124:340–43.

11. Newnham RE. The role of boron in human nutrition. *J Applied Nutr* 1994; 46:81–5.

12. Travers RL, Rennie GC, Newnham RE. Boron and arthritis: The results of a double-blind pilot study. *J Nutr Med* 1990;1:127–32.

13. Altman R, Gray R. Inflammation in osteoarthritis. *Clin Rheum Dis* 1985; 11:353.

14. Kaufman W. The use of vitamin therapy for joint mobility. Therapeutic reversal of a common clinical manifestation of the 'normal' aging process. *Conn State Med J* 1953;17(7):584–89.

15. Kaufman W. The use of vitamin therapy to reverse certain concomitants of aging. *J Am Geriatr Soc* 1955;11:927.

16. Hoffer A. Treatment of arthritis by nicotinic acid and nicotinamide. *Can Med Assoc J* 1959;81:235–38.

17. Jonas WB, Rapoza CP, Blair WF. The effect of niacinamide on osteoarthritis: A pilot study. *Inflamm Res* 1996;45: 330–34.

18. Balagot RC, Ehrenpreis S, Kubota K, et al. Analgesia in mice and humans by D-phenylalanine: Relation to inhibition of enkephalin degradation and enkephalin levels. *Adv Pain Res Ther* 1983;5:289–93.

19. Kerzberg EM, Roldan EJA, Castelli G, Huberman ED. Combination of glycosaminoglycans and acetylsalicylic acid in knee osteoarthritis. *Scand J Rheum* 1987; 16:377.

20. Nielson FH, Hunt CD, Mullen LM, Hunt JR. Effect of dietary boron on mineral, estrogen, and testosterone metabolism in postmenopausal women. *FASEB J* 1987;1:394–97.

21. Bingham R, Bellew BA, Bellew JG. Yucca plant saponin in the management of arthritis. *J Appl Nutr* 1975; 27:45–50.

Osteoporosis

1. Feskanich D, Willett WC, Stampfer MJ, Colditz GA. Protein consumption and bone fractures in women. *Am J Epidemiol* 1996;143:472–79.

2. Abelow BJ, Holford TR, Insogna KL. Cross-cultural associations between dietary animal protein and hip fracture: A hypothesis. *Calcif Tissue Int* 1992; 50:14–18.

3. Zarkadas M, Geougeon-Reyburn R, Marliss EB, et al. Sodium chloride supplementation and urinary calcium excretion in postmenopausal women. *Am J Clin Nutr* 1989;50:1088–94.

4. Hernandez-Avila M, Colditz GA, Stampfer MJ, et al. Caffeine, moderate alcohol intake, and risk of fractures of the hip and forearm in middle-aged women. *Am J Clin Nutr* 1991;54:157–63.

5. Wyshak G, Frisch RE. Carbonated beverages, dietary calcium, the dietary calcium/phosphorus ratio, and bone fractures in girls and boys. *J Adolescent Health* 1994;15:210–15.

6. Smith S, Swain J, Brown EM, et al. A preliminary report of the short-term effect of carbonated beverage consumption on calcium metabolism in normal women. *Arch Intern Med* 1989;149: 2517–19.

7. Hopper JL, Seeman E. The bone density of female twins discordant for tobacco use. *N Engl J Med* 1994;330: 387–92.

8. Chow R, Harrison JE, Notarius C. Effect of two randomised exercise programmes on bone mass of healthy postmenopausal women. *BMJ* 1987;295: 1441–44.

9. Lloyd T, Triantafyllou SJ, Baker ER, et al. Women athletes with menstrual irregularity have increased musculoskeletal injuries. *Med Sci Sports Exercise* 1986; 18(4):374–79.

10. Reid IR, Ames RW, Evans MC, et al. Long-term effects of calcium supplementation on bone loss and fractures in postmenopausal women: A randomized

controlled trial. *Am J Med* 1995;98: 331–35.

11. Nordin BEC, Baker MR, Horsman A, Peacock M. A prospective trial of the effect of vitamin D supplementation on metacarpal bone loss in elderly women. *Am J Clin Nutr* 1985;42(3):470–74.

12. Lips P, Graafmans WC, Ooms ME, et al. Vitamin D supplementation and fracture incidence in elderly persons. *Ann Intern Med* 1996;124:400–6.

13. Cohen L, Laor A, Kitzes R. Magnesium malabsorption in postmenopausal osteoporosis. *Magnesium* 1983;2:139–43.

14. Sahap Atik O. Zinc and senile osteoporosis. *J Am Geriatr Soc* 1983; 31:790–91.

15. Eaton-Evans J, McIlrath EM, Jackson WE, et al. Copper supplementation and bone-mineral density in middle-aged women. *Proc Nutr Soc* 1995;54:191A.

16. Nielson FH, Hunt CD, Mullen LM, Hunt JR. Effect of dietary boron on mineral, estrogen, and testosterone metabolism in postmenopausal women. *FASEB J* 1987;1:394–97.

17. Raloff J. Reasons for boning up on manganese. *Science News* Sep 27, 1986:199.

18. Carlisle EM. Silicon localization and calcification in developing bone. *Fed Proc* 1969;28:374.

19. McCaslin FE, Janes JM. The effect of strontium lactate in the treatment of osteoporosis. *Proc Staff Meetings Mayo Clinic* 1959;34(13):329–34.

20. Strause L, Saltman P, Smith KT, et al. Spinal bone loss in postmenopausal women supplemented with calcium and trace minerals. *J Nutr* 1994;124:1060–64.

21. Gaby AR. *Preventing and Reversing Osteoporosis*. Rocklin, CA: Prima Publishing, 1994.

22. Hart JP. Circulating vitamin K1 levels in fractured neck of femur. *Lancet* 1984;ii:283 (letter).

23. Knapen MHJ, Hamulyak K, Vermeer C. The effect of vitamin K supplementation on circulating osteocalcin (Bone Gla protein) and urinary calcium excretion. *Ann Intern Med* 1989; 111: 1001–5.

Pap Smear (Abnormal)

1. Palan PR et al. Plasma levels of antioxidant beta-carotene and alpha-tocopherol in uterine cervix dysplasias and cancer. *Nutr Cancer* 1991;15:13–20.

2. Dawson EB et al. Serum vitamin and selenium changes in cervical dysplasia. *Fed Proc* 1984;43:612.

3. Wassertheil-Smoller S et al. Dietary vitamin C and uterine cervical dysplasia. *Am J Epidemiol* 1981;114:714–724.

4. Romney SL et al. Retinoids and the prevention of cervical dysplasias. *Am J Obstet Gynecol* 1981;141:890–94.

5. Butterworth CE et al. Improvement in cervical dysplasia associated with folic acid therapy in users of oral contraceptives. *Am J Clin Nutr* 1982;35:73–82.

6. Zarcone R, Bellini P, Carfora E, et al. Folic acid and cervix dysplasia. *Minerva Ginecol* 1996;48:397–400.

7. Butterworth CE, Hatch KD, Soong S-J, et al. Oral folic acid supplementation for cervical dysplasia: A clinical intervention trial. *Am J Obstet Gynecol* 1992; 166:803–9.

8. Butterworth CE Jr et al. Folate deficiency and cervical dysplasia. *JAMA* 1992; 267:528–33.

Peptic Ulcer

1. Katchinski BD, Logan RFA, Edmond M, Langman MJS. Duodenal ulcer and refined carbohydrate intake: A case-control study assessing dietary fiber and refined sugar intake. *Gut* 1990;31:993–96.

2. Yudkin J. Eating and ulcers. *BMJ* Feb 16, 1980:483 (letter).

3. Sonnenberg A. Dietary salt and gastric ulcer. *Gut* 1986;27:1138–42.

4. Cheney G. Rapid healing of peptic ulcers in patients receiving fresh cabbage juice. *Cal Med* 1949;70:10.

5. Doll R, Pygott F. Clinical trial of Robaden and of cabbage juice in the treatment of gastric ulcer. *Lancet* 1954;ii:1200.

6. Grimes DS, Goddard J. Gastric emptying of wholemeal and white bread. *Gut* 1977;18:725–29.

7. Rydning A, Berstad A, Aadland E, Odegaard B. Prophylactic effect of dietary fiber in duodenal ulcer disease. *Lancet* 1982;ii:736–39.

8. Sikka KK, Singhai CM, Vajpeyi GN, et al. Efficacy of dried raw banana powder in the healing of peptic ulcer. *J Assoc Phys India* 1988;36(1):65 (abstract).

9. Kern RA, Stewart G. Allergy in duodenal ulcer: Incidence and significance of food hypersensitivities as observed in 32 patients. *J Allergy* 1931;3:51.

10. Reimann HJ, Lewin J. Gastric mucosal reactions in patients with food allergy. *Am J Gastroenterol* 1988;83: 1212–19.

11. Allison MC, Howatson AG, Caroline MG, et al. Gastrointestinal damage associated with the use of nonsteroidal antiinflammatory drugs. *N Engl J Med* 1992;327:749–54.

12. Lenz HJ, Ferrari-Taylor J, Isenberg JI. Wine and five percent ethanol are potent stimulants of gastric acid secretion in humans. *Gastroenterol* 1983;85: 1082–87.

13. Cohen S, Booth GH Jr. Gastric acid secretion and lower-esophageal-sphincter pressure in response to coffee and caffeine. *N Engl J Med* 1975; 293:897–99.

14. Feldman EJ, Isenberg JI, Grossman MI. Gastric acid and gastrin response to decaffeinated coffee and a peptone meal. *JAMA* 1981;246:248–50.

15. Dubey P, Sundram KR, Nundy S. Effect of tea on gastric acid secretion. *Dig Dis Sci* 1984;29:202–6.

16. Korman MG, Hansky J, Eaves ER, Schmidt GT. Influence of cigarette smoking on healing and relapse in duodenal ulcer disease. *Gastroenterol* 1983; 85:871–74.

17. Patty I, Benedek S, Deak G, et al. Controlled trial of vitamin A therapy in gastric ulcer. *Lancet* 1982;ii:876 (letter).

18. Frommer DJ. The healing of gastric ulcers by zinc sulphate. *Med J Aust* 1975;2:793.

19. Shive W, Snider RN, DuBilier B, et al. Glutamine in treatment of peptic ulcer. *Texas State J Med* Nov 1957:840.

20. Beil W, Birkholz C, Sewing KF. Effects of flavonoids on parietal cell acid secretion, gastric mucosal prostaglandin production and *Helicobacter pylori* growth. *Arzneim-Forsch Drug Res* 1995; 45:697–700.

21. Wendt P, Reiman H, et al. The use of flavonoids as inhibitors of histidine decarboxylase in gastric diseases: Experimental and clinical studies. *Naunyn-Schmeidbergs Arch Pharmakol* 1980; 313(suppl):238.

22. Goso Y, Ogata Y, Ishihara K, Hotta K. Effects of traditional herbal medicine on gastric mucin against ethanol-induced gastric injury in rats. *Comp Biochem Physiol* 1996;113C:17–21.

23. Beil W, Birkholz W, Sewing KF. Effects of flavonoids on parietal cell acid secretion, gastric mucosal prostaglandin production and Helicobacter pylori growth. *Arzneim Forsch* 1995;45:697–700.

24. Brogden RN, Speight TM, Avery GS. Deglycyrrhizinated licorice: A report of its pharmacological properties and therapeutic efficacy. *Drugs* 1974;8:330–39.

Photosensitivity

1. Cripps DJ. Diet and alcohol effects on the manifestation of hepatic porphyrias. *Fed Proc* 1987;46:1894–1900.

2. Mathews-Roth MM, Pathak MA, Fitzpatrick TB, et al. Beta-carotene as an oral photoprotective agent in erythropoietic protoporphyria. *JAMA* 1974; 228:1004–8.

3. Nordlund JJ, Klaus SN, Mathews-Roth MM, Pathak MA. New therapy for polymorphous light eruption. *Arch Dermatol* 1973;108:710–12.

4. Mathews-Roth MM, Pathak MA, Fitzpatrick TB, et al. Beta-carotene as a photoprotective agent in erythropoietic protoporphyria. *N Engl J Med* 1970; 282:1231–34.

5. Mathews-Roth MM. Photoprotection by carotenoids. *Fed Proc* 1987; 46:1890–93 (review).

6. Ayres S Jr, Mihan R. Porphyrea cutanea tarda: Response to vitamin E. *Cutis* 1978;22:50.

7. Werninghaus K, Meydani M, Bhawan J, et al. Evaluation of the photoprotective effect of oral vitamin E supplementation. *Arch Dermatol* 1994; 130:1257–61.

8. Kaufman G. Pyridoxine against amiodarone-induced photosensitivity. *Lancet* 1984;I:51–52 (letter).

9. Ross JB, Moss MA. Relief of the photosensitivity of erythropoietic protoporphyria by pyridoxine. *J Am Acad Dermatol* 1990;22:340–42.

10. Neuman R et al. Treatment of polymorphous light eruption with nicotinamide: A pilot study. *Brit J Dermatol* 1986;115:77–80.

11. Gajdos A. AMP in porphyria cutanea tarda. *Lancet* 1974;I:163 (letter).

Pregnancy Support

1. Barnes B, Bradley SG. *Planning for a Healthy Baby*. London: Ebury Press, 1990.

2. Price, WA. *Nutrition and Physical Degeneration*, 50th anniv. ed. New Canaan, CT: Keats Publishing, Inc., 1989.

3. Gold S, Sherry L. Hyperactivity, learning disabilities, and alcohol. *J Learn Disabil* 1984;17(1):3–6.

4. Northrup C. *Women's Bodies, Women's Wisdom.* New York: Bantam, 1994, 613.

5. Haglund B et al. Cigarette smoking as a risk factor for sudden infant death syndrome. *Am J Publ Health* 1990;80: 29–32.

6. Fenster I et al. Caffeine consumption during pregnancy and fetal growth. *Am J Public Health* 1991;81:458–61.

7. Truswell AS. ABC of nutrition. Nutrition for pregnancy. *Br Med J* 1985;291: 263–66.

8. MRC Vitamin Study Research Group. Prevention of neural tube defects: Results of the Medical Research Council Vitamin Study. *Lancet* 1991;338:131–7.

9. Tamura T, Goldenberg R, Freeberg L, et al. Maternal serum folate and zinc concentrations and their relationships to pregnancy outcome. *Am J Clin Nutr* 1992: 56;365–70.

10. Doyle W et al. The association between maternal diet and birth dimensions. *J Nutr Med* 1990;1:9–17.

11. Truswell AS. ABC of nutrition. Nutrition for pregnancy. *Br Med J* 1985; 291:263–66.

12. Villar J, Repke JT. Calcium supplementation during pregnancy may reduce preterm delivery in high-risk populations. *Am J Obstet Gynecol* 1990;163: 1124–31.

13. Gladstar R. *Herbal Healing for Women.* New York: Simon and Schuster, 1993, 176.

14. Gladstar R. *Herbal Healing for Women.* New York: Simon and Schuster, 1993, 177.

15. Gladstar R. *Herbal Healing for Women.* New York: Simon and Schuster, 1993, 177.

Premenstrual Syndrome

1. Rossignol AM, Bonnlander H. Prevalence and severity of the pre-menstrual syndrome. Effects of foods and beverages that are sweet or high in sugar content. *J Reprod Med* 1991;36:131–36.

2. Halliday A, Bush B, Cleary P, et al. Alcohol abuse in women seeking gynecologic care. *Obstet Gynecol* 1986;68;322.

3. Rossignol AM, Zhang J, Chen Y, Xiang Z. Tea and pre-menstrual syndrome in the People's Republic of China. *Am J Public Health* 1989;79:67–69.

4. Rossignol AM. Caffeine-containing beverages and pre-menstrual syndrome in young women. *Am J Public Health* 1985; 75(11):1335–37.

5. Rossignol AM, Bonnlander H. Caffeine-containing beverages, total fluid consumption, and pre-menstrual syndrome. *Am J Public Health* 1990; 80:1106–10.

6. Werbach MR. *Nutritional Influences on Illness, 2d ed.* Tarzana, CA: Third Line Press, 1993, 540–41 (review).

7. Prior JC, Vigna Y, Sciarretta D, et al. Conditioning exercise decreases premenstrual symptoms: A prospective, controlled 6-month trial. *Fert Steril* 1987; 47(3):402–8.

8. Barr W. Pyridoxine supplements in the pre-menstrual syndrome. *Practitioner* 1984;228:425–27.

9. Gunn ADG. Vitamin B6 and the premenstrual syndrome. *Int J Vit Nutr Res* 1985;suppl 27:213–24 (review).

10. Kleijnen J, Riet GT, Knipshcild P. Vitamin B6 in the treatment of the premenstrual syndrome—a review. *Brit J Obstet Gynaecol* 1990;97:847–52 (review).

11. Williams MJ, Harris RI, Deand BC. Controlled trial of pyridoxine in the treatment of pre-menstrual syndrome. *J Int Med Res* 1985;13:174–79.

12. Brush MG, Perry M. Pyridoxine and the pre-menstrual syndrome. *Lancet* 1985;i:1399 (letter).

13. Dorsey JL, Debruyne LK, Rady SJ. The effect of vitamin B6 therapy on premenstrual acne and tension. *Fed Proc* 1983;42(3):556 (abstract).

14. Malgren R, Collings A, Nilsson C-G. Platelet serotonin uptake and effects of vitamin B6-treatment in pre-menstrual tension. *Neuropsychobiology* 1987;18: 83–88.

15. Hagen I, Nesheim B-I, Tuntland T. No effect of vitamin B6 against pre-menstrual tension. *Acta Obstet Gynecol Scand* 1985;64:667–70.

16. Collin C. Etudes controlees de l'administration orale de progestagenes, d'un antioestrogene et de vitamine B6 dans le traitement des mastodynies. *Rev Med Brux* 1982;3:605–9.

17. Biskind MS. Nutritional deficiency in the etiology of menorrhagia, metrorrhagia, cystic mastitis and pre-menstrual tension: Treatment with vitamin B-complex. *J Clin Endocrinol Metabol* 1943; 3:227–34.

18. Biskind MS, Biskind GR, Biskind LH. Nutritional deficiency in the etiology of menorrhagia, metrorrhagia, cystic mas-titis and pre-menstrual tension. *Surg Gynecol Obstet* 1944;78:49.

19. Piesse JW. Nutritional factors in the pre-menstrual syndrome. *Intl Clin Nutr Rev* 1984;4(2):54–80 (review).

20. Horrobin DF, Manku MS, Brush M, et al. Abnormalities in plasma essential fatty acid levels in women with pre-menstrual syndrome and with nonmalignant breast disease. *J Nutr Med* 1991; 2:259–64.

21. Puolakka J, Makarainen L, Viinikka L, Ylikorkola O. Biochemical and clinical effects of treating the pre-menstrual syndrome with prostaglandin synthesis precursors. *J Reprod Med* 1985; 30:149–53.

22. Ockerman PA, Bachrack I, Glans S, Rassner S. Evening primrose oil as a treatment of the pre-menstrual syndrome. *Rec Adv Clin Nutr* 1986;2:404–5.

23. Massil H, O'Brien PMS, Brush MG. A double blind trial of Efamol evening primrose oil in pre-menstrual syndrome. *2nd International Symposium on PMS*, Kiawah Island, Sep 1987.

24. Casper R. A double blind trial of evening primrose oil in pre-menstrual syndrome. *2nd International Symposium on PMS*, Kiawah Island, Sep 1987.

25. Khoo SK, Munro C, Battisutta D. Evening primrose oil and treatment of pre-menstrual syndrome. *Med J Austral* 1990; 153:189–92.

26. Collins A, Cerin A, Coleman G, Landgren B-M. Essential fatty acids in the treatment of pre-menstrual syndrome. *Obstet Gynecol* 1993;81:93–98.

27. McFayden IJ, Forest AP, et al. Cyclical breast pain—some observations and the difficulties in treatment. *Brit J Clinical Practice* 1992;46:161–64.

28. Abraham GE, Lubran MM. Serum and red cell magnesium levels in patients with pre-menstrual tension. *Am J Clin Nutr* 1981;34:2364–66.

29. Sherwood RA, Rocks BF, Stewart A, Saxton RS. Magnesium and the pre-menstrual syndrome. *Ann Clin Biochem* 1986;23:667–70.

30. Nicholas A. Traitement du syndrome pre-menstruel et de la dysmenorrhee par l'ion magnesium. In *First International Symposium on Magnesium Deficit in Human Pathology*, ed. J Durlach. Paris: Springer-Verlag, 1973, 261–63.

31. Facchinetti F, Borella P, Sances G, et al. Oral magnesium successfully relieves

pre-menstrual mood changes. *Obstet Gynecol* 1991;78:177–81.

32. Werbach MR. Pre-menstrual syndrome: Magnesium. *Internat J Alternative Complementary Med* Feb 1994:29 (review).

33. Rossignol AM, Bonnlander H. Pre-menstrual symptoms and beverage consumption. *Am J Obstet Gynecol* 1993; 168:1640 (letter).

34. Thys-Jacobs S, Ceccarelli S, Bierman A, et al. Calcium supplementation in pre-menstrual syndrome. *J Gen Intern Med* 1989;4:183–89.

35. Penland JG, Johnson PE. Dietary calcium and manganese effects on menstrual cycle symptoms. *Am J Obstet Gynecol* 1993;168:1417–23.

36. Panth M, Raman L, Ravinder P, Sivakumar B. Effect of vitamin A supplementation on plasma progesterone and estradiol levels during pregnancy. *Internat J Vit Nutr Res* 1991;61:17–19.

37. Block E. The use of vitamin A in pre-menstrual tension. *Acta Obstet Gynecol Scand* 1960;39:586–92.

38. Argonz J, Abinzano C. Pre-menstrual tension treated with vitamin A. *J Clin Endocrinol* 1950;10:1579–89.

39. Chuong CJ, Dawson EB, Smith ER. Vitamin E levels in pre-menstrual syndrome. *Am J Obstet Gynecol* 1990;163: 1591–95.

40. London RS, Sundaram GS, Murphy L, Goldstein PJ. The effect of alpha-tocopherol on pre-menstrual symptomatology: A double blind study. *J Am Coll Nutr* 1983;2(2):115–22.

41. London RS, Bradley L, Chiamori NY. Effect of a nutritional supplement on pre-menstrual symptomatology in women with pre-menstrual syndrome: A double-blind longitudinal study. *J Am Coll Nutr* 1991;10:494–99.

42. Stewart A. Clinical and biochemical effects of nutritional supplementation on the pre-menstrual syndrome. *J Reprod Med* 1987;32:435–41.

43. Böhnert KJ, Hahn G. Phytotherapy in gynecology and obstetrics—Vitex agnus castus. *Erfahrungsheilkunde* 1990; 39: 494–502.

44. Dittmar FW, Böhnert KJ, et al. Pre-menstrual syndrome: Treatment with a phytopharmaceutical. *Therapiwoche Gynäkol* 1992;5:60–68.

45. Qi-bing M, Jing-yi T, Bo C. Advance in the pharmacological studies of radix Angelica sisnensis (oliv) diels (Chinese danggui). *Chin Med J* 1991;104: 776–81.

Pritikin Diet Program

1. Heaton KW et al. Treatment of Crohn's disease with an unrefined carbohydrate, fibre-rich diet. *Br Med J* 1979; 2:764–66.

Psoriasis

1. Poikolainen K, Reunala T, Karvonen J, et al. Alcohol intake: A risk factor for psoriasis in young and middle aged men? *BMJ* 1990;300:780–83.

2. Monk BE, Neill SM. Alcohol consumption and psoriasis. *Dermatologica* 1986;173:57–60.

3. Douglas JM. Psoriasis and diet. *Western J Med* 1980;133:450 (letter).

4. Michaelsson G, Gerden B. How common is gluten intolerance among patients with psoriasis? *Acta Derm Venereol* 1991;71:90.

5. Bittiner SB, Tucker WFG, Cartwright I, Bleehen SS. A double-blind, randomised, placebo-controlled trial of fish oil in psoriasis. *Lancet* 1988;I:378–80.

6. Kojima T, Terano T, Tanabe E, et al. Long-term administration of highly purified eicosapentaenoic acid provides improvement of psoriasis. *Dermatologica* 1991;182:225–30.

7. Kojima T, Ternao T, Tanabe E, et al. Effect of highly purified eicosapentaenoic acid on psoriasis. *J Am Acad Dermatol* 1989;21:150–51.

8. Dewsbury CE, Graham P, Darley CR. Topical eicosapentaenoic acid (EPA) in the treatment of psoriasis. *Brit J Dermatol* 1989;120:581–84.

9. Soyland E, Funk J, Rajka G, et al. Effect of dietary supplementation with very-long-chain n-3 fatty acids in patients with psoriasis. *N Engl J Med* 1993; 328:1812–16.

10. Ashley JM, Lowe NJ, Borok ME, Alfin-Slater RB. Fish oil supplementation results in decreased hypertriglyceridemia in patients with psoriasis undergoing etretinate or acitretin therapy. *J Am Acad Dermatol* 1988;19:76–82.

11. Morimoto S, Yoshikawa K, Kozuka T, et al. An open study of vitamin D3 treatment in psoriasis vulgaris. *Brit J Dermatol* 1986;115:421–29.

12. Morimoto S, Yoshikawa K. Psoriasis and vitamin D3 *Arch Dermatol* 1989;125:231–34.

13. Kragballe K. Treatment of psoriasis by the topical application of the novel cholecalciferol analogue Calcipotriol (MC 903). *Arch Dermatol* 1989; 125:1647–52.

14. Smith EL, Pincus SH, Donovan L, Holick MF. A novel approach for the evaluation and treatment of psoriasis. *J Am Acad Dermatol* 1988;19:516–28.

15. Kragballe K, Beck HI, Sogaard H. Improvement of psoriasis by a topical vitamin D3 analogue (MC 903) in a double-blind study. *Brit J Dermatol* 1988;119: 223–30.

16. Henderson CA, Papworth-Smith J, Cunliffe WJ, et al. A double-blind, placebo-controlled trial of topical 1,25-dihydroxycholecalciferol in psoriasis. *Brit J Dermatol* 1989;121:493–96.

17. Van de Kerkhof PCM, Van Bokhoven M, Zultak M, Czarnetzki BM. A double-blind study of topical 1 alpha,25-dihydroxyvitamin D3 in psoriasis. *Brit J Dermatol* 1989;120:661–64.

18. Kolbach DN, Nieboer C. Fumaric acid therapy in psoriasis: Results and side effects of 2 years of treatment. *J Am Acad Dermatol* 1992;27:769–71.

19. Altmeyer PJ, Matthes U, Pawlak F, et al. Antipsoriatic effect of fumaric acid derivatives. *J Am Acad Dermatol* 1994; 30:977–81.

20. Hoffman D. *The Herbal Handbook: A User's Guide to Medical Herbalism.* Rochester, VT: Healing Arts Press, 1988, 23–4 (review).

21. Bradley PR, ed. *British Herbal Compendium*, vol. 1. Bounemouth, Dorset, UK: British Herbal Medicine Association, 1992, 194–96 (review).

Rheumatoid Arthritis

1. Anonymous. Effects of dietary fat on virus-induced autoimmune disease. *Nutr Rev* 1983;41:128–30 (review).

2. Jacobson I et al. Correlation of fatty acid composition of adipose tissue lipids and serum phosphatidylcholine and serum concentrations of micronutrients with disease duration in rheumatoid arthritis. *Ann Rheum Dis* 1990;49:901–5.

3. Lucas CP, Power L. Dietary fat aggravates active rheumatoid arthritis. *Clin Res* 1981;29:754A (abstract).

4. Skoldstram L. Fasting and vegan diet in rheumatoid arthritis. *Scand J Rheumatol* 1987;15:219–21.

5. Nenonen M, Helve T, Hanninen O. Effects of uncooked vegan food—"living food"—on rheumatoid arthritis, a three month controlled and randomised study. *Am J Clin Nutr* 1992;56:762 (abstract #48).

6. Kjeldsen–Kragh J, Haugen M, Borchgrevink CF, et al. Controlled trial of fasting and one-year vegetarian diet in rheumatoid arthritis. *Lancet* 1991; 338:899–902.

7. Warmbrand M. *How Thousands of My Arthritis Patients Regained Their Health.* New York: Arco Publishing, 1974.

8. Panush RS, Carter RL, Katz P, et al. Diet therapy for rheumatoid arthritis. *Arthrit Rheum* 1983;26:462–71.

9. Childers NF. A relationship of arthritis to the solanaceae (nightshades). *J Internat Acad Pre Med* Nov 1982:31–37.

10. Zeller M. Rheumatoid arthritis—food allergy as a factor. *Ann Allerg* 1949; 7:200–05,239.

11. Darlington LG, Ramsey NW, Mansfield JR. Placebo-controlled, blind study of dietary manipulation therapy in rheumatoid arthritis. *Lancet* 1986; I:236–38.

12. Beri D et al. Effect of dietary restrictions on disease activity in rheumatoid arthritis. *Ann Rheum Dis* 1988;47:69–72.

13. Panush RS. Possible role of food sensitivity in arthritis. *Ann Allerg* 1988; 61(part 2):31–35.

14. Taylor MR. Food allergy as an etiological factor in arthropathies: A survey. *J Internat Acad Prev Med* 1983;8:28–38 (review).

15. Darlington LG, Ramsey NW. Diets for rheumatoid arthritis. *Lancet* 1991; 338:1209 (letter).

16. Kay DR, Webel RB, Drisinger TE, et al. Aerobic exercise improves performance in arthritis patients. *Clin Res* 1985;33:919A (abstract).

17. Harkcom TM, Lampman RM, Banwell BF, Castor CW. Therapeutic value of graded aerobic exercise training in rheumatoid arthritis. *Arthrit Rheum* 1985; 28:32–38.

18. Fairburn K, Grootveld M, Ward RJ, et al. Alpha-tocopherol, lipids and lipoproteins in knee-joint synovial fluid and serum from patients with inflammatory joint disease. *Clin Sci* 1992; 83:657–64.

19. Scherak O, Kolarz G. Vitamin E and rheumatoid arthritis. *Arthrit Rheum* 1991;34:1205–6 (letter).

20. Barton-Wright EC, Elliott WA. The pantothenic acid metabolism of rheumatoid arthritis. *Lancet* 1963; ii:862–63.

21. General Practitioner Research Group. Calcium pantothenate in arthritic conditions. *Practitioner* 1980;224:208–11.

22. Simkin PA. Oral zinc sulphate in rheumatoid arthritis. *Lancet* 1976; ii:539–42.

23. Peretz A, Neve J, Jeghers O, Pelen F. Zinc distribution in blood components, inflammatory status, and clinical indexes of disease activity during zinc supplementation in inflammatory rheumatic diseases. *Am J Clin Nutr* 1993;57: 690–94.

24. Job C, Menkes CJ, de Gery A, et al. Zinc sulphate in the treatment of rheumatoid arthritis. *Arthrit Rheum* 1980;23: 1408.

25. Simkin PA. Treatment of rheumatoid arthritis with oral zinc sulfate. *Agents Actions* 1981;8(suppl):587–96.

26. DiSilvestro RA, Marten J, Skehan M. Effects of copper supplementation on ceruloplasmin and copper-zinc superoxide dismutase in free-living rheumatoid arthritis patients. *J Am Coll Nutr* 1992;11: 177–80.

27. Medical News. Copper boosts activity of anti-inflammatory drugs. *JAMA* 1974;229:1268–69.

28. Sorenson JRJ. Copper complexes—a unique class of anti-arthritic drugs. *Progress Med Chem* 1978;15: 211–60 (review).

29. Walker WR, Keats DM. An investigation of the therapeutic value of the 'copper bracelet'—dermal assimilation of copper in arthritic/rheumatoid conditions. *Agents Actions* 1976;6:454–59.

30. Blake DR, Lunec J. Copper, iron, free radicals and arthritis. *Brit J Rheumatol* 1985;24:123–27 (editorial).

31. Kremer JM, Jubiz W, Michalek A, et al. Fish-oil fatty acid supplementation in active rheumatoid arthritis. *Ann Int Med* 1987;106(4):497–503.

32. Kremer JM, Lawrence DA, Jubiz W, et al. Dietary fish oil and olive oil supplementation in patients with rheumatoid arthritis. *Arthrit Rheum* 1990 33(6): 810–20.

33. Geusens P, Wouters C, Nijs J, et al. Long-term effect of omega-3 fatty acid supplementation in active rheumatoid arthritis. *Arthrit Rheum* 1994;37:824–29.

34. van der Tempel H, Tulleken JE, Limburg PC, et al. Effects of fish oil supplementation in rheumatoid arthritis. *Ann Rheum Dis* 1990;49:76–80.

35. Cleland LG, French JK, Betts WH, et al. Clinical and biochemical effects of dietary fish oil supplements in rheumatoid arthritis. *J Rheumatol* 1988; 151471–75.

36. Kremer JM, Lawrence DA, Petrillow GF, et al. Effects of high-dose fish oil on rheumatoid arthritis after stopping nonsteroidal antiinflammatory drugs. *Arthrit Rheum* 1995;38:1107–14.

37. Lee TH, Hoover RL, Williams JD, et al. Effect of dietary enrichment with eicosapentaenoic and docosahexaenoic acids on in vitro neutrophil and monocyte leukotriene generation and neutrophil function. *N Engl J Med* 1985;312(19): 1217–24.

38. Brzeski M, Madhok R, Capell HA. Evening primrose oil in patients with rheumatoid arthritis and side-effects of non-steroidal anti-inflammatory drugs. *Brit J Rheumatol* 1991;30:370–72.

39. Leventhal LJ, Boyce EG, Zurier RB. Treatment of rheumatoid arthritis with gammalinolenic acid. *Ann Intern Med* 1993;119:867–73.

40. Leventahn LJ, Boyce EG, Zuerier RB. Treatment of rheumatoid arthritis with blackcurrant seed oil. *Brit J Rheumatol* 1994;33:847–52.

41. Jantti J, Seppala E, Vapaatalo H, Isomaki H. Evening primrose oil and olive oil in treatment of rheumatoid arthritis. *Clin Rheumatol* 1989;8:238–44.

42. Belch JJF, Ansell D, Madhok R, et al. Effects of altering dietary essential fatty acids on requirements for nonsteroidal anti-inflammatory drugs in patients with rheumatoid arthritis: A double blind placebo controlled study. *Ann Rheum Dis* 1988;47:96–104.

43. Newnham RE. Arthritis or skeletal fluorosis and boron. *Int Clin Nutr Rev* 1991;11:68–70 (letter).

44. Balagot RC, Ehrenpreis S, Kubota K, et al. Analgesia in mice and humans by D-phenylalanine: Relation to inhibition of enkephalin degradation and enkephalin levels. *Adv Pain Res Ther* 1983; 5:289–93.

45. Singh GB, Singh S, Bani S. New phytotherapeutic agent for the treatment of arthritis and allied disorders with novel mode of action. *4th International Con-*

gress on Phytotherapy, Munich, Germany, Sep 10–13, 1992.

46. Kulkarni RR, Patki VP, et al. Treatment of osteoarthritis with a herbomineral formulation: A double-blind, placebo-controlled, cross-over study. *J Ethnopharm* 1991;33:91–95.

47. Deal CL, Schnitzer TJ, Lipstein E, et al. Treatment of arthritis with topical capsaicin: A double-blind trial. *Clin Ther* 1991;13:383–95.

Urinary Tract Infection

1. Avorn J, Monane M, Gurwitz JH, et al. Reduction of bacteriuria and pyuria after ingestion of cranberry juice. *JAMA* 1994;271:751–54.

2. Sobota AE. Inhibition of bacterial adherence by cranberry juice: Potential use for the treatment of urinary tract infections. *J Urol* 1984;131:1013–16.

3. Sanchez A, Reeser JL, Lau HS, et al. Role of sugars in human neutrophilic phagocytosis. *Am J Clin Nutr* 1973; 26:1180–4.

4. MacGregor RR. Alcohol and immune defense. *JAMA* 1986;256(11):1474.

5. Barone J et al. Dietary fat and natural-killer-cell activity. *Am J Clin Nutr* 1989;50:861–67.

6. Horesh AJ. Allergy and infection. *J Asthma Res* 1967;4:269.

7. Rudolph JA. Allergy as a cause of frequent recurring colds and coughs in children. *Dis Chest* 1940;6:138.

8. Berman BA. Pseudomononucleosis of allergic origin: A new clinical entity. *Ann Allerg* 1964;22:403.

9. Randolph TG, Hettig RA. The coincidence of allergic disease, unexplained fatigue, and lymphadenopathy; possible diagnostic confusion with infectious mononucleosis. *Am J Med Sci* 1945; 209:306.

10. Anderson R. Effects of ascorbate on normal and abnormal leucocyte functions. *Intl J Vit Nutr Res* Supplement #23:23.

11. Gerber WF et al. Effect of ascorbic acid, sodium salicylate, and caffeine on the serum interferon level in response to viral infection. *Pharmacol* 1975;13:228.

12. Axelrod DR. Ascorbic acid and urinary pH. *JAMA* 1985;254(10):1310.

13. Hussey GD, Klein M. A randomized, controlled trial of vitamin A in children with severe measles. *N Engl J Med* 1990;323:160–64.

14. Mori S, Ojima Y, Hirose T, et al. The clinical effect of proteolytic enzyme containing bromelain and trypsin on urinary tract infection evaluated by double blind method. *Acta Obstet Gynaec Jap* 1972;19:147–53.

15. Chandra RK. Effect of vitamin and trace-element supplementation on immune responses and infection in elderly subjects. *Lancet* 1992;340:1124–27.

16. Sun DX, Abraham SN, Beachey EH. Influence of berberine sulfate on synthesis and expression of pap fimbrial adhesin in uropathogenic Escherichia c oli. *Antimicr Agents Chemother* 1988; 32:1274–77.

17. European Scientific Cooperative for Phytotherapy. *Proposal for European Monographs,* vol. 3. Bevrijdingslaan, Netherlands: ESCOP Secretariat, 1992.

Vitiligo

1. Ortonne JP, Bose SK. Vitiligo: Where do we stand? *Pigment Cell Res* 1993; 6:61–72.

2. Montes LF, Diaz ML, Lajous J, Garcia NJ. Folic acid and vitamin B12 in vitiligo: A nutritional approach. *Cutis* 1992; 50:39–42.

3. Siddiqui AH, Stolk LM, Bhaggoe R, et al. L-phenylalanine and UVA irradiation in the treatment of vitiligo. *Dermatology* 1994;188:215–18.

4. Schulpis CH, Antoniou C, Michas T, Strarigos J. Phenylalanine plus ultraviolet light: Preliminary report of a promising treatment for childhood vitiligo. *Pediatr Dermatol* 1989;6:332–35.

5. Francis HW. Achlorhydria as an etiological factor in vitiligo, with report of four cases. *Nebraska State M J* 1931; 16:25–26.

6. Sieve BF. The clinical effects of a new B-complex factor, para-aminobenzoic acid, on pigmentation and fertility. *South Med Surg* Mar 1942;104:135–39.

7. Abdel-Fattah, Aboul-Enein MN, et al. An approach to the treatment of vitiligo by khellin. *Dermatologica* 1982; 165:136–40.

8. Brown DJ. *Herbal Prescriptions for Better Health*. Rocklin, CA: Prima Publishing, 1996, 294–95.

Weight Loss and Obesity

1. Biancardi G, Palmiero L, Ghirardi PE. Glucomannan in the treatment of overweight patients with osteoarthritis. *Curr Ther Res* 1989;46:908–12.

2. Muls E, Kempen K, Vansant G, et al. Is weight cycling detrimental to health? A review of the literature in humans. *Int J Obes* 1995;19(3):S46–S50.

3. Horton TJ, Geissler CA. Effect of habitual exercise on daily energy expenditure and metabolic rate during standardized activity. *Am J Clin Nutr* 1994; 59:13–19.

4. Page TG, Ward TL, Southern LL. Effect of chromium picolinate on growth and carcass characteristics of growing-finishing pigs. *J Animal Sci* 1991; 69:356.

5. Lefavi R, Anderson R, Keith R, et al. Efficacy of chromium supplementation in athletes: Emphasis on anabolism. *Int J Sport Nutr* 1992;2:111–22.

6. McCarty MF. The case for supplemental chromium and a survey of clinical studies with chromium picolinate. *J Appl Nutr* 1991;43:59–66.

7. Rogers MA. *Med Sci Sports Exercise* 1996;28(2).

8. Lowenstein JM. Effect of (-)-hydroxycitrate on fatty acid synthesis by rat liver in vivo. *J Biol Chem* 1971;246(3): 629–32.

9. Triscari J, Sullivan AC. Comparative effects of (-)-hydroxycitrate and (=)-allo-hydroxycitrate on acetyl CoA carboxylase and fatty acid and cholesterol synthesis in vivo. *Lipids* 1977;12(4):357–63.

10. Cheema-Dhadli S, Harlperin ML, Leznoff CC. Inhibition of enzymes which interact with citrate by (-)hydroxycitrate and 1,2,3,-tricarboxybenzene. *Eur J Biochem* 1973;38:98–102.

11. Sullivan AC, Hamilton JG, Miller ON, et al. Inhibition of lipogenesis in rat liver by (-)-hydroxycitrate. *Arch Biochem Biophys* 1972;150:183–90.

12. Greenwood MRC, Cleary MP, Gruen R, et al. Effect of (-)-hydroxycitrate on development of obesity in the Zucker obese rat. *Am J Phys* 1981;240:E72–8.

13. Sullivan AC, Triscari J. Metabolic regulation as a control for lipid disorcers. *Am J Clin Nutr* 1977;30:767–76.

14. Sullivan AC, Triscari J, Hamilton JG, et al. Effect of (-)-hydroxycitrate upon the accumulation of lipid in the rat: I. Lipogenesis. *Lipids* 1974;9:121–128.

15. Sullivan AC, Triscari J, Hamilton JG, et al. Effect of (-)-hydroxycitrate upon the accumulation of lipid in the rat: II. Appetite. *Lipids* 1974;9(2):129–34.

16. Sergio W. A natural food, malabar tamarind, may be effective in the treatment of obesity. *Medi Hyp* 1988;27:40.

17. Stanko RT, Tietze DL, Arch JE. Body composition, energy utilization, and nitrogen metabolism with a 4.25-MJ/d low-energy diet supplemented with pyruvate. *Am J Clin Nutr* 1992; 56(4):630–5.

18. Stanko RT, Reynolds HR, Hoyson R, et al. Pyruvate supplementation of a low-cholesterol, low-fat diet: Effects on plasma lipid concentration and body composition in hyperlipidemic patients. *Am J Clin Nutr* 1994;59:423–7.

19. Ivy JL, Cortez MY, Chandler RM, et al. Effects of pyruvate on the metabolism and insulin resistance of obese Zucker rats. *Am J Clin Nutr* 1994;59: 331–7.

20. Becher EW, Jakober B, Luft D, et al. Clinical and biochemical evaluations of the alga spirulina with regard to its application in the treatment of obesity. A double-blind cross-over study. *Nutr Rep Intl* 1986;33(4):565–73.

21. Sterns DM, Belbruno JJ, Wetterhahn. A prediction of chromium (III) accumulation in humans from chromium dietary supplements. *FASEB J* 1995;9: 1650–57.

22. Sterns DM, Wise JP, Patierno SR, Wetterhahn KE. Chromium (III) picolinate produces chromosome damage in Chinese hamster ovary cells. *FASEB J* 1995;9:1643–49.

23. Johnson PE, Shubert LE. Accumulation of mercury and other elements by spirulina (cyanophyceae). *Nutr Rep Intl* 1986;34(6):1063–71.

24. Leung A, Foster S. *Encyclopedia of Common Natural Ingredients Used in Food, Drugs, and Cosmetics*, 2d ed. New York: John Wiley & Sons, 1996, 293–94.

25. Breum L, Pedersen JK, Ahlstrom F, et al. Comparison of an ephedrine/caffeine combination and dexfenfluramine in the treatment of obesity. A double-blind multi-centre trial in general practice. *Int J Obes Rel Met Dis* 1994;18(2):99–103.

26. Toubro S, Astrup A, Breum L, et al. The acute and chronic effects of ephedrine/caffeine mixtures on energy expenditure and glucose metabolism in humans. *Int J Obes Rel Met Dis* 1993; 17(suppl 3):73–77.

Wilson's Disease

1. Hoogenraad TU, Van den Hammer CJA, Van Hattum J. Effective treatment of Wilson's disease with oral zinc sulphate: Two case reports. *BMJ* 1984;289:273–76.

2. Cossack ZT. The efficacy of oral zinc therapy as an alternative to penicillamine for Wilson's disease. *N Engl J Med* 1988;318:322–23 (letter/review).

3. Brewer GJ, Yuzbasiyan-Gurkan V. The use of zinc-copper metabolic interactions in the treatment of Wilson's disease. *J Am Coll Nutr* 1989;8:452 (abstract #103).

4. Brewer GJ, Hill GM, Dick RD, Nostrant TT, et al. Treatment of Wilson's disease with zinc. III. Prevention of reaccumulation of hepatic copper. *J Lab Clin Med* 1987;109:526–31.

5. Brewer GJ, Yuzbasiyan-Gurkan V. Use of zinc-copper metabolic interactions in the treatment of Wilson's disease. *J Am Coll Nutr* 1990;9:487–91.

6. Brewer JG, Yuzbasiyan-Gurkan V, Lee D-Y, Appelman H. Treatment of Wilson's disease with zinc. VI. Initial treatment studies. *J Lab Clin Med* 1989; 114:633–38.

7. Van den Hamer CJA, Hoogenraad TU. Copper deficiency in Wilson's disease. *Lancet* 1989;ii:442 (letter).

8. van Caillie-Bertrand M, Degenhart HJ, Visser HKA, et al. Oral zinc sulphates for Wilson's disease. *Arch Dis Child* 1985; 60:656.

9. Brewer JG, Yuzbasiyan-Gurkan V, Lee D-Y, Appelman H. Treatment of Wilson's disease with zinc. VI. Initial treatment studies. *J Lab Clin Med* 1989;114: 633–38.

Yeast Infection

1. Horowitz BJ, Edelstein SW, Lippman L. Sugar chromatography studies in recurrent candida vulvovaginitis. *J Reproduc Med* 1984;29(7):441.

2. Heidrich F, Berg A, Gergman R, et al. Clothing factors and vaginitis. *J Fam Pract* 1984;19:491–94.

3. Kudelco N. Allergy in chronic monilial vaginitis. *Ann Allergy* 1971;29: 266–67.

4. Hilton E, Isenberg HD, et al. Ingestion of yogurt containing Lactobacillus acidophilus as prophylaxis for candidal vaginitis. *Ann Intern Med* 1992;116: 353–57.

5. Neri A, Sabah G, Samra Z. Bacterial vaginosis in pregnancy treated with yogurt. *Acta Obstet Gynecol Scand* 1993; 72:17–19.

6. Eschenback H. Vaginal infection. *Clin Ob Gyn* 1983;26:186–202.

7. Vincent J, Voomett R, and Riley R. Antibacterial activity associated with Lactobaccillus acidophilus. *J Bact* 1959; A78:477–84.

8. Jovanovic R et al. Antifungal agents vs. boric acid for treating chornic mycotic vulvovaginitis. *J Reprod Med* 1977;36(8): 593–97.

9. Pena EO. *Melaleuca alternifolia* oil. Uses for trichomonal vaginitis and other vaginal infections. *Obstet Gynecol* 1962; 19:793–95.

10. Hughes BG, Lawson LD. Antimicrobial effects of *Allium sativum* L. (garlic), *Allium ampeloprasum* L. (elephant garlic) and *Allium cepa* L. (onion), garlic compounds and commercial garlic supplement products. *Phytother Res* 1991; 5:154–58.

11. Guiraud P, Steiman R, et al. Comparison of the antibacterial and antifungal activities of lapachol and beta-lapachone. *Planta Med* 1994; 60:373–74.

12. Coeugniet E, Kuhnast R. Recurrent candidiasis: Adjuvant immunotherapy with different formulations of Echinacin. *Therapiewoche* 1986;36:3352–58.

13. Duke JA. *CRC Handbook of Medicinal Herbs*. Boca Raton, FL: CRC Press, 1985, 470–71 (review).

Yellow Nail Syndrome

1. Norton L. Further observations on the yellow nail syndrome with therapeutic effects of oral alpha-tocopherol. *Cutis* 1985;36:457–62.

2. Ayres S Jr, Hihan R. Yellow nail syndrome: Response to vitamin E. *Arch Dermatol* 1973;108:267–68.

3. Ayres S Jr. Yellow nail syndrome controlled by vitamin E therapy. *J Am Acad Dermatol* 1986;15:714–16 (letter).

4. Williams HC, Buffham R, du Vivier A. Successful use of topical vitamin E solution in the treatment of nail changes in yellow nail syndrome. *Arch Dermatol* 1991;127:1023–28.

Nutritional Supplements

Introduction

1. Buffoni F, et al. 3-hydrazinopyridazine derivates in inhibitoin of pyridoxalphosphate dependent enzymes. *Farmaco (Edizione Scientifica)* Oct 1980: 848–55.

Acidophilus (Probiotics) and Fructo-Oligosaccharides

1. Smirnov VV, Reznik SR, V'iunitskaia VA, et al. The current concepts of the mechanisms of the therapeutic-prophylactic action of probiotics from bacteria in the genus bacillus. *Mikrobiolohichnyi Zhurnal* 1993;55(4):92–112.

2. Mel'nikova VM, Gracheva NM, Belikov GP, et al. The chemoprophylaxis and chemotherapy of opportunistic infections. *Antibiotiki i Khimioterapiia* 1993; 38:44–48.

3. De Simone C, Vesely R, Bianchi SB, et al. The role of probiotics in modulation of the immune system in man and in animals. *Int J Immunother* 1993;9:23–28.

4. Veldman A. Probiotics. *Tijdschrift voor Diergeneeskunde* 1992; 117(12): 345–48.

5. Kawase K. Effects of nutrients on the intestinal microflora of infants. *Jpn J Dairy Food Sci* 1982;31:A241–43.

6. Rasic JL. The role of dairy foods containing bifido and acidophilus bacteria in nutrition and health. *N Eur Dairy J* 1983;4:80–88.

7. Barefoot SF, Klaenhammer TR. Detection and activity of lactacin B, a bacteriocin produced by lactobacillus acidophilus. *Appl Environ Microbiol* 1983; 45:1808–15.

8. Hilton E, Isenberg HD, Alperstein P, et al. Ingestion of yogurt containing lactobacillus acidophilus as prophylaxis for candidal vaginitis. *Ann Int Med* 1992; 116:353–57.

9. Reid G et al. Implantation of lactobacillus casei var rhamnosus into vagina. *Lancet* 1994;344:1229.

10. Elmer GW, Surawicz CM, McFarland LV. Biotherapeutic agents. *JAMA* 1996;275(11):870–76.

11. Scarpignato C, Rampal P. Prevention and treatment of traveler's diarrhea: A clinical pharmacological approach. *Chemotherapy* 1995;41:48–81.

12. Loizeau E. Can antibiotic-associated diarrhea be prevented? *Annales de Gastroenterologie et d' Hepatologie* 1993; 29(1):15–18.

13. McDonough FE, Hitchins AD, Wong NP, et al. Modification of sweet acidophilus milk to improve utilization by lactose-intolerant persons. *Amer J Clin Nutr* 1987;45:570–74.

14. Newcomer AD, Park HS, O'Brian PC, et al. Response of patients with irritable bowel syndrome and lactase deficiency using unfermented acidophilus milk. *Amer J Clin Nutr* 1983;38:257–63.

15. Williams CH, Witherly SA, Buddington, RK. Influence of dietary neosugar on selected bacterial groups of the human faecal microbiota. *Microb Ecol Health Dis* 1994;7:91–97.

Arginine

1. Park KGM. The immunological and metabolic effects of l-arginine in human cancer. *Proc Nutr Soc* 1993;52:387–401.

2. Takeda Y, Tominga T, Tei N, et al. Inhibitory effect of L-arginine on growth of rat mammary tumors induced by 7,12,Dimethylbenz(a)anthracine. *Cancer Res* 1975;35:2390–3.

BCAAs (Branched-Chain Amino Acids)

1. Plaitakis A, Smith J, Mandeli J, et al. Pilot trial of branched-chain amino acids in amyotrophic lateral sclerosis. *Lancet* May 7, 1988:1015–18.

2. Wahren J, Denis J, Desurmont P, et al. Is intravenous administration of branched chain amino acids effective in the treatment of hepatic encephalopathy? A multicenter study. *Hepatology* 1983; 3(4):475–80.

3. Kelly GS. Sports nutrition: A review of selected nutritional supplements for bodybuilders and strength athletes. *Alt Med Rev* 1997;2 (3):184–201.

4. MacLean DA, Graham TE, Satlin B. Branched-chain amino acids augment ammonia metabolism while attenuating protein breakdown during exercise. *Am J Physiol* 1994;267:E1010–22.

5. Blomstrand E, Hassmen P, Ek S, et al. Influence of ingesting a solution of branched-chain amino acids on perceived exertion during exercise. *Acta Physiol Scand* 1997;159:41–49.

6. Van Hall G, Rasymakers JSH, Saris WHM, Wagenmakers AJM. Supplementation with branched-chain amino acids (BCAA) and tryptophan has no effect on performance during prolonged exercise. *Clin Sci* 1994;87:52 (abstract #75).

Betaine Hydrochloride

1. Giannella RA, Broitman SA, Zamcheck N. Influence of gastric acidity on bacterial and parasitic enteric infections. *Ann Int Med* 1973;78:271–76.

2. Giannella RA, Broitman SA, Zamcheck N. Influence of gastric acidity on bacterial and parasitic enteric infections. *Ann Int Med* 1973;78:271–76.

3. Kokkonen J, Simila S, Herva R. Impaired gastric function in children with cow's milk intolerance. *Eur J Ped* 1979; 132:1–6.

4. Gillespie M. Hypochlorhydria in asthma with specific reference to the age incidence. *Quart J Med* 1935;4:397–405.

5. Fravel RC. The occurrence of hypochlorhydria in gall-bladder disease. *Am J Med Sci* 1920;159:512–17.

6. Murray MJ, Stein N. A gastric factor promoting iron absorption. *Lancet* 1968; 1:614.

7. Russell RM et al. Correction of impaired folic acid (Pte Glu) absorption by orally administered HCl in subjects with gastric atrophy. *Am J Clin Nutr* 1984; 39:656.

8. Ivanovich P et al. The absorption of calcium carbonate. *Ann Intern Med* 1967; 66:917.

Bioflavonoids

1. Vinson JA, Bose P. Comparative bioavailability to humans of ascorbic acid alone or in a citrus extract. *Am J Clin Nutr* 1988;48:601–4.

2. Vinson JA, Bose P. Comparative bioavailability of synthetic and natural vitamin C in Guinea pigs. *Nutr Rep Intl* 1983;27(4):875.

Biotin

1. Said HM, Redha R, Nylander W. Biotin transport in the human intestine: Inhibition by anticonvulsant drugs. *Am J Clin Nutr* 1989;49:127–31.

2. Coggeshall JC et al. Biotin status and plasma glucose in diabetics. *Ann NY Acad Sci* 1985;447:389.

3. Koutsikos D, Agroyannis B, Tzanatos-Exarchou H. Biotin for diabetic peripheral neuropathy. *Biomed Pharmacother* 1990;44:511–14.

4. Hochman LG, Scher RK, Meyerson MS. Brittle nails: Responses to daily biotin supplementation. *Cutis* 1993;51(4): 303–5.

5. Somer E. *The Essential Guide to Vitamins and Minerals.* New York: Harper, 1995, 70–72.

Boron

1. Nielsen FH. Facts and fallacies about boron. *Nutr Today* May/Jun 1992: 6–12.

2. Nielsen FH, Hunt CD, Mullen LM, Hunt JR. Effect of dietary boron on mineral, estrogen, and testosterone metabolism in postmenopausal women. *FASEB J* 1987;1:394–97.

Brewer's Yeast

1. Eng RHK, Dehmel R, Smith SM, Goldstein EJC. Saccharomyces cerevisiae infections in man. *Sabouraudia* 1984; 22:403–7.

Calcium

1. Heaney RP, Recker RR, Weaver CM. Absorbability of calcium sources: The limited role of solubility. *Calcific Tissue Int* 1990;46:300–4.

2. Miller J, Smith D, Flora L, et al. Calcium absorption from calcium carbonate and a new form of calcium (CCM) in healthy male and female adolescents. *Am J Clin Nutr* 1988;48:1291–94.

3. Mortensen L, Charles P. Bioavailability of calcium supplements and the effect of vitamin D: Comparisons between milk, calcium carbonate, and calcium carbonate plus vitamin D. *Am J Clin Nutr* 1996;63:354–57.

4. Sheikh M, Santa Ana C, Nicar M, et al. Gastrointestinal absorption of calcium from milk and calcium salts. *New Engl J Med* 1987;317:532–36.

5. Kohls K, Kies C. Calcium bioavailability: A comparison of several different commercially available calcium supplements. *J Appl Nutr* 1992;44:50–62.

Carnitine

1. Giamberardino MA et al. Effects of prolonged L-carnitine administration on delayed muscle pain and CK release after eccentric effort. *Int J Sports Med* 1996; 17:320–24.

2. Dipalma JR. Carnitine deficiency. *Am Family Phys* 1988;38:243–51.

3. Kendler BS. Carnitine: An overview of its role in preventive medicine. *Prev Med* 1986;15:373–90.

4. Del Favero A. Carnitine and gangliosides. *Lancet* 1988;ii:337 (letter).

Cartilage

1. Prudden FJ, Allen J. The clinical acceleration of healing with a cartilage application. *JAMA* 1965;192:352–56.

2. Prudden JF, Wolarsky E. The reversal by cartilage of the steroid-induced inhibition of wound healing. *Surg Gyn Obset* 1967;125(7):109–13.

3. Prudden JF. The treatment of human cancer with agents prepared from bovine cartilage. *J Biol Res Mod* 1985; 4:551–84.

4. Lee A, Langer R. Shark cartilage contains inhibitors of tumor angiogenesis. *Science* 1983;221:1185–87.

5. Lane IW, Contreras E Jr. High rate of bioactivity (reduction in gross tumor size) observed in advanced cancer patients treated with shark cartilage material. *J Naturopathic Med* 1992;3:86–8.

6. Prudden JF. The treatment of human cancer with agents prepared from bovine cartilage. *J Biol Resp Modif* 1985; 4:551–84.

Chlorophyll

1. Rudolph C. The therapeutic value of chlorophyll. *Clin Med Surg* 1930; 37:119–21.

2. Chernomorsky SA, Segelman AB. Biological activities of chlorophyll derivatives. *N J Med* 1988;85:669–73.

3. Gruskin B. Chlorophyll—its therapeutic place in acute and suppurative disease. *Am J Surg* 1940;49:49–56.

4. Hayatsu H, Negishi T, Arimoto S, et al. Porphyrins as potential inhibitors against exposure to carcinogens and mutagens. *Mutat Res* 1993;290:79–85.

Chondroitin Sulfate

1. Izuka K, Murata K, Nakazawa K, et al. Effects of chondroitin sulfates on serum lipids and hexosamines in atherosclerotic patients: With special reference to thrombus formation time. *JpnHeart J* 1968;9:453–60.

2. Morrison LM, Bajwa GS, Alfin-Slater RB, Ershoff BH. Prevention of vascular lesions by chondroitin sulfate A in the coronary artery and aorta of rats induced by a hypervitaminosis D, cholesterol-containing diet. *Atherosclerosis* 1972;16:105–18.

3. Morrison LM, Branwood AW, Ershoff BH, et al. The prevention of coronary arteriosclerotic heart disease with chondroitin sulfate A: Preliminary report. *Exp Med Surg* 1969;27:278–89.

4. Morrison LM, Enrick NL. Coronary heart disease: Reduction of death rate by chondroitin sulfate A. *Angiology* 1973; 24:269–82.

5. Moss M, Kruger GO, Reynolds DC. The effect of chondroitin sulfate on bone healing. *Oral Surg Oral Med Oral Pathol* 1965;20:795–801.

6. Kerzberg EM, Roldan EJA, Castelli G, Huberman ED. Combination of glycosaminoglycans and acetylsalicylic acid in knee osteoarthritis. *Scand J Rheum* 1987;16:377.

Chromium

1. Page TG, Ward TL, and Southern LL. Effect of chromium picolinate on growth and carcass characteristics of growing-finishing pigs. *J Animal Sci* 1991; 69:356.

2. Lefavi R, Anderson R, Keith R, et al. Efficacy of chromium supplementation in athletes: Emphasis on anabolism. *Int J Sport Nutr* 1992;2:111–22.

3. McCarty MF. The case for supplemental chromium and a survey of clinical studies with chromium picolinate. *J Appl Nutr* 1991;43:59–66.

4. Hallmark MA, Reynolds TH, DeSouza CA, et al. Effects of chromium and resistive training on muscle strength and body composition. *Medicine and Science in Sports and Exercise* 1996;28:139–44.

5. Sterns DM, Belbruno JJ, Wetterhahn KE. A prediction of chromium (III) accumulation in humans from chromium dietary supplements. *FASEB J* 1995;9: 1650–57.

6. Sterns DM, Wise JP, Patierno SR, Wetterhahn KE. Chromium (III) picolinate produces chromosome damage in Chinese hamster ovary cells. *FASEB J* 1995;9:1643–49.

7. Garland M, Morris JS, Colditz GA, et al. Toenail trace element levels and breast cancer. *Am J Epidemiol* 1996; 144:653–60.

8. Offenbacher EG. Promotion of chromium absorption by ascorbic acid. *Trace Elements Electrolytes* 1994;11: 178–81.

Creatine

1. Greenhaff PL, Bodin K, Soderlund K, et al. Effect of oral creatine supplementation on skeletal muscle phosphocreatine resynthesis. *Am J Physiol* 1994; 266:E725–30.

2. Greenhaff PL. Creatine and its application as an ergogenic aid. *Int J Sport Nutr* 1995;5:94–101.

3. Earnest CP, Snell PG, Rodriguez R, et al. The effect of creatine monohydrate ingestion on anaerobic power indices, muscular strength, and body composition. *Acta Physiol Scand* 1995;153:207–9.

4. Kelly GS. Sports nutrition: A review of selected nutritional supplements for bodybuilders and strength athletes. *Alt Med Rev* 1997;2(3):184–201.

Cysteine

1. Salim AS. Sulfhydryl-containing agents in the treatment of gastric bleeding induced by nonsteroidal anti-inflammatory drugs. *Can J Surgery* 1993;36:53–58.

2. Droge W, Eck HP, Gander H, Mihm S. Modulation of lymphocyte functions and immune responses by cysteine and cysteine derivatives. *Am J Med* 1991; 91(suppl 3C):140S–44S.

3. Eck HP, Gander H, Hartmann M, et al. Low concentrations of acid-soluble thiol (cysteine) in the blood plasma of HIV-1 infected patients. *Biol Chem Hoppe Seyler* 1989;370:101–8.

4. Droge W, Eck HP, Mihm S. HIV-induced cysteine deficiency and T-cell dysfunction—a rationale for treatment with N-acetylcysteine. *Immunol Today* 1992; 13:211–14.

5. Droge W. Cysteine and glutathione deficiency in AIDS patients: A rationale for the treatment with N-acetyl-cysteine. *Pharmacol* 1993;46:61–65.

Dehydroepiandrosterone (DHEA)

1. Labrie F, Belanger A, Simard J, et al. DHEA and peripheral androgen and estrogen formation: Intracrinology. *Ann NY Acad Sci* 1995;774:16–28.

2. Ebeling P, Koivisto VA. Physiological importance of dehydroepiandrosterone. *Lancet* 1994;343:1479–81.

3. Weinstein RE, Lobocki CA, Gravett S, et al. Decreased adrenal sex steroid in the absence of glucocorticoid suppression in postmenopausal asthmatic women. *J Allerg Clin Immol* 1996;97:1–8.

4. Wolkowitz OM, Reus VI, Roberts E, et al. Antidepressant and cognition-enhancing effects of DHEA in major depression. *Ann NY Acad Sci* 1995;774:337–39.

5. Gaby AR. Research review. *Nutr Healing* Jun 1997:8.

6. Casson PR, Faquin LC, Stentz FB, et al. Replacement of dehydroepiandrosterone enhances T-lymphocyte insulin binding in postmenopausal women. *Fertil Steril* 1995;63:1027–31.

7. Zumoff B et al. Abnormal 24-hr mean plasma concentrations of dehydroisoandrosterone and dehydroandrosterone sulfate in women with primary operable breast cancer. *Canc Res* 1981; 41:3360–63.

Proteolytic Enzymes

1. Oelgoetz AW, Oelgoetz PA, Wittenkind J. The treatment of food allergy and indigestion of pancreatic origin with pancreatic enzymes. *Am J Dig Dis Nutr* 1935;2:422–26.

2. McCann M. Pancreatic enzyme supplement for treatment of multiple food allergies. *Ann Allerg* 1993;71:269 (abstract #17).

3. Ambrus JL, Lassman HB, DeMarchi JJ. Absorption of exogenous and endogenous proteolytic enzymes. *Clin Pharmacol Ther* 1967;8:362–68.

4. Avakian S. Further studies on the absorption of chymotrypsin. *Clin Pharmacol Ther* 1964;5:712–15.

5. Izaka K, Yamada M, Kawano T, Suyama T. Gastrointestinal absorption and anti-inflammatory effect of bromelain. *Japan J Pharmacol* 1972;22:519–34.

6. Deitrick RE. Oral proteolytic enzymes in the treatment of athletic injuries: A double-blind study. *Pennsylvania Med J* Oct 1965:35–37.

7. Seligman B. Bromelain: An anti-inflammatory agent. *Angiology* 1962;13:508–10.

8. Cichoke AJ. The effect of systemic enzyme therapy on cancer cells and the immune system. *Townsend Letter for Doctors and Patients* Nov 1995:30–32 (review).

9. Wolf M, Ransberger K. *Enzyme Therapy*. New York: Vantage Press, 1972, 135–220 (review).

10. Kleine MW, Stauder GM, Beese EW. The intestinal absorption of orally administered hydrolytic enzymes and their effects in the treatment of acute herpes zoster as compared with those of oral acyclovir therapy. *Phytomedicine* 1995; 2:7–15.

11. Heinicke R, van der Wal L, Yokoyama M. Effect of bromelain (Ananase) on human platelet aggregation. *Experientia* 1972;28:844–45.

12. Gullo L. Indication for pancreatic enzyme treatment in non-pancreatic digestive diseases. *Digestion* 1993;54(suppl 2):43–47.

13. Gaby AR. The story of bromelain. *Nutr Healing* May 1995:3,4,11.

14. Layer P, Groger G. Fate of pancreatic enzymes in the human intestinal lumen in health and pancreatic insufficiency. *Digestion* 1993;54(suppl 2):10–14.

Evening Primrose Oil

1. Horrobin DF. The importance of gamma-linolenic acid and prostaglandin E1 in human nutrition and medicine. *J Holistic Med* 1981;3:118–39.

2. Horrobin DF, Manku M, Brush M, et al. Abnormalities in plasma essential fatty acid levels in women with pre-menstrual syndrome and with non-malignant breast disease. *J Nutr Med* 1991;2:259–64.

3. Kleen H, Payan J, Allawi J, et al. Treatment of diabetic neuropathy with gamma-linolenic acid. *Diabetes Care* 1993;16:8–15 (reviews).

4. Manku MS, Horrobin DF, Morse NL, et al. Essential fatty acids in the plasma phospholipids of patients with atopic eczema. *Brit J Derm* 1984;110:643.

Fish Oil

1. Braden LM, Carroll KK. Dietary polyunsaturated fat in relation to mammary carcinogenesis in rats. *Lipids* 1986; 21(4):285.

2. O'Connor TP et al. Effect of dietary intake of fish oil and fish protein on the development of L-azaserine-induced preneoplastic lesions in the rat pancreas. *J Natl Cancer Inst* 1985;75(5):959–62.

3. Gonzalez MJ. Fish oil, lipid peroxidation and mammary tumor growth. *J Am Coll Nutr* 1995;14:325.

4. Zhu ZR, Mannisto JAS, Pietinene P, et al. Fatty acid composition of breast adipose tissue in breast cancer patients and patients with benign breast disease. *Nutr Cancer* 1995;24:151–60.

5. Leaf A, Weber PC. Cardiovascular effects of n-3 fatty acids. *N Engl J Med* 1988;318:549–57.

6. Malasanos TH, Stacpoole PW. Biological effects of omega-3 fatty acids in diabetes mellitus. *Diabetes Care* 1991; 14:1160–79.

7. Schectman G, Kaul S, Kassebah AH. Effect of fish oil concentrate on lipoprotein composition in NIDDM. *Diabetes* 1988; 37:1567–73.

8. Toft I, Bonaa KH, Ingebretsen OC, et al. Effects of n-3 polyunsaturated fatty acids on glucose homeostasis and blood pressure in essential hypertension. *Ann Intern Med* 1995;123:911–18.

9. Harris WS, Zucker ML, Dujovne CA. Omega-3 fatty acids in type IV hyperlipidemia: Fish oils vs methyl esters. *Am J Clin Nutr* 1987;45(4):858 (abstract).

10. Clarke JTR, Cullen-Dean G, Reglink E, et al. Increased incidence of epistaxis in adolescents with familial hypercholesterolemia treated with fish oil. *J Pediatr* 1990;116:139–41.

11. Piche LA, Draper HH, Cole PD. Malondialdehyde excretion by subjects consuming cod liver oil vs a concentrate of n-3 fatty acids. *Lipids* 1988;23:370–71.

12. Wander RC, Du S-H, Ketchum SO, Rowe KE. Effects of interaction of RRR-a-tocopheryl acetate and fish oil on low-density-lipoprotein oxidation in postmenopausal women with and without hormone-replacement therapy. *Am J Clin Nutr* 1996;63:184–93.

13. Luostarinen R, Wallin R, Wibell L, et al. Vitamin E supplementaion counteracts the fish oil-induced increase of blood glucose in humans. *Nutr Res* 1995;15:953–68.

14. Dunstan DW, Burke V, Mori TA, et al. The independent and combined effects of aerobic exercise and dietary fish intake on serum lipids and glycemic control in NIDDM. *Diabetes Care* 1997;20:913–21.

15. Sheehan JP, Wei IW, Ulchaker M, Tserng K-Y. Effect of high fiber intake in fish oil-treated patients with non-insulin-dependent diabetes mellitus. *Am J Clin Nutr* 1997;66:1183–7.

16. Adler AJ, Holub BJ. Effect of garlic and fish oil supplementation on serum lipid and lipoprotein concentrations in hypercholesterolemic men. *Am J Clin Nutr* 1997; 65:445–50.

Flaxseed Oil

1. de Lorgeril M, Renaud S, Maelle N, et al. Mediterranean alpha-linolenic acid-rich diet in secondary prevention of coronary heart disease. *Lancet* 1994; 343:1454–59.

2. Rice RD. Mediterranean diet. *Lancet* 1994;344:893–94 (letter).

3. Kelley DS, Nelson GJ, Love JE, et al. Dietary a-linolenic acid alters tissue fatty acid composition, but not blood lipids, lipoproteins or coagulation status in humans. *Lipids* 1993;28:533–37.

4. Abbey M, Clifton P, Kestin M, et al. Effect of fish oil on lipoproteins, lecithin:cholesterol acyltransferase, and lipid transfer protein activity in humans. *Arterioscler* 1990;10:85–94.

5. Chan JK, Bruce VM, McDonald BE. Dietary a-linolenic acid is as effective as oleic acid and linoleic acid in lowering blood cholesterol in normolipidemic men. *Am J Clin Nutr* 1991;53:1230–34.

6. James MJ, Rheumatology Unit, Royal Adelaid Hospital, South Australia. Correspondence Nov 15, 1994.

7. Singer P, Jaeger W, Berger I, et al. Effects of dietary oleic, linoleic and a-linolenic acids on blood pressure, serum lipids, lipoproteins and the formation of eicosanoid precursors in patients with mild essential hypertension. *J Human Hypertension* 1990;4:227–33.

8. Sanders TAB, Roshanai F. The influence of different types of omega 3 polyunsaturated fatty acids on blood lipids and platelet function in healthy volunteers. *Clin Sci* 1983;64:91.

9. Mantzioris E, James MJ, Gibson RA, Cleland LG. Dietary substitution with alpha-linolenic acid-rich vegetable oil increases eicosapentaenoic acid concentrations in tissues. *Am J Clin Nutr* 1994; 59:1304–9.

10. Indu M, Ghafoorunissa. n-3 fatty acids in Indian diets: Comparison of the effects of precursor (alpha-linolenic acid) vs product (long-chain n-3 polyunsaturated fatty acids). *Nutr Res* 1992;12:569–82.

Folic Acid

1. Daly LE, Kirke PN, Molloy A, et al. Folate levels and neural tube defects. *JAMA* 1995;274:1698–1702.

2. Shaw GM, O'Malley CD, Wasserman CR, et al. Maternal periconceptional use of multivitamins and reduced risk for conotruncal heart defects and limb deficiencies among offspring. *Am J Med Genetics* 1995;59:536–45.

3. Tolarova M. Periconceptional supplementation with vitamins and folic acid to prevent recurrence of cleft lip. *Lancet* 1982;ii:217 (letter).

4. Shaw GM, Lammer EJ, Wasserman CR, et al. Risks of orofacial clefts in children born to women using multivitamins containing folic acid periconceptionially. *Lancet* 1995;345:393–96.

5. Hayes C, Werler MM, Willett WC, Mitchell AA. Case-control study of periconceptional folic acid supplementation and oral clefts. *Am J Epidemiol* 1996; 143:1229–34.

6. Russel RM. A minimum of 13,500 deaths annually from coronary artery disease could be prevented by increasing folate intake to reduce homocysteine levels. *J Am Med Assoc* 1996;275:1828–29.

7. Butterworth CE Jr, Tamura T. Folic acid safety and toxicity: A brief review. *Am J Clin Nutr* 1989;50:353–58.

8. Wald NJ, Bower C. Folic acid, pernicious anaemia, and prevention of neural tube defects. *Lancet* 1994;343:307.

9. Russell RM, Golner BB, Krasinski SD, et al. Effect of antacid and H2 receptor antagonists on the intestinal absorption of folic acid. *J Lab Clin Med* 1988; 112:458–63.

10. Russell RM, Dutta SK, Oaks EV, et al. Impairment of folic acid absorption by oral pancreatic extracts. *Dig Dis Sci* 1980; 25:369–73.

Gamma Oryzanol

1. Rosenbloom C, Millard-Stafford M, Lathrop J. Contemporary ergogenic aids used by strength/power athletes. *J Am Diet Assoc* 1992;92(10):1264–65.

Histidine

1. Gerber DA et al. Specificity of a low free histidine concentration for rheumatoid arthritis. *J Chron Dis* 1977;30:115.

Hydroxycitric Acid

1. Lowenstein JM. Effect of (-)-hydroxycitrate on fatty acid synthesis by rat liver in vivo. *J Biol Chem* 1971; 246(3):629–32.

2. Triscari J, Sullivan AC. Comparative effects of (-)-hydroxycitrate and (=)-allo-hydroxycitrate on acetyl CoA carboxylase and fatty acid and cholesterol synthesis in vivo. *Lipids* 1977;12(4):357–63.

3. Cheema-Dhadli S, Harlperin ML, Leznoff CC. Inhibition of enzymes which interact with citrate by (-)hydroxycitrate and 1,2,3,-tricarboxybenzene. *Eur J Biochem* 1973;38:98–102.

4. Sullivan AC, Hamilton JG, Miller ON, et al. Inhibition of lipogenesis in rat liver by (-)-hydroxycitrate. *Arch Biochem Biophys* 1972;150:183–90.

5. Greenwood MRC, Cleary MP, Gruen R, et al. Effect of (-)-hydroxycitrate on development of obesity in the Zucker obese rat. *Am J Phys* 1981;240:E72–78.

6. Sullivan AC, Triscari J. Metabolic regulation as a control for lipid disorders. *Am J Clin Nutr* 1977;30:767–76.

7. Sullivan AC, Triscari J, Hamilton JG, et al. Effect of (-)-hydroxycitrate upon the accumulation of lipid in the rat: I. Lipogenesis. *Lipids* 1974;9:121–28.

8. Sullivan AC, Triscari J, Hamilton JG, et al. Effect of (-)-hydroxycitrate upon

the accumulation of lipid in the rat. II. Appetite. *Lipids* 1974;9(2):129–34.

9. Sergio W. A natural food, malabar tamarind, may be effective in the treatment of obesity. *Medi Hyp* 1988;27:40.

Inosine

1. Starling RD, Trappe TA, Short KR, et al. Effect of inosine supplementation on aerobic and anaerobic cycling performance. *Med Sci Sports Ex* 1996;28(9): 1193–98.

2. Rosenbloom D, Millard-Stafford M, Lathrop J. Contemporary erogenic aids used by strength/power athletes. *J Am Diet Assoc* 1992;92(10):1264–66.

3. Starling RD, Trappe TA, Short KR, et al. Effect of inosine supplementation on aerobic and anaerobic cycling performance. *Med Sci Sports Ex* 1996;28(9): 1193–98.

Iodine

1. Mu L, Derun L, Chengyi Q, et al. Endemic goiter in central China caused by excessive iodine intake. *Lancet* 1987; ii:257–59.

2. Pennington JA. A review of iodine toxicity reports. *J Am Dietet Assoc* 1990; 1571–81.

3. Barker DJP, Phillips DIW. Current incidence of thyrotoxicosis and past prevalence of goiter in 12 British towns. *Lancet* 1984;ii:567–70.

4. Williams ED, Doniach I, Bjarnason O, et al. Thyroid cancer in an iodide rich area. *Cancer* 1977;39:215–22.

Ionized Air

1. Gualtierotti R, Solimene U, Tonoli D. Ionized air respiratory rehabilitation technics. *Minerva Medica* 1977; 68:3383–89.

2. Jones DP, O'Connor SA, Collins JV, et al. Effect of long-term ionized air treatment on patients with bronchial asthma. *Thorax* 1976;31(4):428–32.

3. JG Llaurado, A Sances, JH Battocletti. Biologic and clinical effects of low-frequency magnetic and electric fields. Springfield, IL: Charles C. Thomas, 1974.

4. Soyka F, Edmonds A. *The Ion Effect*. New York: Bantam, 1977.

5. Jonathan V Wright, MD, personal correspondence with author. April 1997.

Iron

1. Sullivan JL. Stored iron and ischemic heart disease. *Circulation* 1992;86:1036 (editorial).

2. Cutler P. Deferoxamine therapy in high-ferritin diabetes. *Diabetes* 1989; 38:1207–10.

3. Stevens RG, Graubard BI, Micozzi MS, et al. Moderate elevation of body iron level and increased risk of cancer occurrence and death. *Int J Cancer* 1994; 56:364–69.

4. Weinberg ED. Iron withholding: a defense against infection and neoplasia. *Am J Physiol* 1984;64:65–102.

5. Oh VMS. Iron dextran and systemic lupus erythematosus. *BMJ* 1992;305:1000 (letter).

6. Dabbagh AJ, Trenam CW, Morris CJ, Blake DR. Iron in joint inflammation. *Ann Rheum Dis* 1993;52:67–73.

7. Hunt JR, Gallagher SK, Johnson LK. Effect of ascorbic acid on apparent iron absorption by women with low iron stores. *Am J Clin Nutr* 1994;59:1381–85.

8. Suharno D, West CE, Muhilal, et al. Supplementation with vitamin A and iron for nutritional anemia in pregnant women in West Java, Indonesia. *Lancet* 1993; 342:1325–28.

9. Semba RD, Muhilal, West KP Jr, et al. Impact of vitamin A supplementation on hematological indicators of iron metabolism and protein status in children. *Nutr Res* 1992;12:469–78.

Lactase

1. Gudmand-Hoyer E. The clinical significance of disaccharide maldigestion. *Am J Clin Nutr* 1994;59(3):735S–41S.

2. Ratner D, Shoshani E, Dubnov B. Milk protein-free diet for nonseasonal asthma and migraine in lactase-deficient patients. *Israel J Med Sci* 1983;19(9): 806–9.

3. Wheadon M, Goulding A, Barbezat GO, et al. Lactose malabsorption and calcium intake as risk factors for osteoporosis in elderly New Zealand women. *New Zea Med J* 1991;104:417–19.

Leucine

1. Bruzzone P, Siegel JH, Chiarla C, et al. Leucine dose response in the reduction of urea production from septic proteolysis and in the stimulation of acute-phase proteins. *Surgery* 1991;109:768–78.

2. Berry HK, Brunner RL, Hunt MM, White PP. Valine, isoleucine, and leucine. A new treatment for phenylketonuria. *Am J Dis Child* 1990;144:539–43.

3. Zello GA, Wykes LF, Ball RO, et al. Recent advances in methods of assessing

dietary amino acid requirements for adult humans. *J Nutr* 1995;125:2907–15.

Lycopene

1. Giovannucci E, Ascherio A, Rimm EB, et al. Intake of carotenoids and retinol in relation to risk of prostate cancer. *JNCI* 1995;87:1767–76.

2. Mills PK, Beeson WL, Phillips RL, Fraser GE. Cohort study of diet, lifestyle, and prostate cancer in Adventist men. *Cancer* 1989;64:598–604.

3. Carter HB, Coffey DS. The prostate: An increasing medical problem. *Prostate* 1990;16:39–48.

4. Hsing AW, Comstock GW, Abbey H, Polk F. Serologic precursors of cancer. Retinol, carotenoids, and tocopherol and risk of prostate cancer. *JNCI* 1990;82: 941–46.

5. Levy J, Bosin E, Feldman B, Giat Y, et al. Lycopene is a more potent inhibitory of human cancer cell proliferation than either beta-carotene or beta-carotene. *Nutr Cancer* 1995;24:257–66.

6. Franceshci S, Bidoli E, La Vecchia C, et al. Tomatoes and risk of digestive-tract cancers. *Int J Cancer* 1994;59:181–84.

7. Van Eenwyk J, Davis FG, Bowne PE. Dietary and serum carotenoids and cervical intraepithelial neoplasia. *Int J Cancer* 1991;48:34–38.

8. Wahlqvist ML et al. Changes in serum carotenoids in subjects with colorectal adenomas after 24 months of beta-carotene supplementation. Australian Polyp Prevention Investigators. *Am J Clin Nutr* 1994;60:936–43.

Lysine

1. Civitelli R, Villareal DT, Agneusdei D, et al. Dietary L-lysine and calcium metabolism in humans. *Nutrition* 1992; 8:400–4.

2. Pauling L. Case report: Lysine/ascorbate-related amelioration of angina pectoris. *J Orthomol Med* 1991;6:144–46.

3. Kritchevsky D, Weber MM, Klurfeld DM. Gallstone formation in hamsters: Influence of specific amino acids. *Nutr Rep Internat* 1984;29:117.

4. Leszczynski DE, Kummerow FA. Excess dietary lysine induces hypercholesterolemia in chickens. *Experientia* 1982; 38:266–67.

Manganese

1. Freeland-Graves JH. Manganese: An essential nutrient for humans. *Nutr Today* 1989;23:13–19 (review).

2. Krieger D, Krieger S, Jansen O, et al. Manganese and chronic hepatic encephalopathy. *Lancet* 1995;346:270–74.

Medium Chain Triglycerides

1. Jeukendrup AE, Saris WHM, van Diesen RAJ, et al. Exogenous MCT oxidation from carbohydrate-medium chain triglyceride supplements during moderate intensity exercise. *Clin Sci* 1994;87:33.

Melatonin

1. Zhadanova IV, Wurtman RJ, Lynch HJ, et al. Sleep-inducing effects of low doses of melatonin ingested in the evening. *Clin Pharmacol Ther* 1995;57:552–58.

2. Waldhauser F, Saletu B, Trinchard-Lugan I. Sleep laboratory investigations on hypnotic properties of melatonin. *Psychopharmacology* 1990;100(2):222–26.

3. Petrie K, Dawson AG, Thompson L, et al. A double-blind trial of melatonin as a treatment for jet lag in international cabin crew. *Bio Psych* 1993;33(7):526–30.

4. Samples RJ et al. Effect of melatonin on intraocular pressure. *Curr Eye Res* 1988;7:649–53.

5. Haimov I, Laudon M, Zisapel N, et al. Sleep disorders and melatonin rhythms in elderly people. *BMJ* 1994;309:167.

6. Singer C, McArthur A, Hughes R, et al. Melatonin and sleep in the elderly. *J Am Geriatr Soc* 1996;44:51 (abstract #A1).

7. Attenburrow MEJ, Dowling BA, Sharpley AL, Cowen PJ. Case-control study of evening melatonin concentration in primary insomnia. *BMJ* 1996;312:1263–64.

8. Folkard S, Arendt J, and Clark M. Can melatonin improve shift workers' tolerance of the night shift? Some preliminary findings. *Chronobio Intern* 1993;10(5):315–20.

9. Garfinkel D, Laudon M, Nof D, Zisapel N. Improvement of sleep quality in elderly people by controlled-release melatonin. *Lancet* 1995;346:541–44.

Methionine

1. Garrison R, Somer E. *The Nutrition Desk Reference*. New Canaan, CT: Keats Publishing, 1995, 41.

2. Toborek M, Hennig B. Is methionine an atherogenic amino acid? *J Opt Nutr* 1994;3(2):80–83.

N-Acetyl Cysteine

1. de Quay B, Malinverni R, Lauterburg BH. Glutathione depletion in HIV-infected patients: Role of cysteine deficiency and effect of oral N-acetylcysteine. *AIDS* 1992;6:815–19.

2. Kleinveld HA, Demacker PNM, Stalenhoef AFH. Failure of N-acetylcysteine to reduce low-density lipoprotein oxidizability in healthy subjects. *Eur J Clin Pharmacol* 1992;43:639–42.

3. Brumas V, Hacht B, Filella M, Berthon G. Can N-acetyl-L-cysteine affect zinc metabolism when used as a paracetamol antidote? *Agents Actions* 1992;36:278–88.

Ornithine

1. Bucci LR, Hickson JF, Wolinsky I, et al. Ornithine supplementation and insulin release in bodybuilders. *Int J Sport Nutr* 1992;2:287–91.

2. Varanasi RV, Saltzman JR. Ornithine oxoglutarate therapy improves nutrition status. *Nutr Rev* 1995;53(4):96–102.

Ornithine Alpha-Ketoglutarate

1. Jeevanandam M, Holaday NJ, Petersen SR. Ornithine-alpha-ketoglutarate (OKG) supplementation is more effective than its component salts in traumatized rats. *J Nutr* 1996;126(9):2141–50.

2. Le Bricon T, Cynober L, Baracos VE. Ornithine alpha-ketoglutarate limits muscle protein breakdown without stimulating tumor growth in rats bearing Yoshida ascites hepatoma. *Met Clin Exp* 1994;43(7):899–905.

PABA

1. Wiesel LL et al. The synergistic action of para-aminobenzoic acid and cortisone in the treatment of rheumatoid arthritis. *Am J Med Sci* 1951;222:243–48.

2. Sieve BF. The clinical effects of a new B-complex factor, para-aminobenzoic acid, on pigmentation and fertility. *South Med Surg* 1942(March);104:135–39.

3. Zarafonetis CJD. The treatment of scleroderma: Results of potassium para-aminobenzoate therapy in 104 cases. In *Inflammation and Diseases of Connective Tissue*, ed. LC Mills, JH Moyer. W. B. Saunders Co., 1961, 688–96.

4. Zarafonetis CJD et al. Retrospective studies in scleroderma: Effect of potassium para-aminobenzoate on survival. *J Clin Epidemiol* 1988;41:193–205.

5. Grace WJ et al. Therapy of scleroderma and dermatomyositis. *NY State J Med* 1963;63:140–44.

6. Zarafonetis CJD. Treatment of Peyronie's disease with potassium para-aminobenzoate. *J Urol* 1959;81:770–72.

7. Zarafonetis CJD et al. Treatment of pemphigus with potassium para-aminobenzoate. *Am J Med Sci* 1956;231:30–50.

8. Zarafonetis CJD. Darkening of gray hair during para-amino-benzoic acid therapy. *J Invest Dermatol* 1950;15:399–401.

Pantothenic Acid

1. Fidanza A. Therapeutic action of pantothenic acid. *Int J Vit Nutr Res* 1983; suppl 24:53–67 (review).

Phenylalanine

1. Sabelli HC. Clinical studies on the phenylethylamine hypothesis of affective disorder: Urine and blood phenylacetic acid and phenylalanine dietary supplements. *J Clin Psychiatry* 1986;47:66–70.

2. Fischer E et al. Therapy of depression by phenylalanine. *Arzneimittelforsch* 1975;25:132.

3. Heller B et al. Therapeutic action of D-phenylalanine in Parkinson's disease. *Arzneimittelforsch* 1976;26:577–79.

4. Budd K. Use of D-phenylalanine, an enkephalinase inhibitor, in the treatment of intractable pain. *Adv Pain Res Ther* 1983;5:305–8.

5. Anonymous. Phenylalanine fails to help chronic back pain patients. *Family Pract News* 1987;17(3):37.

Phosphatidylserine

1. Crook TH, Tinklenberg J, Yesavage J, et al. Effects of phosphatidylserine in age-associated memory impairment. *Neurology* 1991;41:644–49.

2. Crook T et al. Effects of phosphatidylserine in Alzheimer's disease. *Psychopharmacol Bull* 1992;28:61–66.

Proanthocyanidins

1. Mitcheva M et al. Biochemical and morphological studies on the effects of anthocyans and vitamin E on carbon tetrachloride induced liver injury. *Cell Mol Bio* 1993;39(4):443–48.

2. Maffei F et al. Free radical scavenging action and anti-enzyme activities of procyanidines from *Vitis vinifera*. A mechanism for their capillary protective action. *Arzn Forsch* 1994;44:592–601.

Pyruvate

1. Stanko RT, Tietze DL, Arch JE. Body composition, energy utilization, and nitro-

gen metabolism with a 4.25-MJ/d low-energy diet supplemented with pyruvate. *Am J Clin Nutr* 1992;56(4):630–35.

2. Stanko RT, Reynolds HR, Hoyson R, et al. Pyruvate supplementation of a low-cholesterol, low-fat diety: Effects on plasma lipid concentration and body composition in hyperlipidemic patients. *Am J Clin Nutr* 1994;59:423–27.

3. Ivy JL, Cortez MY, Chandler RM, et al. Effects of pyruvate on the metabolism and insulin resistance of obese Zucker rats. *Am J Clin Nutr* 1994;59:331–37.

4. Stanko RT, Robertson RJ, Galbreath RW, et al. Enhanced leg exercise endurance with a high-carbohydrate diet and dihyroxyacetone and pyruvate. *J Appl Phys* 1990;69(5):1651–56.

5. Stanko RT, Robertson RJ, Spina RJ, et al. Enhancement of arm exercise endurance capacity with dihydroxyacetone and pyruvate. *J Appl Phys* 1990;68(1):119–24.

6. Deboer LWV, Bekx PA, Han L, et al. Pyruvate enhances recovery of rat hearts after ischemia and reperfusion by preventing free radical generation. *Am J Physiol* 1993;265:H1571–76.

7. Cicalese L, Subbotin V, Rastellini C, et al. Acute rejection of small bowel allografts in rats: Protection afforded by pyruvate. *Trans Proc* 1996;28(5):2474.

8. Cicalese L, Lee K, Schraut W, et al. Pyruvate prevents ischemia-reperfusion mucosal injury of rat small intestine. *Am J Surg* 1996;171:97–101.

9. Stanko RT, Mullick P, Clarke MR, et al. Pyruvate inhibits growth of mammary adenocarcinoma 13762 in rats. *Can Res* 1994;54:1004–7.

Quercetin

1. Ishikawa M, Oikawa T, Hosokawa M, et al. Enhancing effect of quercetin on 3-methylcholanthrene carcinogenesis in C57B1/6 mice. *Neoplasma* 1985; 43:435–41.

2. Hertog MGL, Feskens EJM, Hollman PCH, et al. Dietary flavonoids and cancer risk in the Zutphen elderly study. *Nutr Cancer* 1994;22:175–84.

3. Castillo MH, Perkins E, Campbell JH, et al. The effects of the bioflavonoid quercetin on squamous cell carcinoma of head and neck origin. *Am J Surg* 1989; 351–55.

4. Stavric B. Quercetin in our diet: From potent mutagen to probably anticarcinogen. *Clin Biochem* 1994;27:245–48.

Resveratrol

1. Bertelli AA, Giovanninni L, Bernini W, et al. Antiplatelet activity of cis-resveratrol. *Drugs Exp Clin Res* 1996; 22(2):61–63.

2. Chen CK, Pace-Asciak CR. Vasorelaxing activity of resveratrol and quercetin in isolated rat aorta. *Gen Pharm* 1996;27(2):363–66.

3. Pace-Asciak CR, Rounova O, Hahn SE, et al. Wines and grape juices as modulators of platelet aggregation in healthy human subjects. *Clin Chim Acta* 1996; 246(1–2):163–82.

4. Jang M, Cai L, Udeani GO, et al. Cancer chemopreventive activity of resveratrol, a natural product derived from grapes. *Science* 1997;275:218–20.

5. Jang M, Cai L, Udeani GO, et al. Cancer chemopreventive activity of resveratrol, a natural product derived from grapes. *Science* 1997;275:218–20.

6. Soleas GJ, Diamandis EP, Goldberg DM. Resveratrol: A molecule whose time has come? And gone? *Clin Biochem* 1997;30(2):91–113.

Selenium

1. Clark LC, Combs GF, Turnbull BW, et al. Effects of selenium supplementation for cancer prevention in patients with carcinoma of the skin. *JAMA* 1996; 276:1957–63.

Soy

1. Wei H et al. Antioxidant and antipromotional effects of the soybean isoflavone genistein. *Proc Soc Exp Biol Med* 1995;208:124–29.

2. Messina MJ et al. Soy intake and cancer risk: A review of the in vitro and in vivo data. *Nutri Cancer* 1994;21:113–31.

3. Adlercreutz H et al. Plasma concentrations of phyto-oestrogens in Japanese men. *Lancet* 1993;342:1209–10.

4. Lee HP et al. Dietary effects on breast-cancer risk in Singapore. *Lancet* 1991;337:1197–200.

5. Anderson JW et al. Meta-analysis of the effects of soy protein intake on serum lipids. *New Engl J Med* 1995;333:276–82.

6. Murkies AL et al. Dietary flour supplementation decreases post-menopausal hot flushes: Effect of soy and wheat. *Maturitas* 1995;21(3):189–95.

7. Cassidy A, Bingham S, Setchell KDR. Biological effects of a diet of soy protein rich isoflavones on the menstrual cycle of premenopausal women. *Am J Clin Nutr* 1994;60:333–40.

8. Messina M. To recommend or not to recommend soy foods. *J Am Diet Assoc* 1994;94:(11):1253–54.

9. Divi RL, Chang HC, Doerge DR. Antithyroid isoflavones from soybean. *Biochem Pharmacol* 1997;54:1087–96.

Spirulina

1. Johnson PE, Shubert LE. Accumulation of mercury and other elements by spirulina (cyanophyceae). *Nutr Rep Intl* 1986;34(6):1063–71.

Taurine

1. Franconi F, Bennardini F, Mattana A, et al. Plasma and platelet taurine are reduced in subjects with insulin-dependent diabetes mellitus: Effects of taurine supplementation. *Am J Clin Nutr* 1995;61:1115–19.

Tyrosine

1. Gelenberg AJ, Gibson CJ, Wojcik JD. Neurotransmitter precursors for the treatment of depression. *Psychopharmacol Bull* 1982;18:7–18.

2. Meyer JS, Welch KMA, Deshmuckh VD, et al. Neurotransmitter precursor amino acids in the treatment of multi-infarct dementia and Alzheimer's disease. *J Am Ger Soc* 1977;7:289–98.

3. Banderet LE, Lieberman HR. Treatment with tyrosine, a neurotransmitter precursor, reduces environmental stress in humans. *Brain Res Bull* 1989;22:759–62.

4. Koch R. Tyrosine supplementation for phenylketonuria treatment. *Am J Clin Nutr* 1996;64:974–75.

5. Chiaroni P, Azorin JM, Bovier P, et al. A multivariate analysis of red blood cell membrane transports and plasma levels of L-tyrosine and L-tryptophan in depressed patients before treatment and after clinical improvement. *Neuropsychobiol* 1990;23:1–7.

6. Alvestrand A, Ahlberg M, Forst P, Bergstrom J. Clinical results of long-term treatment with a low protein diet and a new amino acid preparation in patients with chronic uremia. *Clin Nephrol* 1983;19:67–73.

Vanadium

1. Boden G, Chen X, Ruiz J, et al. Effects of vanadyl sulfate on carbohydrate and lipid metabolism in patients with non-insulin-dependent diabetes mellitus. *Metab Clin Exp* 1996;45(9):1130–35.

References

2. Naylor GJ. Vanadium and manic depressive psychosis. *Nutr Health* 1984; 3:79–85 (review).

3. Chakraborty A, Ghosh R, Roy K, et al. Vanadium: A modifier of drug metabolizing enzyme patterns and its critical role in cellular proliferation in transplantable murine lymphoma. *Oncology* 1995;52: 310–14.

Vitamin A and Beta-Carotene

1. Bendich A, Langseth L. Safety of vitamin A. *Am J Clin Nutr* 1989;49:358–71.

2. Xu MJ, Plezia PM, Alberts DS, et al. Reduction in plasma or skin alpha-tocopherol concentration with long-term oral administration of beta-carotene in humans and mice. *J Natl Cancer Inst* 1992; 84:1559–65.

3. Mejia LA, Chew F. Hematological effect of supplementing anemic children with vitamin A alone and in combination with iron. *Am J Clin Nutr* 1988;48: 595–600.

Vitamin B1

1. Cheraskin E, Ringsdorf WM, Medford FH, Hicks BS. The "ideal" daily vitamin B1 intake. *J Oral Med* 1978;33:77-9.

Vitamin B2

1. Bhat KS. Nutritional status of thiamine, riboflavin and pyridoxine in cataract patients. *Nutr Rep Internat* 1987; 36:685–92.

2. Prchal JT, Conrad ME, Skalka HW. Association of presenile cataracts with heterozygosity for galactosaemic states and with riboflavin deficiency. *Lancet* 1978;12–13.

3. Varma RN, Mankad VN, Phelps DD, et al. Depressed erythrocyte glutathione reductase activity in sickle cell disease. *Am J Clin Nutr* 1983;38:884–87.

Vitamin B6

1. Gaby AR. Literature review and commentary. *Townsend Letter for Doctors and Patients* Jun 1990;338–39.

2. Parry G, Bredesen DE. Sensory neuropath with low-dose pyridoxine. *Neurology* 1985;35:1466–68.

3. Schaumburg H, Kaplan J, Windebank A, et al. Sensory neuropathy from pyridoxine abuse. *N Engl J Med* 1983; 309(8):445–48.

Vitamin C

1. Hemila H. Does vitamin C alleviate the symptoms of the common cold? A review of current evidence. *Scand J Infect Dis* 1994;26:1–6.

2. Sandstead HH. Copper bioavailability and requirements. *Am J Clin Nutr* 1982;35:809–14 (review).

3. Finley EB, Cerklewski FL. Influence of ascorbic acid supplementation on copper status in young adult men. *Am J Clin Nutr* 1983;37:553–56.

Vitamin E

1. Rimm EB, Stampfer MJ, Ascherio A, et al. Vitamin E consumption and the risk of coronary heart disease in men. *N Engl J Med* 1993;328:1450–56.

2. Stampfer MJ, Hennekens CH, Manson JE, et al. Vitamin E consumption and the risk of coronary heart disease in women. *N Engl J Med* 1993;328:1444–49.

3. Stephens NG, Parsons A, Schofield PM, et al. Randomised controlled trial of vitamin E in patients with coronary disease: Cambridge Heart Antioxidant Study (CHAOS). *Lancet* 1996;347:781–86.

4. Christen S, Woodall AA, Shigenaga MK, Southwell-Keely, Duncan MW, Ames BN. Gamma-tocopherol traps mutagenic electrophiles such as NO+ and complements alpha-tocopherol: Physiological implications. *Proc Natl Acad Sci* 1997; 94:3217–22.

Zinc

1. Mossad SB, Macknin ML, Medendorp SV, et al. Zinc gluconate lozenges for treating the common cold. *Ann Int Med* 1996;125:81–88.

2. Cherry FF, Sandstead HH, Rojas P, et al. Adolescent pregnancy: Associations among body weight, zinc nutriture, and pregnancy outcome. *Am J Clin Nutr* 1989; 50:945–54.

3. Goldenberg RL, Tamura T, Neggers Y, et al. The effect of zinc supplementation on pregnancy outcome. *JAMA* 1995;274: 463–68.

4. Prasad A. Discovery of human zinc deficiency and studies in an experimental human model. *Am J Clin Nutr* 1991; 53:403–12 (review).

5. Chandra RK. Excessive intake of zinc impairs immune responses. *JAMA* 1984;252(11):1443.

6. Bush AI, Pettingell WH, Multhaup G, et al. Rapid induction of alzheimer A8 amyloid formation by zinc. *Science* 1994;265:1464–65.

7. Potocnik FCV, vanRensburg ST, Park C, et al. Zinc and platelet membrane microviscosity in Alzheimer's disease. *S Afr Med J* 1997;87:1116–9.

8. Broun ER, Greist A, Tricot G, Hoffman R. Excessive zinc ingestion—a reversible cause of sideroblastic anemia and bone marrow depression. *JAMA* 1990; 264:1441–43.

9. Resiser S et al. Effect of copper intake on blood cholesterol and its lipoprotein distribution in men. *Nutr Rep Internat* 1987;36(3):641–49.

10. Sandstead HH. Requirements and toxicity of essential trace elements, illustrated by zinc and copper. *Am J Clin Nutr* 1995;61(suppl):621S–24S (review).

11. Fischer PWF, Giroux A, Labbe MR. Effect of zinc supplementation on copper status in adult man. *Am J Clin Nutr* 1984;40(4):743–46.

12. Dawson EB, Albers J, McGanity WJ. Serum zinc changes due to iron supplementation in teen-age pregnancy. *Am J Clin Nutr* 1990;50:848–52.

13. Crofton RW, Gvozdanovic D, Gvozdanovic S, et al. Inorganic zinc and the intestinal absorption of ferrous iron. *Am J Clin Nutr* 1989;50:141–44.

14. Argiratos V, Samman S. The effect of calcium carbonate and calcium citrate on the absorption of zinc in healthy female subjects. *Er J Clin Nutr* 1994; 48:198–204.

15. Spencer H, Norris C, Williams D. Inhibitory effects of zinc on magnesium balance and magnesium absorption in man. *J Coll Nutr* 1994;13:479–84.

16. Brumas V, Hacht B, Filella M, Berthon G. Can N-acetyl-L-cysteine affect zinc metabolisms when used as a paracetamol antidote? *Agents Actions* 1992;36: 278–88.

Herbs

Alfalfa

1. Briggs C. Alfalfa. *Canadian Pharm J* Mar 1994:84,85,115.

2. Castleman M. *The Healing Herbs.* Emmaus, PA: Rodale Press, 1991, 37–39.

3. Leung AY, Foster S. *Encyclopedia of Common Natural Ingredients Used in Food, Drugs, and Cosmetics,* 2d ed. New York: John Wiley & Sons, 1996, 13–15.

4. Story JA. Alfalfa saponins and cholesterol interactions. *Am J Clin Nutr* 1984; 39:917–29.

5. Foster S. *Herbs for Your Health.* Loveland, CO: Interweave Press, 1996, 2–3.

6. Malinow MR, Bardana EJ, Profsky B, et al. Systemic lupus erythematosus-like syndrome in monkeys fed alfalfa sprouts: Role of a nonprotein amino acid. *Science* 1982;216:415–17.

Aloe

1. Pennies NS. Inhibition of arachidonic acid oxidation in vitro by vehicle components. *Acta Derm Venerol Stockh* 1981;62:59–61.

2. Bruce W. Investigations of the antibacterial activity in the aloe. *S Afr Med J* 1967;41:984.

3. Schmidt JM, Greenspoon JS. Aloe vera dermal wound gel is associated with a delay in wound healing. *Ob Gyn* 1991; 78:115–17.

Asian Ginseng

1. Shibata S, Tanaka O, et al. Chemistry and pharmacology of Panax. In *Economic and Medicinal Plant Research,* vol. 1, ed. H Wagner, H Hikino, NR Farnsworth. London: Academic Press 1985, 217–84.

2. Tomoda M, Hirabayashi K, et al. Characterisation of two novel polysaccharides having immunological activities from the root of *Panax ginseng. Biol Pharm Bull* 1993;16:1087–90.

Astragalus

1. Leung AY, Foster S. *Encyclopedia of Common Natural Ingredients Used in Food, Drugs, and Cosmetics,* 2d ed. New York: John Wiley & Sons, 1996, 50–53.

2. Foster S, Chongxi Y. *Herbal Emissaries: Bringing Chinese Herbs to the West.* Rochester, VT: Healing Arts Press, 1992, 27–33.

3. Shu HY. *Oriental Materia Medica: A Concise Guide.* Palos Verdes, CA: Oriental Healing Arts Press, 1986, 521–23.

Bilberry

1. Salvayre R, Braquet P, et al. Comparison of the scavenger effect of bilberry anthocyanosides with various flavonoids. *Proceed Intl Bioflavonoids Symposium,* Munich, 1981, 437–42.

Bitter Melon

1. Duke JA. *CRC Handbook of Medicinal Herbs.* Boca Raton, FL: CRC Press, 1985, 315–16.

2. Raman A, Lau C. Anti-diabetic properties and phytochemistry of *Momordica charantia* L (Curcurbitaceae). *Phytomed Res* 1996;2:349–62.

3. Zhang QC. Preliminary report on the use of *Momordica charantia* extract by HIV patients. *J Naturopath Med* 1992; 3:65–69.

Black Cohosh

1. Leung AY, Foster S. *Encyclopedia of Common Natural Ingredients Used in Food, Drugs, and Cosmetics,* 2d ed. New York: John Wiley & Sons, 1996, 88–89.

2. Castleman M. *The Healing Herbs.* Emmaus, PA: Rodale Press, 1991, 75–78.

3. Foster S. *Herbs for Your Health.* Loveland, CO: Interweave Press, 1996, 12–13.

4. Düker EM, Kopanski L, Jarry H, Wuttke W. Effects of extracts from *Cimicifuga racemosa* on gonadotropin release in menopausal women and ovariectomized rats. *Planta Medica* 1991;57:420–24.

5. Bradley PR, ed. *British Herbal Compendium,* vol 1. Bournemouth, Dorset, UK: British Herbal Medicine Association, 1992, 34–36.

6. Murray MT. *The Healing Power of Herbs.* Rocklin, CA: Prima Publishing, 1995, 376.

Blessed Thistle

1. Lust JB. *The Herb Book.* New York: Bantam Books, 1974, 343.

2. Bradley PR, ed. *British Herbal Compendium,* vol 1. Bournemouth, Dorset, UK: British Herbal Medicine Association, 1992, 126–27.

Boswellia

1. Safyhi H, Sailer ER, Amnon HPT. 5-lipoxygenase inhibition by acetyl-11-keto-b-boswellic acid. *Phytomed* 1996;3:71–72.

2. Singh GB, Atal CK. Pharmacology of an extract of salai guggal ex-*Boswellia serrata,* a new non-steroidal anti-inflammatory agent. *Agents Actions* 1986;18: 407–12.

Burdock

1. Hoffman D. *The Herbal Handbook: A User's Guide to Medical Herbalism.* Rochester, VT: Healing Arts Press, 1988, 23–24.

2. Leung AY, Foster S. *Encyclopedia of Common Natural Ingredients Used in Food, Drugs, and Cosmetics,* 2d ed. New York: John Wiley & Sons, 1996, 107–8.

3. Morita K, Kada T, Namiki M. A desmutagenic factor isolated from burdock (*Arctium lappa Linne*). *Mutation Res* 1984;129:25–31.

4. Wichtl M. *Herbal Drugs and Phytopharmaceuticals.* Boca Raton, FL: CRC Press, 1994, 9–101.

5. Newall CA, Anderson LA, Phillipson JD. *Herbal Medicines: A Guide for Health-Care Professionals.* London: Pharmaceutical Press, 1996, 52–53.

Butcher's Broom

1. Grieve M. *A Modern Herbal,* vol I. New York: Dover Publications, 1971, 128–29.

2. Weiss RF. *Herbal Medicine.* Gothenburg, Sweden: Ab Arcanum, 1988, 117–18.

3. Bouskela E, Cyrino FZGA, Marcelon G. Inhibitory effect of the Ruscus extract and of the flavonoid heperidine methylchalcone on increased microvascular permeability induced by various agents in the hamster cheek pouch. *J Cardiovasc Pharmacol* 1993;22:225–30.

4. Bouskela E, Cyrino FZGA, Marcelon G. Effects of Ruscus extract on the internal diameter of arterioles and venules of the hamster cheek pouch microcirculation. *J Cardiovasc Pharmacol* 1993; 22:221–24.

Calendula

1. Leung A, Foster S. *Encyclopedia of Common Natural Ingredients Used in Food, Drugs, and Cosmetics,* 2d ed. New York: John Wiley & Sons, 1996, 113–14.

2. Weiss RF. *Herbal Medicine.* Gothenburg, Sweden: Ab Arcanum, 1988, 344.

3. Della Loggia R, Tubaro A, Sosa S, et al. The role of triterpenoids in the topical anti-inflammatory activity of *Calendula officinalis* flowers. *Planta Med* 1994; 60:516–20.

Carob

1. Greally P, Hampton FJ, MacFadyen UM, Simpson H. Gaviscon and Carobel compared with cisapride in gastroesophageal reflux. *Arch Dis Child* 1992; 67:618–21.

Cascara

1. Castleman M. *The Healing Herbs.* Emmaus, PA: Rodale Press, 1991, 99–100.

2. Leung AY, Foster S. *Encyclopedia of Common Natural Ingredients Used in Food, Drugs, and Cosmetics,* 2d ed. New York: John Wiley & Sons, 1996, 128–30.

3. Bradley PR, ed. *British Herbal Compendium,* vol 1. Bournemouth, Dorset, UK: British Herbal Medicine Association, 1992, 52–54.

Catnip

1. Tyler VE. *Herbs of Choice.* Binghamton, NY: Pharmaceutical Products Press, 1994, 120–21.

2. Duke JA. *CRC Handbook of Medicinal Herbs.* Boca Raton, FL: CRC Press, 1985, 325–26.

3. Weiss RF. *Herbal Medicine.* Gothenburg, Sweden: Ab Arcanum, 1988, 282.

4. Sherry CJ, Hunter PS. The effect of an ethanol extract of catnip (*Nepeta cataria*) on the behavior of the young chick. *Experientia* 1979;35:237–38.

Cat's Claw

1. Foster S. *Herbs for Your Health.* Loveland, CO: Interweave Press, 1996, 18–19.

2. Keplinger H. Oxyindole alkaloids having properties stimulating the immunologic system and preparation containing same. US Patent no. 5,302,611, April 12, 1994.

3. Aquino R, De Feo V, De Simone F, et al. Plant metabolites, new compounds and antiinflammatory activity of *Uncaria tomentosa. J Nat Prod* 1991;54:453–59.

4. Rizzi R, Re F, Bianchi A, et al. Mutagenic and antimutagenic activities of *Uncaria tomentosa* and its extracts. *J Ethnopharmacol* 1993;38:63–77.

Cayenne

1. Lynn B. Capsaicin: Actions on nociceptive C-fibers and therapeutic potential. *Pain* 1990;41:61–69.

Chamomile

1. Wichtl M. *Herbal Drugs and Phytopharmaceuticals.* Boca Raton, FL: CRC Press, 1994, 322–25.

2. Jakolev V, Isaac O, et al. Pharmacological investigations with compounds of chamomile. II. New investigations on the antiphlogistic effects of (-)-a-bisabolol and bisabolol oxides. *Planta Med* 1979; 35:125–40.

3. Jakolev V, Isaac O, Flaskamp E. Pharmacological investigations with compounds of chamomile. VI. Investigations on the antiphlogistic effects of chamazulene and matricine. *Planta Med* 1983; 49:67–73.

4. Della Loggia R, Tubaro A, et al. The role of flavonoids in the antiinflammatory activity of *Chamomilla recutita.* In *Plant Flavonoids in Biology and Medicine: Biochemical, Pharmacological, and Structure-Activity Relationships,* ed. V Cody, E Middleton, JB Harborne. New York: Alan R. Liss, 1986, 481–84.

5. Achterrath-Tuckerman U, Kunde R, et al. Pharmacological investigations with compounds of chamomile. V. Investigations on the spasmolytic effect of compounds of chamomile and Kamillosan on the isolated guinea pig ileum. *Planta Med* 1980;39:38–50.

Chickweed

1. Duke JA. *CRC Handbook of Medicinal Herbs.* Boca Raton, FL: CRC Press, 1985, 458–59.

2. Weiss RF. *Herbal Medicine.* Gothenburg, Sweden: Ab Arcanum, 1988, 265.

Cranberry

1. Sobota AE. Inhibition of bacterial adherence by cranberry juice: Potential use for the treatment of urinary tract infections. *J Urol* 1984;131:1013–16.

2. Zafiri D, Ofek I, et al. Inhibitory activity of cranberry juice on adherence of type 1 and type P fimbriated *Esherichia coli* to eucaryotic cells. *Antimicrob Agents Chemother* 1989;33:92–98.

Damiana

1. Bradley PR, ed. *British Herbal Compendium,* vol 1. Bournemouth, Dorset, UK: British Herbal Medicine Association, 1992, 71–72.

2. Duke JA. *CRC Handbook of Medicinal Herbs.* Boca Raton, FL: CRC Press, 1985, 492.

3. Bradley PR, ed. *British Herbal Compendium,* vol 1. Bournemouth, Dorset, UK: British Herbal Medicine Association, 1992, 71–72.

4. Mills SY. *Out of the Earth: The Essential Book of Herbal Medicine.* Middlesex, UK: Viking Arkana, 1991, 516–17.

Dandelion

1. Wichtl M. *Herbal Drugs and Phytopharmaceuticals.* Boca Raton, FL: CRC Press, 1994, 486–89.

2. Bradley PR, ed. *British Herbal Compendium,* vol 1. Bournemouth, Dorset, UK: British Herbal Medicine Association, 1992, 73–75.

3. Racz-Kotilla E, Racz G, Solomon A. The action of *Taraxacum officinale* extracts on body weight and diuresis of laboratory animals. *Planta Med* 1974; 26:212–17.

4. Kuusi T, Pyylaso H, Autio K. The bitterness properties of dandelion. II. Chemical investigations. *Lebensm-Wiss Technol* 1985;18:347–49.

5. Bühm K. Choleretic action of some medicinal plants. *Arzneim-Forsch Drug Res* 1959;9:376–78.

6. Foster S. *Herbs for Your Health.* Loveland, CO: Interweave Press, 1996, 26–27.

Devil's Claw

1. Tyler, VE. *The Honest Herbal,* 3d ed. Binghamton, NY: Pharmaceutical Products Press, 1993, 111–12.

2. Weiss RF. *Herbal Medicine.* Gothenburg, Sweden: Ab Arcanum, 1988, 238–39.

3. Leung AY, Foster S. *Encyclopedia of Common Natural Ingredients Used in Food, Drugs, and Cosmetics,* 2d ed. New York: John Wiley & Sons, 1996, 208–10.

4. Whitehouse LW, Znamirouska M, Paul CJ. Devil's claw (*Harpogophytum procumbens*): No evidence for antiinflammatory activity in the treatment of arthritic disease. *Can Med Assoc J* 1983; 129:249–51.

5. Grahame R, Robinson BV. Devil's claw (*Harpogophytum procumbens*): Pharmacological and clinical studies. *Ann Rheum Dis* 1981;40:632.

Dong Quai

1. Foster S, Chongxi Y. *Herbal Emissaries.* Rochester, VT: Healing Arts Press, 1992, 65–72.

2. Qi-bing M, Jing-yi T, Bo C. Advance in the pharmacological studies of radix *Angelica sinensis* (Oliv) Diels (Chinese danggui). *Chin Med J* 1991;104:776–81.

Echinacea

1. Leuttig B, Steinmüller C, et al. Macrophage activation by the polysaccharide arabinogalactan isolated from plant cell cultures of *Echinacea purpurea. J Natl Cancer Inst* 1989;81:669–75.

Elderberry

1. Duke JA. *CRC Handbook of Medicinal Herbs.* Boca Raton, FL: CRC Press, 1985, 423.

2. Serkedjieva J, Manolova N, Zgórniak-Nowosielska I, et al. Antiviral activity of the infusion (SHS-174) from flowers of *Sambucus nigra* L., aerial parts of *Hypericum perforatum* L., and roots of *Saponaria officinalis* L. against influenza and herpes simplex viruses. *Phytother Res* 1990;4:97–100.

3. Zakay-Rones Z, Varsano N, Zlotnik M, et al. Inhibition of several strains of influenza virus in vitro and reduction of symptoms by an elderberry extract (*Sambucus nigra* L.) during an outbreak of influenza B Panama. *J Alt Compl Med* 1995; 1:361–69.

4. Mascolo N, Autore G, Capasso G, et al. Biological screening of Italian medicinal plants for anti-inflammatory activity. *Phytother Res* 1987;1:28–31.

Eleuthero

1. Collisson RJ. Siberian ginseng (*Eleutheroecoccus senticosus*). *Brit J Phytother* 1991;2:61–71.

2. Farnsworth NR, Kinghorn AD, Soejarto DD, Waller DP. Siberian ginseng (*Eleutheroecoccus senticosus*): Current status as an adaptogen. In *Economic and Medicinal Plant Research,* vol 1, ed. H Wagner, HZ Hikino, NR Farnsworth. London: Academic Press, 1985, 155–215.

3. Hikino H, Takahashi M, et al. Isolation and hypoglycemic activity of eleutherans A, B, C, D, E, F and G: Glycans of *Eleutheroecoccus senticosus* roots. *J Natural Prod* 1986;49:293–97.

4. Wagner H, Nörr H, Winterhoff H. Plant adaptogens. *Phytomed* 1994; 1:63–76.

5. Farnsworth NR, Kinghorn AD, Soejarto DD, Waller DP. Siberian ginseng (*Eleutheroecoccus senticosus*): Current status as an adaptogen. In *Economic and Medicinal Plant Research,* vol 1, ed. H Wagner, HZ Hikino, NR Farnsworth. London: Academic Press, 1985, 155–215.

6. Asano K, Takahashi T, et al. Effect of Eleutherococcus senticosus extract on human working capacity. *Planta Medica* 1986;37:175–77.

7. McNaughton L. A comparison of Chinese and Russian ginseng as ergogenic aids to improve various facets of physical fitness. *Inter Clin Nutr Rev* 1989;9:32–35.

8. Collisson RJ. Siberian ginseng (*Eleutheroecoccus senticosus*). *Brit J Phytother* 1991;2:61–71.

9. Ben-Hur E, Fulder S. Effect of *P. ginseng saponins* and *Eleutherococcus S.* on survival of cultured mammalian cells after ionizing radiation. *Am J Chin Med* 1981; 9:48–56.

Ephedra

1. Foster S. *Herbs for Your Health.* Loveland, CO: Interweave Press, 1996, 37–38.

2. Tyler, VE. *The Honest Herbal,* 3d ed. Binghamton, NY: Pharmaceutical Products Press, 1993, 119–21.

3. Leung AY, Foster S. *Encyclopedia of Common Natural Ingredients Used in Food, Drugs, and Cosmetics,* 2d ed. New York: John Wiley & Sons, 1996, 227–29.

Eyebright

1. Weiss RF. *Herbal Medicine.* Gothenburg, Sweden: Ab Arcanum, 1988, 339–40.

2. Hoffman D. *The Herbal Handbook: A User's Guide to Medical Herbalism.* Rochester, VT: Healing Arts Press, 1988, 136–37.

3. Wichtl M. *Herbal Drugs and Phytopharmaceuticals.* Boca Raton, FL: CRC Press, 1994, 195–96.

4. Commission E. Monograph, *Euphrasia, Bundesanzeiger,* August 29, 1992.

Fennel

1. Duke JA. *CRC Handbook of Medicinal Herbs.* Boca Raton, FL: CRC Press, 1985, 145–46.

2. Mills SY. *Out of the Earth: The Essential Book of Herbal Medicine.* Middlesex, UK: Viking Arkana, 1991, 424–26.

3. Tanira MOM, Shah AH, Mohsin A, et al. Pharmacological and toxicological investigations on *Foeniculum vulgare* dried fruit extract in experimental animals. *Phytother Res* 1996;10:33–36.

Fenugreek

1. Escot N. Fenugreek. *ATOMS* 1994/5;summer:7–12.

2. Sauvaire Y, Ribes G, Baccou JC, Loubatieres-Mariani MM. Implication of steroid saponins and sapogenins in the hypocholesterolemic effect of fenugreek. *Lipids* 1991;26:191–97.

3. Ribes G, Sauvaire Y, Da Costa C, et al. Antidiabetic effects of subfractions from fenugreek seeds in diabetic dogs. *Proc Soc Exp Biol Med* 1986;182:159–66.

Feverfew

1. Makheja AN, Bailey JM. A platelet phospholipase inhibitor from the medicinal herb feverfew (*Tanacetum parthenium*). *Prostagland Leukotrienes Med* 1982; 8:653–60.

2. Hepinstall S, White A, et al. Extracts of feverfew inhibit granule secretion in blood platelets and polymorphonuclear leukocytes. *Lancet* 1985;i:1071–74.

Fo-Ti

1. Foster S, Chongxi Y. *Herbal Emissaries: Bringing Chinese Herbs to the West.* Rochester, VT: Healing Arts Press, 1992, 79–85.

2. Foster S, Chongxi Y. *Herbal Emissaries: Bringing Chinese Herbs to the West.* Rochester, VT: Healing Arts Press, 1992, 79–85.

3. Foster S. *Herbal Renaissance.* Layton, Utah: Gibbs Smith, 1993, 40–41.

4. Foster S, Chongxi Y. *Herbal Emissaries: Bringing Chinese Herbs to the West.* Rochester, VT: Healing Arts Press, 1992, 79–85.

Garlic

1. Kleijnen J, Knipschild P, Ter Riet G. Garlic, onion and cardiovascular risk factors: A review of the evidence from human experiments with emphasis on commercially available preparations. *Br J Clin Pharmacol* 1989;28:535–44.

2. Legnani C, Frascaro M, et al. Effects of a dried garlic preparation on fibrinolysis and platelet aggregation in healthy subjects. *Arzneim-Forsch Drug Res* 1993; 43:119–22.

3. Hughes BG, Lawson LD. Antimicrobial effects of *Allium sativum* L. (garlic), *Allium ampeloprasum* L. (elephant garlic) and *Allium cepa* L. (onion), garlic compounds and commercial garlic supplement products. *Phytother Res* 1991;5:154–58.

4. Dorant E, vander Brandt PA, et al. Garlic and its significance for the prevention of cancer in humans: A critical review. *Br J Cancer* 1993;67:424–29.

Gentian

1. Duke JA. *CRC Handbook of Medicinal Herbs.* Boca Raton, FL: CRC Press, 1985, 207–8.

2. Weiss RF. *Herbal Medicine.* Gothenburg, Sweden: Ab Arcanum, 1988, 40–42.

3. Kondo Y, Takano F, Hojo H. Suppression of chemically and immunologically induced hepatic injuries by gentiopicroside in mice. *Planta Med* 1994; 60:414–16.

Ginger

1. Tyler VE. *Herbs of Choice: The Therapeutic Use of Phytomedicinals.* Binghamton, NY: Pharmaceutical Products Press, 1994, 39–42.

2. Bradley PR, ed. *British Herbal Compendium,* vol 1. Bournemouth, Dorset, UK: British Herbal Medicine Association, 1992, 112–14.

3. Yamahara J, Huang Q, et al. Gastrointestinal motility enhancing effect of

ginger and its active constituents. *Chem Pharm Bull* 1990;38:430–31.

4. Al-Yahya MA, Rafatullah S, et al. Gastroprotective activity of ginger in albino rats. *Am J Chinese Med* 1989;17: 51–56.

5. Holtmann S, Clarke AH, et al. The anti-motion sickness mechanism of ginger. *Acta Otolaryngol (Stockh)* 1989; 108:168–74.

6. Suekawa M, Ishige A, et al. Pharmacological studies on ginger. I. Pharmacological actions of pungent constituents, (6)-gingerol and (6)-shogaol. *J Pharm Dyn* 1984;7:836–48.

7. Verma SK, Singh J, et al. Effect of ginger on platelet aggregation in man. *Indian J Med Res* 1994;98:240–42.

Ginkgo Biloba

1. Drieu K. Preparation and definition of Ginkgo biloba extract. In *Rokan (Ginkgo biloba): Recent Results in Pharmacology and Clinic,* ed. EW Fünfgeld. Berlin: Springer-Verlag, 1988, 32–36.

2. Krieglstein J. Neuroprotective properties of *Ginkgo biloba*—constituents. *Zeitschrift Phytother* 1994;15:92–96.

3. Bruno C, Cuppini R, et al. Regeneration of motor nerves in bilobalide-treated rats. *Planta Medica* 1993; 59:302–7.

4. Clostre F. From the body to the cellular membranes: The different levels of pharmacological action of *Ginkgo biloba* extract. In *Rokan (Ginkgo biloba): Recent Results in Phamacology and Clinic,* ed. EW Fünfgeld. Berlin: Springer-Verlag, 1988, 180–98.

5. Jung F, Mrowietz C, et al. Effect of *Ginkgo biloba* on fluidity of blood and peripheral microcirculation in volunteers. *Arzneim-Forsch Drug Res* 1990;40: 589–93.

6. Ferrandini C, Droy-Lefaix MT, Christen Y, ed. *Ginkgo biloba Extract (EGb 761) As a Free Radical Scavenger.* Paris: Elsevier, 1993.

7. Harman D. Free radical theory of aging: A hypothesis on pathogenesis of senile dementia of the Alzheimer's type. *Age* 1993;16:23–30.

8. Lamant V, Mauco G, et al. Inhibition of the metabolism of platelet activating factor (PAF-acether) by three specific antagonists from *Ginkgo biloba. Biochem Pharmacol* 1987;36:2749–52.

9. Kroegel C. The potential pathophysiological role of platelet-activating factor in human disease. *Klin Wochenschr* 1988; 66:373–78.

10. Kroegel C, Kortsik C, et al. The pathophysiological role and therapeutic implications of platelet activating factor in diseases of aging. *Drugs Aging* 1992;2: 345–55.

11. Krieglstein J. Neuroprotective properties of *Ginkgo biloba*—constituents. *Zeitschrift Phytother* 1994; 15:92–96.

Goldenseal

1. Hahn FE, Ciak J. Berberine. *Antibiotics* 1976;3:577–88.

Gotu Kola

1. Duke JA. *CRC Handbook of Medicinal Herbs.* Boca Raton, FL: CRC Press, 1985, 110–11.

2. Kartnig T. Clinical applications of *Centella asiatica* (L) Urb. In *Herbs, Spices, and Medicinal Plants: Recent Advances in Botany, Horticulture, and Pharmacology,* vol. 3., ed. LE Craker, JE Simon. Phoenix, AZ: Oryx Press, 1986, 145–73.

Green Tea

1. Graham HN. Green tea composition, consumption, and polyphenol chemistry. *Prev Med* 1992;21:334–50.

2. Kono S, Shinchi K, Ikeda N, et al. Green tea consumption and serum lipid profiles: A cross-sectional study in Northern Kyushu, Japan. *Prev Med* 1992; 21:526–31.

3. Yamaguchi Y, Hayashi M, Yamazoe H, et al. Preventive effects of green tea extract on lipid abnormalities in serum, liver and aorta of mice fed an atherogenic diet. *Nip Yak Zas* 1991;97(6):329–37.

4. Sagesaka-Mitane Y, Milwa M, Okada S. Platelet aggregation inhibitors in hot water extract of green tea. *Chem Pharm Bull* 1990;38(3):790–93.

5. Stensvold I, Tverdal A, Solvoll K, et al. Tea consumption. Relationship to cholesterol, blood pressure, and coronary and total mortality. *Prev Med* 1992;21:546–53.

6. Stoner GD, Mukhtar H. Polyphenols as cancer chemopreventive agents. *J Cell Bioch* 1995;22:169–80.

7. You SQ. Study on feasibility of Chinese green tea polyphenols (CTP) for preventing dental caries. *Chin J Stom* 1993; 28(4):197–99.

8. Hamilton-Miller JM. Antimicrobial properties of tea (*Camellia sinensis* L.). *Antimicro Ag Chemo* 1995; 39(11): 2375–77.

Guaraná

1. Duke JA. *CRC Handbook of Medicinal Herbs.* Boca Raton, FL: CRC Press, 1985, 349.

2. Leung AY, Foster S. *Encyclopedia of Common Natural Ingredients Used in Food, Drugs, and Cosmetics,* 2d ed. New York: John Wiley & Sons, 1996, 293–94.

3. Galduroz JC, Carlini EA. The effects of long-term administration of guarana on the cognition of normal, elderly volunteers. *Rev Paul Med* 1996; 114:1073–78.

Guggul

1. Satyavati GV. Gum guggul (*Commiphora mukul*)—The success of an ancient insight leading to a modern discovery. *Indian J Med* 1988;87:327–35.

2. Nityanand S, Kapoor NK. Hypocholesterolemic effect of *Commiphora mukul* resin (Guggal). *Indian J Exp Biol* 1971; 9:367–77.

3. Mester L, Mester M, Nityanand S. Inhibition of platelet aggregation by guggulu steroids. *Planta Med* 1979;37:367–69.

Gymnema

1. Mhasker KS, Caius JF. A study of Indian medicinal plants. II. *Gymnema sylvestre* R.Br. *Indian Medical Research Memoirs* 1930;16:2–75.

2. Shanmugasundaram KR, Panneerselvam C, Sumudram P, Shanmugasundaram ERB. Insulinotropic activity of *G. sylvestre,* R.Br. and Indian medicinal herb used in controlling diabetes mellitus. *Pharmacol Res Commun* 1981;13:475–86.

3. Bishayee A, Chatterjee M. Hypolipidemic and antiatherosclerotic effects of oral *Gymnema sylvestre* R.Br. leaf extract in albino rats fed on a high fat diet. *Phytother Res* 1994;8:118–20.

4. Gymnema. *Lawrence Review of Natural Products,* Aug 1993 (monograph).

5. Fushiki T, Kojima A, Imoto T, et al. An extract of *Gymnema sylvestre* leaves and purified gymnemic acid inhibits glucose-stimulated gastric inhibitory peptide secretion in rats. *J Nutr* 1992; 122:2367–73.

6. Baskaran K, Ahmath BK, Shanmugasundaram KR, Shanmugasundaram ERB. Antidiabetic effect of a leaf extract from *Gymnema sylvestre* in non-insulin-dependent diabetes mellitus patients. *J Ethnopharmacol* 1990;30:295–305.

Hawthorn

1. Rewerski VW, Piechoscki T, et al. Some pharmacological properties of oligomeric procyanidin isolated from hawthorn (*Crataegus oxyacantha*). *Arzneim-Forsch Drug Res* 1967;17:490–91.

2. Weikl A, Noh HS. The influence of *Crataegus* on global cardiac insufficiency. *Herz Gefabe* 1993;11:516–24.

3. Bahorun T, Trotin F, et al. Antioxidant activities of *Crataegus monogyna* extracts. *Planta Med* 1994;60:323–28.

Hops

1. Weiss RF. *Herbal Medicine*. Gothenburg, Sweden: Ab Arcanum, 1988, 285–86.

2. Foster S. *Herbs for Your Health*. Loveland, CO: Interweave Press, 1996, 56–57.

3. Wichtl M. *Herbal Drugs and Phytopharmaceuticals*. Boca Raton, FL: CRC Press, 1994, 305–8.

Horse Chestnut

1. Chandler RF. Horse chestnut. *Canadian Pharm J* Jul/Aug 1993:297, 300.

2. Diehm C, Trampish HJ, Lange S, Schmidt C. Comparison of leg compression stocking and oral horse chestnut seed extract therapy in patients with chronic venous insufficiency. *Lancet* 1996;347: 292–94.

3. Guillaume M, Padioleau F. Veinotonic effect, vascular protection, antiinflammatory and free radical scavenging properties of horse chestnut extract. *Arzneim-Forsch Drug Res* 1994;44:25–35.

4. Tyler VE. *Herbs of Choice: The Therapeutic Use of Phytomedicinals*. Binghamton, NY: Pharmaceutical Products Press, 1994, 112–13.

5. Weiss RF. *Herbal Medicine*. Gothenburg, Sweden: Ab Arcanum, 1988, 188–89.

Horseradish

1. Grieve M. *A Modern Herbal*, vol 2. New York: Dover Publications, 1971, 417–19.

2. Weiss RF. *Herbal Medicine*. Gothenburg, Sweden: Ab Arcanum, 1988, 207.

Horsetail

1. Leung AY, Foster S. *Encyclopedia of Common Natural Ingredients Used in Food, Drugs, and Cosmetics*, 2d ed. New York: John Wiley & Sons, 1996, 306–8.

2. Castleman M. *The Healing Herbs*. Emmaus, PA: Rodale Press, 1991, 219–21.

3. Weiss RF. *Herbal Medicine*. Gothenburg, Sweden: Ab Arcanum, 1988, 238–39.

4. Seaborn CD, Nielsen FH. Silicon: A nutritional beneficence for bones, brains and blood vessels? *Nutr Today* 1993; 28:13–18.

5. Fabre B, Geay B, Beaufils P. Thiaminase activity in *Equisetum arvense* and its extracts. *Plant Med Phytother* 1993; 26:190–97.

Juniper

1. Duke JA. *CRC Handbook of Medicinal Herbs*. Boca Raton, FL: CRC Press, 1985, 256.

2. Tyler VE. *Herbs of Choice: The Therapeutic Use of Phytomedicinals*. Binghamton, NY: Pharmaceutical Products Press, 1994, 76–77.

3. Markkanen T, Markinen ML, Nikoskelainen J, et al. Antiherpetic agent from juniper tree (*Juniperus communis*), its purification, identification and testing in primary human amnion cell cultures. *Drugs Exptl Clin Res* 1981;7:691–97.

Kava

1. Bone K. Kava: A safe herbal treatment for anxiety. *Brit J Phytother* 1994; 3:145–53.

2. Buckley JP, Furgiulel AR, O'Hara MJ. Pharmacology of kava. In *Ethnopharmacological Search for Psychoactive Drugs*, ed. DH Efron, B Holmstedt, NS Kline. New York: Raven Press, 1979, 141–51.

3. Holm E, Staedt U, et al. Studies on the profile of the neurophysiological effects of D,L-kavain: Cerebral sites of action .and sleep-wakefulness-rhythm in animals. *Arzneim-Forsch Drug Res* 1991; 41:673–83.

Kudzu

1. Foster S. Kudzu root monograph. *Quart Rev Nat Med* 1994;winter:303–8.

2. Zhao SP, Zhang YZ. Quantitative TLC-densitometry of isoflavones in *Pueraria lobata* (Willd.) Ohwi. *Yaoxue Xuebao* 1985;20:203.

3. Keung WM, Vallee BL. Daidzin and daidzein suppress free-choice ethanol intake by Syrian Golden hamsters. *Proc Natl Acad Sci USA* 1993;90:10008–12.

4. Leung AY, Foster S. *Encyclopedia of Common Natural Ingredients Used in Food, Drugs, and Cosmetics*, 2d ed. New York: John Wiley & Sons, 1996, 333–36.

Lemon Balm

1. Weiss RF. *Herbal Medicine*. Gothenburg, Sweden: Ab Arcanum, 1988, 31,286.

2. Auf'mkolk M, Ingbar JC, Kubota K, et al. Extracts and auto-oxidized constituents of certain plants inhibit the receptor-binding and the biological activity of Graves' immunoglobulins. *Endocrinol* 1985;116(5):1687–93.

3. Wöhlbling RH, Leonhardt K. Local therapy of herpes simplex with dried extract of Melissa officinalis. *Phytomed* 1994;1(1):25–31.

4. Leach EH, Lloyd JPF. Experimental ocular hypertension in animals. *Trans Ophthalm Soc UK* 1956;76:453–60.

Licorice

1. Steinberg D, Sgan-Cohen HD, Stabholz A, et al. The anticariogenic activity of glycyrrhizin: Preliminary clinical trials. *Isr J Dent Sci* 1989;2:153–57

2. Soma R, Ikeda M, Morise T, et al. Effect of glycyrrhizin on cortisol metabolism in humans. *Endocrin Regulations* 1994;28:31–34.

Maitake

1. Hobbs C. *Medicinal Mushrooms*. Santa Cruz, CA: Botanica Press, 1995, 110–15.

2. Nanba H, Hamaguchi AM, Kuroda H. The chemical structure of an antitumor polysaccharide in fruit bodies of *Grifola frondosa* (maitake). *Chem Pharm Bull* 1987;35:1162–68.

3. Yamada Y, Nanba H, Kuroda H. Antitumor effect of orally administered extracts from fruit body of *Grifola frondosa* (maitake). *Chemotherapy* 1990;38: 790–96.

4. Nanba H. Immunostimulant activity in-vivo and anti-HIV activity in vitro of 3 branched b-1-6-glucans extracted from maitake mushrooms (*Grifola frondosa*). Abstract, VIII International Conference on AIDS, Amersterdam, 1992.

Marshmallow

1. Nosal'ova G, Strapkova A, Kardosova A, et al. Antitussive action of extracts and polysaccharides of marshmallow (*Althea officinalis* L., var. robusta). *Pharmazie* 1992;47:224–26 [in German].

2. Tomoda M, Shimizu N, Oshima Y, et al. Hypoglycemic activity of twenty plant mucilages and three modified products. *Planta Med* 1987;53:8–12.

Milk Thistle

1. Wagner H, Horhammer L, Munster R. The chemistry of silymarin (silybin), the active principle of the fruits of *Silybum marianum* (L.) Gaertn. *Arzneim-Forsch Drug Res* 1968;18:688–96.

2. Hikino H, Kiso Y, et al. Antihepatotoxic actions of flavonolignans from silybum marianum fruits. *Planta Medica* 1984;50:248–50.

3. Faulstich H, Jahn W, Wieland T. Silibinin inhibition of amatoxin uptake in the perfused rat liver. *Arzneim-Forsch Drug Res* 1980;30:452–54.

4. Tuchweber B, Sieck R, Trost W. Prevention by silibinin of phalloidin induced hepatotoxicity. *Toxicol Appl Pharmacol* 1979;51:265–75.

5. Feher J, Lang I, et al. Free radicals in tissue damage in liver diseases and therapeutic approach. *Tokai J Exp Clin Med* 1986;11:121–34.

6. Sonnenbichler J, Zetl I. Stimulating influence of a flavonolignan derivative on proliferation, RNA synthesis and protein synthesis in liver cells. In *Assessment and Management of Hepatobiliary Disease,* ed. L Okolicsanyi, G Csomos, G Crepaldi. Berlin: Springer-Verlag, 1987, 265–72.

Mullein

1. Hoffman D. *The Herbal Handbook: A User's Guide to Medical Herbalism.* Rochester, VT: Healing Arts Press, 1988, 67.

2. Grieve M. *A Modern Herbal,* vol 2. New York: Dover Publications, 1971, 562–66.

3. Wichtl M. *Herbal Drugs and Phytopharmaceuticals.* Boca Raton, FL: CRC Press, 1994, 18–19.

4. Tyler VE. *The Honest Herbal,* 3d ed. Binghamton, NY: Pharmaceutical Products Press, 1993, 219–20.

Myrrh

1. Leung AY, Foster S. *Encyclopedia of Common Natural Ingredients Used in Food, Drugs, and Cosmetics,* 2d ed. New York: John Wiley & Sons, 1996, 382–83.

2. Mills SY. *Out of the Earth: The Essential Book of Herbal Medicine.* Middlesex, UK: Viking Arkana, 1991, 500–2.

3. Al-Harbi MM, Qureshi S, Raza M, et al. Anticarcinogenic effect of *Commiphora molmol* on solid tumors induced by Ehrlich carcinoma cells in mice. *Chemotherapy* 1994;40:337–47.

4. Dolara P, Luceri C, Ghelardini C, et al. Analgesic effects of myrrh. *Nature* 1996;376:29.

Nettle

1. Obertreis B, Giller K, Teucher T, et al. Antiphlogistic effects of Urtica dioica folia extract in comparison to caffeic malic acid. *Arzneim Forsch Drug Res* 1996; 46:52–56.

2. Hirano T, Homma M, Oka K. Effects of stinging nettle root extracts and their steroidal components on the Na+,K+-ATPase of the benign prostatic hyperplasia. *Planta Med* 1994;60:30–33.

Oats

1. Weiss RF. *Herbal Medicine.* Gothenburg, Sweden: Ab Arcanum, 1988, 287–88.

2. Mills SY. *Out of the Earth: The Essential Book of Herbal Medicine.* Middlesex, UK: Viking Arcana, 1991, 510–12.

3. Wichtl M. *Herbal Drugs and Phytopharmaceuticals.* Boca Raton, FL: CRC Press, 1994, 96–98.

Passion Flower

1. Foster S. *Herbs for Your Health.* Loveland, CO: Interweave Press, 1996, 68–69.

2. Meier B. *Passiflora incarnata* L.— Passion flower: Portrait of a medicinal plant. *Zeits Phytother* 1995;16:115–26.

3. Wichtl M. *Herbal Drugs and Phytopharmaceuticals.* Boca Raton, FL: CRC Press, 1994, 363–65.

Pau d'Arco

1. Duke JA. *CRC Handbook of Medicinal Herbs.* Boca Raton, FL: CRC Press, 1985, 470–71.

2. Guiraud P, Steiman R, Campos-Takaki GM, et al. Comparison of antibacterial and antifungal activities of lapachol and beta-lapachone. *Planta Med* 1994; 60:373–74.

3. Tyler VE. *Herbs of Choice: The Therapeutic Use of Phytomedicinals.* Binghamton, NY: Pharmaceutical Products Press, 1994, 180.

4. Oswald EH. Lapacho. *Brit J Phytother* 1993/4;3:112–17.

5. Duke JA. *CRC Handbook of Medicinal Herbs.* Boca Raton, FL: CRC Press, 1985, 470–71.

6. Oswald EH. Lapacho. *Brit J Phytother* 1993/4;3:112–17.

Peppermint

1. Foster S. *Herbs for Your Health.* Loveland, CO: Interweave Press, 1996, 72–73.

2. Rees W, Evans B, Rhodes J. Treating irritable bowel syndrome with peppermint oil. *Brit Med J* 1979;ii:835–36.

3. Bradley PR, ed. *British Herbal Compendium, Vol. 1.* British Herbal Medicine Association, Bournemouth, Dorset, 1992, 174–76.

4. Tyler VE. *Herbs of Choice: The Therapeutic Use of Phytomedicinals.* New York: Pharmaceutical Products Press, 1994, 56–57.

5. Göbel H, Schmidt G, Dwoshak M, et al. Essential plant oils and headache mechanisms. *Phytomed* 1995;2:93–102.

Phyllanthus

1. Bharatiya VB. *Selected Medicinal Plants of India.* Bombay: Tata Press, 1992, 235–37.

2. Nadkarmi KM. *India Materia Medica,* vol 1. Bombay: Popular Prakashan Private Ltd, 1993, 947–48.

3. Thyagarajan SP, Subramanian S, Thirunalasundar T, et al. Effect of *Phyllanthus amarus* on chronic carriers of hepatitis B virus. *Lancet* 1988: ii:764–66.

4. Meixa W, Haowei C, Yanjin L, et al. Herbs of the genus *Phyllanathus* in the treatment of chronic hepatitis B: Observation with three preparations from different geographic sites. *J Lab Clin Med.* 1995; 126:350–52.

Psyllium

1. Leung AY, Foster S. *Encyclopedia of Common Natural Ingredients Used in Food, Drugs, and Cosmetics,* 2d ed. New York: John Wiley & Sons, 1996, 427–29.

Pygeum

1. Murray MT. *The Healing Power of Herbs.* Rocklin, CA: Prima Publishing, 1995, 286–93.

Red Clover

1. Leung AY, Foster S. *Encyclopedia of Common Natural Ingredients Used in Food, Drugs, and Cosmetics,* 2d ed. New York: John Wiley & Sons, 1996, 177–78.

2. Leung AY, Foster S. *Encyclopedia of Common Natural Ingredients Used in Food, Drugs, and Cosmetics,* 2d ed. New York: John Wiley & Sons, 1996, 177–78.

3. Yanagihara K, Toge T, Numoto M, et al. Antiproliferative effects of

isoflavones on human cancer cell lines established from the gastrointestinal tract. *Cancer Res* 53:5815–21.

Red Raspberry

1. Lust JB. *The Herb Book*. New York: Bantam Books, 1974, 328–29.

2. Tyler VE. *Herbs of Choice: The Therapeutic Use of Phytomedicinals.* Binghamton, NY: Pharmaceutical Products Press, 1994, 52, 139.

Reishi

1. Leung AY, Foster S. *Encyclopedia of Common Natural Ingredients Used in Food, Drugs, and Cosmetics,* 2d ed. New York: John Wiley & Sons, 1996, 255–60.

2. Jones K. *Reishi: Ancient Herb for Modern Times*. Issaquah, WA: Sylvan Press, 1990, 6.

3. Willard T. *Reishi Mushroom: Herb of Spiritual Potency and Wonder.* Issaquah, WA: Sylvan Press, 1990, 11.

4. Shu HY. *Oriental Materia Medica: A Concise Guide.* Palos Verdes, CA: Oriental Healing Arts Press, 1986, 640–41.

5. Hobbs C. *Medicinal Mushrooms*. Santa Cruz, CA: Botanica Press, 1995, 96–107.

Sandalwood

1. Duke JA. *CRC Handbook of Medicinal Herbs.* Boca Raton, FL: CRC Press, 1985, 426–27.

2. Okazai K, Oshima S. Antibacterial activity of higher plants. XXIV. Antimicrobial effect of essential oils (5). *J Pharm Soc Japan* 1953;73:344–47.

3. Okugawa H, Ueda R, Matsumoto K, et al. Effect of alpha-santalol and beta-santalol from sandalwood on the central nervous system in mice. *Phytomed* 1995; 2:119–26.

Sarsaparilla

1. Duke JA. *CRC Handbook of Medicinal Herbs.* Boca Raton, FL: CRC Press, 1985, 446.

2. Bradley PR, ed. *British Herbal Compendium,* vol 1. Bournemouth, Dorset, UK: British Herbal Medicine Association, 1992, 194–96.

3. Ageel AM, Mossa JS, Al-Yahya MA, et al. Experimental studies on antirheumatic crude drugs used in Saudi traditional medicine. *Drugs Exp Clin Res* 1989;15:369–72.

4. Rafatullah S, Mossa JS, Ageel AM, et al. Hepatoprotective and safety evaluation studies on sarsaparilla. *Int J Pharmacognosy* 1991;29:296–301.

5. Bradley PR, ed. *British Herbal Compendium,* vol 1. Bournemouth, Dorset, UK: British Herbal Medicine Association, 1992, 194–96.

Saw Palmetto

1. Champault G, Bonnard AM, et al. The medical treatment of prostatic adenoma in a controlled study: PA-109 versus placebo in 110 patients. *Ann Urol* 1984; 6:407–10.

2. Tasca A, Barulli M, et al. Treatment of obstructive symptomology caused by prostatic adenoma with an extract of *Serenoa repens*: Double-blind clinical study vs. placebo. *Minerva Urol Nefrol* 1985; 37:87–91.

3. Braeckman J. The extract of *Serenoa repens* in the treatment of benign prostatic hyperplasia: A multicenter open study. *Curr Ther Res* 1994;55:776–85.

4. Romics I, Wschmitz H, Frang D. Experience in treating benign prostatic hypertrophy with Sabal serrulata for one year. *Inter Urol Nephrol* 1993;25:565–69.

5. Dathe G, Schmid H. Phytotherapy of benign prostatic hyperplasia (BPH) with extractum *Serenoa repens*. *Urologe* 1991; 31:220–23.

Schisandra

1. Leung AY, Foster S. *Encyclopedia of Common Natural Ingredients Used in Food, Drugs, and Cosmetics,* 2d ed. New York: John Wiley & Sons, 1996, 469–72.

2. Shu HY. *Oriental Materia Medica: A Concise Guide.* Palos Verdes, CA: Oriental Healing Arts Press, 1986, 624–25.

3. Foster S, Chongxi Y. *Herbal Emissaries: Bringing Chinese Herbs to the West.* Rochester, VT: Healing Arts Press, 1992, 146–52.

Scullcap

1. Hoffman D. *The Herbal Handbook: A User's Guide to Medical Herbalism.* Rochester, VT: Healing Arts Press, 1988, 77.

2. Foster S. *Herbs for Your Health*. Loveland, CO: Interweave Press, 1996, 86–87.

3. Newall CA, Anderson LA, Phillipson JD. *Herbal Medicines: A Guide for Health-Care Professionals.* London: Pharmaceutical Press, 1996, 239–40.

Senna

1. Leng-Peschlow E. Dual effect of orally administered sennosides on large intestinal transit and fluid absorption in the rat. *J Pharm Pharmacol* 1986;38: 606–10.

2. Mengs U. Reproductive toxicological investigations with sennosides. *Arzneim Forsch Drug Res* 1986;36:1355–58.

3. Faber P, Strenge-Hesse A. Relevance of rhein excretion into breast milk. *Pharmacol* 1988;36(suppl 1):212–20.

Shiitake

1. Jones K. *Shiitake: The Healing Mushroom*. Rochester, VT: Healing Arts Press, 1995.

2. Hobbs C. *Medicinal Mushrooms*. Santa Cruz, CA: Botanica Press, 1995, 125–28.

Slippery Elm

1. Duke JA. *CRC Handbook of Medicinal Herbs.* Boca Raton, FL: CRC Press, 1985, 495–96.

2. Wren RC, Williamson EM, Evans FJ. *Potter's New Cyclopedia of Botanical Drugs and Preparations.* Essex, UK: CW Daniel Company, 1988, 252.

St. John's Wort

1. Weiss RF. *Herbal Medicine*. Gothenburg, Sweden: Ab Arcanum, 1988, 295–97.

2. Hö J. Constituents and mechanism of action of St. John's wort. *Zeitscrhift Phytother* 1993;14:255–64.

3. Suzuki O, Katsumata Y, Oya M. Inhibition of monoamine oxidase by hypericin. *Planta Med* 1984;50:272–74.

4. Hö J, Demisch L, Gollnik B. Investigations about antidepressive and mood changing effects of *Hypericum perforatum*. *Planta Med* 1989;55:643.

5. Reichert RG. St. John's Wort for depression. *Quart Rev Nat Med* 1994; summer:17–18.

Tea Tree

1. Carson CF, Riley TV. Antimicrobial activity of the essential oil of *Melaleuca alternifolia*—A review. *Lett Appl Microbiol* 1993;16:49–55.

2. Carson CF, Cookson BD, Farrelly HD, Riley T. Susceptibility of methicillin-resistant *Staphylococcus aureus* to the essential oil of *Melaleuca alternifolia*. *J Antimicrobial Chemother* 1995;35: 421–24.

Turmeric

1. Sreejayan N, Rao MNA. Free radical scavenging activity of curcuminoids. *Arzneim Forsch Drug Res* 1996; 46:169–71.

2. Arora RB, Basu N, Kapoor V, Jain AP. Anti-inflammatory studies on *Curcuma longa* (turmeric). *Ind J Med Res* 1971;59:1289–95.

3. Kiso Y, Suzuki Y, Watanabe N, et al. Antihepatotoxic principles of *Curcuma longa* rhizomes. *Planta Med* 1983;49: 185–87.

4. Srivastava R, Dikshit M, Srimal RC, Dhawan BN. Anti-thrombotic effect of curcumin. *Thromb Res* 1985;40:413–17.

Uva Ursi

1. Jahodar L, Jilek P, Pakova M, Dvorakova V. Antimicrobial effect of arbutin and an extract of the leaves of *Arctostaphylos uva-ursi* in vitro. *Ceskoslov Farm* 1985;34:174–78.

2. Matsuda H, Nakamura S, Tanaka T, Kubo M. Pharmacological studies on leaf of *Arctostaphylos uva-ursi* (L) Spreng. V. Effect of water extract from *Arctostaphylos uva-ursi* (L) Spreng (bearberry leaf) on the antiallergic and antiinflammatory activities of dexamethasone ointment. *J Pharm Soc Japan* 1992; 112:673–77.

Valerian

1. Mennini T, Bernasconi P, et al. In vitro study on the interaction of extracts and pure compounds from *Valeriana officinalis* roots with GABA, benzodiazepine and barbiturate receptors. *Fitoterapia* 1993;64:291–300.

Vitex

1. Monograph *Agni casti fructus* (Chaste tree fruits). *Bundesanzeiger* May 15, 1985 (no. 90), Dec 2, 1992 (no. 226).

2. Sliutz G, Speiser P, et al. Agnus castus extracts inhibit prolactin secretion of rat pituitary cells. *Horm Metab Res* 1993; 25:253–55.

White Willow

1. Weiss RF. *Herbal Medicine*. Gothenburg, Sweden: Ab Arcanum, 1988, 31, 303.

2. Bradley PR, ed. *British Herbal Compendium,* vol 1. Bournemouth, Dorset, UK: British Herbal Medicine Association, 1992, 224–26.

Wild Cherry

1. Leung AY, Foster S. *Encyclopedia of Common Natural Ingredients Used in Food, Drugs, and Cosmetics,* 2d ed. New York: John Wiley & Sons, 1996, 155–56.

2. Mills SY. *Out of the Earth: The Essential Book of Herbal Medicine*. Middlesex, UK: Viking Arkana, 1991, 314.

Wild Yam

1. Lust JB. *The Herb Book*. New York: Bantam Books, 1974, 401.

2. Iwu MM, Okunji CO, Ohiaeri GO, et al. Hypoglycaemic activity of dioscoretine from tubers of *Dioscorea dumetorum* in normal and alloxan diabetic rabbits. *Planta Med* 1990;56:264–67.

3. Araghiniknam M, Chung S, Nelson-White T, et al. Antioxidant activity of dioscorea and dehydroepiandrosterone (DHEA) in older humans. *Life Sci* 1996; 11:147–57.

4. Araghiniknam M, Chung S, Nelson-White T, et al. Antioxidant activity of dioscorea and dehydroepiandrosterone (DHEA) in older humans. *Life Sci* 1996; 11:147–57.

5. Dollbaum CM. Lab analyses of salivary DHEA and progesterone following ingestion of yam-containing products. *Townsend Letter for Doctors and Patients* Oct 1995:104.

Witch Hazel

1. Duke JA. *CRC Handbook of Medicinal Herbs*. Boca Raton, FL: CRC Press, 1985, 221.

2. Bernard P, Balansard P, Balansard G, Bovis A. Venotonic pharmacodynamic value of galenic preparations with a base of hamamelis leaves. *J Pharm Belg* 1972; 27:505–12.

3. Korting HC, Schafer-Korting M, Hart H, et al. Anti-inflammatory activity of Hamamelis distillate applied topically to the skin. *Eur J Clin Pharmacol* 1993; 44:315–18.

Wormwood

1. Leung AY, Foster S. *Encyclopedia of Common Natural Ingredients Used in Food, Drugs, and Cosmetics,* 2d ed. New York: John Wiley & Sons, 1996, 1–3.

2. Leung AY, Foster S. *Encyclopedia of Common Natural Ingredients Used in Food, Drugs, and Cosmetics,* 2d ed. New York: John Wiley & Sons, 1996, 1–3.

3. Weiss RF. *Herbal Medicine*. Gothenburg, Sweden: Ab Arcanum, 1988, 79–81.

4. Leung AY, Foster S. *Encyclopedia of Common Natural Ingredients Used in Food, Drugs, and Cosmetics,* 2d ed. New York: John Wiley & Sons, 1996, 1–3.

Yohimbe

1. Duke JA. *CRC Handbook of Medicinal Herbs*. Boca Raton, FL: CRC Press, 1985, 351.

2. Riley AJ. Yohimbine in the treatment of erectile disorder. *Br J Clin Pract* 1994; 48:133–36.

3. Cappiello A, McDougle CJ, Maleson RT, et al. Yohimbine augmentation of fluvoxamine in refractory depression: A single-blind study. *Biol Psych* 1995; 38:765–67.

Yucca

1. Bingham R, Bellew BA, Bellew JG. Yucca plant saponin in the management of arthritis. *J Appl Nutr* 1975;27:45–50.

2. Foster S, Duke JA. *A Field Guide to Medicinal Plants: Eastern and Central North America*. Boston: Houghton Mifflin Co., 1990.

INDEX

Apis mellifica
  for benign prostatic hyperplasia, 20, 336
  for eye conditions, 352–353
  for herpes zoster, 357
  for herpex simplex, 356
  for insect bites, 362
  for osteoarthritis, 99, 370
  for rashes, 374
Arbutin, 121, 315–316
Arctium lappa. See Burdock
Arctostaphylos uva-ursi. See Uva ursi
Argentum nitricum
  for anxiety, 333
  for conjunctivitis, 347
  for diarrhea, 46, 350
  for impotence, 358
  for infertility (male), 79
Arginine, 137–138
  and congestive heart failure, 31
  for infertility (male), 77, 78
  ornithine and, 190
Arnica
  for backache, 334
  for broken bone support, 338
  for dental support, 349
  for eye conditions, 352
  for hemorrhoids, 61, 355
  for injuries, 361
  in pregnancy, 109, 373
  for rheumatoid arthritis, 118, 378
  for surgery recovery, 378
  for varicose veins, 383
Arsenicum album
  for canker sores, 23, 341
  for diarrhea, 46, 350
  for herpes zoster, 357
  for indigestion and gas, 360
  for influenza, 360
  for insomnia, 81, 363
  for Raynaud's phenomenon, 375
Artemisia absinthium. See Wormwood
Arterial disease. *See* Atherosclerosis
Arthritis. *See* Osteoarthritis; Rheumatoid arthritis
Ascorbic acid. *See* Vitamin C
Ashwagandha for Alzheimer's disease, 7, 8
Asian ginseng, 30, 232–233
  for Alzheimer's disease, 7–8
  for atherosclerosis, 13
  for athletic performance, 16
  for chemotherapy support, 27
  for common colds, 29, 30
  for diabetes, 43
  for fibromyalgia, 54

Aspirin, peptic ulcers and, 104
Asteraceae family, 22, 46, 83, 105
Asthma, 9–11
  dietary changes for, 9–10
  herbs for, 10–11
  nutrients helping, 10
Astragalus, 233–234
  for Alzheimer's disease, 7, 8
  for chemotherapy support, 27
  for common colds, 29
  for immune function, 74
Atherosclerosis, 11–13. *See also*
    Diabetes; High cholesterol; Hypertriglyceridemia
  chondroitin sulfate and, 149
  dietary changes for, 12
  herbs for, 13
  homocysteine and, 12–13
  lifestyle changes and, 12
  nutrients for, 12–13
  obesity and, 12
  Pritikin diet program and, 112
  smoking and, 12
  type A behavior and, 12
Athletic performance, 14–16
  herbs for, 16
  pyruvic acid and, 200
Autism, 17
  nutrients for, 17
Avena sativa. See Oats
Ayurvedic medicine, 71
  alfalfa in, 230
  ginger in, 267
  gotu kola in, 271
  guggul in, 274
  for peptic ulcers, 103
  phyllanthus in, 298–299
  turmeric in, 314

B

Bach's Rescue Remedy, 358
Backache, homeopathic remedies for, 334–335
Bacteriocins, 135
Bananas for peptic ulcers, 103
BCAAs (branched-chain amino acids), 138
  athletic performance and, 15, 16
  whey protein and, 223
B-complex vitamins, 210–211. *See also*
    Multiple vitamin/mineral supplements; specific vitamins
  athletic performance and, 14, 16
  brewer's yeast and, 143–144

for infertility (female), 76
  for osteoporosis, 101
  for premenstrual syndrome (PMS), 110
  for vitiligo, 122
Bearberry. *See* Uva ursi
Belladonna
  for boils, 337
  for bursitis, 21, 340
  for chicken pox, 344
  for colic, 346
  for ear infections, 49, 351
  for gout, 353
  for migraine headaches, 92, 367
  for mumps, 369
  for osteoarthritis, 99, 370
  for teething pain, 379–380
  for urinary tract infections, 121, 382
Bell's palsy, homeopathic remedies for, 335
Benign prostatic hyperplasia, 18–20
  herbs for, 19–20
  homeopathic remedies for, 20, 336
  nutrients for, 18–19
Benzoyl peroxide for acne, 6
Berberine, 40
  for urinary tract infections, 121
Beta-carotene, 134, 180, 209–210
  as antioxidant, 9
  for cataracts, 24, 25
  macular degeneration and, 86
  Pap smears (abnormal) and, 102
  photosensitivity and, 106
Betaine hydrochloride (HCl), 139–140
  for asthma, 10
  for diarrhea, 45
  for gallstones, 56
  proteolytic enzymes and, 157
  for vitiligo, 122, 123
Beta-lapachone, 297
Beta-sitosterol, BPH and, 19
Bible, garlic in, 265
Bifidobacteria for diarrhea, 45
Bifidobacterium bifidum, 134–135
Bilberry, 140–141, 234–235
  as antioxidant, 9
  for atherosclerosis, 13
  for cataracts, 25
  for diabetes, 43–44
  for macular degeneration, 86
  for night blindness, 96
Bilobalide, 269
Bioflavonoids, 140–141. *See also*
    Anthocyanosides; Quercetin
  for gingivitis, 57

for glaucoma, 59
for hay fever, 60
for high cholesterol, 64
menopause and, 87, 88
for peptic ulcers, 104
Biotin, 141–142
diabetes and, 41
Bitter melon, 235–236
for diabetes, 43, 44
for psoriasis, 114
Bitter principles, 253
Blackberry leaves/root for diarrhea, 46
Black cohosh, 236–237
for menopausal symptoms, 88
Black currant seed oil, 158–159
for eczema, 49
for rheumatoid arthritis, 116
Bladder gravel, 249
Bladder infections. *See* Urinary tract
infections
Blepharitis, eyebright for, 260
Blessed thistle, 237–238
Blindness. *See* Glaucoma; Macular
degeneration; Night blindness
Blueberry leaves for diarrhea, 46
Blue-green algae. *See* Spirulina
Boils, homeopathic remedies for,
337–338
Bones. *See also* Osteoporosis
broken bone support, homeopathic
remedies for, 338–339
Borage oil, 158–159
for eczema, 49
for rheumatoid arthritis, 116
Borax for canker sores, 23, 341
Boric acid capsules for yeast
infections, 128
Boron, 142–143
for osteoarthritis, 98
for osteoporosis, 101
for rheumatoid arthritis, 116, 117
Boswellia, 238–239
for bursitis, 21
for osteoarthritis, 99
for rheumatoid arthritis, 117
Bran, kidney stones and, 84
Branched-chain amino acids. *See* BCAAs
Breast tenderness. *See* Fibrocystic breast
disease
Brewer's yeast, 143–144
diabetes and, 41, 43
for diarrhea, 45
for high cholesterol, 64, 65
inosine in, 169
Brittle bone disease. *See* Osteoporosis
Broken bone support, homeopathic

remedies for, 338–339
Bromelain, 156–157
Bronchial asthma. *See* Asthma
Bruises, homeopathic remedies
for, 361
Bryonia
for chicken pox, 344
for colic, 346
for influenza, 361
for migraine headaches, 92, 367
for osteoarthritis, 99, 371
for rheumatoid arthritis, 118, 377
Bugleweed, 286
Burdock, 239–240
for acne, 6
for eczema, 50, 51
for psoriasis, 113–114
for rheumatoid arthritis, 117
Burns
aloe for, 231–232
homeopathic remedies for, 339
Bursitis, 20–21
herbs for, 21
homeopathic remedies for, 21, 340
nutrients for, 20
Butcher's broom, 240–241
for atherosclerosis, 13
for hemorrhoids, 61, 241

C

Cabbage juice for peptic ulcers, 103
Cadmium, 8
Cadmium sulfuricum for chemotherapy
support, 28, 343
Caffeine
depression and, 36
diarrhea and, 45
eczema and, 49
fibrocystic breast disease and, 51–52
with ginseng, 8
high cholesterol and, 63
hypertension and, 67
infertility (female) and, 75
insomnia and, 79–80
kidney stones and, 83
osteoporosis and, 100
peptic ulcers and, 104
pregnancy and, 107–108
premenstrual syndrome (PMS)
and, 109
in weight loss program, 125–126
Calcarea carbonica
for menopausal symptoms, 88, 365
for mumps, 369–370

for osteoporosis, 101, 371
for teething pain, 380
Calcarea fluorica
for gout, 353
for hemorrhoids, 61, 355
Calcarea phosphorica for osteoporosis,
101, 371
Calcium, 144–145
best form of, 145
for gingivitis, 57
for high cholesterol, 64, 65
for hypertension, 68
kidney stone formation and, 84, 85
for migraine headaches, 92
for osteoporosis, 100, 101
in pregnancy, 108
for premenstrual syndrome
(PMS), 110
rickets and, 118–119
vitamin D and, 219
vitamin K and, 222
zinc and, 19, 225
Calcium ascorbate, 10
Calcium citrate, 84
Calcium citrate/malate (CCM), 145
Calcium magnesium, boron and, 142
Calcium oxalate stone formation. *See*
Kidney stones
Calendula, 241–242
for eczema, 50, 51
Calendula MT
for burns, 339
for dental support, 349
Camellia sinensis. See Green tea
Cancer. *See also* Chemotherapy support; Pap smears (abnormal);
specific cancers
curcumin and, 315
garlic and, 266
lycopene and, 180–181
Pritikin diet program and, 112
selenium and, 203
vitamin D and, 219
Candida albicans, 43, 45. *See also* Yeast
infections
Canker sores, 21–23
dietary changes for, 21–22
herbs for, 22
homeopathic remedies for, 23, 341–342
lifestyle changes for, 21
nutrients for, 22
Cantharis
for burns, 339
for insect bites, 362–363
for urinary tract infections, 121,
381–382

ABOUT THE AUTHORS

Schuyler "Skye" W. Lininger, Jr., D.C., Contributor and Editor-in-Chief

Dr. Skye Lininger is a nutritionally oriented chiropractor who has been involved with computer technology since 1966. He has authored or coauthored a dozen computer books and written over fifty articles for various computer magazines. Since 1986, he has published *HealthNotes*, a newsletter used by over 1,000 natural food stores. He is a regular contributor to *HealthNotes, Let's Live,* and *Nutrition Insights.* As founder of the "Natural Medicine Forum" on CompuServe, he heads up the most popular on-line service on this topic. A former instructor in preventive nutrition at Western States Chiropractic College, he gives regular seminars in both the U.S. and England.

Jonathan V. Wright, M.D., Contributor and Editorial Review

Dr. Jonathan Wright practices nutritional medicine at the Tahoma Clinic in Kent, Washington. He is regarded as one of the world's finest preventive medical doctors. He is the author of *Dr. Wright's Book of Nutritional Therapy* (Rodale, 1979), *Dr. Wright's Guide to Healing with Nutrition* (Keats, 1990), and *Natural Hormone Replacement for Women Over 45* (Smart, 1997). He contributes regularly to *Health-Notes* and coauthors a newsletter called *Nutrition and Healing.*

Steve Austin, N.D., Contributor and Section Editor of Conditions and Nutritional Supplements

Dr. Steve Austin is a naturopathic physician in private practice at the Center for Natural Medicine in Portland, Oregon. Known as the "naturopaths' educator," he is former Professor of Nutrition at the National College of Naturopathic Medicine. Dr. Austin has also headed the nutrition departments at Bastyr University and Western States Chiropractic College. He is the coauthor of *Breast Cancer: What You Should Know (But May Not Be Told) About*

Prevention, Diagnosis, and Treatment (Prima, 1994). He is a contributor to the *Textbook of Natural Medicine* and a regular contributor to *HealthNotes.* He is nutrition editor for the *Quarterly Review of Natural Medicine.*

Donald J. Brown, N.D., Contributor and Section Editor of Herbs

Dr. Donald Brown is a naturopathic physician who is on the faculty of Bastyr University of Natural Health Sciences where he teaches nutrition and herbal medicine. He writes frequently about herbal medicine for *HealthNotes, HerbalGram,* and *Nutrition Science News* and is the author of *Herbal Prescriptions for Better Health* (Prima, 1996). Dr. Brown founded Natural Products Research Consultants in 1992. NPRC is dedicated to furthering education and research in natural medicine and is the publisher of the *Quarterly Review of Natural Medicine.*

Alan R. Gaby, M.D., Contributor

Dr. Alan Gaby, an expert in nutritional therapies, is the Medical Editor of the *Townsend Letter for Doctors* and *Holistic Medicine.* He served as a member of the Ad-Hoc Advisory Panel of the National Institutes of Health Office of Alternative Medicine. He is the author of *Vitamin B6: The Natural Healer* (Keats, 1987) and *Preventing and Reversing Osteoporosis* (Prima, 1994). With Dr. Wright, he conducts nutritional seminars for physicians and has collected over 30,000 scientific papers related to the field of nutritional medicine. He is currently the Endowed Professor of Nutrition at Bastyr University, Seattle, Washington, and is a frequent contributor to *Health-Notes* and coauthor of a newsletter called *Nutrition and Healing.*

Eric Yarnell, N.D., Contributor

Dr. Eric Yarnell works as a naturopathic physician in Sedona, Arizona, at a multidisciplinary clinic. He is a founding member and current secretary of the board of the Botanical Medicine Academy and writes regularly for *Alternative and Complimentary Therapies*.

Ronald G. Reichert, N.D., Contributor

An expert in European phytotherapy, Dr. Ronald Reichert resides in Vancouver, B.C., where he has an active medical practice. He contributes regular articles to lay and professional publications in Canada. In addition to his regular herbal research columns, he provides professional review of German translations for the *Quarterly Review of Natural Medicine*.

Tori Hudson, N.D., Contributor

Dr. Tori Hudson is a nationally known expert on women's health. Her column appears in the *Townsend Letter for Doctors*. A popular speaker, she is a regular contributor to *HealthNotes* and is currently working on a book called *Women's Health and Natural Medicine* for Keats.

Shane McCamey, Contributor and Section Editor of Homeopathic Remedies

Mr. Shane McCamey is a certified homeopath and a graduate of the Pacific Academy of Homeopathic Medicine. He wrote *Fifty Favorite Homeopathic Prescriptions for First Aid and Acute Care*. He lectures extensively and has appeared on both radio and television and has been a study group leader for the National Center for Homeopathy in the United States.

Victoria Dolby, Managing Editor

Ms. Victoria Dolby writes about health issues, with a special focus on nutritional supplements. Her articles appear regularly in many magazines, including *Natural Living Today, Better Nutrition, Let's Live*, and *Vitamin Retailer*. She is the coauthor of *The Green Tea Book* (Avery, 1998) and author of *Natural Therapies for Arthritis* (Keats, 1997). She has been the managing editor for all versions of *HealthNotes Online*.

Rick Wilkes, Technical Director

Mr. Rick Wilkes is an independent consultant and Internet specialist from Deep Creek Lake, Maryland. His first computer work was at age 14 when he wrote a communications system for his county's high school students. An electrical engineer with a degree from Johns Hopkins University, he has focused for the past 20 years on building supportive online communities and helping to make complex issues more understandable and accessible through electronic publishing.

Continue the "natural" experience

Two outstanding offers from the publishers of *HealthNotes Online*

HealthNotes monthly newsletter

Subscribe now to a four-page monthly nutrition newsletter with articles by the same team of authors who created this book. Keep up-to-date with the latest scientific research written in plain language you can understand. Learn how to stay healthy, reduce your chances of serious illness, and use natural remedies to help yourself, your family, and your friends.

For more than twelve years, *HealthNotes* has been the natural information choice for almost 100,000 readers a month in the United States, Canada, and England. Join this informed group by subscribing today. One year of *HealthNotes* delivered to your door each month for only $18.00 per year (£18.00 in the UK).

HealthNotes Online personal CD-ROM software

HealthNotes Online, a popular computer database used by many health food stores, pharmacies, grocery stores, and physicians, is now available for personal use in an inexpensive CD-ROM version.

The content of this exciting electronic database forms the basis for the text in this book. With *HealthNotes Online*, you will enjoy the latest version of the software, including up-to-date information, colorful graphics, and award-winning photography by noted herbalist Steven Foster—all hyper-linked together for instant access to this highly regarded database of complementary and alternative medicine. Preview a demo of this outstanding program at http://www.healthnotes.com.

This personal CD-ROM is available for $49.95 plus $5 shipping (£49 in the UK includes shipping). *HealthNotes Online* does not require a telephone connection. It runs on PCs (using Windows 3.11 or Windows 95) or Macs under any frames-aware Internet browser (such as Internet Explorer 3.0 or Netscape Navigator 3.0 or later).

(The personal version is licensed *only* for personal use by an individual and may *not* be used in a retail, sales, or professional business of any kind. For information on a retail or professional license, contact Virtual Health, LLC at the address below.)

Yes, I want to be kept up-to-date! Please send me the following:

❑ *HealthNotes* monthly four-page newsletter. One year $18 (£18.00 in the UK).

❑ *HealthNotes Online* personal CD-ROM software. $49.95 plus $5 shipping (£49 in the UK includes shipping).

❑ I have a retail store or am a sales or health professional and would like information on licensing *HealthNotes Online* for business or professional use.

Name _____ Address _____

City, State, Zip _____ Phone _____

Visa/Mastercard number _____ Expiration date _____

Signature (for credit card purchase) _____

Mail, fax, or email check, money order, or Visa/Mastercard information to: *HealthNotes*, 1125 SE Madison, Suite 209, Portland, OR 97214; fax +1-503-234-4052; email *info@healthnotes.com*.